Physical Activity

T0144460

Physical activity and its relationship to health is one of the great issues of our age. The causes of, and solutions to, physical inactivity are complex and multi-dimensional, and therefore the subject needs to be studied and understood from a variety of perspectives. This is the first textbook to provide a truly multi-disciplinary introduction to physical activity studies.

Offering a complete foundation to the subject, it covers the basics of every core discipline, from biochemistry, public health and biomechanics to physiology, sport psychology and sociology. It introduces a full range of topics across the physical activity curriculum, including behaviour change, motor skill development, nutrition, exercise prescription, public health policy, and physical education, providing a well-balanced and international perspective on each important issue. There is also a strong emphasis throughout the book on the practical, applied dimensions of physical activity, including innovative approaches to promotion and intervention tailored to every age range and environment.

Physical Activity: A Multi-disciplinary Introduction is an indispensable companion to any course or degree programme with an emphasis on physical activity and health. A variety of exclusive eResources to aid teaching and learning are also available via the Routledge website.

Nick Draper is Professor of Sport and Exercise Science at the University of Canterbury, Christchurch, New Zealand. His teaching is in the area of exercise physiology and he is Programme Director for the Master of Sport Science programme. His research interests focus on psychophysiology in relation to rock climbing, rugby performance and physical activity. He is Chair of SESNZ, the national organisation for Sport and Exercise Science in New Zealand, and a founder member of the International Rock Climbing Research Association.

Gareth Stratton is Head of the School of Sport and Exercise Sciences and Director of the Applied Sports Technology Exercise and Medicine (A-STEM) Research Centre at Swansea University, UK. He is also Adjunct Professor at the University of Western Australia. Professor Stratton began his career as a physical education teacher. This led him to his main areas of academic interest: children, maturation and physical activity, and physical activity, fitness and health. He has been involved in physical activity measurement studies for nearly 30 years and he continues his interest in the development of novel sensor technologies to detect and stimulate changes in physical activity and sedentary behaviour.

Physical Activity

A Multi-disciplinary Introduction

Edited by Nick Draper and Gareth Stratton

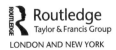

LONDON AND NEW YORK

First published 2019
by Routledge
2 Park Square, Milton Park, Abingdon, Oxon OX14 4RN

and by Routledge
711 Third Avenue, New York, NY 10017

Routledge is an imprint of the Taylor & Francis Group, an informa business

British Library Cataloguing-in-Publication Data
A catalogue record for this book is available from the British Library

Library of Congress Cataloging-in-Publication Data
A catalog record has been requested for this book

ISBN: 978-1-138-69661-7 (hbk)
ISBN: 978-1-138-69662-4 (pbk)
ISBN: 978-1-315-52385-9 (ebk)

Typeset in Perpetua
by Apex CoVantage, LLC

Visit the eResources: www.routledge.com/9781138696624

Contents

Figures

Tables

Part I

Foundations in physical activity

1 Physical activity

A multi-disciplinary introduction

Nick Draper and Gareth Stratton

Keywords: Physical activity, exercise, physical fitness, multi-disciplinary, high-intensity interval training

Changes in the structure of society in many countries around the world, as well as the on-going industrial and technological revolutions, have had a dramatic impact on the way we live our lives and our inherent daily physical activity. Unlike the hunter-gatherers of our past physical activity has been engineered out from many of our daily lives and is now something we have to find time to add into busy schedules. As is described in more detail in Chapter 3 (Historical aspects of physical activity) knowledge regarding the benefits of physical activity for health goes back at least as far as early Greek, Roman, Chinese and Indian civilisations. Yet despite this knowledge, a major health and economic concern facing many societies around the world is how to re-engineer physical activity, with all its associated health benefits, back into the everyday lives of increasingly technology-engaged populations.

As working definitions for the textbook we refer back to the work of Caspersen, Powell and Christenson (1985), who defined **physical activity** as "as any bodily movement produced by skeletal muscles that results in energy expenditure." As such, physical activity includes activities such as recreation, active transport, movement during/as part of work, household activities and sports participation. They further defined **exercise**, as a sub-category of physical activity, as representing physical activity that is "planned, structured, repetitive, and purposive in the sense that improvement or maintenance of one or more components of physical fitness is an objective" and **physical fitness** as a set of "attributes that people have or achieve."

Physical activity: A multi-disciplinary introduction brings together contributions from researchers across a wide range of sport and exercise science disciplines, along with public health specialists. The aim of the textbook is to examine the extent and direction of physical activity research and knowledge in each respective field. The textbook, as an introduction, is designed as a starting point in regard to physical activity knowledge development. In addition, however, it brings together research from across a range of disciplines and consequently provides an opportunity for researchers in any discipline to easily capture a flavour of physical activity research (and its counterpart, physical inactivity) outside their own specialisation. This is an important additional consideration, given the complex multi-factorial activates that have led to the global increases in physical inactivity and the consequential implications for individual health and wellbeing, as well as the economic costs to a nation.

While a vast range of physical activity knowledge and research will be highlighted in the chapters to follow, it is perhaps pertinent in this opening chapter, to highlight a number of foundational studies that have shaped, and will continue to shape, the direction of physical activity research in years to come. The first, which is referred to in several chapters in the textbook, is the series of studies published by Professor Jeremy Morris and colleagues (1953, 1958, 1973 etc.). In particular Morris et al.'s seminal work published in 1953, highlighted in Chapter 3, where the team importantly elucidated the role of physical activity in the reduction of coronary heart disease development for postal and bus workers.

The second relates to the work of one of the contributors to this textbook, Professor Neil Armstrong (Chapter 11, Paediatric physical activity and aerobic fitness). Beginning in the 1980s, Armstrong and colleagues examined physical activity levels and fitness in children. While highlighting low levels of habitual physical activity in his early work, Armstrong and co-workers – controversially at the time, but later confirmed in subsequent studies – suggested that habitual physical activity levels in UK secondary school children in the 1990s had stabilised, rather than continued to decline (Armstrong, Balding, Gentle & Kirby, 1990; Welsman & Armstrong, 2000).

The third relates to the series of papers published in 2012 by the Lancet Physical Activity Series Working Group in the *Lancet*. In respect of the impact on the medical profession this may represent a watershed in the understanding of the risk factors associated with, and health and economic costs of, physical inactivity. In these papers the rise in physical inactivity was referred to as a pandemic (Lee, Shiroma, Lobelo, Puska, Blair & Katzmarzyk, 2012). Three years prior to this Blair, one of the authors of these papers, referred to physical inactivity as the biggest public health issue of the 21st century. Furthermore, increasing awareness of the significance of physical inactivity as a mortality risk factor led Blair and co-workers to coin the term 'smokadiabesity' in relation to their finding mortality risk factors for a large cohort study in the US (Blair, 2009). In this paper Blair highlighted that physical inactivity was a more significant risk factor for mortality than smoking, diabetes and obesity put together.

While these important studies have developed our knowledge and understanding in the field, there remains much work to be done. A recent paper by Lewis and colleagues (2017) identified three key areas as future directions for physical activity research. These included focusing not only in increasing PA, but also on decreasing sedentary behaviour, the use of technology for understanding PA habits and changes through interventions, and the need for future research to maximise public health impact through changes in dissemination approaches. While we support these intentions the authors have perhaps missed a vital aspect in regard to physical activity, namely, that future research should take a multi-disciplinary approach. Given the causes of increased physical inactivity are multi-factorial, to develop the most informed interventions requires us as professionals to work in collaborative teams and create more far impactful solutions.

An example of the need to take such an approach can be found in regard to research relating to high intensity interval training (HIIT). As a physical activity promotion intervention for general population, HIIT has received an increasing research focus since the late 1990s. The rise in interest in this type of intervention arose primarily due to the potential time-saving benefits of HIIT.

In the early 2000s a number of studies highlighted the physiological adaptations that could be brought about through HIIT for young active males and clinical populations in a laboratory setting (Burgomaster et al., 2008; Tjonna et al., 2008; Wisloff et al., 2007; Gibala et al. 2006; Warburton, Nicol, & Bredin, 2006). At that stage though, there had not been a controlled trial investigating the potential of HIIT for inactive participants in the general population for a study conducted in a real-world setting. A 12-week intervention by Lunt and co-workers provided data for such a study (Lunt et al., 2014). The research conducted in New Zealand found that for the obese, previously inactive participants who took part in the study two different forms of HIIT (maximal volitional interval training and aerobic interval training) were non-inferior, in regard to cardiorespiratory improvements, to lower intensity endurance training (LIET), but in this real-world setting, benefits were modest in comparison to previous research.

As a consequence of these findings, Draper and co-workers developed a six-month real-world follow-up study investigating adherence to HIIT over a longer time period and with decreasing group support (activity/session leaders). From data to be published in 2018, Draper and co-workers found a number of key psychological factors that are of importance when planning physical activity interventions. Firstly, the six-month intervention, which began 12 weeks after the Lunt et al. (2014) study included 20 participants who had taken part in the earlier Lunt et al. study. Of these dual-study participants, despite being encouraged to continue activity between the two studies, virtually all of these previously inactive participants ceased physical activity. The dual-study participants waited until the next study to continue with their physical activity sessions.

Secondly, while in the Lunt et al. (2014) study each exercise group had two activity leaders throughout the 12-week study, during the Draper et al. follow-up intervention the level of support for participants was reduced through the duration of the study. In the first two months participants had three supported sessions in each week, in the second two months they received two supported sessions per week and in the final two months they received one supported session per week. The intention of the reducing support by group leaders was to (a) examine the adherence to the sessions with reduced support and (b) to prepare participants to being active independently at the end of the research period. In regard to the intervention, given the equality in benefits of the three previous intervention modalities (maximal volitional interval training and aerobic interval training and LIET) participants were required to complete one session of each exercise form each week, providing a total of three sessions per week which matched the intervention volume in the Lunt et al. (2014) study. Results of the study indicated that when given a choice participants avoided completing the maximal volitional intensity session (4×30 seconds all out efforts) when unsupported. The reason behind this was due to the motivation required to work at that intensity. While the session was more time efficient there was greater adherence to the lower intensity session and this lack of adherence outweighed the time-saving benefits of HIIT in this real-world context.

These findings from a real-world physical activity intervention highlight the need for multi-disciplinary interventions. While many conferences continue to host discipline-specific sessions, biochemists and physiologists are in one room developing knowledge as to the mechanisms behind why HIIT works as a time-saving intervention, while in another room psychologists are discussing why, due to adherence and motivational considerations, there are limitations to HIIT as a physical activity intervention with the general population. Never has the need for multi-disciplinary research interventions been more apparent. Intentionally ***Physical activity: A multi-disciplinary introduction*** takes a discipline-specific approach to examine the development of physical activity research to date for each discipline. This textbook is intended though as a starting point for future research and we appeal to all reading this text to look at research across disciplines and to seek multi-disciplinary approaches in planning future interventions to increase physical activity and decrease physical inactivity and sedentary behaviour. In so doing we are more likely to find real solutions for this multi-factorial real-world problem.

Physical activity: A multi-disciplinary introduction is divided into three parts, the first (Chapters 2–7) covers foundations in physical activity knowledge, from recapping physical activity-related aspects of anatomy and physiology, to contrasting the health effects of physical inactivity and physical activity and finishing by examining a basis for physical activity measurement and prescription. The second section (Chapters 8–17) has a focus on research by discipline including aspects such as physiology, biochemistry, psychology and motor skill development. In the final section (Chapters 18–25) we examine applied physical activity research from a schools, public health, health promotion and international perspective.

Lastly, having written and finished editing this chapter, and indeed the textbook, it has given us the impetus to get away from the standing desks and get active outside, hope you will do the same after and in between reading chapters from this text. Right, off for a climb/mountain bike, respectively. . . .

Chapter summary

- Regular physical activity is essential for maintaining physical and mental health.
- In many countries there has been a decline in daily physical activity volumes and intensities as a result of changes in the way we live our lives.
- To be successful, solutions to increasing physical activity participation will likely require multi-disciplinary approaches.
- This textbook, as well as providing an introductory text for physical activity specialists, also provides an easily accessible avenue through which to learn about research developments in fields other than their own.

References

Armstrong, N., Balding, J., Gentle, P. & Kirby, B.J. (1990). Patterns of physical activity amongst 11 to 16 year old British children. *British Medical Journal, 301*, 203–205.

Blair, S.N. (2009). Physical inactivity: the biggest public health problem of the 21st century. *British Journal of Sports Medicine, 43*(1), 1–2.

Burgomaster, K.A., Howarth, K.R., Phillips, S.M., Rakobowchuk, M., MacDonald, M. J., McGee, S. L. & Gibala, M.J. (2008). Similar metabolic adaptations during exercise after low volume sprint interval and traditional endurance training in humans. *The Journal of Physiology, 586*(1), 151–160.

Caspersen, C.J., Powell, K.E. & Christenson, G.M. (1985). Physical activity, exercise and physical fitness: definitions and distinctions for health-related research. *Public Health Reports, 100*(2): 126–131.

Gibala, M.J., Little, J.P., van Essen, M., Wilkin, G.P., Burgomaster, K.A., Safdar, A., . . . Tarnopolsky, M.A. (2006). Short-term sprint interval versus traditional endurance training: similar initial adaptations in human skeletal muscle and exercise performance. *The Journal of Physiology, 575*(3), 901.

Lee, I.M., Shiroma, E.J., Lobelo, F., Puska, P., Blair, S.N., Katzmarzyk, P.T., & Lancet Physical Activity Series Working Group. (2012). Effect of physical inactivity on major non-communicable diseases worldwide: an analysis of burden of disease and life expectancy. *Lancet* (London, England), *380*(9838), 219–229. https://doi.org/10.1016/S0140-6736(12)61031-9.

Lewis, B.A., Napolitano, M.A., Buman, M.P. Williams D.M. & Nigg, C.R. (2017). Future directions in physical activity intervention research: expanding our focus to sedentary behaviours, technology and dissemination. *Journal of Behavioural Medicine, 40*(1), 112–126.

Lunt, H., Draper, N., Marshall, H.C., Logan, F.J., Hamlin, M.J., Shearman, J.P., Cotter, J.D., Kimber, N.E., Blackwell, G. & Frampton, C.M.A. (2014) High intensity interval training in a real world setting: a randomized controlled feasibility study in overweight inactive adults, measuring change in maximal oxygen uptake. *PLoS ONE, 9*(3): e83256. http://dx.doi.org/10.1371/journal. pone.0083256.

Morris, J.N., Chave, S.P., Adam, C., Sirey, C., Epstein, L. & Sheehan, D.J. (1973). Vigorous exercise in leisure-time and the incidence of coronary heart-disease. *Lancet, 301*(7799), 333–339.

Morris, J.N. & Crawford, M.D. (1958). Coronary heart disease and physical activity of work: evidence of a national necropsy survey. *British Medical Journal, 2*(5111), 1485–1496.

Morris, J.N., Heady, J.A., Raffle, P.A.B., Roberts, C.G. & Parks J.N. (1953). Coronary heart disease and physical activity of work. *Lancet, 2*(6795), 1053–1057.

Tjonna, A.E., Lee, S.J., Rognmo, O., Stolen, T.O., Bye, A., Haram, P.M., . . . Wisløff, U. (2008). Aerobic interval training versus continuous moderate exercise as a treatment for the metabolic syndrome: a pilot study. *Circulation, 118*(4), 346.

Warburton, D.E.R., Nicol, C.W., & Bredin, S.S.D. (2006). Health benefits of physical activity: the evidence. *Canadian Medical Association Journal, 174*(6), 801–809.

Welsman, J.R. & Armstrong, N. (2000). Physical activity patterns in secondary schoolchildren. *European Journal of Physical Education, 5*, 147–157.

Wisloff, U., Stoylen, A., Loennechen, J.P., Bruvold, M., Rognmo, O., Haram, P.M., . . . Skjaerpe, T. (2007). Superior cardiovascular effect of aerobic interval training versus moderate continuous training in heart failure patients: a randomized study. *Circulation, 115*(24), 3086.

2 Foundations in the science of physical activity

Helen Marshall and Louise Sheppard

Keywords: Anatomy, physiology, neuroendocrine, musculoskeletal, cardiorespiratory

INTRODUCTION

Life begins from two single cells that contain all the information needed to grow a full-sized human being. By adulthood those two cells will have reproduced several trillion times to produce 32 individual teeth, thousands of kilometres of blood vessels, and a digestive tract with the surface area equivalent to half a badminton court (Helander & Fändriks, 2014). All of this from two tiny cells.

The study of the human body is divided into the twin disciplines of **anatomy** and **physiology**. Anatomy is concerned with the **structure** of the body – the form of the individual components that make it up. Physiology is concerned with the **function** of the body – how the individual components work together to perform a specific function. Structure and function are always linked, in what is termed the '**complementarity of structure and function**'. The way a body part is designed (the structure) is always related to the job it is required to do (the function). For example, bones are made from tissue that is very strong, but still relatively light and the walls of the lungs are thin to allow oxygen easy access to the blood stream.

Understanding both the structure and the function of the body allows us to optimise performance – for example a personal trainer working on a strengthening programme with a client in the gym, or a health coach explaining the benefits of staying physically active with age. A good grasp of anatomy and physiology also aids understanding when things go wrong, in the case of injury or disease – for example a health promotor explaining the benefits of physical activity for maximising bone health or a physiotherapist helping rehabilitate an ankle sprain.

For ease, the study of the human body is often divided into different systems or individual processes. While this approach can aid understanding, in reality the human body is a complex interaction of all its different parts. The remainder of this chapter will review those aspects of anatomy and physiology of most interest to the study of physical activity – body structure and life processes, the neuroendocrine system, the musculoskeletal system and the cardiorespiratory system.

BODY STRUCTURE AND LIFE PROCESSES

The field of anatomy and physiology has a language all of its own. Anatomical and physiological terms are often derived from Latin or Greek words, which can make learning them challenging.

There is a particular way anatomists discuss where something is located within the human body, using specialised terms to explain where things are in relation to each other. This allows different professions interested in the human body to develop a common understanding of where a structure is located. The **directional terms** of the body describe locations in relation to a standard **anatomical position**, which is defined as standing erect, facing forward, with the palms of the hands visible.

- In this position, structures located closer to the head are **superior**, while those located further towards the feet are **inferior**. *For example, the collar bone is superior to the breast bone, but inferior to the eyes.*
- Structures located closer to the mid line of the body are **medial**, whereas those further away from the midline are **lateral**. *For example, the inside of the leg is lateral to the spine, but medial to the outside of the leg.*
- Structures located closer to the attachment of a limb are **proximal**, whereas those further along a limb are **distal**. *For example, the knee is distal to the hip, but proximal to the ankle.*
- Structures located closer to the front of the body are **anterior**, whereas those closer to the back of the body are **posterior**. *For example, the heart is posterior to the breast bone, but anterior to the shoulder blades.*

The body also has several distinct compartments or **cavities** that can be used to describe the location of a structure. The **cranial cavity** is surrounded by the bones of the skull – the brain is located within the cranial cavity. The **thoracic cavity** is formed by the ribs and breast bone ('sternum') anteriorly and by the ribs and spine posteriorly – the lungs and heart are two of the major structures located in the thoracic cavity. The **abdominopelvic cavity** is located below the thoracic cavity and is formed by the abdominal muscles anteriorly, the back muscles and spine posteriorly and the pelvis inferiorly. The diaphragm, a large dome-shaped muscle important for breathing, divides the thoracic and abdominopelvic cavities. The intestines, liver, bladder and reproductive organs are some of the major structures located within the abdominopelvic cavity.

While showing the same overall form, the human body also shows a large amount of 'anatomical variation' – individual differences in the shape and size of anatomical structures. For example, some people have limbs that are short, or feet that are large relative to their overall height, while others have an extra 'knee cap' in the back of their knee, called the 'fabella' (Driessen et al., 2014). Some people have their internal organs on the opposite side from their normal position, a condition called 'Situs Inversus'. Just as people come in all shapes and sizes so do their bones, muscles and organs.

Cells, tissues and systems

In order to understand the human body, it is necessary to look at the building blocks that together form systems.

Cells

The smallest functional units of the body are **cells**.

There are many different types of cells found in different locations within the body. Each cell type has a specialised function, and therefore is structurally different. For example, nerve cells (neurons) need to conduct electrical signals across large distances, such as from the big toe to the spinal cord. Neurons are therefore long thin cells, allowing them to cover distances of up to 1–2m. In contrast, skin cells provide a protective barrier over the external surface of the body. They are therefore much smaller in size, some are shaped like floor tiles and they are laid in layers to fulfil this covering function.

Tissues

Groups of similar cells working together form what is called a **tissue**.

The entire human body is constructed of four main types of tissue. **Epithelial tissue** is a type of lining tissue found on both the external and internal surfaces of the body. The skin and the lining of the gut are examples of epithelial tissue. **Connective tissue** is a group of tissues that binds the body together to give it integrity. Bone, cartilage and the layer of tissue tying the skin down to the underlying muscle are examples of connective tissues. **Nervous tissue** is a specialised tissue that is able to conduct electrical signals (nerve impulses) around the body. The brain and spinal cord are good examples of nervous tissue. The final type of tissue found in the body is **muscular tissue**. The main function of this tissue type is to contract to produce movement, whether to help food move toward the stomach, the legs to move when walking or the heart to beat.

Systems

All the organs of the body are comprised of several different tissue types. Organs work together as a **system** to perform a particular function.

The 11 systems of the body and their major functions are:

1. **Nervous system** – regulates bodily functions
2. **Endocrine system** – works in conjunction with the nervous system to regulate bodily functions
3. **Muscular system** – produces movement
4. **Skeletal system** – provides support and protection for the body, bones act as levers for bodily movement
5. **Cardiovascular system** – transports blood around the body
6. **Respiratory system** – exchanges gas between the environment and the body
7. **Lymphatic system** – returns proteins and fluids to the blood stream and aids in immunity
8. **Reproductive system** – allows reproduction to occur
9. **Digestive system** – processes food to supply the body with energy
10. **Integumentary system** – protects the body and senses the external environment
11. **Urinary system** – removes waste from the body

The systems of most interest to the study of physical activity are the muscular, skeletal, nervous, endocrine, respiratory and cardiovascular systems. Each of these systems is discussed in more detail in the remainder of this chapter.

Homeostasis

While all having individual functions, ultimately all 11 body systems contribute to maintaining **homeostatic balance** within the body.

Homeostasis is defined as "the condition of equilibrium (balance) in the body's internal environment due to the constant interaction of the body's many regulatory processes" (Tortora & Derrickson, 2014). A loss of homeostasis within the body can result in disease, illness or ultimately, death.

Humans are reasonably sensitive creatures, with finely tuned 'set points' and narrow tolerance for change. For example, the normal temperature of the body is between 36.5 and 37.5 °C (97.7–99.5 °F). Any variation of more than a degree or two outside this range is a sign that things have gone wrong. The normal calcium concentration of the blood is between 9 and 11mg/100mL (Tortora & Derrickson, 2014). If blood calcium varies outside of this 2mg/100mL range, death can result.

The body has inbuilt systems to detect changes within the body and rectify these. For example, if for some reason there was a significant increase in temperature, specialised **receptors** (called thermoreceptors) would detect this rise. These receptors would then communicate this change to a **control centre** (in this case located in the brain). The control centre is then able to communicate with various tissues (**effectors**) in the body to address the rise in temperature. In this case the control centre would signal the blood vessels to open up sending more blood to the surface of the body and would instruct sweat glands to start producing sweat. This **homeostatic feedback loop** would result in a loss of heat from the body, dropping temperature and thereby restoring homeostasis. Homeostasis is one of the most important concepts within the study of anatomy and physiology.

This process of maintaining homeostasis within the body (termed '**allostasis**'), while generally helpful, comes at a cost to the body. The concept of **allostatic load** refers to the 'wear and tear' on the body of constantly adjusting and returning to baseline (McEwen & Wingfield, 2003). Allostatic load increases when the body is exposed to repeated or chronic stress. Allostatic overload has been implicated in many chronic diseases such as diabetes and cardiovascular disease (McEwen, 2005).

Metabolism

One of the most important basic life processes the human body performs is **metabolism**.

The term metabolism refers to all the chemical reactions that occur within the body, allowing the body to build, maintain and repair itself. Metabolism comprises the two opposite processes of **catabolism**, the process of breaking down complex chemical structures into their basic components, and **anabolism**, the synthesis of new complex chemical structures from these basic building blocks. The digestive system is heavily involved in the catabolism of the carbohydrates, fats and proteins we ingest, providing the raw materials needed for all 11 systems of the body to function.

While catabolic reactions release or liberate energy, anabolic reactions use or consume it. The energy released during catabolic reactions can be used to power activities such as moving substances in and out of the cell, assembling chains of amino acids into proteins or muscular contraction.

The main energy currency of the cell is **adenosine triphosphate** (ATP) which comprises three phosphate groups attached to a single adenosine molecule. During catabolism, one of the phosphate groups is split off from ATP to form adenosine diphosphate (ADP) and energy is released. This energy is then used by the cell to power all cellular activity.

Because ATP is an unstable molecule, it is not able to be stored in the cells in any great quantity. Cells therefore have different ways of converting other stored substances (such as glucose or fat) to ATP as it is needed. Tissues with high energy needs, such as skeletal muscle and the brain, are particularly well equipped to manufacture ATP.

There are two main ways cells can produce ATP. During **aerobic metabolism**, fat and/or glucose is completely broken down by catabolic reactions in the **presence of oxygen** to produce carbon dioxide, water and ATP. Aerobic metabolism is like lighting a fire and getting a bed of embers glowing – while the process takes a while to get going it can produce a lot of energy over a long period of time. Aerobic metabolism is primarily responsible for powering low to moderate intensity physical activity lasting a few minutes or longer, such as taking a dog for a walk or running a marathon. During **anaerobic metabolism**, glucose is partially broken down in a series of catabolic reactions in the **absence of oxygen** into pyruvic acid and ATP. Anaerobic glycolysis is more akin to striking a match – the process can create energy very quickly, but it is reasonably short-lived. One of the by-products of this system is lactic acid, which can quickly build up in the muscles and blood, limiting the process. Anaerobic metabolism powers short, intense bouts of physical activity lasting up to about 90 seconds, such as a 100m sprint or a deadlift in the gym.

NEUROENDOCRINE SYSTEM

Together, the nervous system and the endocrine system work collaboratively to control every function of the human body; from growth and development, to metabolism, to the use of our five senses, to every body movement and the beating of the heart. Due to the multitude of functions, disorders of the neuroendocrine system can lead to many varied health issues, such as multiple sclerosis, depression and diabetes mellitus, to name just a few. The healthy functioning of the neuroendocrine system is crucial for the health of the other nine body systems, and therefore the ability to lead an independent, fulfilling and flourishing life. Thanks to the extremely rapid electrical impulses of the nervous system, combined with the slower, yet longer lasting hormonal influences of the endocrine system, the body's internal environment can be maintained within narrow homeostatic ranges, allowing for optimal physiological functioning.

Nervous system

The nervous system is the faster, but more short-lived, of the two systems, transmitting information via rapid electrical impulses and chemical signalling. During physical activity, the nervous system plays a multitude of roles. Information received from the joints and skeletal muscles, along with environmental input, determines all body movements, coordination, reaction and decision making. Additionally, the nervous system initiates the increase in heart rate to meet the increased demand for oxygen during activity, and the increased heat dissipation as body temperature rises during muscular activity. These responses to physical activity occur due to three stages of neural stimulation: sensory input (**receptors** monitor change within, or external to, the body, e.g. rise in body temperature when active); integration (**control centre** processes and interprets information and decides on action); and motor output (activation of **effectors** to generate response, e.g. sweat glands activated to increase sweat production). Together, these three stages function during activity to make decisions and generate body movement, and to return the body to homeostasis.

Nervous system divisions

The nervous system has both structural and functional divisions (Figure 2.1). Structurally, it is divided in two; the central nervous system (CNS) and the peripheral nervous system (PNS). The CNS includes the brain and the spinal cord, while the PNS includes the remainder of the nervous system. The PNS is further divided functionally, into two major divisions; the autonomic nervous system (ANS) and the somatic nervous system (SNS). The ANS controls cardiac muscle, smooth muscle and glands, resulting in involuntary changes to the internal organs and environment. In contrast, the SNS is responsible for all body movement through the voluntary control of skeletal muscle.

A final functional division is found in the ANS: the sympathetic nervous system and the parasympathetic nervous system. Through changes in the activity of these two ANS

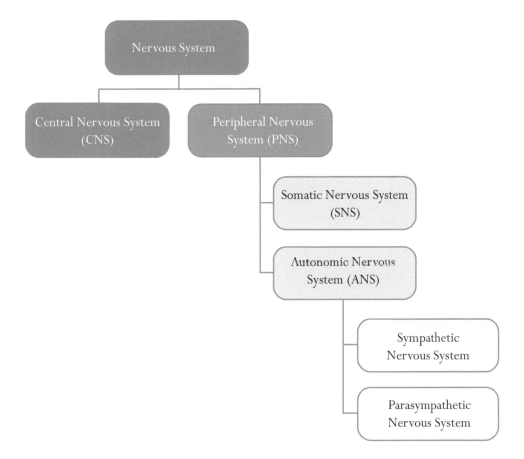

Figure 2.1   Divisions of the nervous system

subdivisions, the nervous system is able to prepare the body for the expenditure of energy (***the fight-or-flight response***), as occurs during activity, or the conservation of energy (***rest and digest***), such as during times of rest. The sympathetic nervous system drives changes conducive to exercise, including the dilation of airways, an increase in heart rate, dilation of skeletal muscle blood vessels and an increase in sweating. In contrast, parasympathetic activity stimulates energy conservation through rest and repair activities such as digestion and the synthesis of glycogen (a form of carbohydrate stored within the body). The sympathetic and parasympathetic nervous systems function in an opposite fashion, with activation of the sympathetic nervous system accompanied by downregulation of the parasympathetic nervous system, and vice versa. The dominant division depends on the current stressors at any given time.

Nervous tissue

Nervous tissue is composed of two main cell types: neurons (nerve cells) and neuroglia (glial cells). As the basic unit of the nervous system, neurons are electrically excitable cells allowing for the extremely rapid transmission of information within the nervous system or between the nervous system and its effectors (cardiac, smooth or skeletal muscle, or glands). Neuroglia include a variety of different non-excitable cell types which, together, function to structurally and metabolically support the neurons.

Neurons

The body contains billions of neurons. In general all neurons consist of three distinct parts: dendrites, a cell body and an axon (Figure 2.2). The dendrites are processes on the neuron that receive incoming information, which can be either excitatory or inhibitory. This information is passed to the cell body which processes the information. Should the excitatory input exceed the inhibitory input, an action potential (or nerve impulse) is generated at the axon hillock and conducted away from the cell body toward the axon terminals. The axons of many neurons have a whitish, electrically insulating layer called a myelin sheath (Figure 2.2). The myelin is produced by the supportive neuroglia and functions to increase the speed of action potential transmission. These high rates of information transfer allow for the incredibly fast reactions demonstrated during sport and physical activity.

Neurons responsible for transmitting information from the environment or the tissues within the body to the CNS are referred to as sensory (or afferent) neurons and, along with specialised receptors, are responsible for the sensory input function of the nervous system. In contrast, motor (or efferent) neurons transmit information from the CNS to the appropriate body tissue, to generate the response required (motor output). Some neurons transmit information from one neuron to another and, as such, are referred to as interneurons. In the body, neurons are grouped together to form nerves. The longest nerve in the human body is the sciatic nerve which is found running from the lower spine, down the leg to the foot.

Neuroglia

Neuroglia are much smaller than neurons and are the most abundant cell type within nervous tissue. Four types of neuroglia are found in the CNS and two in the PNS. The primary function of the oligodendrocytes (CNS) and the Schwann cells (PNS) is the formation of the myelin

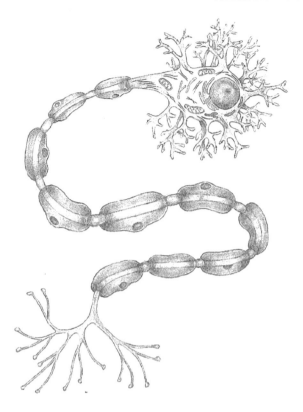

Figure 2.2 Myelinated neuron

sheath found surrounding many neurons (Figure 2.2). Within the CNS, the areas of myelinated neurons can be seen as white matter, whereas the grey matter includes the unmyelinated neurons.

Signal transmission

Neurons can differ in structure, length and purpose. Functionally, however, they all transmit information in the same manner, through the movement of positive sodium ions (Na^+) and positive potassium ions (K^+) across the axon plasma membrane (axolemma). At rest the inside of the neuron is negative to the outside and is in a *polarised* state. It is this difference in charge that allows for the generation and propagation of an electrical current, known as an action potential. Excitation of a neuron stimulates **Na^+** to rapidly **enter** the axon resulting in *depolarisation* (membrane potential becomes positive). Following this, **K^+ leaves** the axon until the negative resting membrane potential is regained. This stage is known as *repolarisation*.

The initial action potential in unmyelinated neurons stimulates the depolarisation, and subsequent action potential, of the adjacent region of the plasma membrane and so forth, resulting in the propagation of the action potential along the length of the axon to the axon terminals. This wave of depolarisation along the axon, at ~ 1–2 m.s^{-1}, is known as continuous conduction. The insulative properties of myelin, however, result in the much faster propagation of action potentials (up to 40 m.s^{-1}) along myelinated neurons. Myelin surrounds the axon in segments with the small gaps between these segments called Nodes of Ranvier (Figure 2.2). It is only at these nodes that an electrical current is able to be generated, hence the action potential appears to 'jump' along the axon (saltatory conduction), greatly increasing the speed of information transfer.

In the majority of situations, neurons transmit information to another neuron or an effector cell by chemical signalling, with the junction between the cells known as a synapse. Neurotransmitters (chemical messages), released from the axon terminal upon arrival of the action potential, bind to specific receptors on the membrane of the effector cell. This binding initiates the development of an action potential in the effector cell. As such, the electrical message has passed from the neuron to the effector cell, be it another neuron, a muscle cell or a gland cell. The neuromuscular junction is an example of a chemical synapse between a neuron and a muscle fibre.

Endocrine system

The endocrine system is the body's second control system, functioning alongside the nervous system to control the other body systems. In contrast to the rapid electrical messaging of the nervous system, the endocrine system utilises hormones as the messenger and hence is slower to generate responses (seconds to minutes) due to the time taken for the hormone to travel in the bloodstream from the site of release to the target cells. The response, however, is longer-lived (seconds to days) than that of the nervous system. The endocrine system is the main regulator of growth and development, metabolism, reproductive processes and homeostasis (see 'Homeostasis' above, p. 11).

Hormones are released by endocrine organs, of which there are 10 in the human body: hypothalamus, pituitary, pineal, thyroid, parathyroid, thymus, adrenal, pancreas, ovary and testes. The hypothalamus, located in the brain, is the controller of endocrine function, and the integral link between the nervous and endocrine systems. Due to this link, the hypothalamus is classed as a neuroendocrine organ.

In general, the endocrine organs produce, store and secrete one or more hormones, which subsequently produce specific responses in target cells. For example, during exercise the adrenal glands are stimulated by nerve impulses to release epinephrine (also known as adrenaline) which, along with the nervous system, plays a role in elevating heart rate to accommodate the increased oxygen demand of skeletal muscle. Simultaneously, a reduction in blood glucose due to the increased muscle contraction, stimulates the release of glucagon by the pancreas, resulting in the mobilisation of muscle and liver glycogen stores (glycogenolysis) and the formation of glucose (gluconeogenesis) by the liver. These combined responses return blood glucose concentration to its homeostatic level. The role of the endocrine system during sport and physical activity becomes clear when you consider the increased cardiovascular, metabolic and substrate demands, all of which involve hormonal messaging. Table 2.1 gives a summary of the key hormones involved in the physiological response to physical activity.

The dysfunction of endocrine organs can result in multiple disorders, from hyperthyroidism, to Cushing's syndrome, to, perhaps the most well-known, diabetes mellitus. These disorders are the result of hormone overproduction, underproduction or abnormal sensitivity

Table 2.1   Key hormones involved in the physiological response to physical activity

Organ	Hormone	Function relating to physical activity
Adrenal medulla	Epinephrine & norepinephrine	Enhance the 'fight-or-flight' response initiated by the sympathetic nervous system; increase heart rate and force of contraction, increase blood flow to skeletal muscle, dilate airways, increase glycogenolysis and lipolysis (fat breakdown)
Adrenal cortex	Cortisol	Increases gluconeogenesis in the liver during prolonged endurance activity
	Aldosterone	Conserves blood sodium (Na^+) and water
Pituitary gland	Antidiuretic hormone	Conserves body water
	Endorphins	Reduces the perception of pain
Pancreas	Insulin	Decreases blood glucose concentration
	Glucagon	Increases blood glucose concentration (glycogenolysis and gluconeogenesis)

of target cells, with the majority due to non-modifiable factors. Type 2 diabetes, however, is termed a lifestyle disease with suboptimal nutrition and an increasingly sedentary lifestyle contributing to its development over many years. Physical inactivity leads to the development of insulin resistance which results in a chronically elevated blood glucose concentration. Type 2 diabetes has multiple co-morbidities, hence health and quality of life can be severely impacted by this condition. Incorporating physical activity within our everyday lives reduces insulin resistance and lowers resting insulin levels, helping to prevent or manage this potentially debilitating condition.

MUSCULOSKELETAL SYSTEM

The musculoskeletal system – comprising the **muscular system** and the **skeletal system** – is of particular interest to the study of physical activity. Together these two systems afford us the ability to walk, run, jump for joy and dance the night away. Disorders of the musculoskeletal system are common, and represent a large burden for the healthcare system. Musculoskeletal conditions range from **acute injuries** (such as fractures, bruises, strains and sprains), to **chronic, overuse injuries** (such as bursitis or tendinitis) and clinical conditions such as muscular dystrophy, osteoporosis and arthritis.

Skeletal system

The main functions of the skeletal system are to provide **support** for the other structures of the body, to provide attachment points for muscles so that **movement** can occur, and to provide **protection** for organs such as the lungs and brain. The skeleton also provides **storage** of minerals and triglycerides, and **manufactures blood cells** in a process called 'haemopoiesis'.

The adult human skeleton (Figure 2.3) is made up of a total of 206 bones, ranging in size from the large long bone of the thigh (the *femur*), to the individual *vertebrae* that comprise the spine to the tiny *stapes* (or *stirrup*) bone found in the inner ear. At birth, the number of bones in the skeleton is

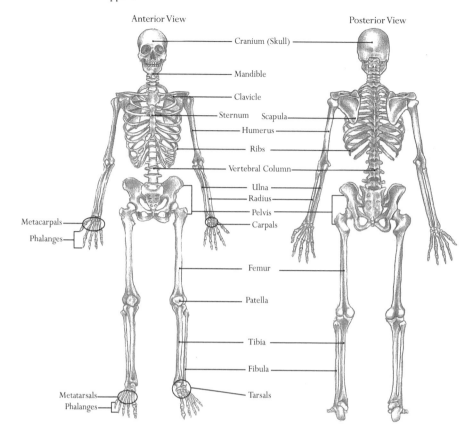

Figure 2.3 Anterior (a) and posterior (b) views of the human skeleton

higher, at approximately 300. Many of these bones will fuse together later in life (for example, the 22 bones that will make up the skull), bringing the adult total to 206.

The skeleton is divided in to two main divisions – the **axial skeleton** (80 bones), acts as the 'axis' or central component to which the four limbs (**appendicular skeleton, 126 bones**) are attached via the shoulder (or pectoral) and hip (or pelvic) girdles.

All of the 206 bones of the skeleton can be classified into one of five main types based on shape:

- **Short bones**, e.g. carpal bones of wrist
- **Long bones**, e.g. femur, tibia, radius
- **Irregular bones**, e.g. facial bones, vertebrae
- **Flat bones**, e.g. scapular, sternum
- **Sesamoid bones**, e.g. patella

The shape of a bone influences the function – for example, an irregular bone such as the vertebrae has many projections that provide places for muscles to attach, whereas a flat bone covers a large surface area to provide protection while also remaining light.

It is common to think of the skeleton as a passive, inactive structure, however the skeleton is very much alive and is under the process of continuous turnover. For this process of replacing old bone tissue with new (**bone remodelling**) to occur, the skeleton needs to be exposed to the right amount of external force, as well as have the right levels of vitamins and minerals. Bone remodelling is under the control of the neuroendocrine system.

Astronauts spending long periods of time in space (more than a few weeks) can lose a significant amount of bone density, as their skeletons are no longer exposed to the bone building effects of gravity (NASA, 2004). Even on earth bone needs movement and impact to remain healthy. If you are unwell enough to be confined to bed rest for a period of time, your skeleton starts to show changes after just several days. Regular, weight-bearing physical activity helps to maintain bone health.

Bone tissue

Each bone of the skeleton is an individual organ, made up of several tissues – **bone, cartilage** (a tough but flexible type of connective tissue that lines joint surfaces), **periosteum** (a thin lining over the surface of bone) and other structures such as **nerves**.

There are two main types of bone tissue. **Spongy bone**, also called **cancellous** bone, appears to have a honeycomb structure as it is made of thin plates of bone called 'trabeculae' with spaces in between. Spongy bone is designed to be light but still strong and is found mainly in short, flat and irregular bones, and at the ends (**epiphyses**) of long bones. **Compact bone**, as the name suggests, is comprised of a hard layer of dense bone tissue designed to resist stress. Compact bone forms the shaft (**diaphysis**) of long bones, and the outside layer of all bones.

Both spongy and compact bone are made up at a cellular level by different types of bone cells (**osteocytes, osteoblasts** and **osteoclasts**) sitting within a matrix made of collagen fibres (the 'organic' component), mineral salts (the 'inorganic' component) and water. This design allows bone to resist both tension (the organic component) and compression (the inorganic component). Together the two components allow bone to resist bending, allowing the skeleton to fulfil its functions of support and protection.

Joints

For the skeleton to be able to move, bones meet at highly specialised junctions called **joints** (or **articulations**).

Structurally, there are three main types of joints found within the human body. Joints are a good example of the **complementarity of structure and function** – each joint is designed differently for the specific job it is required to do. **Fibrous joints** are rigid, allowing very little movement to provide a high level of protection (e.g. the suture joints between the bones of the skull) whereas **cartilaginous joints** (e.g. the joints between each of the vertebrae of the spine) allow a small amount of movement, but still provide some protection. The large, mobile joints of the body are **synovial joints**, which are designed for maximum mobility.

The specific structure of a synovial joint determines the movements available at that joint. For example, a synovial **hinge** joint, just like the hinge on a door, only allows movement in one direction. The elbow is a good example of a hinge joint. The most mobile joints in the human body are the shoulder and hip joint, which are **ball and socket** synovial joints. The

Table 2.2   Main movements at synovial joints

Flexion	A decrease in the angle between two bones
Extension	The opposite of flexion, an increase in the angle between two bones
Abduction	The movement of a bone away from the midline of the body
Adduction	The opposite of abduction, movement of a bone towards the midline of the body
Rotation	The twisting of a bone around its own longitudinal axis
Circumduction	The movement of the end of a bone – a combination of flexion, extension, abduction and adduction
Dorsiflexion	A specialised movement of the ankle, lifting the toes upwards
Plantarflexion	The opposite of dorsiflexion, a specialised movement of the ankle, pointing the toes downwards
Supination	A specialised movement of the forearm, turning the palm to face upwards
Pronation	The opposite of supination, a specialised movement of the forearm, turning the palm to face downwards

design of these joints allows movement through nearly 360 degrees so that you can reach around to scratch your back as well as perform a layup in basketball. Other types of synovial joints include **planar** joints, **saddle** joints, **pivot** joints and **condyloid** joints.

To gain such a large amount of movement, synovial joints sacrifice some of their stability, meaning they can be vulnerable to injury (e.g. shoulder dislocation). To make up for this, synovial joints have a large number of specialised accessory (or 'extra') structures, such as **ligaments**, a joint capsule and **menisci**, that help increase the stability of the joint. These structures can be injured when a joint is forced beyond its normal range of motion, resulting in the sprains and tears commonly seen on the sports field.

Anatomists have specialised terms to describe the different movements that occur at synovial joints. The main movements are shown in Table 2.2.

While these movements occur at the joints, which are part of the skeletal system, without the contribution of the muscular system, movement would not be possible.

Muscular system

The primary function of the muscular system is to **produce movement** but it also assists in temperature homeostasis by **producing heat** and **moves substances around the body** (e.g. moving food down the digestive tract).

Muscle tissue

Each muscle of the body is also an individual organ, made up of several tissues, including **muscle tissue, connective tissue, blood vessels** and **nerves**.

There are three main types of muscle tissue found in the human body. **Skeletal muscle** is the most prevalent. Skeletal muscle makes up the muscles visible on the external surface of the body under the skin, muscles such as the biceps and 'pecs'. Less familiar is **cardiac muscle**, which is found exclusively in the heart and **smooth muscle** which is found in the walls of hollow structures inside the body (such as the bladder, digestive tract and blood vessels). The nervous system controls the three different types of muscle tissue in different ways – skeletal muscle is under voluntary control (somatic nervous system), while cardiac and smooth muscle are involuntary (autonomic nervous system). This explains why you can choose when to lift your arms over your head, but you are unable to consciously decide how quickly to digest the pasta you ate for lunch, or how much to increase heart rate during physical activity.

Surprisingly, there is some debate over the total number of muscles in the human body. Most textbooks estimate the number to be somewhere between 600 and 700, the vast majority of which are skeletal muscles. As with other systems, there is some anatomical variation between people – for example up to 63% of people are missing the *palmaris longus* muscle on the palmar surface of the wrist (Ioannis, Anastasios, Konstantinos, Lazaros, & Georgios, 2015). Some muscles are not easy to separate from their neighbours, leading people to argue as to whether or not they should be named separately, and there is debate on how to include cardiac and smooth muscle in the count.

Figure 2.4 shows the main skeletal muscles of the body. As the muscular system is arranged in layers, with deep muscles underneath the more superficial ones, it is not possible to see all of the skeletal muscles on one picture. Skeletal muscles vary in size from the large *gluteus maximus* to the small muscles that control the eye and fine movements of the fingers.

Muscle physiology

At a cellular level muscle is made up of individual muscle cells called **myocytes** bundled together in functional teams called **motor units**, to form a **muscle belly**. The muscle belly is attached to a different bone on each side of the joint via a strong band of connective tissue

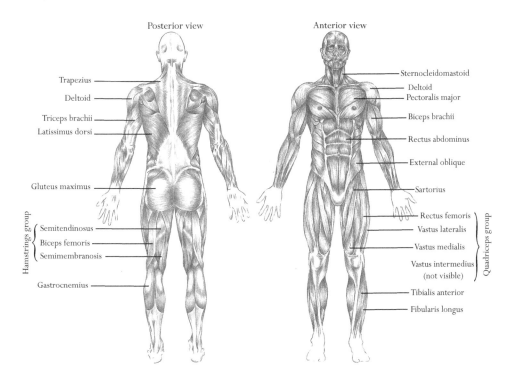

Figure 2.4 Anterior (a) and posterior (b) views of the superficial skeletal muscles of the body

called a **tendon**. The attachment onto the proximal bone is called the muscle's **origin**, whereas the attachment onto the more distal bone is referred to as the muscle's **insertion**. The most well-known tendon in the body is the Achilles tendon, which attaches the *gastrocnemius* (calf) muscle to its insertion on the heel bone (calcaneus).

Each individual myocyte (also called a **muscle fibre**) is made up of smaller units called **myofibrils** which themselves are made up of the contractile proteins that cause muscle contraction. These proteins alternate between bands of 'thick' **myosin** filaments, and bands of 'thin' **actin, troponin and tropomyosin** filaments. This arrangement of alternating thick and thin bands is what makes skeletal muscle appear stripy under a microscope.

Originally it was thought that muscles contracted by folding on themselves like an accordion. However, in the mid 1950s, development of the first electron micrographs of skeletal muscle revealed that the thick and thin filaments actually slide across and past one another in a process termed the **Sliding Filament Mechanism** (Tortora & Derrickson, 2014).

At a microscopic level, the myosin filaments have small 'heads'. In response to a nerve impulse arriving at the **neuromuscular junction**, these heads are able to reach out and form 'cross bridges' with the actin filaments and are able to 'walk' their way along them, sliding the thick and thin filaments past each other, thereby shortening the muscle fibre. When this process occurs in several muscle fibres at once, the force produced is strong enough to pull on the insertion point via the attached tendon, thereby creating movement of a joint. When neural stimulation ceases, the muscle relaxes – the myosin heads detach from the actin filaments and the bands return to the resting position, lengthening the muscle again and returning the joint to its original position. The Sliding Filament Mechanism works most efficiently when there is optimal overlap between the actin and myosin filaments. If a muscle is in an extremely stretched or shortened position, fewer cross bridges are possible resulting in decreased force production and reduced strength.

This alternating contraction and relaxation of muscle fibres is what allows us to move. Even at rest, a small number of muscle fibres remain in a state of contraction, giving the muscle its **muscle tone**, assisting the body to stand up against gravity and resist external perturbations.

Skeletal muscles work functionally in pairs to produce the movements at joints shown in Table 2.2 (main movements at synovial joints), with one muscle contracting while the other one is relaxing.

During a particular movement, the muscle that is contracting and producing force is called the **agonist** or **prime mover**. The opposing muscle, often on the opposite side of the joint, that has to relax to let this movement occur is called the **antagonist**. For example, during elbow flexion the biceps acts as the agonist, while the triceps is the antagonist. During elbow extension, this pairing reverses: the triceps become the agonist, contracting to create the movement, and the biceps becomes the antagonist, relaxing and lengthening to allowing the elbow to straighten.

While strength training in the gym, it is common to train agonist/antagonist pairs together – for example doing an exercise for the quadriceps, and then immediately after another one for the hamstrings. Resistance, or strength training in the gym, results in **hypertrophy** (growth) of the individual muscle fibres, thereby increasing the bulk of muscle, increasing its size.

Commonly, as a muscle produces force (contracts) it will shorten in length. This type of muscle contraction is termed a **concentric contraction** (for example, the biceps contract *concentrically* as the elbow flexes when performing a bicep curl). Alternatively, a muscle can produce force as it lengthens, a type of contraction termed an **eccentric contraction** (for example, the biceps contract *eccentrically* as the elbow extends when slowly lowering the weight back down during a bicep curl). A muscle can also produce force while remaining the same length, called an **isometric contraction** (for example, the biceps contract *isometrically* when pausing at the top of the bicep curl).

Ageing and the musculoskeletal system

The musculoskeletal system undergoes many structural and functional changes with age, such as a progressive loss of stature (height), reduction in flexibility of the joints, and a loss of muscle mass. In addition, there is a progressive reduction in bone density, which can result in a condition called **osteoporosis**. Together, these changes increase the risk of falls, and therefore acute injuries of the musculoskeletal system, such as fractures and contusions ('bruises'), meaning the musculoskeletal system is potentially vulnerable with increasing age.

Fortunately, a lot of these changes can be delayed or minimised with regular physical activity – staying active with age slows the loss of muscle mass and bone density and reduces the risk of injurious falls. Physical activity also has a large part to play in the management of many musculoskeletal disorders, such as arthritis and low back pain, which both respond well to appropriate regular physical activity.

CARDIORESPIRATORY SYSTEM

To continue functioning, the cells of the body require oxygen (O_2) for aerobic metabolism and subsequent energy production. This energy is required for a multitude of processes such as growth and repair, and muscle contraction. Together, the cardiovascular and respiratory systems function to transport oxygen from the atmosphere to the individual cells of the body, adjusting the rate of oxygen delivery as demands change. During physical activity, the additional oxygen required to meet the enhanced energy demands of skeletal muscle is achieved through an increase in breathing (ventilation) and heart rate. Alongside oxygen delivery, the circulating blood carries carbon dioxide (CO_2), a waste product of metabolism, from the body's cells to the lungs for removal.

Many factors influence the efficiency of the cardiorespiratory system including genetics, the environment and physiological factors. Physiological adaptations, such as improved blood flow to skeletal muscle fibres, occur in response to a chronic demand for increased oxygen, for example, moving from a sedentary to an active lifestyle. This ultimately improves the supply of oxygen to the muscle cells, contributing to an elevated aerobic fitness and improved ability to complete the activities of daily living. In addition, elevated physical activity helps to improve the lipid profile and improves breathing, reducing the risk of developing, or improving the management of, cardiorespiratory diseases (such as atherosclerosis, coronary heart disease and asthma). The negative impact physical inactivity has on our health is discussed in more detail in Chapter 4.

Respiratory system

The main function of the respiratory system is gas exchange between the atmospheric air and the circulating blood. Upon inhalation, air travels through the airways to the lungs, the site of gas exchange. Oxygen diffuses from the lungs into the blood while carbon dioxide diffuses in the opposite direction, from the blood to the lungs, following which it is removed from the body during exhalation. In addition to the primary role of gas exchange, the respiratory system is also influential in functions such as smell, speech, coughing and sneezing.

Anatomy

The respiratory system includes many structures from the nose and mouth, to the alveoli in the lungs. Inhalation moves air through the **conducting zone** (Figure 2.5) to the sites of gas exchange (**respiratory zone**). In addition to forming a passageway through which the air can move, the conducting zone also functions to warm, moisten and filter the incoming air, protecting the respiratory surfaces from temperature extremes, dehydration, debris and pathogens. From the terminal bronchioles, the air enters the **respiratory zone** which includes an extensive area for gas exchange, including the respiratory bronchioles, alveolar ducts and alveoli (the smallest microscopic structures of the lungs and main site of gas exchange). The extensive capillary network surrounding the alveoli maximises the potential for gas exchange.

   The lungs are cone-shaped organs located in the thoracic cavity and protected by the ribs. They extend from the apex, just superior to the clavicle (collar bone), to the wide concave

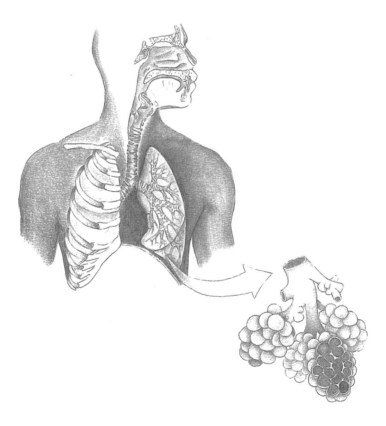

Figure 2.5 Main structures of the respiratory system

base resting on the diaphragm. The right lung is larger, consisting of three lobes, while the smaller left lung consists of two lobes. The medial surface of the left lung has a 'cardiac notch' conforming to the shape of the heart which is located between the lungs.

The lungs are surrounded by a pleural membrane (a double-layered serous membrane) with the outer parietal layer attached to the thoracic wall and the superior surface of the diaphragm, and the inner visceral layer covering the outer surface of the lungs. Pleural fluid is found between these membrane layers, allowing the layers to easily slide over each other while, due to the high surface tension, ensuring the layers remain stuck together. As the lungs contain no muscle, these functions of the pleural membrane are vital to allow the lungs to expand and recoil during ventilation concurrently with the increase and decrease in thoracic volume.

Pulmonary ventilation

Inhalation during resting conditions is reliant on the contraction of the diaphragm and the external intercostal muscles; this is an active process. The increase in lung volume reduces the air pressure within the lung, resulting in air moving from the atmosphere (where the pressure is higher) to the lungs (where the pressure is lower) until pressures become equal once again. In contrast, resting exhalation is a passive process whereby thoracic volume, and hence lung volume, is decreased due to the elastic recoil of the inspiratory muscle fibres. The subsequent increase in lung air pressure (due to decreased lung volume) results in the movement of air from the lungs back to the atmosphere.

Physical activity increases the demand for oxygen by the skeletal muscles, hence inhalation and exhalation become faster, deeper and more forceful, increasing the exchange of oxygen and carbon dioxide between the lungs and the blood. This increase in ventilation requires the contraction of additional muscles in the neck during inhalation. Exhalation becomes an active process, with the contraction of the internal intercostal and abdominal muscles decreasing thoracic and lung volume further, moving more air out of the lungs at a faster rate. The main driver for the increase in ventilation during exercise is the elevation of the partial pressure of carbon dioxide (PCO_2) in the blood. Specialised receptors (chemoreceptors) in the brain and some main arteries relay this information to the respiratory centres in the brain. The respiratory centres subsequently send nerve impulses to the appropriate muscles to induce an increase in ventilation.

Measurement of pulmonary function

A spirometer is used to measure pulmonary function to compare lung volumes and capacities to known healthy values, or to monitor changes, whether a progression of disease or response to treatment. In addition, the analysis of expired air composition at rest and during exercise indicates the efficiency of oxygen and carbon dioxide diffusion into, and out of, the blood, respectively.

Pulmonary function is commonly assessed with the measurement of minute ventilation ($\dot{V}_E$), forced vital capacity (FVC) and forced expiratory volume (FEV). At rest, the average adult breathes 12 times per minute, moving 500 mL of air into and out of the lungs each time. As such, resting $\dot{V}_E$ is around 6 L.min^{-1}. Forced vital capacity is the maximum volume of air exhaled following a full inhalation (average value of 3.1 L (female) or 4.9 L (male)) (Tortora & Derrickson, 2014). The exhalation of air with maximal effort, following full inhalation, is the

FEV. A common measure of lung function is the volume of air exhaled within the first second of FEV, termed FEV_1. This value is reported as a percentage of FVC, with a healthy adult achieving a value around 80%. In practice, a peak flow meter, a cheap and simple alternative to the spirometer, can be used for measuring FEV_1.

Cardiovascular system

The cardiovascular (CV) system is the body's main transport system with the beating of the **heart** functioning to pump the **blood** through a comprehensive network of **blood vessels**. It is the collaboration of this system with the respiratory system that allows for life-giving oxygen to be transported from the atmosphere to the cells of the body. Simultaneously, carbon dioxide is transported to the lungs for removal to the atmosphere. In addition, the blood transports nutrients from the digestive system to the cells, hormones from endocrine organs to target cells and excess heat to the surface of the body for dissipation, all important during physical activity.

Blood

Blood is a fluid connective tissue with an adult volume of 4–5 L in females and 5–6 L in males (Draper & Marshall, 2012). It is composed of a watery fluid portion containing dissolved substances and proteins, called plasma, and a cellular component. The main functions of plasma include transportation (e.g. hormones, nutrients, waste products, oxygen, antibodies) and regulation (pH, temperature). The cellular component of blood contains red blood cells (erythrocytes), white blood cells (leukocytes), and cellular fragments called platelets (thrombocytes). The percentage of blood occupied by cells (haematocrit, Hct) is a common health measure. Males generally present with a higher Hct (40–54%) than females (38–46%) (Tortora & Derrickson, 2014), with a low Hct (anaemia) resulting in general fatigue, weakness and shortness of breath, making physical activity, including everyday tasks, a chore.

With a diameter of only 8 μm, there are approximately 270 million (males) or 240 million (females) erythrocytes in a single drop of blood. Erythrocytes have a biconcave shape and are both flexible and strong, allowing them to fold where necessary when passing through capillaries (the smallest blood vessels, 5–10 μm diameter). The continuous wear on the erythrocyte membrane from travelling through the capillaries results in a short lifespan of around 120 days.

The primary function of erythrocytes is to transport O_2 from the lungs to the cells, with the biconcave shape maximising surface area for O_2 diffusion. A single erythrocyte contains around 280 million haemoglobin molecules, each composed of a protein and four iron-containing haem molecules. Following diffusion from the lungs to the blood, each oxygen molecule binds reversibly to one of the iron ions. As such, each molecule of haemoglobin is able to bind four oxygen molecules. Upon arrival at the tissue, which has a lower O_2 content, haemoglobin releases the O_2 which subsequently diffuses across the capillary wall and into the cells.

The general function of leukocytes is to protect the body from pathogens. There are five different types of leukocyte which function together to combat pathogens through phagocytosis (ingestion and destruction of foreign matter) or immune responses. An increase in leukocyte levels is usually indicative of infection or inflammation. Following injury, platelets play a major role in the clotting of blood.

The heart

The heart is a muscular organ around the size of your fist. It is located between the lungs and rests on the diaphragm, while being protected by the sternum and the ribs. Despite being a muscle, the heart has no chance to rest, beating around 100,000 times every day, equating to ~2.5 billion beats in an average lifetime. It is the beating of the heart that ensures the continuous circulation of blood round all tissues of the body, and subsequent gas exchange to meet the body's metabolic demands.

Anatomy

The heart is surrounded by the pericardium. This includes a fibrous sac which protects the heart and a serous membrane allowing for the increased movement of the heart during activity. The walls of the heart are composed of cardiac muscle (myocardium). There are four chambers within the heart; two superior chambers (atria), and two inferior chambers (ventricles). To ensure the blood flows smoothly in one direction, valves are located between the atria and the ventricles (atrioventricular (AV) valves), and between the ventricles and the blood vessels leaving the heart (semilunar valves). It is the shutting of these valves, and subsequent blood turbulence, that form the two sounds of the heart beat: lubb (AV valves closing) and dupp (semilunar valves closing). Blood leaving the heart flows round one of two circuits: the pulmonary circuit or the systemic circuit. Figure 2.6 illustrates the basic anatomy of the heart, while Figure 2.7 shows the direction of blood flow through the heart and the two circulatory circuits.

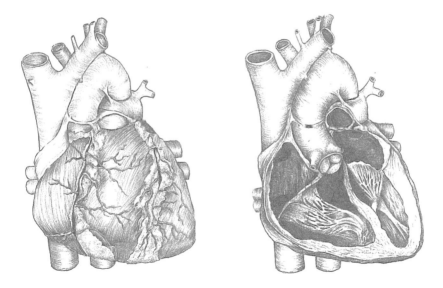

Figure 2.6 Anatomy of the heart: (a) anterior surface structures, (b) anterior view of heart frontal section

Direction of blood flow

To understand the flow of blood through the heart and round the body (Figures 2.6 and 2.7), the journey of a single drop of blood will be considered. The journey will start at the right atrium having just returned from the body's cells where the blood offloaded oxygen and received carbon dioxide. The deoxygenated blood enters the right atrium via the superior vena cava, the inferior vena cava, or the coronary sinus; veins returning blood to the heart from the upper body, lower body and myocardium, respectively. Upon contraction of the heart, blood moves from the right atrium, through the right AV valve (or tricuspid valve), to the right ventricle. From here, the blood is pumped through the right semilunar valve (or pulmonary valve) to the pulmonary trunk – the start of the pulmonary circuit. This then divides to the left and right pulmonary arteries which transport the blood to the left and right lungs, respectively, where the blood is oxygenated and carbon dioxide offloaded (external respiration).

The oxygenated blood returns from the lungs to the left atrium of the heart via one of four pulmonary veins. Contraction of the left atrium then forces the blood through the left AV valve (or bicuspid valve) to the left ventricle. Subsequently, the blood is pumped through the left semilunar valve (or aortic valve) to the aorta (largest artery), the start of the systemic circuit, and round the rest of the body. Upon reaching the body's tissues, gas exchange occurs between the blood and the cells (internal respiration) before the blood is returned to the right atrium where the journey of the blood through the heart and round the body starts again. The left ventricle pumps blood a much greater distance than the right ventricle. Considering the

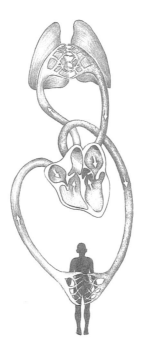

Figure 2.7 Circuits of the circulatory system and direction of blood flow (arrows)

greater pressure required to pump blood round the systemic circuit, i.e. the whole body, the thickness of the left ventricle wall is around three times greater than that of the right ventricle which pumps blood to the lungs located in close proximity (Figure 2.6).

Cardiac conduction

The spontaneous initiation of the heart beat is due to the auto-rhythmic (self-excitable) nature of the sinoatrial (SA) node, commonly referred to as the pacemaker of the heart. This fundamental rhythm ($\sim$ 100 beats.min^{-1}) is modified by the neuroendocrine system, with the parasympathetic division lowering heart rate to $\sim$ 75 (beats.min^{-1}) at rest, and the combined influence of sympathetic stimulation and epinephrine elevating heart rate during activity to meet the increased metabolic demand of skeletal muscle. The SA node, located in the posterior wall of the right atrium, provides the initial stimulus for myocardial contraction. The subsequent spread of electrical activity is coordinated such that the atria contract together, followed by the ventricles.

   Contraction (systole) of the atria is stimulated by the spread of electrical activity from the SA node to the atrioventricular (AV) node (located in the floor of the right atrium), forcing blood from the atria to the ventricles. At this stage of electrical conduction, there is a delay of $\sim$ 0.1 seconds to allow for complete atrial systole before ventricular systole starts. The electrical signal then passes down the conducting fibres of the AV bundle (or Bundle of His) and the bundle branches to the apex of the heart. Specialised Purkinje fibres then propagate the action potential to the ventricular cardiac muscle, resulting in contraction from the apex toward the base, and the ejection of blood from the ventricles. The atria are relaxed (diastole) during ventricular systole, which is followed by ventricular diastole. This cycle of electrical activity, systole and diastole, known as the cardiac cycle, is repeated for each heartbeat.

Recording of heart rate

The electrical activity of the heart described above can be recorded by an electrocardiograph, providing a trace known as an electrocardiogram (ECG). The ECG of a single heart beat includes a P wave, QRS complex and a T wave. Each section of the trace relates to a specific stage of electrical activity and mechanical event during the heartbeat. This sequence of events is outlined in the table below (Table 2.3).

   In reality, an ECG is most commonly used to monitor heart function in a clinical setting to identify any abnormalities in the electrical conduction, and subsequent mechanical function, of the heart. Those monitoring heart rate (HR) during physical activity rely on simple heart rate monitors, with a chest strap detecting the electrical activity of the heart and the use of telemetry to display HR on a watch.

Table 2.3   The electrical and mechanical events of a cardiac cycle

ECG	Electrical event	Mechanical event
P wave	Atrial depolarisation	Atrial systole
QRS complex	Ventricular depolarisation	Ventricular systole
	Atrial repolarisation	Atrial diastole
T wave	Ventricular repolarisation	Ventricular diastole

Cardiac output

Heart rate, and the volume of blood ejected from the heart, varies with changing metabolic needs of the body. At rest, the total volume of blood ejected from the left ventricle each minute is around 5 L.min⁻¹. This **cardiac output ($\dot{Q}$)** is dependent on the **heart rate** and the **stroke volume (SV)**, the volume of blood ejected with each heartbeat. The relationship between these variables is shown below:

$$\dot{Q} = SV \times HR$$

During exercise the cardiac output is elevated through an increase in both HR and SV, meeting the greater metabolic needs of skeletal muscle. The magnitude of cardiac output increase in the average person is 4–5 times resting values, however this can be as great as 7–8 times in elite endurance athletes.

Blood vessels

The vascular system involves an extensive network of blood vessels with arteries leaving the heart, leading to arterioles, capillaries, venules and finally veins returning blood to the heart. The central inside space of these vessels, through which blood flows, is called the lumen. The differing structure of each blood vessel reflects its unique function. The large arteries leaving the heart contain multiple elastic fibres allowing distention to accommodate the blood entering them at high pressure. The recoil of the elastic wall then functions to maintain blood flow during ventricular diastole. Arteries further away from the heart are composed of ~ 75% smooth muscle, allowing for the great ability to vasoconstrict (decrease the size of the lumen) and vasodilate (increase the size of the lumen) to finely adjust blood flow in response to changes in sympathetic stimulation or certain chemicals in the blood. These arteries branch to take blood to all organs of the body, eventually becoming microscopic vessels called arterioles which tightly regulate blood flow to the extensive capillary network (site of internal respiration). The amount of blood flow to the capillaries is controlled by sphincters, with few receiving blood when metabolic demands are low, compared to a full capillary network in skeletal muscle during exercise. Due to the multiple branching and small size of capillaries, they provide a huge surface area for gas exchange. In addition, the one-cell-thick wall allows for rapid exchange of materials.

Blood from a capillary network flows into a venule and the return journey to the heart begins. Venules unite to become veins, distensible thin-walled vessels with a wide lumen, able to accommodate large volumes of blood. Due to the force of gravity, veins in the limbs contain one-way valves, with the contraction of skeletal muscle surrounding the vein forcing blood to move through the one-way valves toward the heart. This process is known as the muscular pump. This explains the need to keep moving following activity, otherwise large volumes of blood entering the veins will pool in the lower limbs, reducing venous return to the heart. Continued movement will ensure the muscular pump aids in blood flow back to the heart.

Blood pressure

As an important predictor of health, blood pressure (BP) is routinely measured by medical practitioners and health researchers. It is measured with a sphygmomanometer and stethoscope or an automated machine. As blood is pumped from the left ventricle to the aorta and round the body, the pressure exerted on the artery walls, during systole and diastole, is recorded as the BP measurement. As such, two readings are obtained: systolic and diastolic BP, with the systolic pressure being the higher of the two numbers. A 'normal' BP, and an indicator of good health, is below 120 mmHg (systolic BP) and 80 mmHg (diastolic BP): written as 120/80.

High blood pressure, or hypertension, is a risk factor for cardiovascular disease and is also one of the risk factors involved with the metabolic syndrome. Hypertension is classified as a BP of 140/90 or higher. This condition can be treated through lifestyle changes, such as increasing physical activity and reducing salt intake, or anti-hypertensive medication.

Chapter summary

- Physical activity is important for physical health.
- Homeostasis is one of the most important concepts within the study of anatomy and physiology.
- The nervous and endocrine systems function to maintain homeostasis and generate movement via electrical impulses and hormone release.
- The muscular and skeletal systems enable us to move our bodies, subsequently maintaining or enhancing the health of these systems.
- The cardiovascular and respiratory systems function together to move oxygen from the atmosphere to the body's cells where it is required for energy production.

References

Draper, N., & Marshall, H. (2012). *Exercise Physiology: For Health and Sports Performance*. Harlow, U.K.: Pearson United Kingdom.

Driessen, A., Balke, M., Offerhaus, C., White, W.J., Shafiz, S., Becher, C., . . . Höher, J. (2014). The fabella syndrome – a rare cause of posterolateral knee pain: a review of the literature and two case reports. *BMC Musculoskelet Disord, 26*, 15–100. doi:10.1186/1471-2474-15-100

Helander, H.F., & Fändriks, L. (2014). Surface area of the digestive tract – revisited. *Scand J Gastroenterol, 49*(6), 681–689. doi:10.3109/00365521.2014.898326

Ioannis, D., Anastasios, K., Konstantinos, N., Lazaros, K., & Georgios, N. (2015). Palmaris longus muscle's prevalence in different nations and interesting anatomical variations: review of the literature. *Journal of Clinical Medicine Research, 7*(11), 825–830. doi:http://doi.org/10.14740/jocmr2243w

McEwen, B.S. (2005). Stressed or stressed out: what is the difference? *Journal of Psychiatry and Neuroscience, 30*(5), 315–318.

McEwen, B.S., & Wingfield, J.C. (2003). The concept of allostasis in biology and biomedicine. *Hormones and Behaviour, 43*(1), 2–15.

NASA. (2004, August 19). *Bones in Space*. Retrieved December 15, 2016, from NASA: www.nasa.gov/audience/foreducators/postsecondary/features/F_Bones_in_Space.html

Tortora, G.J., & Derrickson, B.H. (2014). *Principles of Anatomy and Physiology* (14th ed.). Wiley Global Education.

3 Historical aspects of physical activity

David Broom

Keywords: History, paradigm shift, physical activity, recommendations

Introduction

Modern day *Homo sapiens* have evolved from hunter gatherers for whom physical activity was a daily occurrence to survive and flee or fight off predators. The first part of the chapter highlights issues regarding physical activity throughout the ages up to the 1950s. Systematic research regarding the relationship between physical activity and health only began in the second half of the 20th century so the second part of this chapter discusses landmark studies led by pioneers who have demonstrated the benefits of physical activity on all-cause mortality and for chronic disease. Based on this evidence, national and international organisations, such as the World Health Organization, have recommended an amount of physical activity needed to benefit health. The third part of the chapter explores the evolution of these recommendations from focusing on training for performance and fitness to physical activity for health. Finally, the chapter discusses trends in physical activity over the last 60 years.

Historical context of physical activity from ancient to modern times

> All parts of the body which have a function, if used in moderation and exercised in labours in which each is accustomed, become thereby healthy, well developed and age more slowly, but if unused they become liable to disease, defective in growth and age quickly
>
> Hippocrates, ~450 BC.

In prehistoric times the main motivation for being physically active was to survive by hunting and gathering. Throughout the ages subsistence requirements have changed and consequently the motivation for physical activity has also changed. This first part will highlight the history of physical activity from its primitive beginnings. The timeline and content has been adapted from Dalleck and Kravitz (2002).

Primitive man (pre 10,000 BC)

Hunting and gathering was a daily task of primitive nomadic lifestyles that defined existence. To survive, tribes would embark on one- or two-day hunting journeys to acquire food and water. Physical activity was a fundamental part of daily life and successful hunts were celebrated by visiting neighbouring tribes which again required walking long distances. The celebrations included dancing and active cultural games.

The Neolithic agricultural revolution (10,000–8,000 BC)

Important agricultural developments occurred including the invention of the plough and the domestication of plants and animals. Physical activity decreased as an agrarian society developed and tribes began to concentrate on agriculture and farming. They could obtain food without needing to travel.

Ancient civilisations (2500–200 BC)

Greece

The ancient Greeks believed that the development of the body was as important as the development of the mind. There was an appreciation of the beauty of the body and the importance of health, which was promoted by medical practitioners such as Hippocrates. Although Hippocrates was not the first physician to prescribe exercise for patients, he was the first recorded physician to provide a written exercise prescription of walking for a patient with 'consumption' (Tipton, 2014).

Gymnastics was undertaken in indoor facilities known as palaestras which also had outdoor areas for wrestling and running. Once young boys had reached adulthood they switched to gymnasiums and were supervised by a paedotribe similar to a modern-day personal trainer. The Spartans of Northern Greece promoted physical activity for military purposes meaning young boys entered training from an early age to improve their fighting skills. Females were also required to be active as it was believed they would have stronger offspring.

The ancient Olympic Games were a series of athletic competitions held in the honour of Zeus. The first Olympics is dated to 776 BC and continued when Greece came under Roman rule. They occurred every four years and participants from any Greek city, state or kingdom could participate. They were always held at Olympia and had fewer events than the modern games.

China

The philosophical teachings of Confucius encouraged participation in regular physical activity. Cong Fu gymnastics and exercise programmes consisted of stances and movements characterised by separate foot positions and imitations of different animal fighting styles. Kung Fu (as we know it) is wrongly associated with violent combat and began initially as medical gymnastics which may have been adapted from Yoga practised on the Indian subcontinent (MacAuley, 1994).

India

The religious beliefs of Hinduism and Buddhism warned people against developing their bodies so physical activity was low. Yoga was developed by Hindu priests as its practice conformed to religious beliefs. By copying the movement patterns of animals, they hoped to achieve a balance with nature that animals seemed to possess. Susruta, a physician based at the University of Benares in India is documented as the first to prescribe activity every day to his patients (Tipton, 2014).

Persia

Rulers in the Persian empire implemented rigid training programmes utilising physical activity for military and political purposes. Activity included hunting, marching, riding and javelin throwing to create a more mobile effective army to conquer surrounding nations.

The Romans (200 BC–476 AD)

The health benefits of physical activity continued to be extolled. Claudius Galenus, or Galen, is recognised as the most important physician from Roman times. His influence lasted until the end of the Middle Ages (Tipton, 2014). Galen was an admirer of Hippocrates and agreed that inactivity caused disease but if physical activity was to be prescribed for health reasons, it was to be moderate (Tipton, 2008).

Roman citizens between the ages of 17 and 60 years were eligible for military training and the activity and fitness of the population was at its peak during times of conflict. Their fitness and discipline enabled the Romans to conquer much of the Western World. Fitness and health were part of dietetics, a branch of medicine that included the regulation of food and drink, exercise and bathing (MacAuley, 1994). However, the lavish lifestyle that followed in the pursuit of wealth put an end to the nation's physical activity.

The Dark Ages (476–1000) and Middle Ages (900–1400)

The Romans were conquered by barbarians from Northern Europe who had similar lifestyles to primitive man. Physical activity experienced a revival through hunting, gathering food and rearing cattle (Harris, 1972). This was a time of a succession of kingdoms and empires, invasions and devastating plagues. In medieval Europe, only nobles and mercenaries undertook physical training for military service. The rest of the population (mostly peasants) had to obey their lords by working extremely hard in the fields using rudimentary tools.

The Renaissance (1400–1600)

Greek ideals glorifying the human body were once again accepted and there was an interest in anatomy, biology, health and physical education. In 1420, the Italian, Vittorino da Feltre opened a school where a special emphasis was placed on physical education. Physical educators highlighted that physical activity enhanced intellectual learning so it developed throughout Europe (Hale, 1994).

Europe national period (1700–1860)

Physical education expanded further aligned with feelings of nationalism and independence. Gymnastics became increasingly popular throughout Europe. In Denmark, Franz Nachtegall implemented gymnastic programmes in school systems to increase physical activity. In Germany, Friedrich Jahn earned the title of 'Father of German Gymnastics'. His passion for German nationalism and independence was the driving force behind the gymnastic programmes he developed. He believed that foreign invasion could be prevented through the physical development of the German people. The Turnplatz, an exercise facility like a modern gymnasium, developed throughout Germany.

In Great Britain, medical student Archibald MacLaren advocated the benefits of regular physical activity and his observations are like modern-day physical activity recommendations. He believed the cure for weariness and stress was physical activity and noted recreational exercise found in games and sport was not sufficient for attaining adequate fitness levels. Furthermore, he documented the importance of progression of exercise. In 1849 the first English athletic competition was conducted at the Royal Military Academy. Archibald MacLaren opened a well-equipped gymnasium at the University of Oxford in 1858, where he trained 12 army officers who then implemented his physical training regimen into the British Army.

In Sweden, Per Henrik Ling implemented four different styles of gymnastics – pedagogic, medical, aesthetic, and military – and felt programmes should be devised based on individual differences using science and physiology (Matthews, 1969).

American colonial period (1700–1776)

During the colonial period, no exercise or fitness programmes existed but the struggles of daily life consisting of growing crops, hunting for food, and herding cattle ensured sufficient levels of physical activity.

United States national period (1776–1860)

Throughout the national period in the United States, immigrants from Europe continued their physical activity pursuits but gymnastic programmes did not gain the same level of popularity. President Benjamin Franklin recommended regular physical activity, including running, swimming, and basic forms of resistance training for health purposes. Schools focused on academic subjects rather than physical education for most of the 19th century. Dr J.C. Warren, a medical professor at Harvard University, was a major proponent of physical activity. He had a clear understanding of the necessity for regular exercise, with his recommendations including exercises such as gymnastics and callisthenics. Furthermore, Warren began devising exercises for females.

Outcome of the Industrial Revolution (1865–1900)

The Industrial Revolution resulted in widespread cultural changes throughout the world with advancement in industrial and mechanical technologies replacing labour-intensive jobs. Rural life became urban as people migrated to towns, generally requiring less movement and physical work compared to rural life, consequently decreasing levels of physical activity.

The 20th century (1900–1950)

Military conflicts have a major impact on the physical activity levels of nations. The onset of World War I in 1914 meant hundreds of thousands of military personnel being drafted and trained for combat. Post-war statistics from the United States highlighted that one in three drafted individuals were unfit for combat and many of those drafted were highly unfit prior to military training (Barrow & Brown, 1988). For the United States, World War II followed in 1941 and it became embarrassingly clear yet again that many of those drafted were not fit for combat. When the war was over, it was reported that nearly half of all draftees were rejected or given non-combat positions (Rice, Hutchinson & Lee, 1958).

Thomas K. Cureton at the University of Illinois introduced the application of research to fitness, providing exercise recommendations to individuals. Cureton not only recognised the numerous benefits of regular exercise, but he also strived to expand the body of knowledge regarding physical fitness. He wanted to answer questions such as how much exercise was healthy and what types of exercise were most effective.

1950 onwards

The impacts on health of industrialisation and urbanisation became apparent in the 1950s and 1960s. An epidemic of non-communicable diseases including cardiovascular disease (CVD), cancer, and Type 2 diabetes became leading causes of death. The supposed lifestyle improvements brought in part by the industrial revolution came with unwanted costs to health. This demanded that numerous organisations educate the public about the consequences of physical inactivity based on evidence accumulating regarding the benefits of physical activity from landmark studies led by pioneers in the physical activity and health field.

Pioneers highlighting the benefits of physical activity for health

> Lack of activity destroys the good condition of every human being, while movement and methodical physical exercise save it and preserve it
>
> Plato, date unknown.

Over the last 60 years, thousands of research studies have been published providing greater insight into the benefits of physical exercise for health. Due to space, this part of the chapter will summarise the work of only a few pioneers who have no doubt inspired countless other leading academics globally.

Professor Jeremy Morris

Jeremy Morris undertook the first systematic investigations of the health hazards associated with a sedentary lifestyle, the outcome of which was coronary heart disease (CHD). Morris and colleagues (1953) believed that deaths from CHD might be less among men engaged in physically active work than among those undertaking sedentary jobs. They examined the onset of CHD in 31,000 male transport workers aged 35 to 65 years between 1949 and 1950. Busmen worked an 11-day fortnight, for 50 weeks a year. Their shift was 5.5 hours long during which drivers sat on average for 90% of their shift and conductors less than 10%. The conductor's stair climbing varied considerably with route, time of day, vehicle, and individual, but was predicted they climbed 500–750 stairs per working day. The conductors' mean heart rate during a working shift was 106 beats per minute compared with 91 beats per minute in the drivers. They found that active bus conductors had a lower incidence of CHD compared to sedentary drivers of London double-decker buses.

In the same paper they found similar findings when comparing active postmen with sedentary telephonists and other government workers. Morris hypothesised that men in physically active jobs had less CHD than men in sedentary jobs and that CHD would develop later in life. There were sceptics since this defied the belief that CHD was the result of hypertension, obesity, and hypercholesterolaemia and that physical activity or lack of it had nothing to do with CHD (Paffenbarger, Blair & Lee, 2001). The sceptics were silenced when an analysis of British occupational mortality statistics adjusted for age, social class, and skill showed that CHD death rates were related to the physical demands of jobs (Morris & Crawford, 1958).

If work-based physical activity was contributing to the prevention of CHD, then leisure time physical activity was important too. Morris and colleagues selected a different study group to identify personal characteristics and lifestyle elements for prospective follow-up. The study population was 18,000 male government office personnel aged 40–64 years in the executive middle-management grade with no history of clinical CHD. Physical activity was recorded using a 5-minute interval log recorded on a Monday for the prior Friday and Saturday, a work day and a free day. A sample of these men was divided into thirds by their total activity scores (measured in kilocalories (kcal) per kilogram of body weight per day) which was 40 in the most active group, 38 in the intermediate one, and 33 in the least active. The hypothesis was the frequency of first attacks of CHD would be inversely related to total physical activity outside of work. This was not the case and only vigorous exercise (7.5 kcal per minute) alone was related inversely to future CHD incidence (Morris et al. 1973; Morris, Everitt, Pollard, Chave & Semmence, 1980). The men reporting regular aerobic exercise through fast walking, swimming, cycling, jogging, and callisthenics showed stronger and consistently lower CHD incidence than comparable men reporting equally energetic and frequent heavy work in the garden and in and around the house or on the car.

After 40 years of population studies had shown that physical activity can protect against CHD, Morris' 1994 paper stated that 'Exercise in the prevention of coronary heart disease: today's best buy in public health'. Morris died aged 99 years and his obituary in *The Telegraph* (2009) makes for interesting reading. Morris himself gave up smoking and took up jogging, becoming the first person regularly to run on Hampstead Heath. "People thought I was bananas," Morris recalled. Morris' work is summarised further by Paffenbarger, Blair and Lee (2001).

Professor Ralph Paffenbarger Jr

In the 1970s Ralph Paffenbarger Jr built upon the results of Morris' studies by analysing data collected from longshoremen and college alumni. In 1951 a group of San Francisco longshoremen underwent multiple screening examinations as part of their employment. Paffenbarger and colleagues (1970) reported on their 16-year follow-up of 3,263 men who were 35 to 64 years old at the study onset. During this time, there were 888 deaths, including 291 fatal coronary events and 67 fatal strokes. They found that the most active group of cargo handlers, who expended over 1000 kcal more than other longshoremen, had CHD death rates significantly lower than their sedentary colleagues (59 versus 80 incidents per 10,000 man-years of work) and these differences remained when smoking, body mass index (BMI), and blood pressure were considered.

In 1960, Paffenbarger was involved in the development of one of the most widely cited studies on CHD and physical activity, the college alumni study. Male and female alumni from the University of Pennsylvania and Harvard College who were born between 1896 and 1934 were included in the study population. The Harvard cohort included 36,500 male alumni who enrolled from 1916 to 1950 when it was customary to have a routine physical examination. Participants were followed over time, completing questionnaires and surveys regarding exercise and doctor-diagnosed diseases. Alumni and college records provided information with regards to participation in sports and death certificates were examined for circumstances and cause of death. Paffenbarger, Wing and Hyde (1978) reported a follow-up of 117,680 person-years of observation. They quantified physical activity using standardised measures and attributed kcal per minute expenditures to activities. They created a physical activity index and allocated participants into two groups, low-energy (less than 2,000 kcal per week) and high-energy (more than 2,000 kcal per week). In the 6- to 10-year follow-up period between 1962 or 1966 and 1972, there were 572 first myocardial infarctions (MIs), 215 of which were fatal. There was an inverse relationship between physical activity and risk of CHD, and alumni in the low-energy category on the physical activity index had a 64% increased risk of MI. The finding persisted across all age groups for both fatal and non-fatal MI and angina pectoris, regardless of prior activity level.

Paffenbarger, Hyde, Wing and Hsieh (1986) elaborated on these findings in a 12- to 16-year follow-up of this cohort, accounting for 213,716 person-years of observation. For this analysis, physical activity was divided into tertiles and energy expenditure was divided into 500 kcal increments. An energy expenditure of 2,000 kcal per week was associated with a 28% decrease in all-cause mortality, but was strongest and most significant in relation to CVD. To compare the interrelationship between risk factors, stereograms were created comparing tertiles of energy expenditure (less than 500 kcal per week, 500 to 1,999 kcal per week, and 2,000 or more kcal per week) with tertiles of established risk factors (blood pressure, smoking status, BMI, family history of early death, and college sports activity). For almost every category, higher energy expenditures were increasingly protective. These findings were confirmed using a multivariate analysis, which showed a 31% higher risk of death in sedentary individuals. Based on these results, added longevity emerged, indicating potential benefit up to age 80 years with an energy expenditure of 2,000 or more kcal per week.

Andrade and Ignaszewski (2007) comment that the results of his research influenced Paffenbarger himself. A previously inactive man, with a strong family history of premature CHD, he started running in 1967 at the age of 45 years. By 1993, when he was forced to retire from running at age 71 years, he had competed in 151 marathons and ultramarathons. Paffenbarger died in 2007 and his work and legacy is summarised by Lee, Matthews and Blair (2009).

Professor Steven Blair

Steven Blair has been instrumental in the publication of works from the Aerobics Center Longitudinal Study from the Cooper Institute, Dallas, Texas that has focused on the importance of physical fitness. Blair and colleagues (1989) presented risk of all-cause and cause-specific mortality in 10,224 men and 3,120 women who were given a preventive medical examination and had their physical fitness measured using a maximal treadmill exercise test. Average follow-up was slightly more than 8 years, for a total of 110,482 person-years of observation, and there were 240 deaths in men and 43 deaths in women. Age-adjusted all-cause mortality rates declined across physical fitness quintiles from 64.0 per 10,000 person-years in the least-fit men to 18.6 per 10,000 person-years in the most-fit men. Corresponding values for women were 39.5 per 10,000 person-years to 8.5 per 10,000 person-years. These trends remained after statistical adjustment for age, smoking status, cholesterol, systolic blood pressure, fasting blood glucose, parental history of CHD, and follow-up interval. They concluded that higher levels of physical fitness appear to delay all-cause mortality, primarily due to lowered rates of CVD and cancer.

Blair et al. (1995) examined the relationship between change in physical fitness and risk of mortality in 9,777 men who had undertaken two clinical examinations (mean interval between examinations was 4.9 years) including a maximal fitness test and assessment of health status. During follow-up after the subsequent examination (mean follow-up from subsequent examination was 5.1 years), the main outcome measures were 223 all-cause deaths and 87 deaths from CVD mortality in which the highest age-adjusted all-cause death rate was observed in men who were unfit at both examinations (122.0 per 10,000 man-years). The lowest death rate was in men who were physically fit at both examinations (39.6 per 10,000 man-years). Men who improved from unfit to fit between the first and subsequent examinations had an age-adjusted death rate of 67.7 per 10,000 man-years. This is a reduction in mortality risk of 44% (95% confidence interval, 25% to 59%) relative to men who remained unfit at both examinations. Improvement in fitness was associated with lower death rates after adjusting for age, health status, and other risk factors. For each minute increase in maximal treadmill time between examinations, there was a corresponding 7.9% decrease risk of mortality. Therefore, men who maintained or improved adequate physical fitness were less likely to die from all causes and from CVD during follow-up than persistently unfit men.

Blair currently works in the departments of exercise science and epidemiology and biostatistics at the Arnold School of Public Health, University of South Carolina. He continues to publish articles (now exceeding 400) on the relationship between physical fitness, body composition, and all-cause mortality and chronic disease. Blair (2009) states that physical inactivity is the biggest public health problem of the 21st century.

Due to the research of pioneers like Professors Morris, Paffenbarger and Blair, it is clear being physically active benefits health. This has led to numerous organisations publishing public health recommendations highlighting the specific amounts required, which have evolved throughout history.

The evolution of physical activity recommendations by key organisations

> In today's tyrannical healthcare, nothing is more certain than guidelines, regulation and death
> Abassi, 2015.

Physical activity recommendations in the UK for adults are to aim to be active daily and to undertake 150 minutes of moderate-intensity activity per week in bouts of at least 10 minutes. Comparable benefits can be achieved by undertaking 75 minutes of vigorous-intensity activity or a combination of vigorous and moderate intensity (Chief Medical Officers, 2011). This amount will provide substantial benefits across a broad range of health outcomes. In addition to aerobic activity, people should engage in physical activity to improve strength at least twice a week. There have been substantial changes to present day physical activity recommendations, so here their evolution will be presented and the reasons for such changes discussed.

In 1978 the American College of Sports Medicine (ACSM) published a position statement that summarised studies to date and presented recommendations for the type and amount of exercise needed to improve fitness (ACSM, 1978): frequency should be 3–5 days per week, intensity should be 60–90% HRmax or 50–85% VO$_2$max, duration should be 15–60 minutes per session and the mode should use large muscle groups. A common finding among the studies presented was that higher intensity exercise produced greater gains in fitness. However the volume of exercise was not controlled and was higher for those exercising at a higher intensity because they worked for the same number of minutes per week as those working at a lower intensity for an equivalent amount of time. Studies with this design are unable to isolate the effects of two different exercise intensities at a fixed volume of exercise, so the ACSM updated its position statement in the 1990s since moderate amounts and moderate intensities of exercise produced important physiologic adaptations (ACSM, 1990; ACSM, 1998).

The 1995 report from the Centers for Disease Control and Prevention (CDC) and ACSM (Pate et al., 1995) recommended that every US adult should accumulate 30 minutes or more of moderate-intensity physical activity on most, or preferably all, days of the week. Reports from a National Institutes of Health consensus conference, the US Surgeon General, and the American Heart Association presented very similar recommendations because the evidence was accruing that moderate-intensity activity produces significant improvements in work capacity and that exercising at higher intensities or volumes has only modest additional effects (U.S. Department of Health and Human Services, 1996). This paradigm shift from physical training to improve fitness and performance to recommendations of physical activity to improve health was likely to be achievable by the primary target population and was supported by a large evidence base as being efficacious for disease risk reduction among most persons. Despite this, moderate-intensity recommendations were criticised since some studies only showed protection with vigorous-intensity exercise (Barinaga, 1997). For an insightful review of physical activity recommendations up to this point see Blair, LaMonte and Nichaman (2004).

In 2004, England's Chief Medical Officer published *At Least Five a Week* which stated that for general health benefit, adults should achieve a total of at least 30 minutes a day of at least moderate-intensity physical activity on 5 or more days of the week (Department of Health, 2004). Swain and Franklin (2006) undertook a review of epidemiological studies that evaluated the benefits of physical activity of varying intensity levels and clinical trials that trained individuals at different intensities but kept the energy expenditure constant. They consistently found a greater reduction in CVD risk with vigorous- than with moderate-intensity activity if the total energy expenditure of exercise was held constant. O'Donovan and Shave (2007) examined whether the promotion of moderate-intensity physical activity had created a widespread belief that it offered greater health benefits than vigorous-intensity activity. A nationally representative survey of 1,191 Britons aged 16–65 years took place in 2006. They found that 78% of men and 84% of women interviewed were aware that moderate-intensity activity was recommended for adults. However, 56% of men and 71% of women aged 25–65 years indicated that moderate-intensity activity offered greater health benefits than vigorous-intensity, so it was concluded that British physical activity recommendations should be amended.

American recommendations were updated in 2007 (Haskell et al., 2007) to include vigorous-intensity and in 2011 in the UK (Chief Medical Officers, 2011) to include the recommendation of 75 minutes vigorous-intensity per week or a combination of moderate- and vigorous-intensity. Whereas the previous 2004 recommendations were solely for adults (Department of Health, 2004), the 2011 physical activity recommendations were presented for various age groups throughout the lifespan. For the early years (under 5s) physical activity should be encouraged from birth. Children of pre-school age who are capable of walking unaided should be physically active daily for at least 180 minutes (3 hours), spread throughout the day. Children and young people (5–18 years) should engage in moderate- to vigorous-intensity physical activity for at least 60 minutes and up to several hours every day. Vigorous-intensity activities, including those that strengthen muscle and bone, should be incorporated at least three days a week. Recommendations for adults (19–64 years) have been presented above (p. 39) and these recommendations are the same for older adults (65+ years), except for the inclusion of incorporating physical activity to improve balance and co-ordination on at least two days a week in older adults at risk of falls. There is also recognition that any physical activity will benefit older adults.

In recent years there has been a substantial increase in the number of published papers exploring the effects of sedentary behaviour on health. One of the first was Katzmarzyk et al. (2008) who posited that although moderate- to vigorous-intensity activity is related to premature mortality, the relationship between sedentary behaviours and mortality has not been fully explored. They examined sitting time and mortality in a representative sample of 17,013 Canadians aged 18–90 years. Daily sitting time (almost none of the time, one-fourth of the time, half of the time, three-fourths of the time, almost all of the time), leisure-time physical activity, smoking status, and alcohol consumption were recorded at baseline. Participants were followed prospectively for an average of 12.0 years. During this time there were 1,832 deaths (759 from CVD and 547 from cancer) during 204,732 person-years of follow-up. After adjustment for potential confounders, there was a progressively higher risk of mortality across higher levels of sitting time from all causes but not cancer. Similar results were obtained when stratified by sex, age, smoking status, and BMI. Age-adjusted all-cause mortality rates per 10,000 person-year of follow-up were 87, 86, 105, 130, and 161 (P for trend < 0.0001) in physically inactive participants and 75, 69, 76, 98, and 105 (P for trend < 0.008) in active participants across sitting time categories. The findings show a dose-response association between sitting time and mortality from all causes and CVD, independent of leisure-time physical activity.

Due to increasing evidence regarding the dangers of sedentary behaviour, the 2011 recommendations suggest everyone should minimise the amount of time spent being sedentary (sitting) for extended periods throughout the lifespan (Chief Medical Officers, 2011). Recommendations on how frequently sitting time should be interrupted or the daily maximum duration persons should be sedentary are not provided since the research is still in its infancy. Recommendations for the workplace have been published (Buckley et al., 2015) suggesting that in those occupations which are predominantly desk-based, workers should aim initially to progress towards accumulating two hours per day of standing and light activity (light walking) during working hours and eventually progressing to a total accumulation of four hours per day (prorated to part-time hours). However, high levels of moderate-intensity activity (about 60–75 minutes per day) can eliminate the increased risk of death associated with high sitting time (Ekelund et al., 2016).

Other organisations with a remit for the promotion of physical activity have published recommendations. The World Health Organization (2010) published global recommendations on physical activity for health which are similar to those of both the UK and US. Also in 2010, the British Association of Sport and Exercise Sciences (BASES) convened a panel of experts to review the literature and produce a consensus statement. Rather than adopting a lifespan approach, in the 'ABC of Physical Activity for Health', A is for All healthy adults, B is for Beginners, and C is for Conditioned individuals (O'Donovan et al., 2010).

Key organisations that advocate physical activity recommendations include the Global Advocacy for Physical Activity (GAPA) council and International Society for Physical Activity and Health (ISPAH). GAPA and ISPAH (2010) published the Toronto Charter for Physical Activity which is a call for action and advocacy tool to create sustainable opportunities for physically active lifestyles for all. In 2014, Public Health England launched 'Everybody active, every day' which is a national, evidence-based approach to support all sectors to embed physical activity into daily life. ISPAH (2016) published the Bangkok declaration on physical activity for global health and sustainable development.

Despite the clear benefits of physical activity, the potential dangers associated with sedentary behaviour, and key organisations recommending and advocating specific amounts of activity, there has been a decline in physical activity in the last few decades.

Lifespan physical activity trends in the last 60 years

> Man does not cease to play because he grows old, man grows old because he ceases to play
>
> George Bernard Shaw, date unknown.

In the last 60 years, there has been a large shift towards less physically demanding work which has been accompanied by increasing use of mechanised transportation, a greater prevalence of labour saving technology in the home, and fewer people participating in active hobbies. The supposed fitness boom of the 1980s did not happen with some of the first national surveys including the Canada Fitness Survey (Stephens, Craig & Ferris, 1986) and the Allied Dunbar National Fitness Survey in England (Activity and Health Research, 1992) highlighting low physical activity and fitness levels.

Using historical data on time spent on occupational and domestic work, travel, and leisure activities, Ng and Popkin (2012) estimated that between 1961 and 2005 physical activity levels dropped by around 20% in the UK. The majority falls within occupational and domestic activity and although voluntary active leisure or recreational activities have increased slightly, this did not make up much of the shortfall. Ng and Popkin (2012) also predict that by 2030, time spent in sedentary behaviour will exceed 50 hours per week.

The Health Survey for England reports 67% of adult men and 55% of adult women met the Chief Medical Officers' (2011) physical activity recommendations in 2012 (Joint Health Surveys Unit, 2013). Due to the introduction of these new recommendations there are no long-term trends. Health Survey for England 2008 data have been reanalysed to measure physical activity against the 2011 recommendations which shows that there was no overall change between 2008 and 2012. However, these statistics should be interpreted with caution since they measure physical activity using self-reporting which is prone to over reporting as a subjective measure. A sub-sample of adults wore an accelerometer for a week in the Health Survey for England in 2008 (Health and Social Care Information Centre, 2009) which is more valid as an objective measure. Only 6% of adult men and 4% of adult women met the Department of Health (2004) recommendations, which is alarming.

In England, a higher proportion of boys (21%) than girls (16%) reported meeting recommendations in the 5- to 15-year age group in 2012 (Joint Health Surveys Unit, 2013). Boys in the 8- to 10-year age group had the highest proportion of active children (26%), while for girls it was found in the 5- to 7-year age group (23%). In both boys and girls in England the proportion of children aged 5 to 15 years meeting recommendations fell between 2008 and 2012. The largest declines were at age 13 to 15 years for both sexes.

Physical activity data globally show that physical activity levels decline with age and men are more active than women in 137 of the 146 countries for which data are available (Sallis et al., 2016). There is a large decrease in activity, particularly in sports participation, once young people leave school (Telama et al., 2005).

Since the publication of the first epidemiological studies examining the benefits of physical activity on health, levels have now reached a plateau. History has demonstrated that population levels of physical activity are greatest during times of conflict and when food is not readily available. As it is not ethical to create such conditions in modern times, effective interventions are needed to overcome this.

Chapter summary

- Primitive man was a hunter gatherer who was active daily for survival. Because of the industrial revolution and availability of subsistence, modern man's daily life could be less active.
- Pioneers in the second half of the 20th century published landmark studies that have highlighted the benefits of physical activity for health. This has inspired the publication of thousands of other research studies and many others to become pioneers themselves.
- As the evidence of the benefits of physical activity has increased and the potential dangers of sedentary behaviour have been highlighted, key organisations have used this evidence to recommend and advocate physical activity to the public.
- Despite these recommendations and advocacy, physical activity levels have plateaued and are predicted to decline with a parallel increase in sedentary behaviour demanding effective interventions to overcome this.

References

Abassi, K. (2015). Loosening the grip. *British Medical Journal*. doi: https://doi.org/10.1136/bmj. h5372.

Activity and Health Research (1992). *Allied Dunbar National Fitness Survey. A Report on Activity Patterns and Fitness Levels: Main Findings*. London: Sports Council and Health Education Authority.

American College of Sports Medicine (1978). Position statement on the recommended quantity and quality of exercise for developing and maintaining fitness in healthy adults. *Medicine and Science in Sports and Exercise, 10*, vii–x.

American College of Sports Medicine (1990). Position Stand. The recommended quantity and quality of exercise for developing and maintaining cardiorespiratory and muscular fitness in healthy adults. *Medicine and Science in Sports and Exercise, 22*, 265–274.

American College of Sports Medicine (1998) Position Stand. The recommended quantity and quality of exercise for developing and maintaining cardiorespiratory and muscular fitness, and flexibility in healthy adults. *Medicine and Science in Sports and Exercise, 30*, 975–991.

Andrade, J. & Ignaszewski, A. (2007). Exercise and the heart: a review of the early studies, in memory of Dr R.S. Paffenbarger. *British Canadian Medical Journal, 49*(10), 540–546.

Barinaga, M. (1997). How much pain for cardiac gain? *Science, 276*(5317), 1324–1327.

Barrow, H.M. & Brown, J.P. (1988). *Man and Movement: Principles of Physical Education*. 4th Ed. Philadelphia: Lea & Febiger.

Blair, S.N. (2009). Physical inactivity: the biggest public health problem of the 21st century. *British Journal of Sports Medicine, 43*, 1–2.

Blair, S.N., Kohl, H.W. III, Barlow, C.E., Paffenbarger, R.S. Jr, Gibbons, L.W. & Macera C.A. (1995). Changes in physical fitness and all-cause mortality: a prospective study of healthy and unhealthy men. *Journal of the American Medical Association, 273*, 1093–1098.

Blair, S.N., Kohl, H.W. III, Paffenbarger R.S. Jr, Clark, D.G., Cooper, K.H. & Gibbons, L.W. (1989). Physical fitness and all-cause mortality: a prospective study of healthy men and women. *Journal of the American Medical Association, 262*, 2395–2401.

Blair, S.N, LaMonte, M.J. & Nichaman, M.Z. (2004). The evolution of physical activity recommendations: how much is enough? *American Journal of Clinical Nutrition, 79*(suppl), 913S–920S.

Buckley, J.P., Hedge, A., Yates, T., Copeland, R.J., Loosemore, M., Hamer, M., Bradley, G. & Dunstan, D.W. (2015). The sedentary office: a growing case for change towards better health and productivity. Expert statement commissioned by Public Health England and the Active Working Community Interest Company. *British Journal of Sports Medicine* doi:10.1136/bjsports-2015-094618.

Chief Medical Officers (2011). *Start Active, Stay Active: A Report on Physical Activity for Health from the Four Home Countries' Chief Medical Officers.* London: Department of Health.

Dalleck, L.C. & Kravitz, L. (2002). The history of fitness. *IDEA Health and Fitness Source, 20*(2), 28–33.

Department of Health (2004). *At Least Five a Week. Evidence on the Impact of Physical Activity and its Relationship to Health.* London: Department of Health.

Ekelund, U., Steene-Johannessen, J., Brown, W.J., Fagerland, M.W., Owen, N., Powell, K., Bauman, A. & Lee, I.-M. (2016). Does physical activity attenuate, or even eliminate, the detrimental association of sitting time with mortality? A harmonised meta-analysis of data from more than 1 million men and women. *Lancet, 388*(10051), 1302–1310.

Global Advocacy for Physical Activity Council and International Society for Physical Activity and Health (2010). *The Toronto Charter for Physical Activity: A Global Call to Action.* Retrieved from www.interamericanheart.org/images/PHYSICALACTIVITY/TorontoCharterPhysicalActivityENG.pdf

Hale, J. (1994). *The Civilization of Europe in the Renaissance.* New York: Maxwell Macmillan International.

Harris, H.A. (1972). *Sport in Greece and Rome.* New York: Cornell University Press.

Haskell, W.L., Lee, I.-M., Pate, R.R., Powell, K.E., Blair, S.N., Franklin, B.A., . . . Bauman, A. (2007). Physical activity and public health updated recommendation for adults from the American College of Sports Medicine and the American Heart Association. *Circulation, 116*, 1081–1093.

Health and Social Care Information Centre (2009). *Health Survey for England 2008: Physical Activity and Fitness.* Leeds: The Information Centre.

International Society for Physical Activity and Health (2016). *The Bangkok Declaration on Physical Activity for Global Health and Sustainable Development.* Retrieved from www.rafapana.org/index.php/en/news/721-the-bangkok-declaration-on-physical-activity-for-global-health-and-sustainable-development-2016

Joint Health Surveys Unit (2013). *Health Survey for England 2012: Health, Social Care and Lifestyles.* Leeds: The Information Centre.

Katzmarzyk, P., Church, T.S., Craig, C.L. & Bouchard, C. (2008). Sitting time and mortality from all causes, cardiovascular disease and cancer. *Medicine and Science in Sports and Exercise, 41*(5), 998–1005.

Lee, I.-M., Matthews, C.E. & Blair, S.N. (2009). The legacy of Dr. Ralph Seal Paffenbarger, Jr. – past, present, and future contributions to physical activity research. *President's Council of Physical Fitness and Sports Research Digest, 10*(1), 1–8.

Matthews, D.O. (1969). A historical study of the aims, contents, and methods of Swedish, Danish, and German gymnastics. *Proceedings of the National College Physical Education Association for Men.*

MacAuley, D. (1994). A history of physical activity, health and medicine. *Journal of the Royal Society of Medicine, 87*, 32–35.

Morris, J.N. (1994). Exercise in the prevention of coronary heart disease: today's best buy in public health. *Medicine and Science in Sports and Exercise, 26*(7), 807–814.

Morris, J.N., Chave, S.P., Adam, C., Sirey, C., Epstein, L. & Sheehan, D.J. (1973). Vigorous exercise in leisure-time and the incidence of coronary heart-disease. *Lancet, 301*(7799), 333–339.

Morris, J.N. & Crawford, M.D. (1958). Coronary heart disease and physical activity of work: evidence of a national necropsy survey. *British Medical Journal, 2*(5111), 1485–1496.

Morris, J.N., Everitt, M.G., Pollard, R., Chave, S.P. & Semmence, A.M. (1980). Vigorous exercise in leisure-time: protection against coronary heart disease. *Lancet, 316*(8206), 207–210.

Morris, J.N., Heady, J.A., Raffle, P.A.B., Roberts, C.G. & Parks J.N. (1953). Coronary heart disease and physical activity of work. *Lancet, 2*(6795), 1053–1057.

Ng, S.W. & Popkin, B.M. (2012). Time use and physical activity: a shift away from movement across the globe. *Obesity Reviews, 13*(8), 659–680.

O'Donovan, G., Blazevich, A.J., Boreham, C., Cooper, A.R., Crank, H., Ekelund, U., . . . Stamatakis, E. (2010). The ABC of Physical Activity for Health: a consensus statement from the British Association of Sport and Exercise Sciences. *Journal of Sports Sciences, 28*(6), 573–591.

O'Donovan, G. & Shave, R. (2007). British adults views on the health benefits of moderate and vigorous activity. *Preventive Medicine, 45*, 432–435.

Paffenbarger, R.S. Jr, Blair, S.N. & Lee, I-M. (2001). A history of physical activity, cardiovascular health and longevity: the scientific contributions of Jeremy N Morris. *International Journal of Epidemiology, 30*, 1184–1192.

Paffenbarger, R.S. Jr, Hyde, R.T., Wing, A.L., & Hsieh, C.C. (1986). Physical activity, all-cause mortality, and longevity of college alumni. *New England Journal of Medicine, 314*(10) 605–613.

Paffenbarger, R.S. Jr, Laughlin, M.E., Gima A.S. & Black, R.A. (1970). Work activity of longshoremen as related to death from coronary heart disease and stroke. *New England Journal of Medicine, 282*, 1109–1114.

Paffenbarger, R.S. Jr, Wing, A.L. & Hyde, R.T. (1978). Physical activity as an index of heart attack risk in college alumni. *American Journal of Epidemiology, 108*, 161–175.

Pate, R.R., Pratt, M., Blair, S.N., Haskell, W.L., Macera, C.A., Bouchard, C., . . . Wilmore, J.H. (1995). Physical activity and public health: a recommendation from the Centers for Disease Control and Prevention and the American College of Sports Medicine. *Journal of the American Medical Association, 273*, 402–407.

Rice, E.A., Hutchinson, J.L., & Lee, M. (1958). *A Brief History of Physical Education*. New York: The Ronald Press Co.

Sallis, J.F., Bull, F., Guthold, R., Heath, G.W., Inoue, S., Kelly, P., . . . Hallal, P.C. (2016). Progress in physical activity over the Olympic quadrennium. *Lancet, 388*(10051), 1325–1336.

Stephens, T., Craig, C.L. & Ferris, B.F. (1986). Adult physical activity in Canada: findings from the Canada Fitness Survey I. *Canadian Journal of Public Health, 77*, 285–290.

Swain, D.P. & Franklin, B.A. (2006). Comparison of cardioprotective benefits of vigorous versus moderate intensity aerobic exercise. *American Journal of Cardiology, 97*, 141–147.

Telama, R., Yang, X., Viikari, J., Valimaki, I., Wanne, O. & Raitakari, O. (2005). Physical activity from childhood to adulthood: a 21-year tracking study. *American Journal of Preventive Medicine, 28*(3), 267–273.

The Telegraph (2nd November 2009). *Professor Jeremy Morris*. Retrieved from www.telegraph.co.uk/news/obituaries/medicine-obituaries/6488393/Professor-Jeremy-Morris.html

Tipton, C.M. (2008). Historical perspective: the antiquity of exercise, exercise physiology and the exercise prescription for health. *World Review of Nutrition and Dietetics, 98*, 198–245.

Tipton, C.M. (2014). The history of 'Exercise Is Medicine' in ancient civilizations. *Advances in Physiology Education, 38*(2), 109–117.

U.S. Department of Health and Human Services (1996). *Physical Activity and Health: A Report of the Surgeon General*. Retrieved from www.cdc.gov/nccdphp/sgr/index.htm

World Health Organization (2010). *Global Recommendations on Physical Activity for Health*. Retrieved from http://apps.who.int/iris/bitstream/10665/44399/1/9789241599979_eng.pdf

4 Physical inactivity and ill health

Duck-chul Lee and Laura Ellingson

Keywords: Sedentary behavior, physical inactivity, physical fitness, chronic diseases, mortality

Spectrum of sedentary behavior and physical inactivity

Definitions and differences between sedentarism and physical inactivity

Humans are capable of a wide range of behaviors from sleeping to being vigorously physically active, which all contribute to overall health and wellbeing (Figure 4.1). Two prominent categories within this range, physical inactivity and sedentary time, are distinct risk factors for many chronic health conditions, which can interact to differentially impact health and wellbeing (Benatti & Ried-Larsen, 2015; Dunstan et al., 2012; Dunstan, Thorp & Healy, 2011). Though varying definitions exist, throughout this chapter we will define physical inactivity (<3 METs) as the absence or insufficient accumulation of moderate- to vigorous-intensity physical activity (PA). Sedentary time, on the other hand, will be defined as any waking behavior characterized by a sitting or reclining posture and a low energy expenditure (≤1.5 METs) (Sedentary Behaviour Research Network, 2012). In other words, inactivity refers to not being active enough to meet the current US physical activity guidelines (e.g. 150 minutes of moderate-intensity or 75 minutes of vigorous-intensity aerobic PA per week (U.S. Department of Health and Human Services, 2008), while sedentary time refers to a lack of movement during waking hours, generally while seated. For the purposes of this chapter, sleep will not be included in sedentary time as the psychobiological consequences of this behavior are distinct from those associated with being in a similar posture, while awake.

Current PA guidelines recommend at least moderate-intensity PA (≥3 METs) such as brisk walking for a minimum of 10 minutes at a time, for a total of 150 minutes per week to gain health benefits. This is referred to as *health-enhancing PA* (Figure 4.1) (U.S. Department of Health and Human Services, 2008; World Health Organization, 2010). On the other hand, light-intensity PA, which is considerably more prevalent throughout the day and includes many activities of daily living (e.g., slow walking, standing, etc.) is regarded as *baseline PA*. In other words, activities performed at this lower intensity are often considered insufficient for improving health. Thus, individuals with even significant amount of light-intensity PA are categorized as *physically inactive*. These current PA guidelines are based on evidence from exercise physiology, which demonstrates significant health benefits from PA at moderate-to-vigorous intensities. However, emerging evidence suggests that there may be health benefits associated with light-intensity PA as well, especially when it is in place of sedentary time. This relatively

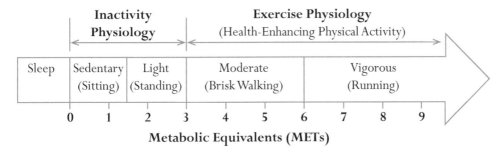

Figure 4.1   Spectrum of sedentary behavior and physical activity

new body of research, called inactivity physiology, relies on understanding the physiological effects of inactivity as well as the health benefits of reducing physical inactivity with light-intensity activity such as breaking up prolonged periods of sitting (Hamilton, Hamilton, & Zderic, 2004).

Prevalence and risk factors of sedentary behavior and physical inactivity

Physical inactivity is highly prevalent in many societies. Recent estimates from the World Health Organization (WHO) suggest that globally 23% of adults, 18 years of age and older are insufficiently active with higher rates of inactivity in Europe and the Americas (World Health Organization, 2016). In the United States, estimates vary widely from ~16–95% depending on whether behavior is measured objectively or using self-report (Bauman et al., 2009; Troiano et al., 2008). While reality is likely somewhere in between these two extremes, it is clear that inactivity is a significant problem facing the world today. General patterns demonstrate that women are more inactive than men and inactivity increases with age. Also, higher income countries had twice the levels of inactivity as lower income countries.

Evidence also demonstrates that sedentary behavior is highly prevalent. Though estimates vary widely, the majority of adults from industrialized nations are accumulating more than 10 hours of sedentary time per day or more than two-thirds of waking hours (Diaz et al., 2016; Healy et al., 2011). Sedentary time is more prevalent in individuals with sedentary occupations and increases with age (Diaz et al., 2016; Gennuso, Thraen-Borowski, Gangnon, & Colbert, 2015). However, leisure time activities account for a large percentage of this time as well, with screen time playing an increasingly greater role (Balboa-Castillo et al., 2011; Chau et al., 2012; van der Ploeg et al., 2013).

There are numerous risk factors and determinants of sedentary behavior and physical inactivity proposed in various populations (Chastin et al., 2016; Deliens, Deforche, De Bourdeaudhuij, & Clarys, 2015; Diaz et al., 2016; Wendel-Vos, Droomers, Kremers, Brug, & van Lenthe, 2007). Risk factors can be classified into two main categories: individual and environmental factors, as shown in Figure 4.2. Individual factors are further broken down into socioeconomic, health, and psychological factors. Environmental factors are divided into four major domains of physical activity such as household, occupational and school, leisure-time, and transportation.

To effectively reduce sedentary behavior and increase PA, it is crucial to adopt and apply multilevel and transdisciplinary approaches targeting both individuals and their surrounding

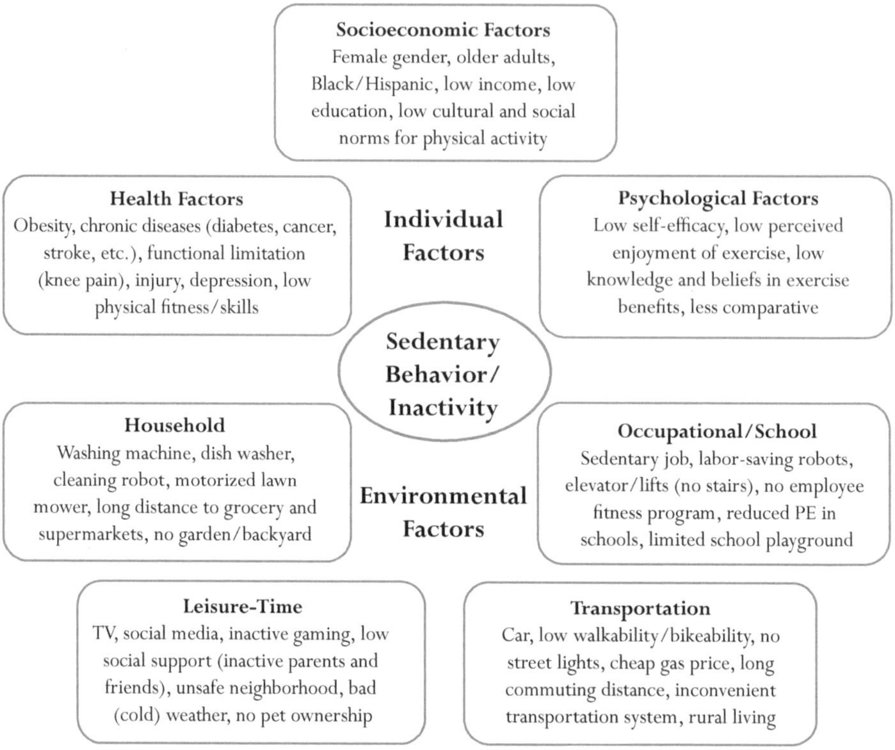

Figure 4.2 Risk factors of sedentary behavior and physical inactivity

environments. For example, interventions targeting factors like self-efficacy in combination with factors like neighborhood safety will be more effective than strategies targeted at either factor in isolation. In addition, to ensure a greater likelihood of success, different sectors of society must work together including business and industry, community recreation (fitness and parks), education, faith-based settings, health care, mass media, public health, sport, and transportation at local, national, and international levels (National Physical Activity Plan Alliance, 2016).

Economic cost of physical inactivity

As inactivity and sedentary behavior impact not just individual health, but also the health of communities and society as a whole, understanding the economic burden of these behaviors is important. This information is critical for helping policy makers quantify the impact of physical inactivity and sedentary behavior specifically on health care costs and losses in productivity to encourage funding for strategies to promote physical activity and reduce sedentary time.

A recent large study based on data collected in 2013 from 142 countries, representing 93% of the world's population, estimated that health care costs attributable to physical inactivity on five major non-communicable diseases (coronary heart disease, stroke, type 2 diabetes, breast cancer, and colon cancer) are $53.8 billion worldwide (Ding et al., 2016).

Further, physical inactivity-related deaths contribute to $13.7 billion in productivity losses, and physical inactivity is responsible for $13.4 million disability-adjusted life-years at the global level. They found that high-income countries bear a larger proportion of economic burden (81% of direct health care cost) because physical inactivity is more prevalent in those countries.

Another approach in the estimation of economic burden of physical inactivity is to link physical inactivity data directly to health care expenditures at the individual level. In a study of over 4,000 adults aged >40 years old in the United States (US), the average annual health care costs were $5,783 in inactive (0 day/week of PA), $4,966 in moderately active (1–3 days/week of PA), and $4,240 in active individuals (≥4 days/week of PA) (Anderson et al., 2005). In another study of 42,520 US Medicare retirees aged ≥65 years, annual medical care costs were $12,450 in inactive (0 day/week of PA), $10,760 in moderately active (1–3 days/week of PA), and $9,764 in active retirees (≥4 days/week of PA) (Wang, McDonald, Reffitt, & Edington, 2005). The total health care charges were lower with higher PA level regardless of age and body mass index. Similarly, in over 7,000 Australian women (50–55 years), the mean annual costs of Medicare-subsidized services were $542 per woman in Australian dollars, and costs were 25% higher in inactive women (<10 min/week of PA), compared with the most active women (≥300 min/week of PA) ($643 vs. $514) (Brown, Hockey, & Dobson, 2008).

Although the economic cost of physical inactivity varies between studies depending on the health care system, the age of individuals, and how physical inactivity is defined, health care costs are about 25–35% higher in inactive individuals, compared with their active peers. These data clearly suggest that there would be significant savings in health care costs by increasing PA, especially in developed (high-income) countries.

Mechanisms linking sedentary behavior to ill health

Much of the research examining the influence of physical inactivity and sedentary behavior on human health has come from cross-sectional studies showing relationships between high amounts of inactivity and/or sedentary time and increased prevalence of chronic diseases. However, an important component of understanding the causal link between these behaviors and health outcomes is examining underlying mechanisms that link these behaviors to physiological changes. While this body of research is relatively new, there is evidence from a series of human and animal studies examining the effects of long periods of bed rest on physiology. This evidence points to a host of changes that occur when individuals become inactive for prolonged periods of time. For example, animal studies that prevented rats from standing on their hind legs found a rapid reduction in the local lipoprotein lipase (LPL) activity, which plays an important role in plasma lipoprotein profile (triglyceride and cholesterol) and fat deposition (Hamilton, Hamilton, & Zderic, 2004). LPL activity is therefore associated with the development of cardiometabolic diseases such as type 2 diabetes, obesity, hypercholesterolemia, and coronary heart diseases (Hamilton, Hamilton, & Zderic, 2007).

Recent research has also begun to explore the physiological effects of sedentary time for the prevention of chronic diseases, specifically metabolic and cardiovascular diseases (Hamilton et al., 2008). Though few studies have been replicated and more research is needed, there is evidence that accumulating high amounts of sedentary time results in a variety of observable physiological changes. These include reductions in glycemic control (Mikus et al., 2012), metabolic function (Chastin, Palarea-Albaladejo, Dontje, & Skelton, 2015; Healy et al. 2008), insulin sensitivity (Yates et al., 2015), attenuated endothelial function (Thosar,

Bielko, Mather, Johnston, & Wallace, 2015), elevated levels of systemic inflammation (Hamer, Poole, & Messerli-Bürgy, 2013; Hamer, Smith, & Stamatakis, 2015; Stubbs et al., 2015; Yates et al., 2012), and telomere shortening, a marker of chromosomal deterioration associated with accelerated aging (Edwards & Loprinzi, 2017; Loprinzi, 2015). These physiological changes are directly linked to increased risk for the development of cardiometabolic conditions (Hamilton, Hamilton, & Zderic, 2007). This body of work underlines the importance of replacing sedentary time with light-intensity PA or exercise for the prevention of chronic diseases. This is an area of increased attention at present and it is expected that our knowledge of sedentary physiology and the link to health consequences will increase dramatically in the coming decade.

Assessment and patterns of sedentary behavior

Assessment of sedentary behavior

Accurately measuring sedentary behavior is critical to understand associated health risks, develop evidence-based guidelines, and assess treatment effects. However, accurate assessment is difficult. Sedentary behavior is defined by three basic features: posture (sitting or lying down), low energy expenditure, and being awake (Sedentary Behaviour Research Network, 2012). In addition to these basic elements, there are also a number of other facets of sedentary behavior which may influence its impact on health. These include the purpose of the activity (e.g., work vs. leisure), environmental influences (e.g., inside vs. outdoors), posture (sitting vs. lying down), social context (e.g., alone vs. with others), associated behaviors that may influence health (e.g., snacking), the functional and psychological status of the individual, the time of day/week and season that the behavior takes place, and the type of behavior (e.g., screen time vs. non-screen time) (Chastin et al., 2016). Thus, measuring this set of behaviors presents unique challenges that require development of new tools and/or significant adaptations of existing PA measurement tools (Celis-Morales et al., 2012).

There are two basic ways of assessing sedentary time: self-report and objective wearable devices. Questionnaires are the most common way of measuring sedentary time, asking participants to estimate total time spent sedentary or inquiring about sedentary time in one or more domains (e.g. hours of television, computer use) (Atkin, Gorely, et al., 2012; Celis-Morales et al., 2012). Currently, summary and surrogate measures are typically used including only one or a small set of questions: for example, "During the last 7 days, how much time did you usually spend sitting on a weekday?" or "On average, how many hours of television do you watch per day?" Tools like these provide useful, but relatively limited information, compared to more detailed questionnaires that assess sedentary time in a more thorough fashion (e.g. different domains, time of day, etc.). However, these more detailed measures also suffer from limitations as sedentary behaviors often co-occur. For example, an individual can watch television while eating, socializing, and using a computer. Thus, sedentary time may be overestimated when using these measures. Strengths of self-report measures include cost-effectiveness, high utility with large populations, a low burden for participants and researchers, and the ability to assess contextual information to inform our understanding of health risks and intervention design. However, a critical limitation of self-report measures is that due to poor recall, cultural norms, and perceived social desirability, they consistently demonstrate poor validity (Atkin, Gorely, et al., 2012; Celis-Morales et al., 2012; Healy et al., 2011).

To address some of the limitations associated with self-reported sedentary behavior, objective methods of measurement are increasingly being used. These include accelerometers and sensors that assess posture. These monitors can be used to estimate the total volume of sedentary behavior through the accumulation of low movement counts at specified cut points or time spent in sedentary postures. They can also be used to detect the length of sedentary bouts as well as breaks in sedentary time, which as you'll read below may have important implications for health. The validity of these monitors is substantially higher than self-report measures. For example, a thigh-worn monitor (the activPAL™) has demonstrated excellent validity for assessing sedentary time under free-living conditions (Lyden, Keadle, Staudenmayer, & Freedson, 2016; Lyden, Kozey Keadle, Staudenmayer, & Freedson, 2012). Further, as the collected information includes a time-stamp, particular segments of the day or week can be isolated, such as waking hours or work time. However, these monitors do not collect potentially valuable contextual information and are influenced by compliance issues with participants wearing the monitors throughout the day. Furthermore, these devices are substantially more expensive than questionnaires and require an increased burden on both participants and researchers.

Much has been learned from surveillance studies that incorporate brief sedentary behavior questionnaires to determine the effects of sedentary time on various health outcomes. However, inclusion of objective measures and more detailed self-report measures will be instrumental for understanding what aspects of sedentary time are most detrimental for health. These data can then be used to inform intervention trials designed to improve health and ultimately to aid in the creation of recommendations similar to those that have been developed for exercise to guide individuals about the safest ways to accumulate sedentary behavior in order to avoid negative health consequences.

Patterns of sedentary behavior and physical activity

Use of objective measures of sedentary time has allowed for the more detailed exploration of different patterns of accumulation with the goal of understanding whether differential patterns influence health outcomes. For example, people may tend towards accumulating sedentary behaviors in prolonged or shorter bouts. This is illustrated by Figure 4.3. As you can see, individuals consistent with patterns 1 and 3 tend to have shorter bouts of sedentary time throughout the day as demonstrated by shorter blocks of white space, while those represented in patterns 2 and 4 tend to have longer bouts (measuring physical activity is covered in further detail in Chapter 6).

Moreover, use of objective measurement tools allows for examination of interactions between sedentary behaviors and PA. As shown in Pattern 2 in Figure 4.3, an individual can be *highly sedentary*, meaning that he or she sits for long periods of time throughout the day and also *vigorously active* by going for an hour-long run or to the gym each morning. This might be a pattern seen in a marathon runner with a desk job. Conversely, an individual can be *low sedentary* and *inactive* if they do not sit often, but also do not exercise regularly. This pattern, illustrated in Figure 4.3 as Pattern 3, may be common in someone with a cashier job who stands for long hours each day, but does not regularly exercise. These different patterns of accumulation of both sedentary behaviors and PA likely have differential influences on human health.

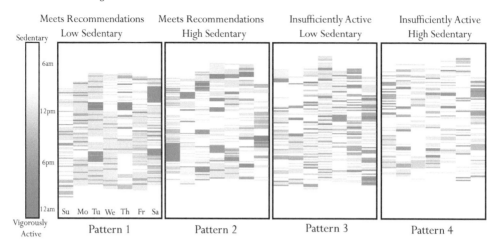

Figure 4.3 A week's worth of data in four individuals with different activity and sedentary behavior patterns. Columns are days of the week and time of day is indicated on the y-axis. The shading within each column indicates the activity intensity recorded by accelerometer from white (sedentary) to black (vigorously active)

Sedentary behavior, physical inactivity, and ill health

High rates of sedentary behavior and physical inactivity are associated with increased risk for the development of chronic health conditions such as cardiovascular diseases and depression, and an increased risk of all-cause mortality (Benatti & Ried-Larsen, 2015; Dunstan et al., 2012). Importantly, there is evidence that the health consequences of these behaviors are independent and also additive. As such, being physically active may mitigate, but may not fully protect against the negative consequences of a sedentary lifestyle. Moreover, physical inactivity combined with high amounts of sedentary behavior has more severe consequences than either behavior alone.

Cardiometabolic diseases

Increasingly, studies are demonstrating that prolonged sedentary time is significantly associated with deleterious health outcomes. A systematic review with meta-analysis from 47 studies revealed that greater sedentary time was associated with 91% increased risk of type 2 diabetes, 14% increased risk of CVD incidence, and 13% increased risk of cancer incidence after adjusting for PA (Biswas et al., 2015). These associations were generally more pronounced at lower levels of PA, indicating that inactivity and sedentary time may interact to influence health. Another large meta-analysis including data from over 1 million adults supports that high levels of PA seem to at least attenuate the increased risk of mortality associated with sedentary behavior (Ekelund et al., 2016). Based on this growing body of evidence on sedentary behavior and cardiometabolic health outcomes, the American Heart Association recently included sedentary behavior as a risk factor for diabetes and CVD (Endorsed by The Obesity Society et al., 2016). Prolonged TV viewing is one of the most common sedentary activities and is associated with cardiometabolic diseases. In a recent review, researchers found that every two hours of TV viewing per day was associated with 20% increased risk of type 2 diabetes and 15% increased risk of CVD (Grøntved & Hu, 2011). Another study suggested that frequent TV viewers (≥3 hours/day) had a significantly higher percentage of body fat in comparison with moderate (2 hours/day) and infrequent (≤1 hour/day) viewers, controlling for body mass index (Tucker & Tucker, 2011).

As mentioned above, there is some evidence that the way in which an individual accumulates sedentary behavior influences health. Early research in this area conducted by Healy and colleagues (2008) showed that introducing regular breaks in sedentary time had positive health benefits, including decreased waist circumference and body mass index and improved triglyceride and plasma glucose profiles. These results were subsequently replicated in a study where participants were asked to break up prolonged bouts of sedentary time with either walking or standing. Results showed that both methods were effective for attenuating post-prandial metabolic responses (glucose, insulin, fatty acids) in overweight or obese women at high risk of type 2 diabetes (Henson et al., 2016). Based on these and similar results, a systematic review was conducted and concluded that the evidence collected to date suggests that breaking up prolonged periods of sedentary time may have a positive effect on glucose metabolism and obesity metrics (Chastin, Egerton, Leask, & Stamatakis, 2015). These results further suggest that replacing sedentary time with light-intensity PA such as standing still could be effective for the prevention of cardiometabolic diseases. Light-intensity PA could also be more appealing and practical for many inactive individuals to replace sitting time since continuous high-intensity exercise is challenging and difficult to maintain.

Mental health

There is an abundance of evidence demonstrating the benefits of PA for mental health and, conversely, the detrimental mental health consequences of an inactive lifestyle. Being inactive is associated with higher levels of depression and anxiety and lower levels of overall well-being for both healthy individuals as well as those with chronic conditions (Schuch et al., 2016). There is also evidence that increasing physical activity levels can be as effective as front-line treatments including medication and cognitive behavioral therapy for improving mental health conditions, suggesting a causal link between activity levels and mental health (Herring, O'Connor, & Dishman, 2010; Mammen & Faulkner, 2013; Rosenbaum, Tiedemann, Sherrington, Curtis, & Ward, 2014).

More recent evidence has begun to suggest a link between sedentary behaviors and various aspects of mental health including diagnosable conditions such as depression, anxiety, and bipolar disorder (Asztalos, Cardon, De Bourdeaudhuij, & De Cocker, 2015; Teychenne, Ball, & Salmon, 2010; Teychenne, Costigan, & Parker, 2015; Vallance et al., 2011; Vancampfort et al., 2016) and subclinical symptoms including stress, poor sleep and lower levels of wellbeing (An, Jang, & Kim, 2015; Atkin, Adams, Bull, & Biddle, 2012; Kline, Krafty, Mulukutla, & Hall, 2016; Rebar, Vandelanotte, van Uffelen, Short, & Duncan, 2014). Adding to this cross-sectional work are several longitudinal investigations showing that sedentary time may be predictive of future mental health and wellbeing (Balboa-Castillo et al., 2011; Lucas et al., 2011; Sanchez-Villegas et al., 2008; Sui et al., 2015). Also, a few short intervention trials demonstrated that changing sedentary behavior results in concomitant changes in mental health-related outcomes (Barwais, Cuddihy, & Tomson, 2013; Ellingson, Meyer, & Cook, 2016; Endrighi, Steptoe, & Hamer, 2015; Pronk, Katz, Lowry, & Payfer, 2012). However, this link has not been universally supported (Hagger-Johnson et al., 2014; van Uffelen et al., 2013) and there is some evidence of reverse causality (Teychenne, Abbott, Ball, & Salmon, 2014). This area of research is currently receiving more attention and our knowledge of the influence of sedentary time on mental health will be expanding in the coming years.

Mortality

The WHO has reported that physical inactivity is the fourth leading global risk factor for premature mortality after high blood pressure, cigarette smoking, and high blood glucose (World Health Organization, 2009). The fifth and sixth leading risk factors for death were overweight/obesity and high cholesterol, suggesting that physical inactivity is relatively more important than obesity and hypercholesterolemia for longevity. The WHO also indicates that risk factors including physical inactivity are responsible for increasing the risk of chronic diseases. A large review study based on international collaborations estimated that physical inactivity caused 9% of premature mortality, or more than 5.3 million deaths worldwide in 2008 (I.-M. Lee et al., 2012). If physical inactivity were decreased by 10% or 25%, more than 533,000 and more than 1.3 million deaths, respectively, could be prevented each year.

Sedentary time has also been noted as a risk factor for premature mortality. A large study in over 220,000 Australian adults examined the relationship of sitting time with all-cause mortality and found that, compared with <4 hours/day of sitting, sitting 8–10 and ≥11 hours/day were associated with 15% and 40% increased risk of all-cause mortality, respectively, after adjusting for PA and other potential confounders (van der Ploeg, Chey, Korda, Banks, & Bauman, 2012). This association was consistent across the sexes, age groups, body mass index, medical conditions, and PA. Regarding life expectancy in relation to sedentary behavior, the analysis from the US national survey data indicated that population life expectancy would be two years higher if adults reduced total sitting time to <3 hours/day, and 1.4 years higher if they reduced TV viewing to <2 hours/day (Katzmarzyk & Lee, 2012). This evidence clearly supports that physical inactivity increases the risk of premature mortality, and reducing sitting time provides significant longevity benefits.

Running is one of the most popular and convenient leisure-time PA and exercise with a consistent growth in most developed countries. A study by Lee et al. examined the relative importance of no running (non-runners), as an example of inactive lifestyle, compared with other common mortality predictors (Lee et al., 2014). As shown in Table 4.1, the authors found that compared with runners, non-runners had 24% and 40% increased risk of all-cause and CVD mortality, respectively, in their population of over 55,000 men and women aged 18–100 years. In addition, based on the estimation of population attributable fractions, being inactive (not running) appeared to be as influential as hypertension, and possibly more influential than being overweight/obese or smoking as an attributable factor to prevent premature mortality, accounting for 16% and 25% of all-cause and CVD mortality, respectively. Moreover, compared with runners, non-runners had 3.0 and 4.1 years shorter life expectancy after controlling for a comprehensive set of confounders including all other mortality predictors included in the analysis in Table 4.1.

Interestingly, the authors also found that even 5–10 minutes of daily running, which is lower than the current minimum vigorous-intensity PA guidelines (≥75 minutes/week), was significantly associated with a 28% lower risk of all-cause and a 58% lower risk of CVD mortality, compared with no running. These findings held after adjusting for potential confounders and other types of PA except running. Similar results were observed in lower weekly

Table 4.1 Hazard ratios, population attributable fractions, and estimated decreased life expectancy by running and other mortality predictors

Mortality Predictor	All-cause mortality*			Cardiovascular disease mortality*		
	HR (95% Confidence Interval)	PAF (%)†	Decreased Life Expectancy (years)‡	HR (95% Confidence Interval)	PAF (%)†	Decreased Life Expectancy (years)‡
Non-runner	1.24 (1.13–1.37)	16	3.0	1.40 (1.18–1.66)	25	4.1
Current smoker	1.67 (1.54–1.80)	11	7.0	1.69 (1.49–1.92)	12	6.3
Overweight or obesity	1.16 (1.08–1.25)	8	2.0	1.43 (1.26–1.63)	20	4.4
Parental CVD	1.20 (1.12–1.29)	7	2.5	1.38 (1.23–1.54)	13	3.9
Abnormal ECG	1.55 (1.42–1.70)	7	6.0	2.43 (2.14–2.77)	17	10.7
Hypertension	1.46 (1.36–1.57)	15	5.2	1.94 (1.72–2.18)	28	8.0
Diabetes	1.36 (1.23–1.51)	3	4.2	1.53 (1.31–1.79)	6	5.1
Hypercholesterolemia	1.06 (0.98–1.13)	2	0.7	1.32 (1.18–1.48)	10	3.4

*Hazard ratio (HR), population attributable fraction (PAF), and decreased life expectancy were adjusted for baseline age, sex, examination year, and all other mortality predictors in the table. The reference category for each HR and PAF analysis includes individuals who did not have the particular mortality predictor.

†PAF was computed as $P_c (1-1/HR_{adj})$, where P_c is the prevalence of the mortality predictor among mortality cases, and HR_{adj} is the multivariable HR for mortality associated with the specified mortality predictor.

‡Decreased life expectancy was compared β coefficients for mortality associated with each year of age with the β coefficients difference in mortality for each mortality predictor using the multivariable Cox proportional hazards model.

ECG=electrocardiogram, CVD=cardiovascular disease, HR=hazard ratio, PAF=population attributable fraction.

running distance (<10 km), frequency (1–2 times), total amount (<506 MET-minutes), and slower speed (<10 km/hour). Further, maintenance of regular running over time was more strongly associated with mortality reduction. These findings clearly suggest that health benefits can be achieved by participating in even low levels of PA that are not sufficient for meeting guidelines.

Low physical fitness and ill health

Low cardiorespiratory fitness and ill health

Current PA guidelines are predominantly based on self-reported PA. However, as mentioned above, self-reported measures are often subject to issues with validity because people tend to over-report their activity levels. One option to minimize this measurement error in PA and health research is to use an objective measure such as cardiorespiratory fitness (CRF). CRF is usually measured by a maximal or submaximal exercise test as an objective marker of recent aerobic PA, which is a well-established health indicator and mortality predictor (Lee, Artero, Sui, & Blair, 2010). Thus, low levels of CRF may be indicative of high levels of inactivity and sedentary behavior.

The Aerobics Center Longitudinal Study (ACLS) demonstrated that low CRF accounts for about 16% of all deaths as the most important leading mortality predictor, followed by hypertension, smoking, obesity, hypercholesterolemia, and diabetes (Blair, 2009), which is very similar to the findings on running shown in Table 4.1 above. In a comprehensive review research from 33 studies comprising over 100,000 participants, each 1-MET increase in CRF (corresponding to roughly 1 km/hour faster running speed) was associated with 13% and 15% lower risks of all-cause mortality and CVD events, respectively (Kodama et al., 2009). The authors explained that a 1-MET higher CRF is equivalent to a 7 cm lower waist circumference, 5 mmHg lower systolic blood pressure, 88 mg/dl lower triglyceride levels, and 18 mg/dl lower fasting glucose.

In another ACLS study investigating the effects of changes in CRF levels on the development of CVD risk factors, results showed that every 1-MET improvement in CRF was associated with 7%, 22%, and 12% lower risk of developing hypertension, metabolic syndrome, and hypercholesterolemia, respectively (Lee et al., 2012). In a similar study on the effects of changes in CRF on mortality, maintaining or improving CRF was associated with 30–40% lower risk of all-cause and CVD mortality (Lee et al., 2011a). The authors also performed an informative analysis on the potential interactions of fitness and fatness with mortality. Compared with individuals who gained fitness and lowered their body mass index (BMI) (expected ideal change), individuals who lost fitness had 65–106% increased risk of all-cause mortality regardless of changes in BMI, after adjusting for potential confounders (Figure 4.4). In additional analyses, results revealed that even an increase in BMI, body weight, or % body fat was not associated with all-cause mortality, when controlling for CRF. Very similar results were observed for CVD mortality. These results have direct public health implications since extensive attention has been given to weight loss, which is very challenging for most overweight and obese individuals. These studies therefore emphasize that preventing fitness loss is important for reducing premature mortality regardless of weight change, and increased attention needs to be placed on maintaining or improving CRF.

There are several possible mechanisms linking CRF to premature mortality. Individuals with moderate-to-high CRF levels generally have improved insulin sensitivity, blood lipid

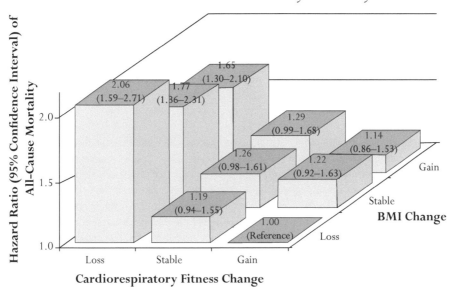

Figure 4.4 Hazard ratios (95% confidence intervals) of all-cause mortality by combinations of changes in cardiorespiratory fitness and body mass index (BMI) in 14,358 men aged 20 years or older (mean age 44 years). All data were adjusted for age, examination year, parental cardiovascular disease, BMI, and maximal METs at baseline, changes in lifestyle factors (smoking status, alcohol intake, and physical activity), changes in medical conditions (abnormal electrocardiogram, hypertension, diabetes, and hypercholesterolemia), and the number of clinic visits between the baseline and last examinations in calculations of changes in fitness and BMI

and lipoprotein profile, body composition, chronic inflammation, blood pressure, and autonomic nervous system, compared with individuals with low CRF levels (Lee et al., 2010). Since CRF is a significant health indicator, the next important question would be how to improve CRF. A recent review described that CRF depends on several modifiable factors including physical activity in addition to non-modifiable factors such as age, gender, and genotype (Lee et al., 2010). There is strong evidence demonstrating a dose-response relationship between PA and improvements in CRF, suggesting that increasing either intensity or volume of PA appears to significantly improve CRF (U.S. Department of Health and Human Services, 2008). Even moderate-intensity PA at 40–55% of peak VO2 is sufficient to improve CRF (Church, Earnest, Skinner, & Blair, 2007). Therefore, in inactive individuals, low- to moderate-intensity PA should be encouraged and included in daily life to reduce and replace sitting time to lower premature mortality risk.

It is possible that some physically active people may have relatively low CRF, due to genetics and other factors unrelated to PA. As such, another interesting and important research question is, what are the independent and combined effects of aerobic PA and CRF on health. This was examined in a large cohort study including over 40,000 adults. Results showed that mortality risk reduction was larger in men with high CRF than in men who met the recommended PA, suggesting that CRF is more strongly associated with all-cause mortality than PA (Lee et al., 2011b). They also reported that the association of PA with mortality was no longer significant after controlling for CRF in men, whereas the association of CRF with mortality remained significant after further adjustment of PA in both men and women. Similar results were reported in another study examining leisure-time running and mortality. Although runners had significantly lower risk of mortality compared with non-runners, this mortality benefit of running was lost after controlling for CRF (Lee et al., 2014). These findings suggest that the effect of PA on mortality is possibly mediated largely by CRF.

Low muscular strength and ill health

Similar to aerobic exercise and PA, the current evidence used for the development of PA guidelines is based on self-reported resistance exercise in large population studies or relatively small intervention studies. This is largely due to the fact that there is still no reliable objective measure of lifestyle muscle-strengthening activities that can be used in large intervention or population studies. However, as muscle strength should improve when an individual regularly resistance trains, one way to resolve this issue is to use an objectively measured muscular strength, as opposed to using self-reported resistance exercise (U.S. Department of Health and Human Services, 2008). Current data mostly focus on the benefits of higher levels of muscular strength, and very limited data exist on the effects of low muscular strength, as an indicator of low resistance exercise (inactivity), on health and mortality. Therefore, we will focus on studies about the effects of higher levels of muscular strength on health here.

Most studies on muscular strength have used handgrip strength as a proxy of total body strength. However, there are studies using measured total body strength including both upper and lower body strength tests. Several studies have demonstrated that the higher levels of muscular strength measured by one repetition maximum of bench and leg presses are associated with lower risks of developing hypertension (Maslow, Sui, Colabianchi, Hussey, & Blair, 2010), metabolic syndrome (Jurca et al., 2005), obesity (Jackson et al., 2010), and reduced risks of premature mortality by cancer (Ruiz et al., 2009), CVD, or any causes after adjusting for potential confounders including age, sex, body fatness, aerobic PA, and even CRF (Ruiz et al., 2008). Also, another study has found that higher muscular strength was associated with lower mortality risk in men even with hypertension (Artero et al., 2011). This study has an important public health message because many people, even physicians, believe that people with hypertension should not participate in resistance exercise due to potential risks associated with breath holding while straining (Valsalva maneuver). A recent review has also shown the cardiovascular health benefits of muscular strength, beyond the health benefits from CRF (Artero et al., 2012). In this review, the authors also indicated that higher levels of muscular strength seem to counteract the adverse effects of obesity on CVD. Furthermore, this study indicated that higher levels of muscular strength have been inversely associated with insulin resistance, clustered cardiometabolic risk, and inflammatory proteins. These studies expand our knowledge and understanding of the health benefits of resistance exercise and muscular strength, independent of aerobic exercise and CRF. Also, these data support the current PA guidelines recommending at least two days of resistance exercise on top of aerobic exercise for additional health benefits that aerobic exercise cannot provide.

Future directions

Although the underlying mechanisms are not fully understood, it is clear that both sedentary behavior and physical inactivity negatively influence human health. Nonetheless, there is much work still to be done to improve our understanding regarding the health consequences of these behaviors. For example, it will be crucial to improve our understanding of the psychobiological consequences of these behaviors as well as how to effectively target reductions while allowing individuals to accomplish necessary activities of daily living that require being seated (e.g. driving). Active pursuit of these lines of investigation will be instrumental for informing public health guidelines specific to sedentary behavior to complement existing PA recommendations. Considering the complete PA spectrum from sitting to vigorous-intensity PA, we now have two strong independent weapons to fight the pandemic of chronic preventable health conditions: reducing sitting time and promoting physical activity.

Summary and practical applications

Knowledge regarding the two health-related behaviors of inactivity and sedentary time is an important step in tackling the health care crisis that is facing much of the developed world. This information will be instrumental for learning how best to modify these behaviors to promote health and wellbeing. For example, there is convincing evidence that prolonged sitting time is detrimental for health. Thus, breaking up longer periods of sedentary time, for example by replacing with light-intensity activities such as standing, has positive benefits on obesity and metabolic health including decreased body fatness, improved glucose metabolism, and enhanced lipid profiles. Evidence collected to data also suggests that health benefits can be achieved by participating in even low amounts of physical activity, below the current minimum guidelines. However, targeting changes in these behaviors is challenging, as there are numerous risk factors and determinants of both sedentary behavior and physical inactivity. Therefore, it is crucial to apply multilevel approaches targeting both individuals and their surrounding environments to reduce sedentary behaviors and increase physical activity. Considering the complete physical activity spectrum from sitting to vigorous-intensity physical activity, we now have two strong independent weapons to fight preventable chronic diseases: reducing sitting time and promoting physical activity.

Chapter summary

- The WHO has reported that physical inactivity is the 4th leading global risk factor for premature mortality, above obesity and hypercholesterolemia.
- High levels of sedentary behavior such as sitting and TV viewing are associated with higher risk of cardiometabolic diseases such as obesity, type 2 diabetes, and heart disease as well as mental health conditions including depression and anxiety.
- Although the economic cost of physical inactivity varies between studies, health care costs are about 25–35% higher in inactive individuals, compared with active individuals.
- Low levels of physical fitness (cardiorespiratory fitness and muscular strength), as an objective marker of sedentary behavior and physical inactivity, are associated with increased risk of chronic diseases and mortality, regardless of body weight.
- Emerging evidence suggests that there may be health benefits associated with even light-intensity physical activity, especially when it is in place of sedentary time.

References

An, K.O., Jang, J.Y., & Kim, J. (2015). Sedentary behavior and sleep duration are associated with both stress symptoms and suicidal thoughts in Korean adults. *The Tohoku Journal of Experimental Medicine,* 237(4), 279–286. https://doi.org/10.1620/tjem.237.279

Anderson, L.H., Martinson, B.C., Crain, A.L., Pronk, N.P., Whitebird, R.R., O'Connor, P.J., & Fine, L.J. (2005). Health care charges associated with physical inactivity, overweight, and obesity. *Preventing Chronic Disease, 2*(4), A09.

Artero, E.G., Lee, D., Lavie, C.J., España-Romero, V., Sui, X., Church, T.S., & Blair, S.N. (2012). Effects of muscular strength on cardiovascular risk factors and prognosis. *Journal of Cardiopulmonary Rehabilitation and Prevention, 32*(6), 351–358. https://doi.org/10.1097/HCR.0b013e3182642688

Artero, E.G., Lee, D., Ruiz, J.R., Sui, X., Ortega, F.B., Church, T.S., . . . Blair, S.N. (2011). A prospective study of muscular strength and all-cause mortality in men with hypertension. *Journal of the American College of Cardiology, 57*(18), 1831–1837. https://doi.org/10.1016/j.jacc.2010.12.025

Asztalos, M., Cardon, G., De Bourdeaudhuij, I., & De Cocker, K. (2015). Cross-sectional associations between sitting time and several aspects of mental health in Belgian adults. *Journal of Physical Activity and Health, 12*(8), 1112–1118. https://doi.org/10.1123/jpah.2013-0513

Atkin, A.J., Adams, E., Bull, F.C., & Biddle, S.J.H. (2012). Non-occupational sitting and mental well-being in employed adults. *Annals of Behavioral Medicine, 43*(2), 181–188. https://doi.org/10.1007/s12160-011-9320-y

Atkin, A.J., Gorely, T., Clemes, S.A., Yates, T., Edwardson, C., Brage, S., . . . Biddle, S.J.H. (2012). Methods of measurement in epidemiology: sedentary behaviour. *International Journal of Epidemiology, 41*(5), 1460–1471. https://doi.org/10.1093/ije/dys118

Balboa-Castillo, T., León-Muñoz, L.M., Graciani, A., Rodríguez-Artalejo, F., & Guallar-Castillón, P. (2011). Longitudinal association of physical activity and sedentary behavior during leisure time with health-related quality of life in community-dwelling older adults. *Health and Quality of Life Outcomes, 9*, 47. https://doi.org/10.1186/1477-7525-9-47

Barwais, F.A., Cuddihy, T.F., & Tomson, L.M. (2013). Physical activity, sedentary behavior and total wellness changes among sedentary adults: a 4-week randomized controlled trial. *Health and Quality of Life Outcomes, 11*, 183. https://doi.org/10.1186/1477-7525-11-183

Bauman, A., Bull, F., Chey, T., Craig, C.L., Ainsworth, B.E., Sallis, J.F., . . . Pratt, M. (2009). The International Prevalence Study on Physical Activity: results from 20 countries. *International Journal of Behavioral Nutrition and Physical Activity, 6*, 21. https://doi.org/10.1186/1479-5868-6-21

Benatti, F.B., & Ried-Larsen, M. (2015). The effects of breaking up prolonged sitting time: a review of experimental studies. *Medicine and Science in Sports and Exercise, 47*(10), 2053–2061. https://doi.org/10.1249/MSS.0000000000000654

Biswas, A., Oh, P.I., Faulkner, G.E., Bajaj, R.R., Silver, M.A., Mitchell, M.S., & Alter, D.A. (2015). Sedentary time and its association with risk for disease incidence, mortality, and hospitalization in adults: a systematic review and meta-analysis. *Annals of Internal Medicine, 162*(2), 123–132. https://doi.org/10.7326/M14-1651

Blair, S.N. (2009). Physical inactivity: the biggest public health problem of the 21st century. *British Journal of Sports Medicine, 43*(1), 1–2.

Brown, W.J., Hockey, R., & Dobson, A.J. (2008). Physical activity, Body Mass Index and health care costs in mid-age Australian women. *Australian and New Zealand Journal of Public Health, 32*(2), 150–155. https://doi.org/10.1111/j.1753-6405.2008.00192.x

Celis-Morales, C.A., Perez-Bravo, F., Ibañez, L., Salas, C., Bailey, M.E.S., & Gill, J.M.R. (2012). Objective vs. self-reported physical activity and sedentary time: effects of measurement method on relationships with risk biomarkers. *PLoS ONE, 7*(5), e36345. https://doi.org/10.1371/journal.pone.0036345

Chastin, S.F.M., De Craemer, M., Lien, N., Bernaards, C., Buck, C., Oppert, J.-M., . . . DEDIPAC consortium, expert working group and consensus panel. (2016). The SOS-framework (Systems of Sedentary behaviours): an international transdisciplinary consensus framework for the study of determinants, research priorities and policy on sedentary behaviour across the life course: a DEDIPAC-study. *The International Journal of Behavioral Nutrition and Physical Activity, 13*, 83. https://doi.org/10.1186/s12966-016-0409-3

Chastin, S.F.M., Egerton, T., Leask, C., & Stamatakis, E. (2015). Meta-analysis of the relationship between breaks in sedentary behavior and cardiometabolic health. *Obesity* (Silver Spring, Md.), *23*(9), 1800–1810. https://doi.org/10.1002/oby.21180

Chastin, S.F.M., Palarea-Albaladejo, J., Dontje, M.L., & Skelton, D.A. (2015). Combined effects of time spent in physical activity, sedentary behaviors and sleep on obesity and cardio-metabolic health markers: a novel compositional data analysis approach. *PLoS ONE, 10*(10), e0139984. https://doi.org/10.1371/journal.pone.0139984

Chau, J.Y., Merom, D., Grunseit, A., Rissel, C., Bauman, A.E., & van der Ploeg, H.P. (2012). Temporal trends in non-occupational sedentary behaviours from Australian Time Use Surveys 1992, 1997 and 2006. *The International Journal of Behavioral Nutrition and Physical Activity, 9*, 76. https://doi.org/10.1186/1479-5868-9-76

Church, T.S., Earnest, C.P., Skinner, J.S., & Blair, S.N. (2007). Effects of different doses of physical activity on cardiorespiratory fitness among sedentary, overweight or obese postmenopausal women with elevated blood pressure: a randomized controlled trial. *JAMA, 297*(19), 2081–2091. https://doi.org/10.1001/jama.297.19.2081

Deliens, T., Deforche, B., De Bourdeaudhuij, I., & Clarys, P. (2015). Determinants of physical activity and sedentary behaviour in university students: a qualitative study using focus group discussions. *BMC Public Health, 15*, 201. https://doi.org/10.1186/s12889-015-1553-4

Diaz, K.M., Howard, V.J., Hutto, B., Colabianchi, N., Vena, J.E., Blair, S.N., & Hooker, S.P. (2016). Patterns of sedentary behavior in US middle-age and older adults: The REGARDS Study. *Medicine and Science in Sports and Exercise, 48*(3), 430–438. https://doi.org/10.1249/MSS.0000000000000792

Ding, D., Lawson, K.D., Kolbe-Alexander, T.L., Finkelstein, E.A., Katzmarzyk, P.T., van Mechelen, W., . . . Lancet Physical Activity Series 2 Executive Committee. (2016). The economic burden of physical inactivity: a global analysis of major non-communicable diseases. *Lancet* (London, England), *388*(10051), 1311–1324. https://doi.org/10.1016/S0140-6736(16)30383-X

Dunstan, D.W., Howard, B., Healy, G.N., & Owen, N. (2012). Too much sitting – a health hazard. *Diabetes Research and Clinical Practice, 97*(3), 368–376. https://doi.org/10.1016/j.diabres.2012.05.020

Dunstan, D.W., Thorp, A.A., & Healy, G.N. (2011). Prolonged sitting: is it a distinct coronary heart disease risk factor? *Current Opinion in Cardiology, 26*(5), 412–419. https://doi.org/10.1097/HCO.0b013e3283496605

Edwards, M.K., & Loprinzi, P.D. (2017). Sedentary behavior, physical activity and cardiorespiratory fitness on leukocyte telomere length. *Health Promotion Perspectives, 7*(1), 22–27. https://doi.org/10.15171/hpp.2017.05

Ekelund, U., Steene-Johannessen, J., Brown, W.J., Fagerland, M.W., Owen, N., Powell, K.E., . . . Lancet Sedentary Behaviour Working Group. (2016). Does physical activity attenuate, or even eliminate, the detrimental association of sitting time with mortality? A harmonised meta analysis of data from more than 1 million men and women. *Lancet* (London, England), *388*(10051), 1302–1310. https://doi.org/10.1016/S0140-6736(16)30370-1

Ellingson, L.D., Meyer, J.D., & Cook, D.B. (2016). Wearable technology reduces prolonged bouts of sedentary behavior. *Translational Journal of the American College of Sports Medicine, 1*(2), 10–17. https://doi.org/10.1249/TJX.0000000000000001

Endorsed by The Obesity Society, Young, D.R., Hivert, M.-F., Alhassan, S., Camhi, S.M., Ferguson, J.F., . . . Physical Activity Committee of the Council on Lifestyle and Cardiometabolic Health; Council on Clinical Cardiology; Council on Epidemiology and Prevention; Council on Functional Genomics and Translational Biology; and Stroke Council. (2016). Sedentary behavior and cardiovascular morbidity and mortality: a science advisory from the American Heart Association. *Circulation, 134*(13), e262–279. https://doi.org/10.1161/CIR.0000000000000440

Endrighi, R., Steptoe, A., & Hamer, M. (2015). The effect of experimentally induced sedentariness on mood and psychobiological responses to mental stress. *The British Journal of Psychiatry: The Journal of Mental Science.* https://doi.org/10.1192/bjp.bp.114.150755

Gennuso, K.P., Thraen-Borowski, K.M., Gangnon, R.E., & Colbert, L.H. (2015). Patterns of sedentary behavior and physical function in older adults. *Aging Clinical and Experimental Research*. https://doi.org/10.1007/s40520-015-0386-4

Grøntved, A., & Hu, F.B. (2011). Television viewing and risk of type 2 diabetes, cardiovascular disease, and all-cause mortality: a meta-analysis. *JAMA, 305*(23), 2448–2455. https://doi.org/10.1001/jama.2011.812

Hagger-Johnson, G., Hamer, M., Stamatakis, E., Bell, J.A., Shahab, L., & Batty, G.D. (2014). Association between sitting time in midlife and common mental disorder symptoms: Whitehall II prospective cohort study. *Journal of Psychiatric Research, 57*, 182–184. https://doi.org/10.1016/j.jpsychires.2014.04.023

Hamer, M., Poole, L., & Messerli-Bürgy, N. (2013). Television viewing, C-reactive protein, and depressive symptoms in older adults. *Brain, Behavior, and Immunity, 33*, 29–32. https://doi.org/10.1016/j.bbi.2013.05.001

Hamer, M., Smith, L., & Stamatakis, E. (2015). Prospective association of TV viewing with acute phase reactants and coagulation markers: English Longitudinal Study of Ageing. *Atherosclerosis, 239*(2), 322–327. https://doi.org/10.1016/j.atherosclerosis.2015.02.009

Hamilton, M.T., Hamilton, D.G., & Zderic, T.W. (2004). Exercise physiology versus inactivity physiology: an essential concept for understanding lipoprotein lipase regulation. *Exercise and Sport Sciences Reviews, 32*(4), 161–166.

Hamilton, M.T., Hamilton, D.G., & Zderic, T.W. (2007). Role of low energy expenditure and sitting in obesity, metabolic syndrome, type 2 diabetes, and cardiovascular disease. *Diabetes, 56*(11), 2655–2667. https://doi.org/10.2337/db07-0882

Hamilton, M.T., Healy, G.N., Dunstan, D.W., Zderic, T.W., & Owen, N. (2008). Too little exercise and too much sitting: inactivity physiology and the need for new recommendations on sedentary behavior. *Current Cardiovascular Risk Reports, 2*(4), 292–298. https://doi.org/10.1007/s12170-008-0054-8

Healy, G.N., Clark, B.K., Winkler, E.A.H., Gardiner, P.A., Brown, W.J., & Matthews, C.E. (2011). Measurement of adults' sedentary time in population-based studies. *American Journal of Preventive Medicine, 41*(2), 216–227. https://doi.org/10.1016/j.amepre.2011.05.005

Healy, G.N., Dunstan, D.W., Salmon, J., Cerin, E., Shaw, J.E., Zimmet, P.Z., & Owen, N. (2008). Breaks in sedentary time: beneficial associations with metabolic risk. *Diabetes Care, 31*(4), 661–666. https://doi.org/10.2337/dc07-2046

Henson, J., Davies, M.J., Bodicoat, D.H., Edwardson, C.L., Gill, J.M.R., Stensel, D.J., . . . Yates, T. (2016). Breaking up prolonged sitting with standing or walking attenuates the postprandial metabolic response in postmenopausal women: a randomized acute study. *Diabetes Care, 39*(1), 130–138. https://doi.org/10.2337/dc15-1240

Herring, M.P., O'Connor, P.J., & Dishman, R.K. (2010). The effect of exercise training on anxiety symptoms among patients: a systematic review. *Archives of Internal Medicine, 170*(4), 321–331. https://doi.org/10.1001/archinternmed.2009.530

Jackson, A.W., Lee, D.-C., Sui, X., Morrow, J.R., Church, T.S., Maslow, A.L., & Blair, S.N. (2010). Muscular strength is inversely related to prevalence and incidence of obesity in adult men. *Obesity* (Silver Spring, Md.), *18*(10), 1988–1995. https://doi.org/10.1038/oby.2009.422

Jurca, R., Lamonte, M.J., Barlow, C.E., Kampert, J.B., Church, T.S., & Blair, S.N. (2005). Association of muscular strength with incidence of metabolic syndrome in men. *Medicine and Science in Sports and Exercise, 37*(11), 1849–1855.

Katzmarzyk, P.T., & Lee, I.-M. (2012). Sedentary behaviour and life expectancy in the USA: a cause-deleted life table analysis. *BMJ Open, 2*(4). https://doi.org/10.1136/bmjopen-2012-000828

Kline, C.E., Krafty, R.T., Mulukutla, S., & Hall, M.H. (2016). Associations of sedentary time and moderate-vigorous physical activity with sleep-disordered breathing and polysomnographic sleep in community-dwelling adults. *Sleep and Breathing*, 1–8. https://doi.org/10.1007/s11325-016-1434-9

Kodama, S., Saito, K., Tanaka, S., Maki, M., Yachi, Y., Asumi, M., . . . Sone, H. (2009). Cardiorespiratory fitness as a quantitative predictor of all-cause mortality and cardiovascular events in healthy men and women: a meta-analysis. *JAMA, 301*(19), 2024–2035. https://doi.org/10.1001/jama.2009.681

Lee, D.C., Artero, E.G., Sui, X., & Blair, S.N. (2010). Mortality trends in the general population: the importance of cardiorespiratory fitness. *Journal of Psychopharmacology* (Oxford, England), *24*(4 Suppl), 27–35. https://doi.org/10.1177/1359786810382057

Lee, D.C., Pate, R.R., Lavie, C.J., Sui, X., Church, T.S., & Blair, S.N. (2014). Leisure-time running reduces all-cause and cardiovascular mortality risk. *Journal of the American College of Cardiology, 64*(5), 472–481. https://doi.org/10.1016/j.jacc.2014.04.058

Lee, D.C., Sui, X., Artero, E.G., Lee, I.-M., Church, T.S., McAuley, P.A., . . . Blair, S.N. (2011a). Long-term effects of changes in cardiorespiratory fitness and body mass index on all-cause and cardiovascular disease mortality in men: the Aerobics Center Longitudinal Study. *Circulation, 124*(23), 2483–2490. https://doi.org/10.1161/CIRCULATIONAHA.111.038422

Lee, D.C., Sui, X., Church, T.S., Lavie, C.J., Jackson, A.S., & Blair, S.N. (2012). Changes in fitness and fatness on the development of cardiovascular disease risk factors hypertension, metabolic syndrome, and hypercholesterolemia. *Journal of the American College of Cardiology, 59*(7), 665–672. https://doi.org/10.1016/j.jacc.2011.11.013

Lee, D.C., Sui, X., Ortega, F.B., Kim, Y.-S., Church, T.S., Winett, R.A., . . . Blair, S.N. (2011b). Comparisons of leisure-time physical activity and cardiorespiratory fitness as predictors of all-cause mortality in men and women. *British Journal of Sports Medicine, 45*(6), 504–510. https://doi.org/10.1136/bjsm.2009.066209

Lee, I.-M., Shiroma, E.J., Lobelo, F., Puska, P., Blair, S.N., Katzmarzyk, P.T., & Lancet Physical Activity Series Working Group. (2012). Effect of physical inactivity on major non-communicable diseases worldwide: an analysis of burden of disease and life expectancy. *Lancet* (London, England), *380*(9838), 219–229. https://doi.org/10.1016/S0140-6736(12)61031-9

Loprinzi, P.D. (2015). Leisure-time screen-based sedentary behavior and leukocyte telomere length: implications for a new leisure-time screen-based sedentary behavior mechanism. *Mayo Clinic Proceedings, 90*(6), 786–790. https://doi.org/10.1016/j.mayocp.2015.02.018

Lucas, M., Mekary, R., Pan, A., Mirzaei, F., O'Reilly, E.J., Willett, W.C., . . . Ascherio, A. (2011). Relation between clinical depression risk and physical activity and time spent watching television in older women: a 10-year prospective follow-up study. *American Journal of Epidemiology, 174*(9), 1017–1027. https://doi.org/10.1093/aje/kwr218

Lyden, K., Keadle, S.K., Staudenmayer, J., & Freedson, P.S. (2016). The activPAL TM accurately classifies activity intensity categories in healthy adults. *Medicine and Science in Sports and Exercise*. https://doi.org/10.1249/MSS.0000000000001177

Lyden, K., Kozey Keadle, S.L., Staudenmayer, J.W., & Freedson, P.S. (2012). Validity of two wearable monitors to estimate breaks from sedentary time. *Medicine and Science in Sports and Exercise, 44*(11), 2243–2252. https://doi.org/10.1249/MSS.0b013e318260c477

Mammen, G., & Faulkner, G. (2013). Physical activity and the prevention of depression: a systematic review of prospective studies. *American Journal of Preventive Medicine, 45*(5), 649–657. https://doi.org/10.1016/j.amepre.2013.08.001

Maslow, A.L., Sui, X., Colabianchi, N., Hussey, J., & Blair, S.N. (2010). Muscular strength and incident hypertension in normotensive and prehypertensive men. *Medicine and Science in Sports and Exercise, 42*(2), 288–295. https://doi.org/10.1249/MSS.0b013e3181b2f0a4

Mikus, C.R., Oberlin, D.J., Libla, J.L., Taylor, A.M., Booth, F.W., & Thyfault, J.P. (2012). Lowering physical activity impairs glycemic control in healthy volunteers. *Medicine and Science in Sports and Exercise, 44*(2), 225–231. https://doi.org/10.1249/MSS.0b013e31822ac0c0

National Physical Activity Plan Alliance. (2016). NPAP. Retrieved January 14, 2017, from www.physicalactivityplan.org/index.html

Pronk, N.P., Katz, A.S., Lowry, M., & Payfer, J.R. (2012). Reducing occupational sitting time and improving worker health: the Take-a-Stand Project, 2011. *Preventing Chronic Disease, 9*, E154. https://doi.org/10.5888/pcd9.110323

Rebar, A.L., Vandelanotte, C., van Uffelen, J., Short, C., & Duncan, M.J. (2014). Associations of overall sitting time and sitting time in different contexts with depression, anxiety, and stress symptoms. *Mental Health and Physical Activity, 7*(2), 105–110. https://doi.org/10.1016/j.mhpa.2014.02.004

Rosenbaum, S., Tiedemann, A., Sherrington, C., Curtis, J., & Ward, P.B. (2014). Physical activity interventions for people with mental illness: a systematic review and meta-analysis. *The Journal of Clinical Psychiatry, 75*(9), 964–974. https://doi.org/10.4088/JCP.13r08765

Ruiz, J.R., Sui, X., Lobelo, F., Lee, D.-C., Morrow, J.R., Jackson, A.W., . . . Blair, S.N. (2009). Muscular strength and adiposity as predictors of adulthood cancer mortality in men. *Cancer Epidemiology, Biomarkers & Prevention: A Publication of the American Association for Cancer Research, Cosponsored by the American Society of Preventive Oncology, 18*(5), 1468–1476. https://doi.org/10.1158/1055-9965. EPI-08-1075

Ruiz, J.R., Sui, X., Lobelo, F., Morrow, J.R., Jackson, A.W., Sjöström, M., & Blair, S.N. (2008). Association between muscular strength and mortality in men: prospective cohort study. *BMJ (Clinical Research Ed.), 337*, a439.

Sanchez-Villegas, A., Ara, I., Guillén-Grima, F., Bes-Rastrollo, M., Varo-Cenarruzabeitia, J.J., & Martínez-González, M.A. (2008). Physical activity, sedentary index, and mental disorders in the SUN cohort study. *Medicine and Science in Sports and Exercise, 40*(5), 827–834. https://doi.org/10.1249/MSS.0b013e31816348b9

Schuch, F., Vancampfort, D., Firth, J., Rosenbaum, S., Ward, P., Reichert, T., . . . Stubbs, B. (2016). Physical activity and sedentary behavior in people with major depressive disorder: A systematic review and meta-analysis. *Journal of Affective Disorders, 210*, 139–150. https://doi.org/10.1016/j.jad.2016.10.050

Sedentary Behaviour Research Network. (2012). Letter to the editor: standardized use of the terms "sedentary" and "sedentary behaviours." *Applied Physiology, Nutrition, and Metabolism = Physiologie Appliquée, Nutrition et Métabolisme, 37*(3), 540–542. https://doi.org/10.1139/h2012-024

Stubbs, B., Gardner-Sood, P., Smith, S., Ismail, K., Greenwood, K., Farmer, R., & Gaughran, F. (2015). Sedentary behaviour is associated with elevated C-reactive protein levels in people with psychosis. *Schizophrenia Research, 168*(1–2), 461–464. https://doi.org/10.1016/j.schres.2015.07.003

Sui, X., Brown, W.J., Lavie, C.J., West, D.S., Pate, R.R., Payne, J.P.W., & Blair, S.N. (2015). Associations between television watching and car riding behaviors and development of depressive symptoms: a prospective study. *Mayo Clinic Proceedings, 90*(2), 184–193. https://doi.org/10.1016/j.mayocp.2014.12.006

Teychenne, M., Abbott, G., Ball, K., & Salmon, J. (2014). Prospective associations between sedentary behaviour and risk of depression in socio-economically disadvantaged women. *Preventive Medicine, 65*, 82–86. https://doi.org/10.1016/j.ypmed.2014.04.025

Teychenne, M., Ball, K., & Salmon, J. (2010). Sedentary behavior and depression among adults: a review. *International Journal of Behavioral Medicine, 17*(4), 246–254. https://doi.org/10.1007/s12529-010-9075-z

Teychenne, M., Costigan, S.A., & Parker, K. (2015). The association between sedentary behaviour and risk of anxiety: a systematic review. *BMC Public Health, 15*, 513. https://doi.org/10.1186/s12889-015-1843-x

Thosar, S.S., Bielko, S.L., Mather, K.J., Johnston, J.D., & Wallace, J.P. (2015). Effect of prolonged sitting and breaks in sitting time on endothelial function. *Medicine and Science in Sports and Exercise, 47*(4), 843–849. https://doi.org/10.1249/MSS.0000000000000479

Troiano, R.P., Berrigan, D., Dodd, K.W., Mâsse, L.C., Tilert, T., & McDowell, M. (2008). Physical activity in the United States measured by accelerometer. *Medicine and Science in Sports and Exercise, 40*(1), 181–188. https://doi.org/10.1249/mss.0b013e31815a51b3

Tucker, L.A., & Tucker, J.M. (2011). Television viewing and obesity in 300 women: evaluation of the pathways of energy intake and physical activity. *Obesity* (Silver Spring, Md.), *19*(10), 1950–1956. https://doi.org/10.1038/oby.2011.184

U.S. Department of Health and Human Services. (2008). Physical Activity Guidelines for Americans. Retrieved from www.health.gov/paguidelines/

Vallance, J.K., Winkler, E.A.H., Gardiner, P.A., Healy, G.N., Lynch, B.M., & Owen, N. (2011). Associations of objectively-assessed physical activity and sedentary time with depression: NHANES (2005–2006). *Preventive Medicine, 53*(4–5), 284–288. https://doi.org/10.1016/j.ypmed.2011.07.013

van der Ploeg, H.P., Chey, T., Korda, R.J., Banks, E., & Bauman, A. (2012). Sitting time and all-cause mortality risk in 222 497 Australian adults. *Archives of Internal Medicine, 172*(6), 494–500. https://doi.org/10.1001/archinternmed.2011.2174

van der Ploeg, H.P., Venugopal, K., Chau, J.Y., van Poppel, M.N.M., Breedveld, K., Merom, D., & Bauman, A.E. (2013). Non-occupational sedentary behaviors: population changes in The Netherlands, 1975–2005. *American Journal of Preventive Medicine, 44*(4), 382–387. https://doi.org/10.1016/j.amepre.2012.11.034

van Uffelen, J.G.Z., van Gellecum, Y.R., Burton, N.W., Peeters, G., Heesch, K.C., & Brown, W.J. (2013). Sitting-time, physical activity, and depressive symptoms in mid-aged women. *American Journal of Preventive Medicine, 45*(3), 276–281. https://doi.org/10.1016/j.amepre.2013.04.009

Vancampfort, D., Firth, J., Schuch, F., Rosenbaum, S., De Hert, M., Mugisha, J., . . . Stubbs, B. (2016). Physical activity and sedentary behavior in people with bipolar disorder: a systematic review and meta-analysis. *Journal of Affective Disorders, 201*, 145–152. https://doi.org/10.1016/j.jad.2016.05.020

Wang, F., McDonald, T., Reffitt, B., & Edington, D.W. (2005). BMI, physical activity, and health care utilization/costs among Medicare retirees. *Obesity Research, 13*(8), 1450–1457. https://doi.org/10.1038/oby.2005.175

Wendel-Vos, W., Droomers, M., Kremers, S., Brug, J., & van Lenthe, F. (2007). Potential environmental determinants of physical activity in adults: a systematic review. *Obesity Reviews: An Official Journal of the International Association for the Study of Obesity, 8*(5), 425–440. https://doi.org/10.1111/j.1467-789X.2007.00370.x

World Health Organization. (2009). *Global health risks: mortality and burden of disease attributable to selected major risks*. Retrieved from http://apps.who.int/iris/handle/10665/44203

World Health Organization. (2010). *Global Recommendations on Physical Activity for Health*. Geneva: World Health Organization. Retrieved from www.ncbi.nlm.nih.gov/books/NBK305057/

World Health Organization. (2016). *WHO | Prevalence of insufficient physical activity*. Retrieved January 14, 2017, from www.who.int/gho/ncd/risk_factors/physical_activity_text/en/

Yates, T., Henson, J., Edwardson, C., Dunstan, D., Bodicoat, D.H., Khunti, K., & Davies, M.J. (2015). Objectively measured sedentary time and associations with insulin sensitivity: importance of reallocating sedentary time to physical activity. *Preventive Medicine, 76*, 79–83. https://doi.org/10.1016/j.ypmed.2015.04.005

Yates, T., Khunti, K., Wilmot, E.G., Brady, F., Webb, D., Srinivasan, B., . . . Davies, M.J. (2012). Self-reported sitting time and markers of inflammation, insulin resistance, and adiposity. *American Journal of Preventive Medicine, 42*(1), 1–7. https://doi.org/10.1016/j.amepre.2011.09.022

5   Physical activity and health

Ian Lahart, George Metsios and Chris Kite

Keywords: Physical activity, exercise, chronic disease, epidemiology, randomised controlled trials

Introduction

In this chapter we aim to present an up-to-date synthesis of the best available evidence for the therapeutic role of physical activity (PA) and exercise for non-communicable diseases (NCDs) and health. Firstly, we examine the epidemiologic evidence for an association between PA and cardiorespiratory fitness (CRF) and premature mortality, and the prevention and management of NCDs. To help readers interpret this type of evidence, we will also explore the limitations of epidemiology and the risk of biases inherent in this type of research. Next, we review randomised controlled trials (RCTs) of the effects of exercise interventions on early death and the prevention and management of some of the most prevalent NCDs for which sufficient data exist (e.g., cardiovascular disease, type 2 diabetes, breast and colorectal cancers, and chronic respiratory diseases). Finally, as in the case with the epidemiologic evidence, RCTs are not without their limitations, and we, therefore, provide an overview of the risk of biases these studies are prone to.

Epidemiological evidence for physical activity

In PA epidemiology, the reduction in risk of developing a particular outcome (e.g., disease incidence) following exposure to PA is typically expressed in terms of relative risk (RR) reduction. We will present RR reductions in this chapter as percentages, and all included RR reductions referred to were statistically significant (i.e. the 95% confidence intervals of the RR reduction do not pass the line of no effect), unless specifically identified as non-significant.

The modern history of PA and disease research arguably began with the seminal work of Jerry Morris and colleagues in the 1950s. Morris and colleagues (1953) observed lower incidences of coronary artery disease (CAD), later onset of CAD, and lower CAD-related mortality in double-decker bus conductors (who climbed on average 500–750 steps/day) compared with sedentary bus drivers. Similar findings were also observed by Morris and his team when comparing postmen who cycled or walked to deliver mail with less active co-workers (e.g., postal supervisors) and sedentary counterparts (e.g., telephonists). Subsequent work of

Morris and colleagues (1973; 1966; 1956) noted that 1) CAD incidence was higher in bus drivers compared with conductors independent of physique and blood pressure, 2) CAD was lower in the most active compared with the least active in three separate social classes (skilled, semi-skilled, and unskilled workers), and 3) civil servants who performed more vigorous leisure-time PA experienced lower rates of fatal CAD events. There is further information in regard to the work of Morris and co-workers in Chapter 3.

Two other often cited classical studies were conducted by Ralph Paffenbarger (see also Chapter 3) and colleagues on San Francisco longshoremen (known as dock workers in the UK) (Paffenbarger, Laughlin, Gima, & Black, 1970) and college alumni (Paffenbarger, Wing, & Hyde, 1978), respectively. In a 16-year follow-up of 3,263 men (aged 35–64 years), Paffenbarger and co-workers (1970) observed that the most active group of longshoremen had fewer CAD deaths than their less active co-workers, regardless of smoking patterns, weight for height, and blood pressure. Similarly, in the Harvard Alumni study, an analysis of nearly 17,000 men followed-up for 16 years revealed an inverse dose-response association between PA and all-cause mortality rates, after controlling for high blood pressure, cigarette smoking, extreme body weight gains, and early parental death (Paffenbarger, Hyde, Wing, & Hsieh, 1986). The rates of all-cause mortality, primarily due to cardiovascular or respiratory causes, were 25–33% lower among participants who expended ≥2000 kcal during PA per week compared to less active alumni.

More recently in one of the largest European-based PA cohort studies, the European Prospective Investigation into Cancer and Nutrition Study (EPIC) investigated whether the association between PA and all-cause mortality was modified by adiposity (Ekelund et al., 2015). In an analysis that consisted of 334,161 men and women followed-up for 12.4 years, the authors (2015) reported that PA was associated with lower all-cause mortality at all levels of body mass index (BMI) and waist circumference. The researchers (2015) estimated that the number of early deaths would theoretically be reduced by ~7% if all inactive individuals were at least moderately inactive, compared with a ~4% reduction in deaths if all individuals with a BMI above 30 kg/m^2 had a BMI below 30.

Many systematic reviews, pooled analyses, and meta-analyses have collated the epidemiological evidence and calculated average RR reductions in all-cause premature mortality and disease incidence and mortality associated with PA. Arem and colleagues (2015) pooled data taken from eight studies (661,137 participants) of the USA National Cancer Institute (NCI) Cohort Consortium. The authors (2015) reported that compared with participants performing no leisure-time moderate-to-vigorous PA (MVPA), participants performing some MVPA but less than the recommended USA PA guidelines (defined as ≥7.5 MET-h/week), and those achieving 1–2, 2–3, and 3–5 times the recommendation had 20%, 31%, 37%, and 39% reductions in all-cause premature mortality risk, respectively (see Figure 5.1). Similarly, based on six studies (654,827 participants) from the same NCI Cohort, compared with no leisure-time activity, PA below recommended levels (0.1–3.74 and 3.74–7.49 MET-h/week), 1–2 times the recommended level (7.5–14.9 MET-h/week), and exceeding 22.5 MET-h/week (or ≥450 min/week of brisk walking) was associated with a gain of 1.8, 2.5, 3.4, and 4.5 years in life expectancy, respectively (Moore et al., 2012). Hupin and co-workers (2015) noted similar findings in a meta-analysis of prospective cohort studies in older adults (≥60 years). Low MVPA (1–499 MET-min/week) was associated with a 22% reduction in all-cause mortality in older adults, whereas following the current PA recommendations (500–999 MET-min/week) and beyond (≥1000 MET-min/week) was related to higher risk reductions of 28% and 35%, respectively, compared with no MVPA.

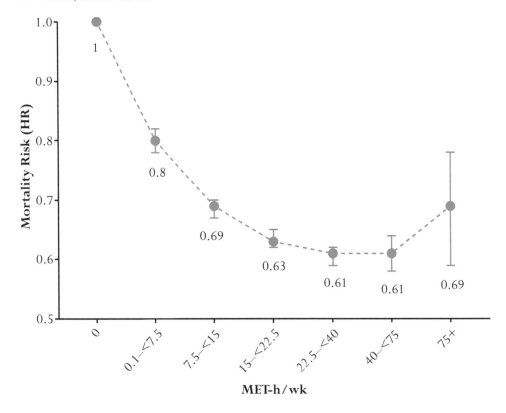

Figure 5.1 Multivariable-adjusted with body mass index hazard ratios (HRs) and 95% confidence
intervals for leisure time moderate- to vigorous-intensity physical activity and premature
mortality risk. Mortality risk is expressed as a HR, which is a measure of relative risk (RR)
over time. An RR is the probability that a member of a group exposed to PA will develop a
disease relative to the probability that a member of an unexposed group will develop that
same disease. If RR = ~1.0, an association between exposure to PA and disease is unlikely
to exist. If RR = >1.0, there is an increased risk of developing that disease in those who
were exposed to PA, and if RR = <1.0, there is a reduced risk of developing that disease
to those who have been exposed to PA. For an example, the RR of 0.69 associated with
7.5 to <15 MET-h/week of MVPA would mean a 31% lower risk of premature mortality.

As well as leisure-time PA, there is evidence of associations between all-cause mortality
and PA performed in other domains. Samitz and colleagues (2011) investigated the association between higher levels of total and domain-specific PA and all-cause mortality in a large
meta-analysis of 80 studies (~1.4 million participants and 118,121 deaths). Comparing the
highest PA group with the lowest, the authors (2011) observed RR reductions of 35% for
total PA, 36% for activities of daily living, 26% for leisure-time PA, and 17% for occupational
activity. Furthermore, each 1-hour increment per week of vigorous- and moderate-intensity
PA was associated with 9% and 4% RR reductions, respectively.

Recently, researchers have suggested that the amount of PA associated with a reduced
risk of early death may be dependent on the amount of sedentary behaviour a person performs. A large harmonised meta-analysis involving over one million participants observed

that high levels of moderate-intensity PA may be needed to protect against the increased risk of premature death associated with high sitting time (Ekelund et al., 2016). Compared with the reference group (<4 hours/day of sitting and >35.5 MET-h/week), the authors (2016) observed that for participants sitting at least 8 hours per day only those who also reported at least 35.5 MET-h/week (~60–75 min/day of moderate PA) were not at an increased risk of early mortality. However, using accelerometer measured PA in over 3,000 participants (5 years follow-up), Fishman and colleagues (2016) found that replacing 30 minutes of sedentary time with light activity or MVPA was associated with respective 20% and 51% reductions in RR of all-cause mortality risk. These two findings have important implications given that evidence suggests that sedentary behaviour is an independent risk factor of NCDs and early death (Owen, Healy, Matthews, & Dunstan, 2010).

A series of systematic reviews and meta-analyses have also examined the association between PA and the risk of developing a NCD and disease-specific mortality. Kyu et al. (2016) included 174 studies (149.2 million total person-years of follow-up) in a Bayesian dose-response meta-analysis aimed at quantifying the association between total PA (i.e. leisure-time, occupation, domestic, and active transportation PA) and risk of five common NCDs (breast cancer, colon cancer, diabetes, CAD, and ischemic stroke). Higher levels of PA were associated with lower risk for all five NCDs, with the greatest risk reduction observed for PA levels up to 3,000–3,600 MET-min/week, or 5–6 times the current World Health Organization recommendation of 600 MET-min/week (WHO, 2010) (see Figure 5.2). When compared with participants who performed below the recommended amount of PA (<600 MET-min/week), those in the highly active category (≥8000 MET-minutes/week) had average RR reductions

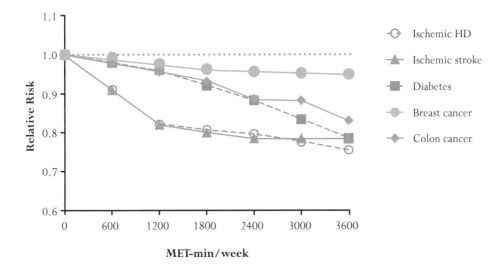

Figure 5.2 Continuous risk curves for association between meeting recommended physical activity guidelines (600 MET-min/week) and above (600 MET-min/week × 2, 3, 4, 5, and 6) and risk of ischemic heart disease (HD), ischemic stroke, diabetes, breast cancer, and colon cancer. Achieving at [3]600 MET-min/week was significantly associated with a reduction in the risk of ischemic HD and diabetes, [3]1800 MET-min/week was significantly associated with lower ischemic stroke risk, [3]2400 MET-min/week was significantly associated with a reduction in colon cancer risk and [3]3000 MET-min/week was significantly associated with a lower breast cancer risk.

of 28% for diabetes, 26% for ischemic stroke, 25% for CAD, 21% for colon cancer, and 14% for breast cancer. Similarly, another meta-analysis (Wahid et al., 2016) found that an increase from being inactive to achieving recommended PA levels (150 min/week of moderate-intensity PA) was associated with a lower risk of type 2 diabetes (26%), CAD (20%), and ischemic stroke (18%), and a lower chance of dying from CAD (20%), after controlling for body weight.

PA is also associated with a reduced risk of developing certain cancers. In a pooled analysis of 12 prospective USA and European cohorts involving 1.44 million participants (186,932 cancer cases), Moore and co-workers (2016) observed that high (90th percentile) versus low (10th percentile) levels of leisure-time PA were associated with lower RRs of oesophageal adenocarcinoma (38%), myeloid leukaemia (15%), myeloma (13%), and cancers of the lung (27%), kidney (16%), head and neck (15%), colon (13%), bladder (12%), rectum (12%), and breast (7%), after adjustments for important risk factors including BMI. Similarly, a recent meta-analysis (Liu et al., 2015) also found an inverse association between cancer incidence and PA, but at a lower dose than Moore et al. (2016). Liu et al. (2015) conducted a large meta-analysis involving 126 studies (199,820 cancer incidences in 7.3 million participants) and examined the association between meeting recommended moderate-intensity PA guidelines (defined as 10 MET-h/week of leisure-time PA) and the risk of developing cancer. Compared with no leisure-time PA, 10 MET-h/week of leisure-time PA was associated with an overall RR reduction in cancer incidence of 7%, which was almost entirely attributable to a 4% reduction in breast cancer risk and an 8% reduction in colorectal cancer risk. The authors (2015) also reported that the protection against cancer associated with PA reached saturation at twice the current PA recommendation.

In addition to reduced cancer incidence, PA has also been associated with a reduced risk of cancer mortality both in the general population and cancer survivors. In a meta-analysis consisting of 71 prospective cohort studies (~4 million participants from the general population and 69,000 patients with cancer), a minimum of 150 min/week of moderate-intensity PA (7.5 MET-hours/week) was associated with a 13% reduction in cancer mortality in the general population, whereas, the same dose of PA was associated with a 14% lower risk of cancer mortality in cancer survivors (Li et al., 2015). Again, most of the observed inverse relationship between PA and cancer mortality was attributed to the associated reductions in breast and colorectal cancer mortality (24% risk reduction for both). The authors also discovered a much stronger association between post-cancer diagnosis PA and cancer mortality compared with pre-diagnosis PA (40% vs. 14% risk reductions). Similar differences in the reductions in mortality risk associated with pre-diagnosis and post-diagnosis PA have been reported for breast cancer (16% vs. 41% risk reduction) and colorectal (25% vs. 39% risk reduction) cancer in two other meta-analyses (Lahart, Metsios, Nevill, & Carmichael, 2015; Schmid & Leitzmann, 2014a).

Based on a recent pooled analysis of 11 British cohorts (63,591 adult respondents), O'Donovan and colleagues (2017) found that meeting PA recommendations (≥150 min/week in moderate-intensity or ≥75 min/week in vigorous-intensity activities from ≥3 sessions) was associated with lower risks of cancer-related mortality (21%) as well as all-cause (35%) and cardiovascular disease (CVD) (61%) mortality, compared to inactive participants. Interestingly, compared with the inactive participants, participants who were categorised as insufficiently active (<150 min/week in moderate-intensity or <7 min/week in vigorous-intensity activities) and those described as 'weekend warriors' (≥150 min/week in moderate-intensity or ≥75 min/week in vigorous-intensity activities from 1–2 sessions) also had lower risks of all-cause (36% and 30%, respectively) and CVD mortality (both 40%), whereas, only insufficiently active participants had a lower risk cancer mortality (17%).

Although, most of the evidence above pertains to PA performed in a recreational, occupational, or active transport setting, evidence now exists for an association between other types of activity and risk of disease and early mortality. In a recent meta-analysis, participation in cycling, swimming, racquet sports, and aerobics was associated with significant reductions in all-cause mortality, whereas participation in swimming, racquet sports, and aerobics was associated with lower CVD mortality risk (Oja et al., 2016). Similarly, an estimated RR reduction in all-cause mortality of 11% and 10% was observed for a standardised dose of 11.25 MET-hours per week of walking and cycling, respectively, in another meta-analysis (Kelly et al., 2014).

Findings of inverse associations between muscular strength and risks of all-cause, CVD, cancer mortality (Artero et al., 2011; Leong et al., 2015; Ortega, Silventoinen, Tynelius, & Rasmussen, 2012; Ruiz et al., 2009; Ruiz et al., 2008), and suicide in male adolescents (Ortega et al., 2012) has led to an increased interest in the potential health benefits of resistance training (also referred to as strength training or weightlifting). In an analysis of data from over 30,000 adults aged 65 years and older who participated in the USA National Interview Survey (followed up for 15 years), Kraschnewski and colleagues (2016) found that older adults who reported meeting guidelines for strength training behaviour (≥2 sessions per week) had 46% lower odds of all-cause mortality than those who did not. Another study, involving 8,772 adults aged at least 20 years, observed a 23% reduced risk of all-cause mortality in those performing any strength training activity (Dankel, Loenneke, & Loprinzi, 2016b). The same authors (2016a) also reported in a dose-response analysis that only individuals performing 8–14 sessions over a 30-day period had a reduced risk of all-cause mortality (30%).

However, a recent study suggests that the outcome (muscular strength) may be more important than the behaviour (resistance training). Dankel and colleagues (2016a) found that despite meeting muscle strengthening activity guidelines (≥2 sessions per week) those participants who were not in highest strength quartile did not have a statistically significant reduction in all-cause mortality risk. However, compared with individuals not meeting muscle strengthening activity guidelines and not in the top quartile for lower-extremity strength, the greatest reduction (72%) in risk of premature all-cause mortality was still observed in those who both met the guideline and were in the top strength quartile.

Epidemiological evidence for cardiorespiratory fitness

The vast majority of the epidemiological evidence discussed above has measured PA via self-report, however, some researchers have argued that CRF, assessed via maximal exercise testing, provides a more objective, precise, and reliable measure (LaMonte & Blair, 2006; Lee, Artero, Sui, & Blair, 2010). Although, CRF is determined in part by factors such as age, gender, smoking, adiposity, health/disease status, and genetics, the principle determinant is recent patterns of PA (Lee et al., 2010). Similar to physical inactivity, low CRF has been associated with risk of NCDs and early mortality (Blair et al., 1989; Kodama et al., 2009; Laukkanen, Kurl, Salonen, Rauramaa, & Salonen, 2004; Sawada et al., 2014; Sui, LaMonte, et al., 2007). Therefore, as well as being an important focus for lifestyle interventions, low CRF may also be an important disease and mortality risk factor (Gupta et al., 2011).

In a landmark study (Blair et al., 1989), the Aerobics Centre Longitudinal Study (ACLS) reported results of an analysis of the relationship between initial levels of CRF and all-cause mortality in 10,224 men and 3,120 women followed for eight years (further information on this study is available in Chapter 3). The authors (1989) observed inverse dose-response relationships between CRF and all-cause mortality, and when compared with the least fit men and women, the most fit men and women had lower risk of all-cause mortality (43% and 53% for men and women, respectively) and CVD mortality (47% and 70% for men and women, respectively). Since the ACLS, similar associations between CRF and the risk of developing several NCDs and early mortality have been observed. In a recent meta-analysis of 33 studies and ~103,000 participants, Kodama and colleagues (2009) reported that for each 1-Metabolic Equivalent (MET) higher level of CRF (equivalent to 1 km/h higher running speed) there was an associated 13% reduction in all-cause mortality and a 15% reduction in CVD events. Encouragingly the greatest reduction in risk of all-cause mortality reported in the literature appears to occur between the least fit and the next-to-least fit groups (McKinney et al., 2016).

As well as all-cause and CVD mortality, CRF is associated with reduced risk of cancer mortality. Schmid and Leitzmann (2014b) combined data from six prospective studies with a total number of 71,654 individuals and 2,002 cases of total cancer mortality (median follow-up time, 16 years), and observed that compared to low CRF, intermediate and high CRF was associated with 20% and 45% lower total cancer mortality, respectively. As well as cancer mortality, high CRF in men has also been associated with a lower risk of lung and colorectal cancer but not prostate cancer (Lakoski et al., 2015). Furthermore, high CRF is associated with more favourable CAD risk factors, lower risk of developing type 2 diabetes (Chow et al., 2016; Sui, Hooker, et al., 2007), metabolic syndrome (Earnest et al., 2013), and dementia (Defina et al., 2013), improved surgical outcomes (Ross et al., 2016), reduced length of stay in hospital after major elective surgery (Snowden et al., 2010), and lower measures of anxiety and depressive symptoms (Dishman et al., 2012; Schuch et al., 2016; Sui et al., 2008; Trivedi et al., 2011).

The majority of studies rely on a single baseline CRF measurement and relate this to subsequent mortality follow-up. Studies that assess the change in CRF over time provide stronger evidence of the importance of CRF in relation to risk of disease and early mortality. Although genetics may contribute towards up to 47% of the improvements in CRF possible (Bouchard et al., 1999), changes in PA can affect CRF. Therefore, individuals may be able to lower their early mortality risk through PA-induced improvements in CRF. At the time of writing, the most recent study (Laukkanen et al., 2016) investigating long-term changes in CRF and premature mortality observed that a 1 ml/kg/min higher change in CRF was associated with a 9% RR reduction in all-cause mortality in a sample of 579 participants followed over 11 years. Similarly, in a study involving 14,345 men followed up for 6.3 years, every 1-MET improvement in CRF was associated with a lower risk of all-cause (15%) and CVD mortality (19%) (Lee et al., 2011). There are currently a lack of studies that have investigated the relationship between CRF change and mortality in women.

Higher CRF may also be protective for those with high levels of adiposity. Previous research has shown that individuals who are obese and have high levels of CRF have a lower risk of all-cause mortality and cardiovascular disease compared to individuals who are lean and have low levels of CRF (Barry et al., 2014; Lee, Blair, & Jackson, 1999). In a systematic review of the literature (36 studies), compared with individuals with normal BMI (18–24.9 kg/m2) and poor CRF, individuals with high BMI (>25 kg/m2) and good CRF had lower risk of all-cause and cardiovascular mortality (Fogelholm, 2009). Similarly, in a recent meta-analysis, Barry and colleagues (2014) found that individuals who were unfit had twice the risk of early mortality regardless of BMI, while fit and overweight and obese individuals had premature mortality risks equivalent to their normal weight counterparts (see Figure 5.3). Furthermore,

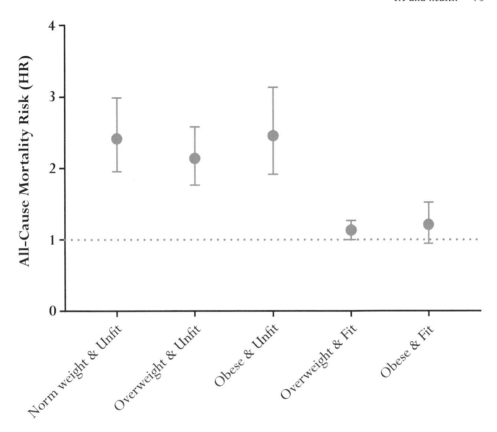

Figure 5.3 Pooled hazard ratio (HR) and 95% confidence intervals for each comparison group (i.e., normal weight unfit, overweight and obese unfit and overweight and obese fit) vs. normal weight fit group. Compared to normal weight and fit individuals, unfit individuals had twice the risk of all-cause mortality regardless of BMI. Fit individuals who were also overweight or obese had similar mortality risks as normal weight and fit individuals.

participants who are overweight or obese with higher CRF also have lower visceral adiposity and in turn, have more favourable cardiometabolic risk profiles (e.g., higher HDL cholesterol, and lower triglycerides, blood pressure, and insulin resistance) compared with BMI-matched participants with low CRF (Arsenault et al., 2009; O'Donovan, Kearney, Sherwood, & Hillsdon, 2012; Rhéaume et al., 2009).

Issues with epidemiological evidence for physical activity

Two reviews of the evidence supporting the Canadian recommended PA guidelines (i.e., accumulate 60 min of daily PA or 30 min of MVPA on at least 4 days/week) reached the following conclusions: 1) the current guidelines appear to be appropriate to reduce the risks of all-cause mortality and the risk of CVD, stroke, hypertension, colon and breast cancer, type 2 diabetes, and osteoporosis (Warburton, Katzmarzyk, Rhodes, & Shephard, 2008); and 2) the evidence supports a dose-response relationship between PA and all-cause mortality and the risk of developing the seven chronic conditions listed above (Warburton, Charlesworth, Ivey, Nettlefold, & Bredin, 2010). The authors of the later review (2010) determined that the level of evidence supporting PA should be considered level 2A based on the presence of overwhelming evidence from observational trials. To be considered level 1A, evidence would be required from RCTs without important limitations showing the action can apply to most individuals in most circumstances and the benefits clearly outweigh risks. To appreciate why the vast amount of epidemiological evidence supporting an inverse association between PA and morbidity and early mortality cannot be regarded as the highest level evidence, an under-standing of the limitations of epidemiological studies is needed.

Statistical associations obtained through observational studies do not necessarily imply casual associations (Kundi, 2006). They may instead represent a spurious (resulting from selec-tion bias, information bias, and chance) or indirect (resulting from confounding) association (Grimes & Schulz, 2002). Epidemiologic research cannot easily (if at all) determine between a spurious, indirect, or causal association (see Hill (1965) for a discussion of the criteria needed to attempt this). Similarly, it is often difficult to establish the direction of the potential causal association between the exposure and the outcome. Reverse causation, which occurs when the outcome may have caused the variation in the exposure, may be particularly relevant to PA observational studies. For example, the association between high PA and low risk of disease may not be because higher PA results in lower incidence of disease, instead, it may be because lower incidences in disease results in higher levels of PA (i.e. people who are free from disease are active because they are healthy). While, it is beyond the scope of this chapter to provide a comprehensive overview of all the limitations (biases) of the epidemiological evidence (see Delgado-Rodriguez & Llorca, 2004; Grimes & Schulz, 2002; Sackett, 1979), we will attempt to briefly summarise some of the key biases in PA epidemiology, namely, selection bias, infor-mation bias, and confounding.

Selection bias can occur in PA observational studies from the inappropriate definition of eligible populations, lack of accuracy of sampling frame, unequal diagnostic procedures in the target population, and during trial implementation because of missing data due to loss of follow-up and non-responses (Delgado-Rodriguez & Llorca, 2004). Among the types of selection biases that can occur are healthcare access bias, competing risks, healthy volunteer effect, uneven diagnostic procedures, and Neyman bias (see Table 5.1).

Information bias, such as regression to the mean, ecological fallacy, and misclassification bias, can influence the findings of observational studies (see Table 5.1) (Grimes & Schulz, 2002). Misclassification bias is particularly important when interpreting PA observational studies. Despite the importance of PA for health and disease there is currently no stan-dardised approach to its measurement. Self-report questionnaires are the most commonly used method to assess PA in epidemiological studies and there are an extensive range of ques-tionnaires available for this purpose. However, despite their widespread use for many years, PA questionnaires still show limited reliability and validity (van Poppel, Chinapaw, Mokkink, Mechelen, & Terwee, 2010). Self-reported PA is at risk of recall bias, observer expectation bias, and reporting bias, such as social desirability bias (see Table 5.1). Misclassification bias combined with the use of a single measurement of PA at baseline can mean that individuals are wrongly categorised as physically active or inactive, which can lead to spurious associations in the literature.

Table 5.1 Examples of biases in epidemiological studies

Types of bias	Definition
Selection bias	When exposed (PA) and unexposed (physically inactive) groups differ in some important factor other than exposure of interest (i.e., PA levels) or when the study population does not represent the target population.
• *Healthcare access bias*	Patients admitted to the study institution are not representative of the typical patient population due to cultural, geographical, or economic reasons.
• *Competing risks*	When two or more outcomes (e.g. causes of death) are mutually exclusive, they compete with each other in the same subject, such as when there are competing causes of death.
• *Healthy volunteer effect*	When the study participants are healthier than the general population.
• *Uneven diagnostic procedures*	If the same diseases are diagnosed differently across studies or time can make comparisons difficult.
• *Neyman bias (incidence-prevalence bias)*	A distorted frequency of the exposure (e.g. smoking) in a sample of cases resulting if the exposure is related to prognostic factors or is a prognostic determinant itself. Can occur if there is a gap in time between exposure (e.g. PA assessment) and selection of study participants.
Informational bias	Results from the inaccurate determination of the exposure or outcome, or both.
• *Regression to the mean*	When a variable that shows an extreme value of one assessment, such as PA assessment, it tends to be closer to the population average on a subsequent assessment. Can occur in trials involving multiple measures of the same variable over time.
• *Misclassification bias*	When the procedure to measure the exposure (e.g. PA) and/or the outcome (e.g. disease diagnosis) is not perfect. Includes:
	• *Recall bias*: where the amount and accuracy of information recalled differs between those exposed and those unexposed.
	• *Observer expectation bias*: when the interviewers knowledge of the hypothesis, health or exposure status influence data recording.
	• *Social desirability bias*: where participants can over report socially desirable behaviours and under report socially undesirable behaviours.
• Ecological fallacy	When findings attained in an ecological (or group level) analysis are used to make inferences at the individual level.
Confounding	When a variable is both associated with the exposure (e.g. PA) and affects the outcome (e.g. early mortality), but is not an intermediate step in the causal pathway between the exposure and the outcome. For example, if a PA cohort study observed that participants in a physically active group had lower rates of CVD compared to an inactive group, but also consumed more alcohol. The higher rate of disease in the inactive group may be explained not by their lack of PA but by the higher levels of alcohol consumption.

Confounding can occur in every epidemiological study (see Table 5.1). Although current epidemiological studies often control for most of the known confounding variables that might influence the association between PA and morbidity and premature mortality, early studies in the field controlled only for a few confounders (such as age, BMI, and smoking) (Warburton et al., 2010). Therefore, early studies and possibly current studies are at risk of omitted variable bias, which occurs when a confounding variable has not been included in the analysis. Differences in the confounding variables controlled for in studies also make the comparisons of RR reductions more difficult. The inability to adequately measure and control for all potential confounding variables is one of the key limitations of epidemiological research.

On a final note, the reporting of risk reductions as RR in the epidemiological literature can be misleading. When the event is rare, even a small change in absolute risk (AR) is likely to produce a large RR estimate. However, when the event is common the same RR reduction

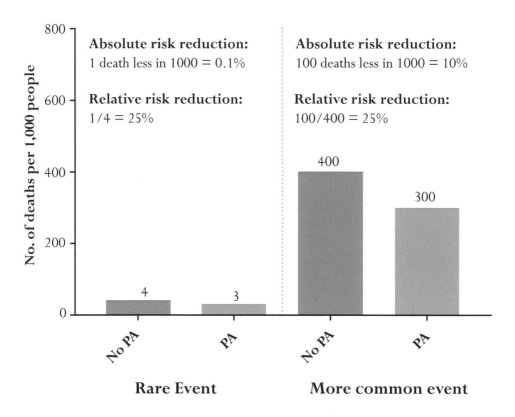

Figure 5.4 In the rare event scenario, a small difference in absolute risk (AR), the number of events in a no physical activity (PA) or PA group divided by the number of people in that group between two groups (AR reduction of 0.1% or 1 death less in 1000 people) still produces a large RR reduction estimate (RR reduction of 25%). In the more common event scenario a far larger AR reduction (10% or 100 less deaths in 1000 people) results in the same RR reduction (25%) as observed in the rare event.

would represent a far larger number of people (see Figure 5.4 for an illustration of this point). Therefore, presenting RR without the underlying AR reductions provides incomplete information (Yueh & Feinstein, 1999). Unfortunately, it is uncommon for observational studies and systematic reviews to report AR reductions, and it is rarer still for these publications to report both RR and AR statistics (Gigerenzer, Wegwarth, & Feufel, 2010; King, Harper, & Young, 2012).

Table 5.2   A non-exhaustive list of chronic physiologic adaptations of human organs/systems to exercise training (mainly endurance exercise)

Organ/system	Adaptations
Brain	• Possible increase in neural activity • Possible increase in cerebral blood flow • Possible increase in brain metabolism • Possible changes at the receptor level • Enhanced or maintained brain size
Lungs	• Increase or no change in blood flow and gas exchange reserve • Increased vital capacity and tidal volume • Increase in maximal inspiratory and expiratory force • Possible increase in capillary surface area
Cardiovascular system	• Increase in cavity size and wall thickness • Improved aortic compliance and reduced stiffness • Enhanced myocardial contractility • Reduced sympathetic tone and increased parasympathetic tone • Improved left ventricle ejection fraction • Normalisation of heart rate variability • Lower resting blood pressure in hypertensives • Prevention of age-related diastolic dysfunction • No change in response or an increase in blood flow and oxygen consumption • Possible improved blood flow distribution • Possible improved oxygen extraction • Increase in blood volume • Increase total red blood cell mass • Reduced haematocrit (via increased plasma volume) • Higher or lower levels of circulating energy substrates • Decreased glycated haemoglobin (Hb1ac) • Favourable changes in circulating serum lipid and amino acid profiles • Increased lipoprotein lipase activity and triglyceride catabolism • Increased arterial diameters • Possible improvement in endothelial function in those with endothelial dysfunction • Increased nitric oxide production • Reduced oxidative stress • Reduced inflammation • Increased capillary density through angiogenesis

(Continued)

Table 5.2   (Continued)

Organ/system	Adaptations
Skeletal muscle	• Muscle hypertrophy • Increased mitochondrial mass and mitochondrial enzyme concentrations and activities • Increased oxygen extraction due to enlarged capillary surface area and longer blood transit time • Improved uptake of substrates, with constant relative contribution of glucose, free fatty acids, and lactate at corresponding relative exercise intensities. • Enhanced skeletal muscle vasodilation capacity • Higher insulin sensitivity and lower insulin resistance • Increases glucose transporter type 4 and 5' AMP-activated protein kinase • Improved calcium handling
Bone	• Possibly improved skeletal blood flow and metabolism • Improved bone mineral content, structure and strength
Liver, pancreas, gut, and kidneys	• Possibly ameliorates insulin resistance in the liver, pancreas, gut, and kidneys • Possibly improved blood flow and metabolism • Greater epinephrine secretion capacity
Adipose tissue	• Reduced fat mass • Decreased size of adipocytes • Reduced inflammation • Reduced oxidative stress • Possibly improved blood flow and metabolism • Transformation of the phenotype of white adipocytes to a more beige or even brown adipocyte phenotype
Skin	• Improved thermoregulation • Enhanced sweating capacity • Possibly improved blood flow

Adapted from Metsios, Stavropoulos-Kalinoglou, and Kitas, 2015; Heinonen et al., 2014; Bonnet and Ferrari, 2010; Gielen, Schuler, and Adams, 2010.

The experimental evidence for exercise

The effect of exercise on different health outcomes has been a topic at the forefront of recent research given the multiple exercise-induced beneficial physiological adaptations that positively impact on health (see Table 5.2). Despite these exercise-induced health benefits, there is still a dearth of relevant research with regards to the effects of exercise on mortality.

The two major RCTs that investigated mortality in relation to increasing PA levels have both been conducted in patients with cardiac disease as well as diabetes. The RAMIT UK study, evaluated the effects of exercise cardiac rehabilitation on cardiovascular mortality, morbidity, and quality of life in patients that experienced a myocardial infarction (West, Jones, & Henderson, 2012). Within its limitations, this trial concluded that exercise cardiac rehabilitation did not have beneficial effects on mortality at two years post-cardiac rehabilitation. Another major USA RCT, the Look Ahead study, investigated the effects of a lifetime intensive lifestyle intervention (caloric restriction and increased PA) on type 2 diabetes patients (Look et al., 2013). This study concluded that the lifetime exercise intervention did not reduce cardiovascular mortality rates at 9.6 years, despite that it improved more important health-related outcomes in the intervention versus control groups.

Current evidence demonstrates that PA can be an effective adjunct intervention to ameliorate and help manage symptoms of the major NCDs. According to the World Health Organization (WHO, 2016), the most prevalent NCDs are: cardiovascular diseases, cancers, respiratory diseases (e.g., asthma and chronic obstructive pulmonary disease) and diabetes, however, the beneficial effects of PA extend to other chronic conditions such as mental health.

Cardiovascular disease

A 2016 meta-analysis of 63 RCTs and 14,486 randomised CVD patients from the Cochrane Collaboration confirms the conclusion of previous reports, and suggests that PA cardiac rehabilitation reduces cardiovascular mortality risk, risk of hospitalisation, and health-related quality of life but not total mortality, risk of myocardial infarction, or revascularisation (Anderson et al., 2016; see Figure 5.5). This review included the RAMIT study mentioned earlier (West et al., 2012), which demonstrated no effects of exercise cardiac rehabilitation on mortality, cardiac or psychological morbidity, risk factors, health-related quality of life or activity. However, the RAMIT study has been in the spotlight due to its methodological limitations, including inadequate sample size, younger patients than is typical, the lack of

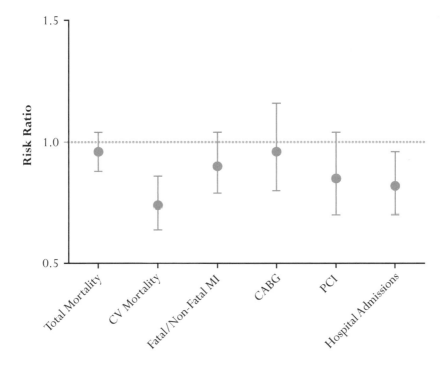

Figure 5.5 Pooled risk ratio (RR) and 95% confidence intervals for the impact of exercise-based cardiac rehabilitation on total and cardiovascular mortality and clinical outcomes, such as fatal and/or non-fatal myocardial infarction (MI), coronary artery bypass graft (CABG), percutaneous coronary intervention (PCI), and hospital admissions across all trials at their longest follow-up (median 12 months). RR of 1.0 equals the line of no effect.

participating patients to adhere to suggested guidelines, as well as issues around sub-optimal medication and the heterogeneity of variance (BACPR, 2012), which put the final conclusions of the RAMIT study into question. Finally, it is worth mentioning that a recent meta-analysis of meta-analyses that compared exercise versus drug interventions (305 RCTs with 339,274 participants), reveals that exercise may have comparative effectiveness with drugs in terms of benefits for mortality (secondary prevention), rehabilitation after stroke, and treatment for heart failure (Naci & Ioannidis, 2015).

Type 2 diabetes

In a systematic review and meta-analysis of screening tests and interventions to prevent the onset of type 2 diabetes in people with pre-diabetes, Barry and colleagues (2017) found that lifestyle (exercise and diet) interventions were associated with a 36% RR reduction in type 2 diabetes over six months to six years. However, the associated reduction in risk was reduced to 20% in the follow-up period after the trials. In terms of the effectiveness of exercise in controlling diabetes symptoms, a 2006 Cochrane Collaboration meta-analysis of 14 RCTs and 377 diabetic patients, demonstrated that compared with the control group, patients that participated in exercise interventions (both aerobic and resistance training) significantly improved glycemic control (Thomas, Elliott, & Naughton, 2006) at a clinically and statistically significant level (Thomas et al., 2006). Regarding which type of exercise improves symptoms more, a recent 2014 meta-analysis in 12 RCTs (624 diabetic patients included in the analysis) revealed that reductions of glycosylated haemoglobin can be achieved by both resistance and aerobic exercise, with neither significantly better than the other (Yang, Scott, Mao, Tang, & Farmer, 2014).

The comprehensive multi-centre Look Ahead RCT (16 centres, and 5,145 overweight or obese patients with type 2 diabetes) evaluated the effects of combined exercise and caloric restriction versus usual care on mortality and cardiovascular events. Unfortunately, this trial was stopped early at 9.6 years because there was no significant differences in these main outcomes between study conditions (Look et al., 2013). The secondary outcomes of the trial, however, indicated that the intervention group achieved greater weight loss, better control of glycated haemoglobin, and greater improvements in CRF and all cardiovascular risk factors assessed, apart from low-density lipoprotein levels.

Cancers

Meta-analysis evidence from 34 RCTs demonstrated that exercise can be effective in reducing BMI and body weight, increasing peak oxygen consumption and peak power output, as well as improved quality of life in breast, colorectal, and endometrial cancer survivors (Fong et al., 2012). A Cochrane Collaboration meta-analysis of 40 trials with 3,694 participants revealed that exercise improves quality of life in survivors from breast, colorectal, head and neck, lymphoma, and other types of cancer (Mishra, Scherer, Geigle, et al., 2012). In addition, another Cochrane Collaboration meta-analysis (56 trials with 4,826 cancer patients) revealed that exercise also has beneficial effects on quality of life of cancer patients undergoing treatment (Mishra, Scherer, Snyder, et al., 2012). Similarly, in an individual patient data meta-analysis, Buffart and co-workers (2016) reported that exercise interventions, particularly those that involved supervised exercise, led to improvements in quality of life and physical function in patients with cancer with different demographic and clinical characteristics during and following treatment. Previous reviews have also reported beneficial effects of aerobic exercise on cancer-related fatigue during or post-adjuvant cancer therapy in patients with breast and prostate cancer but not for those with haematological malignancies (Cramp & Byron-Daniel, 2012), and modest positive effects of fully or partially supervised exercise interventions – particularly those with exercise sessions ≥30 minutes in duration – on depressive symptoms (Craft, Vaniterson, Helenowski, Rademaker, & Courneya, 2011; Vaniterson, Helenowski, Rademaker, & Courneya, 2011).

Meta-analyses of RCTs on specific cancers also exist, with some providing contradictory results from meta-analyses that have assessed different types of cancers together. Specifically, a 2014 meta-analysis on colorectal cancer patients (5 RCTs and 238 patients) revealed no effects of exercise on quality of life or fatigue but a strong beneficial effect on physical fitness levels (Cramer, Lauche, Klose, Dobos, & Langhorst, 2014). For breast cancer, consistent evidence (9 studies with 1,156 patients) reveals that exercise has beneficial effects on fatigue of breast cancer survivors (Meneses-Echavez, Gonzalez-Jimenez, & Ramirez-Velez, 2015), as well as quality of life, CRF, and physical functioning (14 studies with 717 participants, McNeely et al. (2006)). Exercise can also be beneficial during adjuvant treatment for patients with breast cancer. In a recent meta-analysis, Furmaniak and colleagues (2016) found that exercise probably reduces fatigue, improves physical fitness, but has little or no effect on health-related or cancer-specific quality of life and depression in women undergoing adjuvant therapy. For men with prostate cancer, Bourke et al. (2015) found that exercise interventions can improve cancer site-specific quality of life, cancer site-specific fatigue, submaximal CRF, and lower body strength. However, for children and young adults during and after childhood cancer, a Cochrane Collaboration systematic review found less convincing evidence for exercise interventions (Braam et al., 2016), although the authors did report some positive effects of exercise on body composition, flexibility, CRF, muscle strength, and health-related quality of life.

Chronic respiratory diseases

The most common chronic respiratory diseases are chronic obstructive pulmonary disease (COPD) and asthma. The most recent Cochrane Collaboration meta-analysis of 65 RCTs (3,822 participants), including studies consisting of inpatient, outpatient, or home-based rehabilitation programmes of at least four weeks duration, revealed that exercise can relieve dyspnoea, and improve fatigue, emotional function, and the sense of control that individuals have over their condition (McCarthy et al., 2015). With regards to asthma, the most recent meta-analysis (17 studies with 599 participants) reveals that exercise interventions significantly improve asthma symptoms, quality of life, exercise capacity, bronchial hyper-responsiveness, exercise-induced bronchoconstriction, and forced expiratory volume in one second in asthmatic patients (Eichenberger, Diener, Kofmehl, & Spengler, 2013).

Mental health

Anxiety disorders and depressions are the most prevalent mental health problems. A recent review of 37 RCTs on the effects of exercise on both anxiety and depression (Wegner et al., 2014), reported that the anxiolytic effects of exercise are small (42,264 participants); but in contrast, exercise has an overall moderate effect on depressive symptoms (48,207 participants). The same study suggests that exercise seems to benefit patients more rather than participants with non-clinical symptoms. Similarly, a 2013 Cochrane Collaboration review (Cooney et al., 2013) concluded that exercise was moderately more effective than a control intervention for reducing symptoms of depression in adults with depression, but no more effective than psychological or pharmacological therapies.

Other non-communicable diseases and conditions

In addition to the aforementioned NCDs above, there is RCT evidence that exercise interventions illicit favourable effects on other notable NCDs and conditions. Exercise interventions improve muscular strength, CRF, disease-related characteristics, functional ability without exacerbating disease activity, fatigue, and reverses cachexia, and likely reduces CVD risk in rheumatoid arthritis (Cairns & McVeigh, 2009; Cooney et al., 2011; Cramp et al., 2013; Metsios et al., 2007). For patients with osteoarthritis (primarily knee osteoarthritis), exercise can relieve pain, stiffness, muscular strength, and CRF (Tanaka, Ozawa, Kito, & Moriyama, 2015; Uthman et al., 2014). In particular, combined interventions incorporating endurance, strength, and flexibility exercises may be most effective for improving limitations in functional capacity in osteoarthritic populations. A recent systematic review (Kelley, Kelley, & Hootman, 2015), including patients with osteoarthritis, rheumatoid arthritis, and systemic lupus erythematous, found that exercise reduced symptoms of depression, anxiety, pain, quality of life, physical function, CRF, and muscular strength.

Older adults, particularly those who are also frail, are at an increased risk of falls and fall-related injury. Almost one in three people aged 65 years and older and one in two people aged at least 80 years fall at least once a year (NICE, 2013). Evidence from systematic reviews suggests that exercise can reduce the rate of falls in frail older adults living in both community dwellings (Cadore, Rodríguez-Mañas, Sinclair, & Izquierdo, 2013; El-Khoury, Cassou, Charles, & Dargent-Molina, 2013), and care facilities (Lee & Kim, 2016). There is evidence that exercise interventions can result in fewer falls requiring medical attention and prevent injuries caused by falls, including severe falls and those resulting in fracture (El-Khoury et al., 2013). In addition to reducing the risk of fall-related fractures, structured exercise – especially progressive resistance training – can result in small improvements in overall mobility after hip fracture (Diong, Allen, & Sherrington, 2015). Furthermore, exercise interventions – multi-component programmes comprising of endurance, strength, and balance exercises, in particular – have resulted in improved balance, mobility, gait ability, muscle function, physical and functional capacity, CRF, and quality of life in older adults with frailty (Cadore et al., 2013; El-Khoury et al., 2013; Labra, Guimaraes-Pinheiro, Maseda, Lorenzo, & Millán-Calenti, 2015; Theou et al., 2011). Similarly, exercise has been shown to be an effective intervention for older adults with sarcopenia, often linked to the development of frailty, resulting in improved muscular strength and physical performance (Cruz-Jentoft et al., 2014).

Patients with osteoporosis are particularly at an increased risk of fall-related fractures. Exercise interventions (combined with calcium and vitamin D supplementation) may reduce falls in older adults with osteoporosis, and increase bone mineral density and lower the risk of fracture in both older adults (Giangregorio et al., 2013) and postmenopausal women with osteoporosis (Howe et al., 2011). In addition, resistance training can result in improvements in self-reported physical function and activities of daily living in participants with osteoporosis and osteopenia (Wilhelm et al., 2013).

Effects of exercise on risk factors for non-communicable diseases

Experimental studies have also investigated the effects of exercise on well-established risk factors for the development of NCDs, such as the classical CVD risk factors (smoking, hypertension, insulin resistance, hypercholesterolaemia) and other factors that impact on the development of NCDs in general, including obesity and inflammation.

Smoking

A 2014 Cochrane Collaboration meta-analysis of RCTs (20 studies with 5,870 participants) comparing exercise programmes alone or exercise programmes as an adjunct to a smoking cessation programme with a cessation programme, found only two studies offered evidence that exercise can aid long-term smoking cessation (Ussher, Taylor, & Faulkner, 2014). The remaining studies were too small or the exercise intensity was insufficient to result in the desired exercise dose that may have had beneficial effects on smoking cessation.

Blood pressure

The most recent meta-analysis on the effects of exercise lasting more than four weeks on the blood pressure of healthy individuals (93 studies with 5,223 participants) demonstrates clear benefits of exercise on lowering blood pressure (Cornelissen & Smart, 2013). Specifically, the authors concluded that endurance and resistance training can lower both systolic and diastolic blood pressure, but the combination of the two training methods was effective in lowering diastolic blood pressure only – a small number of studies suggested that resistance training could lower systolic blood pressure (Cornelissen & Smart, 2013). However, a more recent meta-analysis, consisting of 11 trials with 302 patients, revealed that isometric resistance exercise lasting more than two weeks can lower both systolic and diastolic blood pressure as well as mean arterial pressure in patients with hypertension (Inder et al., 2016).

Insulin resistance

Meta-analyses exist on the combined effects of exercise and diet on insulin sensitivity, however, this section focuses only on the effects of exercise alone. In healthy adults, a meta-analysis on 78 reports with 2,509 participants confirmed that exercise may have beneficial effects on the prevention of diabetes via improving insulin sensitivity (Conn et al., 2014). In type 2 diabetics, a 2016 meta-analysis of 16 trials with 479 individuals on exercise interventions that included at least three exercise sessions of either continuous or high-intensity intermittent training, demonstrated that regular exercise improves insulin sensitivity in type 2 diabetes patients; the authors also concluded that these exercise-induced effects on insulin sensitivity may persist beyond 72 hours after the last exercise session (Way, Hackett, Baker, & Johnson, 2016).

Cholesterol

A 2014 review that investigated all relevant meta-analysis and RCTs on the effects of exercise on lipids shows that exercise has significant effects on dyslipidaemia as well as on lowering cholesterol levels (Mann, Beedie, & Jimenez, 2014). Endurance exercise appears to be particularly effective in improving high density lipoprotein cholesterol (Pattyn, Cornelissen, Eshghi, & Vanhees, 2013), and reducing triglycerides when the intervention is more than four weeks duration (Kelley, Kelley, & Franklin, 2006).

Adiposity

A 2016 meta-analysis (117 studies with 4,815 participants) on the effects of exercise versus hypocaloric diet on visceral fat, concluded that hypocaloric diets reduced body fat more than exercise, but exercise resulted in a greater visceral fat loss in the absence of weight loss (Verheggen et al., 2016). In individuals who are overweight or obese, another 2015 meta-analysis demonstrated that combining exercise with a dietary intervention facilitates greater improvements in body composition and biomarkers of metabolic issues (Clark, 2015). The authors also noted that resistance training combined with a hypocaloric diet was particularly effective in improving body composition. Specifically, resistance training programmes involving 2–3 sets of 6–10 repetitions of whole body and free-weight exercises performed for at an intensity of ≥75% one repetition maximum appears to be most effective for retaining fat-free mass while reducing body mass and fat mass.

Inflammation

The most recent meta-analysis of RCTs and non-randomised studies (83 studies with 3,769 participants) found that exercise reduced C-Reactive Protein (CRP – an acute phase reactant indicative of inflammatory load) regardless of age and sex, and that greater reductions in CRP occured with decreases in BMI or percentage body fat (Fedewa, Hathaway, & Ward-Ritacco, 2016). In support of this finding, another 2016 meta-analysis involving 3,575 healthy participants and patients with heart disease across 43 trials, concluded that exercise interventions can reduce CRP irrespective of the presence of heart disease (Hammonds, Gathright, Goldstein, Penn, & Hughes, 2016).

Issues with experimental evidence for exercise

The key strength of RCT designs is that, when appropriately conducted, they offer excellent internal validity – the ability of the study to establish the causal relationship between an intervention and the observed outcome. The primary strength of an RCT is that it minimises bias by confounding through adequate randomisation, which aims to ensure that the only difference between study arms is their exposure to the intervention of interest (Booth & Tannock, 2014). However, RCTs, particularly those inadequately conducted, are prone to other biases, such as selection bias, performance bias, detection bias, attrition bias, and reporting bias, which can limit its applicability to practice (see Table 5.3).

Selection bias can be prevented or at least minimised by allocating participants to study arms based on a chance (random) process and concealing this allocation sequence from researchers assigning participants to intervention groups (Higgins & Green, 2011). If the allocation is not concealed, researchers can influence allocation of interventions to participants, which can result in ascertainment bias. Selection bias can also refer to situations where the participants in a trial are not representative of the population of all possible participants (Moher et al., 2010). In a clinical context, this would mean that the trial participants are different from the patients seen in routine practice, which would limit the applicability and

Table 5.3 Examples of biases in randomised controlled trials

Bias	Definition
Selection bias	Systematic differences between baseline characteristics of the study groups being compared
Allocation concealment bias	Intervention groups are assigned differently to the population
Ascertainment bias	Results or conclusions of a study are systematically biased by knowledge of which intervention was received by each participant
Performance bias	Systematic differences in the care or attention that is provided, or in exposure to factors other than the intervention administered
Detection bias	Systematic differences between groups how measurements are made
Compliance bias	Differences in compliance to the intervention affect the trial outcomes
Attrition bias	Withdrawals are systematically different between groups in a study
Reporting bias	Systematic differences between reported and unreported findings
Contamination bias	The control group perform intervention-like activities, which minimises the differences between the study groups.

generalisability of the findings (known as external validity). Readers should read closely the inclusion and exclusion criteria and characteristics of participants to judge the external validity of a study's findings.

A lack of blinding of participants and research personnel to the group allocation of participants can lead to performance bias (Higgins & Green, 2011). Blinding of participants is not possible in exercise trials, and therefore, it is possible that knowledge of the intervention received, rather than the intervention itself, may affect trial outcomes. In addition, not blinding the research personnel carrying out the outcome assessments can lead to them either consciously or unconsciously influencing the test performance of participants (detection bias), particularly, if tests require motivation or are subjective (Higgins & Green, 2011).

To ensure that participants in exercise trials receive an appropriate 'dose' they are required to adhere to the assigned exercise programme. The degree of adherence (compliance) to the exercise programme, therefore, can affect the trial outcomes (compliance bias) (Delgado-Rodriguez & Llorca, 2004). Adherence to long-term exercise programmes is a problem, and previous research has reported levels between 10 and 80% (Balducci, Leonetti, Di Mario, & Fallucca, 2004; Dunstan et al., 2006; Praet et al., 2008). The outcomes of a study can be affected if participants' compliance differs. For example, if the control group in an exercise trial perform intervention-like activities this could minimise the differences between the study groups (contamination bias).

Participant withdrawal from a study results in incomplete outcome data. If withdrawals are systematically different between groups in a study (attrition bias) and the groups differ in a characteristic that is related to study outcomes this can influence the trial's results and conclusions (Higgins & Green, 2011). Attrition bias can be minimised by adopting an intention-to-treat analysis – all enrolled and randomly allocated participants are included in the analysis and analysed in their allocated group. Researchers can also introduce bias by selective reporting of outcomes (reporting bias). For instance, researchers may only choose to report outcomes for which there were statistically significant differences between intervention groups. This type of bias can lead to an underreporting of non-significant findings in published studies, a phenomenon referred to as the file drawer problem.

The list of biases described above and defined in Table 5.3 are not exhaustive. When interpreting RCT evidence, readers should recognise that although RCTs are valuable tools to investigate causal relationships, they can never be completely objective. The accuracy, applicability, and generalisability of exercise RCT results must be interpreted in light of the risks of bias, in addition to other potential limitations, such as validity and reliability of measures, magnitude (clinical vs. statistical meaningfulness) and precision of estimates (width of confidence intervals), and trial sample size.

Summary and practical applications

A vast amount of epidemiologic evidence supports the inverse, dose-response relationship between PA and the risk of premature all-cause and disease-related mortality, and development of NCDs such as CVD, type 2 diabetes, and breast and colon cancer. Although, the greatest risk reductions were observed up to 3–6 times the recommended PA level, clear reductions in early mortality and morbidity risk were found even in the groups who reported at least some PA but less than recommended, compared with the least active group. The epidemiologic evidence for CRF revealed similar findings to those reported for PA, with the greatest associated reduction in all-cause mortality risk occurring between the least fit and next-to-least fit groups. There is currently RCT evidence for the beneficial effects of exercise on premature mortality in CVD, but not type 2 diabetes. Studies that investigated the effects of exercise on mortality in other NCDs are lacking, possibly due to the finances and resources needed to investigate cause-and-effect relationships. Exercise, however, may have beneficial effects on mental health, arthritis, osteoporosis, and risk of falling, in addition to improving high blood pressure, insulin sensitivity, visceral fat loss, and long-term smoking cessation.

Chapter summary

- Epidemiologic evidence supports the inverse, dose-response relationship between both PA and CRF and the risk of premature all-cause and disease-related mortality, and development of non-communicable diseases, such as CVD, type 2 diabetes, and breast and colon cancer.
- Epidemiologic studies need to be interpreted in light of their limitations and the extent that biases, such as selection bias, misclassification bias, and confounding, may have influenced the observed associations.
- There is evidence for the beneficial effects of exercise on premature mortality in CVD, but not type 2 diabetes, but studies investigated the effects of exercise on mortality in other non-communicable diseases are lacking.
- There is a dearth of relevant RCTs on the effects of exercise on disease outcomes for the most prevalent non-communicable diseases, however, exercise may have beneficial effects on mental health, arthritis, osteoporosis, and risk of falling.
- Evidence suggests that exercise may be beneficial in reducing high blood pressure, improving insulin sensitivity, promoting visceral fat loss, and facilitating long-term smoking cessation.
- Although RCTs are valuable tools to investigate causal relationships, they can never be completely objective. The accuracy, applicability, and generalisability of exercise RCT results must be interpreted in light of the risks of bias, validity and reliability of measures, magnitude and precision of estimates, and trial sample size.

References

Anderson, L., Thompson, D.R., Oldridge, N., Zwisler, A.D., Rees, K., Martin, N., & Taylor, R.S. (2016). Exercise-based cardiac rehabilitation for coronary heart disease. *The Cochrane database of systematic reviews, 1*, CD001800. doi:10.1002/14651858.CD001800.pub3

Arem, H., Moore, S.C., Patel, A., Hartge, P., de Gonzalez, A.B., Visvanathan, K., . . . Matthews, C.E. (2015). Leisure time physical activity and mortality: A detailed pooled analysis of the dose-response relationship. *JAMA Internal Medicine, 175*(6), 959–967.

Arsenault, B.J., Cartier, A., Côté, M., Lemieux, I., Tremblay, A., Bouchard, C., . . . Després, J.-P. (2009). Body composition, cardiorespiratory fitness, and low-grade inflammation in middle-aged men and women. *The American Journal of Cardiology, 104*(2), 240–246. doi:10.1016/j.amjcard.2009.03.027

Artero, E.G., Lee, D.C., Ruiz, J.R., Sui, X., Ortega, F.B., Church, T.S., . . . Blair, S.N. (2011). A prospective study of muscular strength and all-cause mortality in men with hypertension. *Journal of the American College of Cardiology, 57*(18), 1831–1837.

BACPR. (2012). British Association for Cardiovascular Prevention and Rehabilitation. The discussion around RAMIT: Summary of the editorials and letters in response to West et al. Retrieved from www.bacpr.com/resources/RAMIT_Trial_Responses_-_Final_Full_Text_website_June_2012. pdf accessed 22/12/2016.

Balducci, S., Leonetti, F., Di Mario, U., & Fallucca, F. (2004). Is a long-term aerobic plus resistance training program feasible for and effective on metabolic profiles in type 2 diabetic patients? *Diabetes Care, 27*(3), 841–842. doi:10.2337/diacare.27.3.841

Barry, E., Roberts, S., Oke, J., Vijayaraghavan, S., Normansell, R., & Greenhalgh, T. (2017). Efficacy and effectiveness of screen and treat policies in prevention of type 2 diabetes: Systematic review and meta-analysis of screening tests and interventions. *BMJ (Clinical research ed.), 356*, BMJ 2017;356:i6538.

Barry, V.W., Baruth, M., Beets, M.W., Durstine, L.J., Liu, J., & Blair, S.N. (2014). Fitness vs. fatness on all-cause mortality: A meta-analysis. *Progress in Cardiovascular Diseases, 56*(4), 382–390. doi:10.1016/j.pcad.2013.09.002

Blair, S.N., Kohl, H.W., 3rd, Paffenbarger, R.S. Jr., Clark, D.G., Cooper, K.H., & Gibbons, L.W. (1989). Physical fitness and all-cause mortality. A prospective study of healthy men and women, *JAMA, 262*(17), 2395–2401.

Bonnet, N., & Ferrari, S.L. (2010). Exercise and the skeleton: How it works and what it really does. *IBMS BoneKEy, 7*, 235–248. doi:10.1138/20100454

Booth, C.M., & Tannock, I.F. (2014). Randomised controlled trials and population-based observational research: Partners in the evolution of medical evidence. *British Journal of Cancer, 110*(3), 551–555.

Bouchard, C., An, P., Rice, T., Skinner, J.S., Wilmore, J.H., Gagnon, J., . . . Rao, D.C. (1999). Familial aggregation of VO2 max response to exercise training: Results from the HERITAGE family study, *Journal of Applied Physiology, 87*(3), 1003–1008.

Bourke, L., Smith, D., Steed, L., Hooper, R., Carter, A., Catto, J., . . . Rosario, D.J. (2015). Exercise for men with prostate cancer: A systematic review and meta-analysis. *European Urology, 69*(4), 693–703.

Braam, K.I., van der Torre, P., Takken, T., Veening, M.A., van Dulmen-den Broeder, E., & Kaspers, G.J. (2016). Physical exercise training interventions for children and young adults during and after treatment for childhood cancer. *The Cochrane database of systematic reviews, 3*.

Buffart, L.M., Kalter, J., Sweegers, M.G., Courneya, K.S., Newton, R.U., Aaronson, N.K., . . . Brug, J. (2016). Effects and moderators of exercise on quality of life and physical function in patients with cancer: An individual patient data meta-analysis of 34 RCTs. *Cancer Treatment Reviews, 52*, 91–104.

Cadore, E.L., Rodríguez-Mañas, L., Sinclair, A., & Izquierdo, M. (2013). Effects of different exercise interventions on risk of falls, gait ability, and balance in physically frail older adults: A systematic review. *Rejuvenation Research, 16*(2), 105–114.

Cairns, A.P., & McVeigh, J.G. (2009). A systematic review of the effects of dynamic exercise in rheumatoid arthritis. *Rheumatology International, 30*(2), 147–158.

Chow, L.S., Odegaard, A.O., Bosch, T.A., Bantle, A.E., Wang, Q., Hughes, J., . . . Schreiner, P.J. (2016). Twenty year fitness trends in young adults and incidence of prediabetes and diabetes: The CARDIA study. *Diabetologia, 59*(8), 1659–1665.

Clark, J.E. (2015). Diet, exercise or diet with exercise: Comparing the effectiveness of treatment options for weight-loss and changes in fitness for adults (18–65 years old) who are overfat, or obese; systematic review and meta-analysis. *J Diabetes Metab Disord, 14*, 31. doi:10.1186/s40200-015-0154-1

Conn, V.S., Koopman, R.J., Ruppar, T.M., Phillips, L.J., Mehr, D.R., & Hafdahl, A.R. (2014). Insulin sensitivity following exercise interventions: Systematic review and meta-analysis of outcomes among healthy adults. *J Prim Care Community Health, 5*(3), 211–222. doi:10.1177/2150131913520328

Cooney, G.M., Dwan, K., Greig, C.A., Lawlor, D.A., Rimer, J., Waugh, F.R., . . . Mead, G.E. (2013). Exercise for depression. *The Cochrane database of systematic reviews, 9*.

Cooney, J.K., Law, R.J., Matschke, V., Lemmey, A.B., Moore, J.P., Ahmad, Y., . . . Thom, J.M. (2011). Benefits of exercise in rheumatoid arthritis. *Journal of Aging Research, 2011*.

Cornelissen, V.A., & Smart, N.A. (2013). Exercise training for blood pressure: A systematic review and meta-analysis. *J Am Heart Assoc, 2*(1), e004473. doi:10.1161/JAHA.112.004473

Craft, L.L., Vaniterson, E.H., Helenowski, I.B., Rademaker, A.W., & Courneya, K.S. (2011). Exercise effects on depressive symptoms in cancer survivors: A systematic review and meta-analysis. *Cancer epidemiology, biomarkers & prevention: A publication of the American Association for Cancer Research, cosponsored by the American Society of Preventive Oncology, 21*(1), 3–19.

Cramer, H., Lauche, R., Klose, P., Dobos, G., & Langhorst, J. (2014). A systematic review and meta-analysis of exercise interventions for colorectal cancer patients. *Eur J Cancer Care (Engl), 23*(1), 3–14. doi:10.1111/ecc.12093

Cramp, F., & Byron-Daniel, J. (2012). Exercise for the management of cancer-related fatigue in adults. *The Cochrane database of systematic reviews, 11*.

Cramp, F., Hewlett, S., Almeida, C., Kirwan, J.R., Choy, E.H., Chalder, T., . . . Christensen, R. (2013). Non-pharmacological interventions for fatigue in rheumatoid arthritis. *The Cochrane database of systematic reviews, 8*, CD008322. doi:10.1002/14651858.CD008322.pub2

Cruz-Jentoft, A.J., Landi, F., Schneider, S.M., Zúñiga, C., Arai, H., Boirie, Y., . . . Cederholm, T. (2014). Prevalence of and interventions for sarcopenia in ageing adults: A systematic review. *Report of the International Sarcopenia Initiative (EWGSOP and IWGS). Age and Ageing, 43*(6), 748–759. doi:10.1093/ageing/afu115

Dankel, S.J., Loenneke, J.P., & Loprinzi, P.D. (2016a). Determining the importance of meeting muscle-strengthening activity guidelines: Is the behavior or the outcome of the behavior (strength) a more important determinant of all-cause mortality? *Mayo Clinic Proceedings, 91*(2), 166–174.

Dankel, S.J., Loenneke, J.P., & Loprinzi, P.D. (2016b). Dose-dependent association between muscle-strengthening activities and all-cause mortality: Prospective cohort study among a national sample of adults in the USA. *Archives of Cardiovascular Diseases, 109*(11), 626–633.

Defina, L.F., Willis, B.L., Radford, N.B., Gao, A., Leonard, D., Haskell, W.L., . . . Berry, J.D. (2013). The association between midlife cardiorespiratory fitness levels and later-life dementia: A cohort study. *Annals of Internal Medicine, 158*(3), 162–168.

Delgado-Rodriguez, M., & Llorca, J. (2004). Bias. *J Epidemiol Community Health, 58*(8), 635–641. doi:10.1136/jech.2003.008466

Diong, J., Allen, N., & Sherrington, C. (2015). Structured exercise improves mobility after hip fracture: A meta-analysis with meta-regression. *British Journal of Sports Medicine, 50*(6), 346–355.

Dishman, R.K., Sui, X., Church, T.S., Hand, G.A., Trivedi, M.H., & Blair, S.N. (2012). Decline in cardiorespiratory fitness and odds of incident depression. *Am J Prev Med, 43*(4), 361–368.

Dunstan, D.W., Vulikh, E., Owen, N., Jolley, D., Shaw, J., & Zimmet, P. (2006). Community center-based resistance training for the maintenance of glycemic control in adults with type 2 diabetes. *Diabetes Care, 29*(12), 2586–2591.

Earnest, C.P., Artero, E.G., Sui, X., Lee, D.C., Church, T.S., & Blair, S.N. (2013). Maximal estimated cardiorespiratory fitness, cardiometabolic risk factors, and metabolic syndrome in the aerobics center longitudinal study. *Mayo Clinic Proceedings, 88*(3), 259–270.

Eichenberger, P.A., Diener, S.N., Kofmehl, R., & Spengler, C.M. (2013). Effects of exercise training on airway hyperreactivity in asthma: A systematic review and meta-analysis. *Sports Med, 43*(11), 1157–1170. doi:10.1007/s40279-013-0077-2

Ekelund, U., Steene-Johannessen, J., Brown, W.J., Fagerland, M.W., Owen, N., Powell, K.E., . . . Sedentary, L. (2016). Does physical activity attenuate, or even eliminate, the detrimental association of sitting time with mortality? A harmonised meta-analysis of data from more than 1 million men and women. *Lancet* (London, England), *388*(10051), 1302–1310.

Ekelund, U., Ward, H.A., Norat, T., Luan, J., May, A.M., Weiderpass, E., . . . Riboli, E. (2015). Physical activity and all-cause mortality across levels of overall and abdominal adiposity in European men and women: The European prospective investigation into cancer and nutrition study (EPIC). *The American Journal of Clinical Nutrition, 101*(3), 613–621.

El-Khoury, F., Cassou, B., Charles, M.A., & Dargent-Molina, P. (2013). The effect of fall prevention exercise programmes on fall induced injuries in community dwelling older adults: Systematic review and meta-analysis of randomised controlled trials. *BMJ (Clinical research ed.), 347*, BMJ 2013;347:f6234.

Fedewa, M.V., Hathaway, E.D., & Ward-Ritacco, C.L. (2016). Effect of exercise training on C-reactive protein: A systematic review and meta-analysis of randomised and non-randomised controlled trials. *Br J Sports Med, 51*(8), 670-676. doi:10.1136/bjsports-2016-095999

Fishman, E.I., Steeves, J.A., Zipunnikov, V., Koster, A., Berrigan, D., Harris, T.A., & Murphy, R. (2016). Association between objectively measured physical activity and mortality in NHANES. *Medicine and Science in Sports and Exercise, 48*(7), 1303–1311.

Fogelholm, M. (2009). Physical activity, fitness and fatness: Relations to mortality, morbidity and disease risk factors. A systematic review. *Obesity Reviews: An Official Journal of the International Association for the Study of Obesity, 11*(3), 202–221.

Fong, D.Y., Ho, J.W., Hui, B.P., Lee, A.M., Macfarlane, D.J., Leung, S.S., . . . Cheng, K.K. (2012). Physical activity for cancer survivors: Meta-analysis of randomised controlled trials. *BMJ, 344*, e70. doi:10.1136/bmj.e70

Furmaniak, A.C., Menig, M., & Markes, M.H. (2016). Exercise for women receiving adjuvant therapy for breast cancer. *The Cochrane Database of Systematic Reviews, 9*.

Giangregorio, L.M., Papaioannou, A., Macintyre, N.J., Ashe, M.C., Heinonen, A., Shipp, K., . . . Cheung, A.M. (2013). Too fit to fracture: Exercise recommendations for individuals with osteoporosis or osteoporotic vertebral fracture. *Osteoporosis International: A Journal established as a result of cooperation between the European Foundation for Osteoporosis and the National Osteoporosis Foundation of the USA, 25*(3), 821–835.

Gielen, S., Schuler, G., & Adams, V. (2010). Cardiovascular effects of exercise training: Molecular mechanisms, *Circulation, 122*(12), 1221–1238. doi:10.1161/CIRCULATIONAHA.110.939959

Gigerenzer, G., Wegwarth, O., & Feufel, M. (2010). Misleading communication of risk. *BMJ (Clinical research ed.), 341*.

Grimes, D.A., & Schulz, K.F. (2002). Bias and causal associations in observational research. *Lancet* (London, England), *359*(9302), 248–252.

Gupta, S., Rohatgi, A., Ayers, C.R., Willis, B.L., Haskell, W.L., Khera, A., . . . Berry, J.D. (2011). Cardiorespiratory fitness and classification of risk of cardiovascular disease mortality. *Circulation, 123*(13), 1377–1388.

Hammonds, T.L., Gathright, E.C., Goldstein, C.M., Penn, M.S., & Hughes, J.W. (2016). Effects of exercise on c-reactive protein in healthy patients and in patients with heart disease: A meta-analysis. *Heart Lung, 45*(3), 273–282. doi:10.1016/j.hrtlng.2016.01.009

Heinonen, I., Kalliokoski, K.K., Hannukainen, J.C., Duncker, D.J., Nuutila, P., & Knuuti, J. (2014). Organ-specific physiological responses to acute physical exercise and long-term training in humans. *Physiology* (Bethesda), *29*(6), 421–436. doi: 10.1152/physiol.00067.2013

Higgins, J.P.T., & Green, S. (2011). Cochrane handbook for systematic reviews of interventions (J.P.T. Higgins & S. Green Eds. 5.1.0 ed.). *The Cochrane Collaboration*: Available from www.handbook.cochrane.org.

Hill, A.B. (1965). The environment and disease: Association or causation? *Proceedings of the Royal Society of Medicine, 58*(5), 295–300.

Howe, T.E., Shea, B., Dawson, L.J., Downie, F., Murray, A., Ross, C., . . . Creed, G. (2011). Exercise for preventing and treating osteoporosis in postmenopausal women. *The Cochrane database of systematic reviews*.

Hupin, D., Roche, F., Gremeaux, V., Chatard, J.-C., Oriol, M., Gaspoz, J.-M., . . . Edouard, P. (2015). Even a low-dose of moderate-to-vigorous physical activity reduces mortality by 22% in adults aged ≥60 years: A systematic review and meta-analysis. *British Journal of Sports Medicine, 49*(19), 1262–1267. doi:10.1136/bjsports-2014-094306

Inder, J.D., Carlson, D.J., Dieberg, G., McFarlane, J.R., Hess, N.C., & Smart, N.A. (2016). Isometric exercise training for blood pressure management: A systematic review and meta-analysis to optimize benefit. *Hypertens Res, 39*(2), 88–94. doi:10.1038/hr.2015.111

Kelley, G.A., Kelley, K.S., & Franklin, B. (2006). Aerobic exercise and lipids and lipoproteins in patients with cardiovascular disease: A meta-analysis of randomized controlled trials. *J Cardiopulm Rehabil, 26*(3), 131–139; quiz 140–141, discussion 142–144.

Kelley, G.A., Kelley, K.S., & Hootman, J.M. (2015). Effects of exercise on depression in adults with arthritis: A systematic review with meta-analysis of randomized controlled trials. *Arthritis Research & Therapy, 17*, doi: 10.1186/s13075-015-0533-5

Kelly, P., Kahlmeier, S., Götschi, T., Orsini, N., Richards, J., Roberts, N., . . . Foster, C. (2014). Systematic review and meta-analysis of reduction in all-cause mortality from walking and cycling and shape of dose response relationship. *The International Journal of Behavioral Nutrition and Physical Activity, 11*, doi: 10.1186/s12966-014-0132-x

King, N.B., Harper, S., & Young, M.E. (2012). Use of relative and absolute effect measures in reporting health inequalities: Structured review. *BMJ (Clinical research ed.), 345*, BMJ 2012;345:e5774.

Kodama, S., Saito, K., Tanaka, S., Maki, M., Yachi, Y., Asumi, M., . . . Sone, H. (2009). Cardiorespiratory fitness as a quantitative predictor of all-cause mortality and cardiovascular events in healthy men and women: A meta-analysis. *JAMA, 301*(19), 2024–2035.

Kraschnewski, J.L., Sciamanna, C.N., Poger, J.M., Rovniak, L.S., Lehman, E.B., Cooper, A.B., . . . Ciccolo, J.T. (2016). Is strength training associated with mortality benefits? A 15 year cohort study of US older adults. *Preventive Medicine, 87*, 121–127.

Kundi, M. (2006). Causality and the interpretation of epidemiologic evidence. *Environmental Health Perspectives, 114*(7), 969–974.

Kyu, H.H., Bachman, V.F., Alexander, L.T., Mumford, J.E., Afshin, A., Estep, K., . . . Forouzanfar, M.H. (2016). Physical activity and risk of breast cancer, colon cancer, diabetes, ischemic heart disease, and ischemic stroke events: Systematic review and dose-response meta-analysis for the global burden of disease study 2013. *BMJ (Clinical research ed.), 354*.

Labra, C. de, Guimaraes-Pinheiro, C., Maseda, A., Lorenzo, T., & Millán-Calenti, J.C. (2015). Effects of physical exercise interventions in frail older adults: A systematic review of randomized controlled trials. *BMC Geriatrics, 15*.

Lahart, I.M., Metsios, G.S., Nevill, A.M., & Carmichael, A.R. (2015). Physical activity, risk of death and recurrence in breast cancer survivors: A systematic review and meta-analysis of epidemiological studies. *Acta Oncologica* (Stockholm, Sweden), *54*(5), 635–654.

Lakoski, S.G., Willis, B.L., Barlow, C.E., Leonard, D., Gao, A., Radford, N.B., . . . Jones, L.W. (2015). Midlife cardiorespiratory fitness, incident cancer, and survival after cancer in men: The Cooper Center longitudinal study. *JAMA Oncology, 1*(2), 231–237.

LaMonte, M.J., & Blair, S.N. (2006). Physical activity, cardiorespiratory fitness, and adiposity: Contributions to disease risk. *Current Opinion in Clinical Nutrition and Metabolic Care, 9*(5), 540–546.

Laukkanen, J.A., Kurl, S., Salonen, R., Rauramaa, R., & Salonen, J.T. (2004). The predictive value of cardiorespiratory fitness for cardiovascular events in men with various risk profiles: A prospective population-based cohort study. *European Heart Journal, 25*(16), 1428–1437.

Laukkanen, J.A., Zaccardi, F., Khan, H., Kurl, S., Jae, S.Y., & Rauramaa, R. (2016). Long-term change in cardiorespiratory fitness and all-cause mortality. *Mayo Clinic Proceedings, 91*(9), 1183–1188. doi:10.1016/j.mayocp.2016.05.014

Lee, C.D., Blair, S.N., & Jackson, A.S. (1999). Cardiorespiratory fitness, body composition, and all-cause and cardiovascular disease mortality in men. *The American Journal of Clinical Nutrition, 69*(3), 373–380.

Lee, D.-c., Artero, E.G., Sui, X., & Blair, S.N. (2010). Mortality trends in the general population: The importance of cardiorespiratory fitness. *Journal of Psychopharmacology, 24*(4S), 27–35.

Lee, D.-c., Sui, X., Artero, E.G., Lee, I.M., Church, T.S., McAuley, P.A., . . . Blair, S.N. (2011). Long-term effects of changes in cardiorespiratory fitness and body mass index on all-cause and cardiovascular disease mortality in men: The Aerobics Center longitudinal study. *Circulation, 124*(23), 2483–2490. doi:10.1161/circulationaha.111.038422

Lee, S.H., & Kim, H.S. (2016). Exercise interventions for preventing falls among older people in care facilities: A meta-analysis. *Worldviews on Evidence-Based Nursing, 14*(1), 74–80.

Leong, D.P., Teo, K.K., Rangarajan, S., Lopez-Jaramillo, P., Avezum, A., Orlandini, A., . . . Urban, P. (2015). Prognostic value of grip strength: Findings from the Prospective Urban Rural Epidemiology (PURE) study. *Lancet* (London, England), *386*(9990), 266–273.

Li, T., Wei, S., Shi, Y., Pang, S., Qin, Q., Yin, J., . . . Liu, L. (2015). The dose-response effect of physical activity on cancer mortality: Findings from 71 prospective cohort studies. *British Journal of Sports Medicine, 50*(6), 339–345.

Liu, L., Shi, Y., Li, T., Qin, Q., Yin, J., Pang, S., . . . Wei, S. (2015). Leisure time physical activity and cancer risk: Evaluation of the WHO's recommendation based on 126 high-quality epidemiological studies. *British Journal of Sports Medicine, 50*(6), 372–378.

Look, A.R.G., Wing, R.R., Bolin, P., Brancati, F.L., Bray, G.A., Clark, J.M., . . . Yanovski, S.Z. (2013). Cardiovascular effects of intensive lifestyle intervention in type 2 diabetes. *N Engl J Med, 369*(2), 145–154. doi:10.1056/NEJMoa1212914

Mann, S., Beedie, C., & Jimenez, A. (2014). Differential effects of aerobic exercise, resistance training and combined exercise modalities on cholesterol and the lipid profile: Review, synthesis and recommendations. *Sports Med, 44*(2), 211–221. doi:10.1007/s40279-013-0110-5

McCarthy, B., Casey, D., Devane, D., Murphy, K., Murphy, E., & Lacasse, Y. (2015). Pulmonary rehabilitation for chronic obstructive pulmonary disease. *The Cochrane database of systematic reviews 2*, CD003793. doi:10.1002/14651858.CD003793.pub3

McKinney, J., Lithwick, D.J., Morrison, B.N., Nazzari, H., Isserow, S.H., Heilbron, B., . . . Krahn, A.D. (2016). The health benefits of physical activity and cardiorespiratory fitness. *BC Medical Journal, 58*(3), 131–137.

McNeely, M.L., Campbell, K.L., Rowe, B.H., Klassen, T.P., Mackey, J.R., & Courneya, K.S. (2006). Effects of exercise on breast cancer patients and survivors: A systematic review and meta-analysis. *CMAJ, 175*(1), 34–41. doi:10.1503/cmaj.051073

Meneses-Echavez, J.F., Gonzalez-Jimenez, E., & Ramirez-Velez, R. (2015). Effects of supervised exercise on cancer-related fatigue in breast cancer survivors: A systematic review and meta-analysis. *BMC Cancer, 15*, 77. doi:10.1186/s12885-015-1069-4

Metsios, G.S., Stavropoulos-Kalinoglou, A., & Kitas, G.D. (2015). The role of exercise in the management of rheumatoid arthritis. *Expert Rev Clin Immunol., 11*(10), 1121–1130. doi: 10.1586/1744666X.2015.1067606

Metsios, G.S., Stavropoulos-Kalinoglou, A., Veldhuijzen van Zanten, J.J., Treharne, G.J., Panoulas, V.F., Douglas, K.M., . . . Kitas, G.D. (2007). Rheumatoid arthritis, cardiovascular disease and physical exercise: A systematic review. *Rheumatology* (Oxford, England), *47*(3), 239–248.

Mishra, S.I., Scherer, R.W., Geigle, P.M., Berlanstein, D.R., Topaloglu, O., Gotay, C.C., & Snyder, C. (2012). Exercise interventions on health-related quality of life for cancer survivors. *The Cochrane database of systematic reviews 8*, CD007566. doi:10.1002/14651858.CD007566.pub2

Mishra, S.I., Scherer, R.W., Snyder, C., Geigle, P.M., Berlanstein, D.R., & Topaloglu, O. (2012). Exercise interventions on health-related quality of life for people with cancer during active treatment. *The Cochrane database of systematic reviews 8*, CD008465. doi:10.1002/14651858.CD008465.pub2

Moher, D., Hopewell, S., Schulz, K.F., Montori, V., Gøtzsche, P.C., Devereaux, P.J., . . . Altman, D.G. (2010). CONSORT 2010 explanation and elaboration: Updated guidelines for reporting parallel group randomised trials. *BMJ (Clinical research ed.), 340*, BMJ 2010;340:c869.

Moore, S.C., Lee, I.M., Weiderpass, E., Campbell, P.T., Sampson, J.N., Kitahara, C.M., . . . Patel, A.V. (2016). Association of leisure-time physical activity with risk of 26 types of cancer in 1.44 million adults. *JAMA Internal Medicine, 176*(6), 816–825.

Moore, S.C., Patel, A.V., Matthews, C.E., Berrington de Gonzalez, A., Park, Y., Katki, H.A., . . . Lee, I.M. (2012). Leisure time physical activity of moderate to vigorous intensity and mortality: A large pooled cohort analysis. *PLoS Medicine, 9*(11), e1001335. doi:10.1371/journal.pmed.1001335

Morris, J.N., Chave, S.P.W., Adam, C., Sirey, C., Epstein, L., & Sheehan, D.J. (1973). Vigorous exercise in leisure-time and the incidence of coronary heart-disease. *The Lancet, 301*(7799), 333–339. doi:10.1016/s0140-6736(73)90128-1

Morris, J.N., Heady, J.A., & Raffle, P.A.B. (1956). Physique of London busmen. *The Lancet, 268*(6942), 569–570. doi:10.1016/s0140-6736(56)92049-9

Morris, J.N., Heady, J.A., Raffle, P.A.B., Roberts, C.G., & Parks, J.W. (1953). Coronary heart-disease and physical activity of work. *The Lancet, 262*(6795), 1053–1057. doi:10.1016/s0140-6736(53)90665-5

Morris, J.N., Kagan, A., Pattison, D.C., Gardner, M.J., & Raffle, P.A.B. (1966). Incidence and prediction of ischæmic heart-disease in London busmen. *The Lancet, 288*(7463), 553–559. doi:10.1016/s0140-6736(66)93034-0

Naci, H., & Ioannidis, J.P. (2015). Comparative effectiveness of exercise and drug interventions on mortality outcomes: Metaepidemiological study. *Br J Sports Med, 49*(21), 1414–1422. doi:10.1136/bjsports-2015-f5577rep

National Institute of Clinical Excellence. (2013). *Falls in older people: Assessing risk and prevention.*

O'Donovan, G., Kearney, E., Sherwood, R., & Hillsdon, M. (2012). Fatness, fitness, and cardiometabolic risk factors in middle-aged white men. *Metabolism, 61*(2), 213–220. doi:10.1016/j.metabol.2011.06.009

O'Donovan, G., Lee, I.M., Hamer, M., & Stamatakis, E. (2017). Association of "weekend warrior" and other leisure time physical activity patterns with risks for all-cause, cardiovascular disease, and cancer mortality. *JAMA Internal Medicine, 177*(3), 335–342.

Oja, P., Kelly, P., Pedisic, Z., Titze, S., Bauman, A., Foster, C., . . . Stamatakis, E. (2016). Associations of specific types of sports and exercise with all-cause and cardiovascular-disease mortality: A cohort study of 80 306 British adults. *British Journal of Sports Medicine, 51*(10), 812–817.

Ortega, F.B., Silventoinen, K., Tynelius, P., & Rasmussen, F. (2012). Muscular strength in male adolescents and premature death: Cohort study of one million participants. *BMJ, 345*, BMJ 2012;345:e7279.

Owen, N., Healy, G.N., Matthews, C.E., & Dunstan, D.W. (2010). Too much sitting: The population-health science of sedentary behavior. *Exercise and Sport Sciences Reviews, 38*(3), 105–113. doi:10.1097/JES.0b013e3181e373a2

Paffenbarger, R.S. Jr, Hyde, R., Wing, A.L., & Hsieh, C.-c. (1986). Physical activity, all-cause mortality, and longevity of college alumni. *New England Journal of Medicine, 314*(10), 605–613. doi:10.1056/nejm198603063141003

Paffenbarger, R.S. Jr, Laughlin, M.E., Gima, A.S., & Black, R.A. (1970). Work activity of longshoremen as related to death from coronary heart disease and stroke. *New England Journal of Medicine, 282*(20), 1109–1114. doi:10.1056/nejm197005142822001

Paffenbarger, R.S. Jr, Wing, A.L., & Hyde, R.T. (1978). Physical activity as an index of heart attack risk in college alumni. *American Journal of Epidemiology, 108*(3), 161–175.

Pattyn, N., Cornelissen, V.A., Eshghi, S.R., & Vanhees, L. (2013). The effect of exercise on the cardio-vascular risk factors constituting the metabolic syndrome: A meta-analysis of controlled trials. *Sports Med, 43*(2), 121–133. doi:10.1007/s40279-012-0003-z

Poppel, M.N. van, Chinapaw, M.J., Mokkink, L.B., van Mechelen, W., & Terwee, C.B. (2010). Physical activity questionnaires for adults: A systematic review of measurement properties. *Sports Medicine* (Auckland, N.Z.), *40*(7), 565–600.

Praet, S.F., van Rooij, E.S.J., Wijtvliet, A., Winter, L.J.M.B.-d., Enneking, T., Kuipers, H., . . . van Loon, L.J.C. (2008). Brisk walking compared with an individualised medical fitness programme for patients with type 2 diabetes: A randomised controlled trial. *Diabetologia, 51*(5), 736–746.

Rhéaume, C., Arsenault, B.J., Bélanger, S., Pérusse, L., Tremblay, A., Bouchard, C., . . . Després, J.-P. (2009). Low Cardiorespiratory fitness levels and elevated blood pressure: What is the contribution of visceral adiposity? *Hypertension, 54*(1), 91–97. doi:10.1161/hypertensionaha.109.131656

Ross, R., Blair, S.N., Arena, R., Church, T.S., Després, J.-P., Franklin, B.A., . . . Wisløff, U. (2016). Importance of assessing cardiorespiratory fitness in clinical practice: A case for fitness as a clinical vital sign: A scientific statement from the American Heart Association. *AHA Scientific Statement, 461*. doi:10.1161/CIR.0000000000000461

Ruiz, J.R., Sui, X., Lobelo, F., Lee, D.C., Morrow, J.R., Jackson, A.W., . . . Blair, S.N. (2009). Muscular strength and adiposity as predictors of adulthood cancer mortality in men. *Cancer epidemiology, biomarkers & prevention: A publication of the American Association for Cancer Research, cosponsored by the American Society of Preventive Oncology, 18*(5), 1468–1476.

Ruiz, J.R., Sui, X., Lobelo, F., Morrow, J.R., Jackson, A.W., Sjöström, M., & Blair, S.N. (2008). Association between muscular strength and mortality in men: Prospective cohort study. *BMJ* (Clinical research ed.), *337*(7661), 92–95.

Sackett, D.L. (1979). Bias in analytic research. *Journal of Chronic Diseases, 32*, 51–63.

Samitz, G., Egger, M., & Zwahlen, M. (2011). Domains of physical activity and all-cause mortality: Systematic review and dose-response meta-analysis of cohort studies. *International Journal of Epidemiology, 40*(5), 1382–1400.

Sawada, S.S., Lee, I.M., Naito, H., Kakigi, R., Goto, S., Kanazawa, M., . . . Blair, S.N. (2014). Cardiorespiratory fitness, body mass index, and cancer mortality: A cohort study of Japanese men. *BMC Public Health, 14*.

Schmid, D., & Leitzmann, M.F. (2014a). Association between physical activity and mortality among breast cancer and colorectal cancer survivors: A systematic review and meta-analysis. *Annals of Oncology, 25*(7), 1293–1311.

Schmid, D., & Leitzmann, M.F. (2014b). Cardiorespiratory fitness as predictor of cancer mortality: A systematic review and meta-analysis. *Annals of Oncology, 26*(2), 272–278. doi:10.1093/annonc/mdu250

Schuch, F.B., Vancampfort, D., Sui, X., Rosenbaum, S., Firth, J., Richards, J., . . . Stubbs, B. (2016). Are lower levels of cardiorespiratory fitness associated with incident depression? A systematic review of prospective cohort studies. *Preventive Medicine, 93*, 159–165.

Snowden, C.P., Prentis, J.M., Anderson, H.L., Roberts, D.R., Randles, D., Renton, M., & Manas, D.M. (2010). Submaximal cardiopulmonary exercise testing predicts complications and hospital length of stay in patients undergoing major elective surgery. *Annals of Surgery, 251*(3), 535–541.

Sui, X., Hooker, S.P., Lee, I.M., Church, T.S., Colabianchi, N., Lee, C.D., & Blair, S.N. (2007). A prospective study of cardiorespiratory fitness and risk of type 2 diabetes in women. *Diabetes Care, 31*(3), 550–555.

Sui, X., Laditka, J.N., Church, T.S., Hardin, J.W., Chase, N., Davis, K., & Blair, S.N. (2008). Prospective study of cardiorespiratory fitness and depressive symptoms in women and men. *J Psychiatr Res, 43*(5), 546–552.

Sui, X., LaMonte, M.J., Laditka, J.N., Hardin, J.W., Chase, N., Hooker, S.P., & Blair, S.N. (2007). Cardiorespiratory fitness and adiposity as mortality predictors in older adults. *JAMA, 298*(21), 2507–2516.

Tanaka, R., Ozawa, J., Kito, N., & Moriyama, H. (2015). Does exercise therapy improve the health-related quality of life of people with knee osteoarthritis? A systematic review and meta-analysis of randomized controlled trials. *Journal of Physical Therapy Science, 27*(10), 3309–3314.

Theou, O., Stathokostas, L., Roland, K.P., Jakobi, J.M., Patterson, C., Vandervoort, A.A., & Jones, G.R. (2011). The effectiveness of exercise interventions for the management of frailty: A systematic review. *Journal of Aging Research*, 2011.

Thomas, D.E., Elliott, E.J., & Naughton, G.A. (2006). Exercise for type 2 diabetes mellitus. *The Cochrane database of systematic reviews 3*, CD002968. doi:10.1002/14651858.CD002968.pub2

Trivedi, M.H., Greer, T.L., Church, T.S., Carmody, T.J., Grannemann, B.D., Galper, D.I., . . . Blair, S.N. (2011). Exercise as an augmentation treatment for nonremitted major depressive disorder: A randomized, parallel dose comparison. *The Journal of Clinical Psychiatry, 72*(5), 677–684.

Ussher, M.H., Taylor, A.H., & Faulkner, G.E. (2014). Exercise interventions for smoking cessation. *The Cochrane database of systematic reviews 8*, CD002295. doi:10.1002/14651858.CD002295.pub5

Uthman, O.A., van der, Jordan, J.L., Dziedzic, K.S., Healey, E.L., Peat, G.M., & Foster, N.E. (2014). Exercise for lower limb osteoarthritis: Systematic review incorporating trial sequential analysis and network meta-analysis. *British Journal of Sports Medicine, 48*(21).

Verheggen, R.J., Maessen, M.F., Green, D.J., Hermus, A.R., Hopman, M.T., & Thijssen, D.H. (2016). A systematic review and meta-analysis on the effects of exercise training versus hypocaloric diet: Distinct effects on body weight and visceral adipose tissue. *Obes Rev, 17*(8), 664–690. doi:10.1111/obr.12406

Wahid, A., Manek, N., Nichols, M., Kelly, P., Foster, C., Webster, P., . . . Scarborough, P. (2016). Quantifying the association between physical activity and cardiovascular disease and diabetes: A systematic review and meta-analysis. *Journal of the American Heart Association, 5*(9).

Warburton, D.E.R., Charlesworth, S., Ivey, A., Nettlefold, L., & Bredin, S.S.D. (2010). A systematic review of the evidence for Canada's physical activity guidelines for adults. *International Journal of Behavioral Nutrition and Physical Activity, 7*(1), 39. doi:10.1186/1479-5868-7-39

Warburton, D.E.R., Katzmarzyk, P.T., Rhodes, R.E., & Shephard, R.J. (2008). Evidence-informed physical activity guidelines for Canadian adults. *Canadian Journal of Public Health = Revue canadienne de sante publique, 98*.

Way, K.L., Hackett, D.A., Baker, M.K., & Johnson, N.A. (2016). The effect of regular exercise on insulin sensitivity in type 2 diabetes mellitus: A systematic review and meta-analysis. *Diabetes Metab J, 40*(4), 253–271. doi:10.4093/dmj.2016.40.4.253

Wegner, M., Helmich, I., Machado, S., Nardi, A.E., Arias-Carrion, O., & Budde, H. (2014). Effects of exercise on anxiety and depression disorders: Review of meta-analyses and neurobiological mechanisms. *CNS Neurol Disord Drug Targets, 13*(6), 1002–1014.

West, R.R., Jones, D.A., & Henderson, A.H. (2012). Rehabilitation after myocardial infarction trial (RAMIT): Multi-centre randomised controlled trial of comprehensive cardiac rehabilitation in patients following acute myocardial infarction. *Heart, 98*(8), 637–644. doi:10.1136/heartjnl-2011-300302

WHO. (2016). *NCD mortality and morbidity*. World Health Organization.

Wilhelm, M., Roskovensky, G., Emery, K., Manno, C., Valek, K., & Cook, C. (2013). Effect of resistance exercises on function in older adults with osteoporosis or osteopenia: A systematic review. *Physiotherapy Canada. Physiotherapie Canada, 64*(4), 386–394.

World Health Organization. (2010). *Global Recommendations on Physical Activity for Health*. Geneva: World Health Organization. Retrieved from www.ncbi.nlm.nih.gov/books/NBK305057/

Yang, Z., Scott, C.A., Mao, C., Tang, J., & Farmer, A.J. (2014). Resistance exercise versus aerobic exercise for type 2 diabetes: A systematic review and meta-analysis. *Sports Med, 44*(4), 487–499. doi:10.1007/s40279-013-0128-8

Yueh, B., & Feinstein, A.R. (1999). Abstruse comparisons: The problems of numerical contrasts of two groups. *Journal of Clinical Epidemiology, 52*(1), 13–18.

6　Measuring physical activity behaviours and outcomes in children and adults

Stuart J. Fairclough, Robert J. Noonan and Whitney B. Curry

Keywords: Energy expenditure, calibration, objective methods, laboratory methods, self-report methods

Introduction

Physical activity (PA) is defined as any bodily movement that results in energy expenditure (EE) above resting levels (Casperson, Powell, & Christenson, 1985), and therefore EE occurs as a result of PA. Estimation of EE through PA is important as both are implicated in the increasing rates of obesity and type 2 diabetes and other forms of non-communicable diseases (Hills, Mokhtar, & Byrne, 2014). Different PA measurement approaches are commonly used to quantify how much and what type of PA people undertake in various settings (Hills et al., 2014). These approaches typically aim to quantify some aspect of PA behaviour, such as frequency, duration, intensity, and type, or estimate the physiological cost of PA (e.g., EE). PA measurement methods are applied in controlled laboratory settings as well as in free-living contexts, and include self-report tools such as diaries and questionnaires, portable monitors worn for extended periods of time, and laboratory-based apparatus that measure the physiological costs of PA. This chapter will outline a range of PA measurement methods and discuss their characteristics, utility, and the evidence underpinning their validity and reliability, as well as emerging issues relevant to their use.

Principles of physical activity measurement

PA measurement approaches capture one or more dimensions of PA behaviour (e.g., movement measured by accelerometer activity counts) that can be analysed and reported in raw form or translated to other units such as EE or minutes spent in moderate-to-vigorous PA (MVPA). This calibration of raw activity data into intensity-related minutes or EE is based on the relationships between PA intensity and EE (Welk, Morrow, & Saint-Maurice, 2017). Algorithms based on these relationships can be built into PA measurement tools to convert raw movement data into more readily interpretable PA and/or EE metrics. One such metric is metabolic equivalents (METs) which equates to oxygen consumption required at rest (assumed to be 3.5 mL/O_2/min per kg body weight). METs are used to express EE or PA intensity as multiples of rest (i.e., 1 MET) and are therefore useful for categorising and prescribing physical activities at different intensities (Schutz, Weinsier, & Hunter, 2001). For adults, light PA (LPA) is defined as ≥1.5 METs, moderate PA (MPA) as 3–6 METs, and vigorous PA (VPA) as ≥6 METs (Figure 6.1).

It is important to note that, due to variations in body composition, METs do not determine the precise energy cost of PA in individuals, (e.g., 1 MET overestimates resting EE in obese adults (Wilms et al., 2014)). Similarly, PA intensities are defined differently in children due to variation in body composition-related resting EE, which is higher than in adults (Harrell et al. 2005). To reflect this, sex-specific adjusted MET thresholds for resting EE, sedentary behaviour, and MVPA have been formulated for children from 8 years upwards (Welk et al., 2017). Sedentary behaviour is defined as any waking behaviour characterised by an energy expenditure ≤1.5 METs, while in a sitting, reclining or lying posture (Tremblay et al., 2017). Recognising that sedentary behaviour and health research is a field of study in its own right, this chapter will focus solely on methods of PA measurement and will not discuss measuring sedentary behaviour in any detail. For interested readers, comprehensive examinations of this topic can be found elsewhere (Byrom et al., 2016; Kang & Rowe, 2015; Rowe & Kang, 2015; Zhu & Owen, 2017).

Many different validated methods of measuring PA are available, which can present uncertainty when deciding which method is most suitable. A common method for comparing measures is to consider their validity (i.e., accuracy) in relation to their feasibility (i.e., ease of use). This relationship is usually inverse with the more accurate methods (e.g., doubly labelled water) tending to be less feasible due to the greater expense, technical complexity, time required, etc. Conversely, more feasible measures such as questionnaires which can be used with large numbers of participants, generally are less accurate at estimating PA levels. The validity/feasibility continuum for PA measures (Welk et al., 2017) is a useful basis for researchers when deciding on

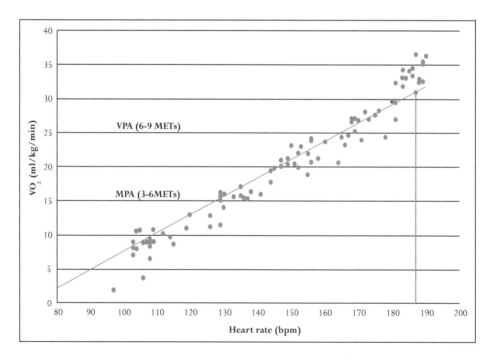

Figure 6.1 Relationship between PA intensity and energy expenditure

the most appropriate PA measurement tools (Dollman et al., 2009) (Figure 6.2). The next sections of this chapter will consider wearable PA monitors, direct observation, laboratory-based PA measurement approaches, and self-report methods. For ease of reference, an overview of the methods discussed in the chapter is presented in Table 6.1.

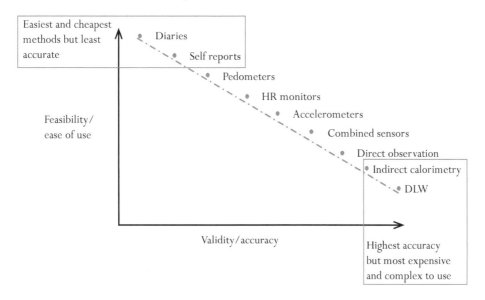

Figure 6.2　Feasibility-validity continuum of PA measurement methods

Table 6.1　Comparison of physical activity measurement methods

Physical activity measurement method	What is measured?	Physical activity outcomes	Strengths	Weaknesses
Wearable monitors				
Accelerometers	Human movement	Movement 'counts' Acceleration (g units) Time spent at PA intensities Time spent active/ inactive/sedentary PA/sedentary bouts Steps	Unobtrusive Large data storage capacity Long battery life High frequency time-stamped data Open source data processing where raw data are available	Expensive Wear location determines which movements are recorded/missed (e.g., upper body movements missed by hip-worn monitor) Cannot guarantee accurate monitor placement Time consuming data handling Large amount of data storage required

(Continued)

Table 6.1 (Continued)

Physical activity measurement method	What is measured?	Physical activity outcomes	Strengths	Weaknesses
Pedometers	Steps Distance covered* Energy cost* PA intensity*	Steps	Low cost Non-invasive Provides feedback Low participant burden Ease of use and interpretation	Does not assess PA intensity Risk of data loss due to tampering Potential reactivity Variable validity and reliability across models
Heart rate monitors	Cardiorespiratory load of PA	Mean heart rate Time spent at PA intensities (e.g., heart rate reserve, percentage maximum HR)	Ease of use Monitor over extended periods of time (especially wrist-worn) Socially acceptable Can be used for water-based activities	Expensive Heart rate influenced by factors other than PA Heart rate response lags behind movement Monitor discomfort Data loss caused by poorly fitting devices
Multi-sensor monitors	Heart rate Human movement Energy expenditure Postural allocation	Time spent at PA intensities Time spent active/inactive/sedentary PA/sedentary bouts Energy expenditure PA mode	More accurate estimation of PA Large data storage capacity Long battery life High frequency time-stamped data	Expensive Monitor discomfort Some devices require skin preparation for successful monitoring Can be obtrusive Time consuming data handling
Consumer-focused monitors	Human movement Heart rate Location Energy expenditure Distance covered Speed/pace of travel	Steps Time spent at PA intensities Time spent active/inactive/sedentary Energy expenditure Mean heart rate	Accurate estimation of steps Provides feedback Comfort and attractive design Low participant burden Widely available and acceptable to wear Linked to smartphone apps or web interface for tracking and social interaction	Limited battery life Lack accuracy for PA intensity and energy expenditure Potential novelty effect as motivational PA tracking tool For researchers, data not straightforward to access for analysis

Physical activity measurement method	What is measured?	Physical activity outcomes	Strengths	Weaknesses
GPS	Location Distance covered Speed/pace of travel	Proxy indication of PA intensity (i.e., speed/pace of travel)	Provides information about where PA takes place Data can be linked to that from other monitors (e.g., accelerometers)	Limited to outdoor PA Limited battery life GPS signal can be interrupted in certain locations Time-consuming data handling, especially when linking with accelerometer data
Life-logging cameras	Digital image of location	Contexts and settings where PA occurs	Multiple PA contexts and settings captured in real time Potential to link to images to time-stamped objectively measured PA data	Low acceptability and feasibility of wearing over extended periods Participant burden Ethical issues Time-consuming data handling
Direct observation	PA behaviour PA mode PA levels Postural allocation Contextual factors	PA intensity Frequency and duration of PA behaviours and modes	Contextually rich data produced Comprehensive Can provide qualitative and quantitative information about factors influencing PA behaviours Applicable to specific settings (e.g., PE classes)	Time consuming High associated costs High observer and participant burden Potential for reactivity Extensive training required PA levels may be overestimated
Laboratory-based methods				
Whole-room calorimetry	Energy expenditure (EE)	Total EE Resting EE PA EE Can be expressed as kcals or METs	Valid and reliable Range of PA activities can be explored Criterion measurement for other methods	Costly Required specialised equipment and knowledge High participant burden Not free-living environment Time consuming

(Continued)

Table 6.1 (Continued)

Physical activity measurement method	What is measured?	Physical activity outcomes	Strengths	Weaknesses
Indirect calorimetry	EE	Total EE Resting EE PA EE Can be expressed as kcals or METs	Less costly than whole room Portable More able to simulate free-living activities Criterion measurement for other methods	Validity and reliability issues Requires specialised equipment and knowledge Somewhat high participant burden Time consuming
Doubly labelled water	EE	Total EE Resting EE PA EE Expressed as kcals	Gold standard of measuring EE in free-living environment Measures habitual PA Valid and reliable Relatively low participant burden	Costly Requires specialised equipment and knowledge Time consuming for researcher and participant Dose and analyses vary depending on body weight of participant
Self-report methods				
Short-term recall questionnaires	Types of PA and behaviour PA levels	Bouts of PA Minutes of PA engagement PA 'scores'	Low cost Low participant burden Can be used in large population studies Captures contextual information	Reliability and validity problems Limited utility with younger children Potential recall bias Misinterpretation of PA due to language, cultural factors
Global questionnaires	Types of PA and behaviour PA levels	Bouts of PA Minutes of PA engagement PA 'scores'	Low cost Low participant burden Can be used in large population studies	Potential recall bias and errors Offer limited contextual information
PA diaries	Types of PA and behaviour PA levels	Bouts of PA Minutes of PA engagement PA 'scores' PA behaviours and modes	Contextually rich data produced Potential to reduce recall errors due to in-situ reports	High participant burden Reactivity Data loss caused by non-compliant behaviour

Physical activity measurement method	What is measured?	Physical activity outcomes	Strengths	Weaknesses
EMA	Types of PA and behaviour PA levels Contextual factors	Bouts of PA Minutes of PA engagement PA 'scores' PA behaviours and modes	Contextually rich data produced Potential to reduce recall errors due to in-situ reports Potential to reduce non-compliant behaviour Can provide qualitative and quantitative information about factors influencing PA behaviours	High participant burden Potential recall bias Software failure Reactivity

*Only available on some models

Measuring PA using wearable monitors and direct observation

Accelerometry is the most widely used objective method of PA measurement and is used in free-living and discrete settings. Accelerometers are valid and reliable tools to measure PA in a range of populations (Freedson, Melanson, & Sirard, 1998; Mackintosh et al., 2012; Phillips, Parfitt, & Rowlands, 2012; Plasqui, Bonomi, & Westerterp, 2013). The basis for accelerometry is the continuous time-stamped measurement of raw accelerations resulting from human movement. In contemporary accelerometers, these accelerations are captured in three orthogonal directions (Troiano et al., 2014). These raw accelerations are translated into relevant and meaningful information about the participant's PA behaviours (e.g., time spent in MVPA) (Sievänen & Kujala, 2017), but this information is dependent on a series of decisions made by the researcher, such as, accelerometer wear location, frequency of recording, criteria to determine valid wear periods, processed data metrics, and thresholds for PA intensities (Migueles et al., 2017). An example accelerometry trace can be seen in Chapter 4, Figure 4.3. Currently, there is no consensus as to how this decision making should be operationalised, which makes comparisons between accelerometer studies challenging. Accelerometers have traditionally been worn on the hip, but wrist-worn monitors are becoming increasingly prevalent (e.g., the ActiGraph GT9X, GENEActiv). This shift towards wrist-worn devices is driven by the growing popularity of wrist-worn consumer-focused wearable activity monitors (Welk et al., 2017), and evidence that participant compliance to wearing the accelerometer is better if worn on the wrist (Fairclough et al., 2016). This transition has been illustrated most significantly by the use of wrist-worn accelerometers since 2011 in the US National Health and Nutrition Examination Survey (Troiano et al., 2014) as well as in other population-level surveillance research (e.g., UK Biobank (Doherty et al., 2017)), and smaller studies (Kim et al., 2017).

The accelerometer 'output' has traditionally been a 'movement count', which is a dimensionless unit calculated from the raw accelerations which are subsequently subjected to a proprietary algorithm on-board the monitor (Figure 6.3). Counts have been calibrated to more meaningful outcomes such as EE and MET values (Welk et al., 2017), to provide estimates of time spent in specific PA intensities. This allows accelerometer counts to be translated to more interpretable metrics that are relevant to public health indicators (e.g., the proportion of individuals achieving daily PA guidelines). In recent years there have been calls for greater transparency of accelerometer data procedures in an attempt to improve the clarity of how accelerometer-derived estimates of PA are calculated (Freedson et al., 2012). These calls have centred on the use of raw acceleration signal processing which theoretically should allow direct comparison of PA outcomes derived from different accelerometer brands and models (Fairclough et al., 2016). Presently though, PA outcomes derived from raw accelerations produced by different brands of device are still not directly comparable, possibly because of technical differences between devices such as the microelectromechanical sensors used and their dynamic ranges, reference voltage, and the analogue-to-digital conversion rate (Rowlands et al., 2015).

Accelerometers are attractive tools for researchers because they provide detailed information about the frequency, intensity, and duration of PA. They are small devices, with capability to store large amounts of data over extended periods. Accelerometers though are relatively costly, ranging from £100 to £350 each and require trained staff with sufficient expertise to process and interpret the data produced. Although use of 24-hour monitoring protocols over extended periods are becoming more common (Troiano et al., 2014), accelerometers will not capture all PA modes. For example, hip-worn devices ignore upper body movements, cycling is notoriously difficult to quantify using waist- or wrist-worn accelerometry, and only accelerometer models that are waterproof allow for water-based PA modes such as swimming to be recorded (Harrison et al., 2017). Moreover, the physiological cost of PA is not captured by accelerometry meaning that PA intensity is underestimated during some ambulatory activities such as stair climbing and walking on inclines, or when similar activities are performed

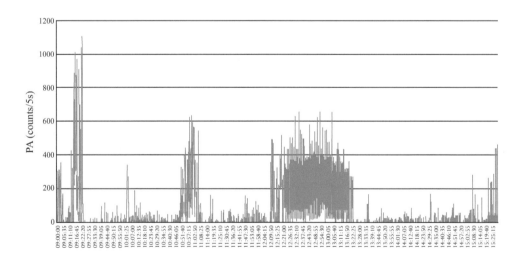

Figure 6.3 Accelerometer count measured PA profile of 10-year-old boy during the school day

by individuals of differing fitness status (e.g., obese vs. healthy weight). These issues can be addressed through the use of novel analytical approaches using machine learning (Clark et al., 2016), which enables movement pattern recognition that can detect specific types of movements and PA modes and intensities (De Vries et al., 2011; Trost et al. 2012). The portable and objective nature of accelerometers, combined with the emergence of new analytical techniques means that these devices offer many advantages to PA researchers (Welk et al., 2017).

Pedometers provide data on the volume of ambulatory activity. Data are expressed as 'step counts' which reflect the number of steps taken over the time the pedometer is worn. Pedometers are worn on the waist and steps are generated in response to the vertical accelerations of the hip that occur during walking and running. In traditional pedometers a spring-suspended lever arm or piezo-electrical mechanism captures the vertical motion of the hip, and this in turn leads to the accumulated step count (Bassett & Strath, 2002). Many of the more modern pedometer models now use an accelerometer to detect steps taken (Welk et al., 2017). Pedometers can also provide the user with data related to distance travelled, cadence, duration of movement, and EE. These metrics are dependent on additional user information such as stride length, weight, and age (Tudor-Locke & Myers, 2001), though the accuracy of EE estimates is often limited (Welk et al., 2017). Although pedometers require little setting up before wear and the data are easily stored in memory or manually recorded at the end of the prescribed wear period, researchers still need to consider decisions within the data collection protocol to ensure that the data collected reflect the intended study outcomes. Such decisions include whether the data are recorded by participants or by researchers, whether the participants should be blinded to their steps counts in an attempt to limit reactivity, and what data collection monitoring frame is most appropriate to ensure the data are representative of typical PA patterns (Tudor-Locke & Myers, 2001). The fact that pedometers display step (and other) output metrics in real time is important for researchers to consider. Such direct and immediate feedback to the user may be positive from a PA promotion perspective as it allows for comparisons against generic or individualised step-count goals. This feedback may be motivational for some users and could be central to positive behavioural change (Tudor-Locke, 2002). It is for these reasons that pedometer-based intervention programmes are known to be effective (Bravata et al., 2007). Alternatively, in studies using unsealed pedometers as a measure of PA, data may be compromised if participants modify their normal or treatment-related PA behaviours in response to pedometer feedback. However, in adults such reactivity may only be sort term when pedometers are worn for more than one week (Clemes & Deans, 2012).

The big advantages of pedometers are that they are simple to use, data are straightforward to interpret, they have strong validity and reliability during walking activities (Beets et al., 2011; Tudor-Locke et al., 2002), and their cost is low (e.g., £20 for a research grade pedometer). Although pedometers are most accurate in assessing total volume of steps, they cannot capture non-ambulatory PA, and have lower levels of accuracy when predicting PA intensity and EE (Welk et al., 2017).

An individual's response to PA can be measured using heart rate, which provides an indication of the stress on the cardiorespiratory system during movement (Armstrong, 1998). As MVPA is primarily aerobic and therefore dependent on oxygen, heart rate monitoring can provide an estimate of PA EE (Casperson et al., 1985). Traditionally, heart rate monitors comprise of a chest strap which detects the electrical signal of the heart and a wrist watch which displays the heart rate data. Data can be collected and stored in the watch memory for extended periods (e.g., one week) and downloaded for subsequent analyses. Converting HR data to meaningful and intensity-specific PA metrics involves use of various thresholds and individualised calibration methods. Individual calibration allows for more accurate estimates of PA, because parameters such as individuals' fitness status, age, sex, etc. can be accounted for. Example calibration methods include percent heart rate reserve, PA heart rate, and flex heart rate (Janz, 2002). It should be noted that such approaches are based on the assumption of linearity between heart rate and EE. While this assumption is true for MVPA, it may not be valid for less intense activity (i.e., LPA (Welk et al., 2017)). Before the widespread use of accelerometers, heart rate monitors were commonly used to study PA behaviours (J. Karvonen & Vuorimaa, 1988; M. Karvonen, Kentela, & Mustala, 1957) but over extended data collection periods, low participant compliance due to discomfort and skin irritability, and data attrition due to poor fitting chest straps can compromise data quality (Janz, 2002). Moreover, the delay in heart rate response after movement can mask the intermittent activity patterns of children (Baquet et al., 2007), which can lead to underestimated PA levels in this population.

Contemporary heart rate monitors often employ optical sensors built into wrist bands or watches. This wrist conductivity approach tracks the number of heart beats per minute and uses existing calibration algorithms to estimate EE and time spent in different PA intensities (Welk et al., 2017). As is the case with traditional heart rate monitors though, the accuracy of these estimations diminishes at lower PA intensities as well as during more vigorous PA (e.g., running speeds >6.0 mph) (Welk et al., 2017). Moreover, heart rate responds to factors other than PA such as ambient temperature, emotional arousal, and hydration level (Janz, 2002) which can compromise the accuracy of resultant PA estimates. For these reasons, heart rate monitors have frequently been used in combination with other measures such as accelerometers to provide a more accurate estimate of PA behaviours across the full intensity spectrum (Brage et al., 2004; Hesketh et al., 2014).

Devices which contain more than one sensor to detect different aspects of PA behaviour have been available for over 10 years. One commonly used multi-sensor monitor is the Actiheart, which has demonstrated strong validity to predict PA EE (Brage et al., 2004). Its design relies on users wearing two ECG electrodes on the chest or a heart rate belt along with an integrated accelerometer. The requirement for direct contact with the chest over prolonged periods may compromise participant compliance and result in data attrition (Costa et al., 2013; Schrack et al., 2016). Other devices use multiple integrated sensors to produce highly sophisticated estimates of daily PA patterns. For example, the Intelligent Device for EE and Activity (IDEEA) gait analysis system uses multiple accelerometers positioned in body locations predetermined by the researchers (e.g., thigh, wrist, chest) which connect wirelessly to a main recorder worn on the hip. Pattern recognition algorithms applied to the accelerometer signals allow EE to be estimated from 35 postures and activities. Though the IDEEA system has demonstrated acceptable accuracy for predicting EE in different contexts, it has limited memory capacity and the number of sensors and their positioning places a significant burden on the participant, which may impact on compliance (Hills et al., 2014). The Sensewear Armband is a single unit multi-sensor monitor worn on the upper arm. This device integrates a bi-axial accelerometer with physiological sensors of EE in the form of a skin temperature sensor, a near body temperature sensor, a heat flux sensor, and a galvanic skin response sensor. The combination of signals from these sensors are applied to proprietary pattern recognition algorithms to estimate EE and the assessment of PA type and intensity. Validation evidence in children and adults demonstrates that the Sensewear Armband can accurately estimate EE (Casiraghi et al., 2013) and PA levels at a range of intensities (Calabró, Welk, & Eisenmann,

2009; Reece et al., 2015). The advent of consumer-focused wearable PA monitors saw the patented technology at the heart of the Sensewear Armband acquired by Jawbone in 2013, and as a result production of the Armband has ceased.

Most PA monitoring devices provide detailed information about the quality of participants' PA in relation to frequency, intensity, and time. Application of pattern recognition algorithms has also enabled time spent in different PA modes to be investigated using devices like the Sensewear Armband. However, using objective measures to investigate the influence of the PA environment and context has received less attention. Objective monitoring of PA contexts has largely been undertaken using global positioning systems (GPS) and to a lesser extent by wearable cameras (Loveday et al., 2016). GPS has been used in conjunction with accelerometers to provide estimates of PA in specific outdoor locations, such as parks, schools, and commuting routes (Cooper et al., 2010; Dac Minh Tuan et al., 2013; Van Kann et al., 2016). While this combination of devices provides a rich degree of novel contextual data, the need for participants to wear two separate monitors increases the burden, and GPS signals are compromised when wearers are indoors. Moreover, harmonisation of GPS and accelerometer data, as well as the need for additional skill sets (e.g., expertise in Geographic Information Systems) are further challenges to GPS use. Wearable cameras, such as the Microsoft Sense-Cam and Vicon Revue provide 'lifelogging' capability by taking digital images of the wearer's immediate front facing environment up to 2,000 times per day. The former device also includes an integrated accelerometer which reduces participant burden of having to wear an additional device. SenseCam data have been used to quantify time spent in different free-living PA contexts and locations (e.g., indoors/outdoors, transport, domestic, occupation) (Doherty, Kelly, et al., 2013) and to estimate time spent in various movement behaviours (e.g., sitting, standing, walking, running) (Kerr et al., 2013). Despite the advantages using wearable cameras in PA research, numerous challenges are also present which relate to device acceptability for users, time-consuming data analysis, and variable quality of digital images produced (Doherty, Hodges, et al., 2013). Ethical and privacy concerns have also been raised, although in response an ethical framework for wearable camera use has been proposed (Kelly et al., 2013). Like other objective PA methods, the relatively high cost of wearable cameras combined with the other challenges of using them are limiting factors. The widespread use of smartphones equipped with high quality cameras does though provide an alternative method of either digitally capturing or storing logged images (Gurrin et al., 2013) that can subsequently be analysed to answer PA research context questions.

Direct observation is another objective PA measurement method which captures context, and therefore warrants discussion. Direct observation involves trained observers using time-sampling methods to classify PA into distinct categories that can be quantified and analysed. A key characteristic of direct observation is its capacity to identify the type of PA and when, where, and with whom it occurs (McKenzie, 2010). Direct observation is most suited for use with small samples in specific settings (e.g., school playtime, physical education classes) (McKenzie, 2002). Most direct observation instruments are used in youth populations (e.g., SOFIT (McKenzie, Sallis, & Nader, 1991), SOPLAY (McKenzie, Marshall, Sallis, & Conway, 2000), SOCARP (Ridgers, Stratton, & McKenzie, 2010)) with fewer focused on adults and others (e.g., SOPARC (McKenzie et al., 2006). Direct observation can also provide information on factors that may influence PA behaviour such as the social or physical environment and can thus aid interpretation of study findings (Warren et al., 2010) (Figure 6.4). Moreover, due to its high internal validity, direct observation has been widely used as a criterion measure for validating other data collection tools such as pedometers and accelerometers

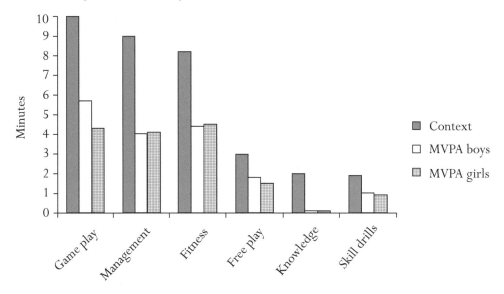

Figure 6.4 SOFIT data depicting MVPA of boys and girls in different Physical Education lesson contexts and time spent in each context

(McKenzie & van der Mars, 2015). However, a limitation is that levels of MVPA may also be overestimated (Hollis et al., 2016; Saint-Maurice et al., 2011) due to the time-sampling nature of the observations and selection of observed participants. Though direct observation is advantageous in that it can provide rich contextual PA data, the cost and time intensive nature of the method, both to train researchers and collect data should be considered (Dollman et al., 2009). Further, to ensure observer competence, observer retraining is required throughout the data collection process to reduce the potential for observers' skills deteriorating over time (McKenzie, 2002).

In recent years, the popularity of consumer-focused wearable PA and health tracking devices has increased dramatically. Brands such as Fitbit, Garmin, Jawbone, Withings, Samsung, Apple, and others have introduced a multitude of predominantly wrist-based monitors designed for consumers to track and monitor their PA and sleep habits as well as other lifestyle behaviours such as dietary patterns. These devices contain a range of sensors to monitor and track PA and other outcomes (e.g., sleep, postural allocation), such as accelerometers, heart rate monitors, GPS, gyroscopes, and inclinometers. Most consumer devices are paired with a mobile application and in some cases an internet interface to give users round the clock access to their data. However, the availability of the research evidence examining the accuracy of these monitors has somewhat lagged behind the boom in market sales. A 2015 systematic review of the validity and reliability evidence of Fitbit and Jawbone wearable monitors found that both devices had higher validity when measuring steps, but lower validity when estimating EE, which was usually underestimated (Evenson, Goto, & Furberg, 2015). In the same year an empirical laboratory study confirmed the accuracy of 10 different activity trackers for measuring steps (Kooiman et al., 2015). During free-living though, when compared to the ActiGraph GT3X+ accelerometer the Fitbit One and Jawbone UP were observed to overestimate steps (8% and 14%, respectively) and underestimate time spent in MVPA by almost 50% (Gomersall et al., 2016). These findings are supported by those of Murakami and colleagues (Murakami et al., 2016) and Chowdhury et al. (2017) who reported significant underestimation of measured EE from a total of 15 different consumer-wearable devices under simulated and free-living conditions. Variation in EE prediction was also highlighted in a recent study which found that Fitbit models One, Zip, and Flex and the Jawbone UP under- and over-estimated EE during a range of simulated sedentary, household, and ambulatory activities (Nelson et al., 2016). In this same study the accuracy of the devices for measuring steps during ambulatory activities was confirmed (Nelson et al., 2016). Most research conducted into the efficacy of consumer-focused wearable monitors has been undertaken with adults, but these devices are increasingly worn by children and adolescents. A recent systematic review identified five studies reporting use of wearables in youth (Ridgers, McNarry, & Mackintosh, 2016). Comfort, style, and feedback were reported to be important features that would influence use among youth. Feedback features may have potential to help PA behaviour change through self-monitoring and goal setting (e.g., steps per day) (Ridgers et al., 2016).

It is clear that consumer-focused monitors provide unprecedented opportunities to measure a range of PA behaviours and outcomes continuously over extended periods (Wright et al., 2017). There is evidence that these devices can contribute to behaviour change strategies by allowing users to self-monitor and adjust their activity behaviours. The accuracy of such monitors when measuring steps is acceptable, but studies comparing consumer monitors to direct, indirect, and field-based measures of EE all conclude that wearables have questionable accuracy, and so should be used with caution by researchers and consumers alike.

Laboratory measures of physical activity

An estimation of the physiological cost of PA (e.g., EE) is important to understanding energy balance and its contribution to health. In its simplest of terms, energy balance is the relationship between energy consumed (e.g., food) and energy expended (e.g., at rest and during PA), and has long been a focus of PA researchers seeking to understand this relationship in order to reduce obesity and improve health outcomes (Brage et al., 2015).

The respiratory system's primary function is the exchange of oxygen for carbon dioxide and during PA the body demands more oxygen and the rapid removal of carbon dioxide. This exchange can be used as an indicator of EE over a specified period of time. One method for measuring respiratory gas exchange is a whole room indirect calorimetry chamber. This is an airtight, environmentally controlled room, typically equipped with a bed, toilet, chair, phone, and exercise equipment such as a treadmill or stationary bike, depending on the activity of interest. The chamber system can measure consumption of oxygen and production of carbon dioxide in real time, with a high level of accuracy. The frequency, duration, intensity, mode, and onset of PA and the associated EE can be calculated with this method (Rothney, Schaefer, Neumann, Choi, & Chen, 2008). This method of measuring EE is also frequently used as a criterion method for validation of other PA measurement methods such as accelerometry and heart rate monitoring.

Specialised equipment and software expertise are required for use of the chamber. There are varying protocols for measurement using the chamber, but an example could be for participants to have resting metabolic rate measured, to stay in the chamber for 23 hours, exercise for a specified period of time, and consume pre-prepared and nutrient-controlled food (Rothney et al., 2008). EE can be expressed as kilocalories or as METs as dictated by the aims of the study (Zhang et al., 2004). When used as a criterion method the same procedures would apply with participants wearing other devices such as an accelerometer or heart rate monitor while in the chamber.

While this method is useful for measuring EE in a carefully controlled environment, it is more ecologically valid to measure EE in a free-living environment. Therefore, portable gas exchange analysers have become an important tool for researchers interested in this area. Portable gas analysers measure the consumption of oxygen and the production of carbon dioxide in the same way as a whole room indirect calorimetry chamber, but are easily used in various environments. A face mask with tubes is connected to a portable gas analyser (some models on a cart, others strapped to the participant) and data can be collected breath-by-breath (Sasaki et al., 2016). As with the chamber, protocols will differ but an example could consist of a familiarisation period for participants to adjust to the device, and the varying lengths of time engaging in the activities of interest to the study, along with rest periods between each activity. Data from portable gas analysers can also be presented as kilocalories or METs.

Respiratory gas analysis has many strengths. Gas analysis is a non-invasive method of collecting data on EE. This method can be used to inform and validate self-report tools and objective measures that are widely used by PA researchers with both adults and children, as both can participate in gas analysis (Sasaki et al., 2016; Trost et al., 2016). Finally, the portability of some gas analysers makes them an attractive option for measuring EE in free-living settings. Although gas exchange analysis has many strengths, there are several limitations to consider. The whole room indirect calorimetry chamber can cost in excess of £1,000,000 and requires a full-time technician to maintain and operate it. Replacement parts can be expensive and the chamber itself can take up a large amount of laboratory space. Portable gas analysers are significantly less expensive, but have limitations such as short battery life and the need for a specially trained operator. There is relatively high participant burden with this method as participants must spend a significant amount of time in the chamber or wear an often uncomfortable mask with the portable version. If researchers want to measure children, they will need a specialised and smaller version depending on age and for the portable version different masks and expertise with the data collection process and analysis. Data analysis can be complex and requires specialised knowledge to produce data that can be easily understood and applied for practical purposes (Sasaki et al., 2016).

Validity and reliability studies of respiratory gas exchange analysis have produced inconsistent findings. Studies have found that different brands of devices cannot be used interchangeably as they do not demonstrate inter-device reliability (Gore, 2000; Jakovljevic et al., 2008; Thoden, 1991). Thus, caution should be used when comparing EE reported by studies using different brands of gas analysers (Jakovljevic et al., 2008). Gas exchange analysers have been validated against the Douglas Bag Method (DBM) as a criterion. Gas analysers have often been found not to be valid during moderate or vigorous exercise without the use of correction equations for oxygen uptake or carbon dioxide production therefore again, caution should be used when selecting a device as well as determining the PA intensity suitable for use with the device (Cooper et al., 2009; Macfarlane & Wong, 2012).

The doubly labelled water (DLW) method is widely accepted as the 'gold standard' in measuring EE of PA under free-living conditions and used for the validation of many other methods of measuring PA (Westerterp, 2009). DLW is water in which oxygen and hydrogen has been tagged or 'labelled' with heavy, non-radioactive isotopes (e.g., deuterium and oxgygen-18). The elimination rate of these isotopes is measured over a period of time via urine sample and gives an estimation of oxygen use and carbon dioxide elimination (Westerterp, 2015). The procedure for the DLW method is highly technical, requiring specialised expertise and laboratory equipment. Typically, EE is measured over 1 to 4 weeks (Butte et al., 2010). Participants provide baseline urine samples, and then consume a body weight specific dose of DLW. Participants subsequently collect a daily urine sample and keep these refrigerated until the end of the specified measurement period. Urine samples are analysed and EE calculated using various equations which account for PA EE, resting EE, diet-induced thermogenesis, and total EE (Brage et al., 2015). Other methods of PA measurement, such as heart rate monitoring and accelerometry can be validated by being worn for comparison during the same DLW testing period (Calabró, Stewart, & Welk, 2013; Hoos, Plasqui, Gerver, & Westerterp, 2003).

Appropriate measurement of EE during PA is essential to understanding the interaction between PA and health outcomes and must provide data over a length of time that represents habitual and normal daily activity. The DLW method is widely regarded as the most valid and reliable method of measuring EE in free-living conditions (Westerterp, 2009). There is minimal participant burden during the testing period and the assessment does not require participants to track their own activity as in other methods. This method can be used with both adults and children (Ekelund et al., 2001; Westerterp, 2009). Despite these advantages, there are also various limitations that researchers should be equally mindful of when considering this method. DLW is expensive, is not always readily available, requires specialised laboratory equipment and training, and requires participants to adhere strictly to providing daily samples while storing these samples until they are collected by the researcher (Hoos, Plasqui, Gerver, & Westerterp, 2003). Although considered the gold standard, there are known validity and reliability issues with the DLW method. When validated against respiratory gas exchange, the method has been shown to have a precision of 2–8% but this depends on the length of testing period, loading dose, and the number of samples taken during the testing period. The agreement between DLW and respiratory gas exchange across nine studies was found to be 0.78% (2–8% SD), which indicates that individual errors within the 95%CI ($\pm$2SD) are likely to be even higher (Butte et al., 2010). This variation has been contributed to physiologic variation (6%) such as participants who are leaner (i.e., higher water-to-body weight ratio). This can be an issue as the dose of DLW is dependent on body weight (Brage et al., 2015). Analytic variation (2%) must also be considered when interpreting any activity monitor validation when using DLW method as a criterion method (Calabró, Stewart, & Welk, 2013).

Self-reported measurement of PA behaviours

Questionnaires are the most widely used measure of PA (Sylvia et al. 2014). Questionnaires are cost-effective, of low burden to the respondent, and provide a versatile, non-invasive, and time-effective way of collecting PA data from participants. Questionnaires can provide contextual information (i.e., location and why the behaviour takes place), which can be valuable for studying specific health associations and developing intervention programmes. Moreover, unlike most objective measures, self-report methods provide understanding of activity domain, including organised (e.g., group-based gym activity, team or individual sport), non-organised (e.g., walking for recreation or exercise, active play), occupational (e.g., work-related EE), domestic (e.g., gardening, house chores), and transportation (e.g., walking or cycling from place to place) (Dollman et al., 2009). Understanding the domain, location, and with whom PA is performed is important for PA assessment and promotion (Welk & Kim, 2015). Such rich contextual information helps to determine when and what types of PA interventions might be needed, and for which population (van Sluijs & Kriemler, 2016). Furthermore, distinguishing between structured and unstructured PA participation, and between nondiscretionary (e.g., incidental walking due to a carless household) and discretionary behaviour (e.g., walking for leisure and health) is important to understand an individual's PA behaviour, and inform mode-specific intervention programmes (e.g., walking; Green, 2009; Troiano et al., 2012).

A broad range of questionnaires have been developed for different populations and age groups, all of which differ in length and recall period. Questionnaires have been used to assess PA prevalence in large-scale surveillance studies (Dai et al., 2015; Dwyer-Lindgren et al., 2013; Ham, Kruger, & Tudor-Locke, 2009; Mindell et al., 2012). They have also been used to evaluate PA intervention programmes (Angelopoulos et al., 2009; Hansen et al., 2012; McNeil et al., 2009), and assess relationships between PA and health outcomes in older adults (Knaeps et al., 2016; Lacey et al., 2015), adults (Macera et al., 2005; Tucker et al., 2016), adolescents and children (Bai et al., 2016). Recall time periods for questionnaires range from between one day to one year. Generally, the longer the recall period the less accurate the data (Ainsworth et al., 2012).

The International PA Questionnaire (IPAQ) is the most extensively used questionnaire for adult and older adult populations (Hurtig-Wennlof, Hagströmer, & Olsson, 2010; Silsbury, Goldsmith, & Rushton, 2015; van Poppel et al. 2010). The IPAQ comes in a variety of formats and languages and has been used worldwide in PA surveillance research (Lee et al., 2011). It is available in short- and long-form. The short-form is used for surveillance, and the long-form is used when more detailed PA information is needed. The IPAQ short-form assesses PA undertaken across various domains including occupation, transportation, housework/gardening, and leisure. Time spent sitting is also assessed to classify sedentary behaviour. Respondents report the number of days per week and time per day spent in moderate and vigorous activity for each of the domains. IPAQ data have been validated using accelerometers, and reliability confirmed across various countries and different languages (Craig et al., 2003). Validation studies have also been conducted on individual questions which have demonstrated lower validity compared to the full questionnaire (van der Ploeg et al., 2010). The IPAQ has been known to overestimate PA compared to accelerometer data (Hagströmer et al., 2010). In a study involving 50 adults, almost half of the respondents reported participating in walking, moderate PA, or vigorous PA when they had not participated in any of them (Rzewnicki et al., 2003). Moreover, the IPAQ has been found to underestimate the strength of relationships between PA and cardiometabolic risk factors compared to accelerometers (Celis-Morales et al., 2012).

The IPAQ (long-form) has been modified for use in adolescents (IPAQ-A; Hagströmer et al., 2008), and used in various European studies (Bergier et al., 2012; Chillón et al., 2011; Vanhelst et al., 2013). Modest correlations between the IPAQ and accelerometry have been reported (Ottevaere et al., 2011). Hagströmer et al. (2008) found significant associations between the IPAQ-A and accelerometers for time spent walking, total PA and moderate and vigorous activities ($r = 0.17$–0.30) among 15–17 year olds, but no significant associations were observed for any of the studied variables for 12–14 year olds. This finding suggests that the IPAQ-A is not a valid measure of young adolescents' PA. Other studies have found that the IPAQ-A underestimates adolescent boys' MVPA relative to accelerometer-derived MVPA estimates (Raask et al., 2017). However, over- and underestimating PA is not limited to the IPAQ, it is a limitation of all self-report questionnaires, especially among children (Chinapaw et al., 2010; Helmerhorst et al., 2012).

Questionnaires hold additional limitations for children because of their lower cognitive, linguistic, and recall abilities (Chinapaw et al., 2010). When using questionnaires with children, it is recommended that questions are clearly structured, sequential, and unambiguous

(Jørgensen et al., 2013). Questionnaires that assess recall of recent PA types or frequencies rather than time spent in PA are known to yield greater accuracy in children (Biddle et al., 2011). The 7-day recall PA Questionnaire for Older Children (PAQ-C) (Kowalski, Crocker, & Donen, 2004) assesses general levels of PA in children aged 8 to 14 years and is the most commonly used child PA questionnaire (Biddle et al., 2011; Saint-Maurice et al., 2014; Thomas & Upton, 2014). While the PAQ-C score cannot be used to estimate PA frequency, duration, or intensity, it is a useful tool to classify active and low active children for surveillance and intervention research (Voss, Ogunleye, & Sandercock, 2013).

A key limitation of all PA questionnaires is their inability to accurately classify time spent in specific PA intensities such as MVPA, which prohibits discussion of a respondent's PA level relative to public health PA guidelines. A favourable approach for improving the accuracy of PA estimates obtained from questionnaires is to calibrate them against objective measures. Researchers have recently demonstrated the utility of calibrating self-report measures against accelerometers to convert questionnaire scores to time spent in PA and sedentary behaviour (Saint-Maurice et al. 2014; Saint-Maurice & Welk, 2014; 2015). Saint-Maurice and Welk (2014) found that the Youth Activity Profile (YAP) tool accurately estimated activity levels in groups of youth when calibrated against objective monitors (Saint-Maurice & Welk, 2015). More recently, YAP-predicted minutes of MVPA and sedentary behaviour provided similar group estimates to that of wrist-worn accelerometers (Saint-Maurice et al., 2017). The YAP therefore holds promise as an alternative to activity monitoring in large groups of youth in the future.

Questionnaires are generally administered in paper-based format but can also be completed electronically on computers or handheld devices. Computerised questionnaires have several advantages over paper-based questionnaires (e.g., cost and time saving, greater anonymity, reduced coding error, automatic data entry, immediate feedback; Warren et al., 2010) and offer great opportunity for large-scale surveillance studies (Bain et al., 2010; Mathew et al., 2011). Several validation studies have been conducted comparing computerised questionnaires with objective measures (Matton et al., 2007; Scheers et al., 2012; Vandelanotte et al., 2005). Scheers et al. (2012) found that all parameters of the Flemish PA computerised questionnaire (FPACQ) were significantly and positively correlated with SenseWear Armband outcomes ($r = 0.21$ to 0.65). However, FPACQ estimates of PA were higher and sedentary time lower compared to the SenseWear Armband data. Similarly, other studies have found acceptable validity for questionnaires when compared against objective accelerometer data even though the questionnaires overestimated PA estimates (Boon et al., 2010; Ekelund et al., 2006; Matton et al., 2007).

Global questionnaires are short, contain few items and are quick to complete. They provide a general measure of PA and are commonly used to classify individuals as active or inactive based on PA guidelines. The Global PA Questionnaire (GPAQ) comprises 16 questions that assess PA in three domains (work, transport, and leisure time) and sedentary time (Bull, Maslin, & Armstrong, 2009). The self-administered version has performed similarly to the interviewer-administered version (Chu et al., 2015), and has demonstrated acceptable reliability and validity in various studies (Herrmann et al., 2014; Hoos et al., 2012; Rivièrea et al., 2016; Wanner et al., 2017). Cleland et al. (2014) reported moderate agreement between the GPAQ and accelerometers for MVPA mins/day ($r = 0.48$) but poor agreement for sedentary behaviour ($r = 0.19$) suggesting that the GPAQ is an appropriate measure of MVPA but not sedentary behaviour. Although global questionnaires are quick to complete and provide little burden to respondents, they offer limited information regarding a person's PA pattern or the context within which their PA takes place.

Short-term recalls which include diaries and previous-day recalls (PDRs) have been recommended as an appropriate alternative to questionnaires (Matthews et al., 2013). Participants record the frequency and/or duration of activities as they occur and provide comprehensive characterisation of PA patterns. PA diaries have the potential to overcome the limitations of questionnaires which request retrospective long-term recall of PA. However, the experience of completing a PA diary can encourage the respondent to change (i.e., increase) their PA behaviour leading to biased estimates of PA. Furthermore, diaries place a significant burden on respondents, with them expected to complete multiple diary entries. Such a burden can lead to significant data loss from missing responses. Bouchard's PA record (B-PAR; Bouchard et al., 1983) is among the most widely used PA diary, and has been used with adults (Wickel, Welk, & Eisenmann, 2006) and adolescents (Martínez-Gómez et al. 2009; 2010). The diary records PA in 15 minute intervals over a period of three days, with activity intensity scored on a scale of 1 to 9 (1 = sedentary, 9 = intense manual work or high-intensity sports) to provide an overall total EE score expressed in METs or as kcal/kg/15 min.

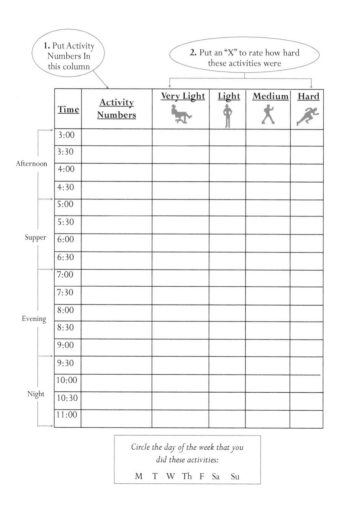

Figure 6.5   Example Previous Day PA Recall questionnaire format (Weston, Petosa, & Pate, 1997)

Other commonly used short-term recall instruments include the Previous Day PA Recall (PDPAR) (Figure 6.5), and the Three-Day PA Recall (3DPAR; Anderson, Hagströmer, & Yngve, 2005; Matthews et al. 2013; McBrearty et al. 2014). The PDPAR is designed specifically for use with young people. The number of recall days used in the Previous Day PA Recall can be increased or decreased based on the cognitive ability of the children. The PDPAR assesses activities undertaken in the after-school period of the previous day. The time between 3:00pm and 11:30pm is divided into 30-minute blocks and children are instructed to recall for each block, the type and intensity of PA undertaken. Clipart images depicting the different intensity categories are used to aid respondents rate the intensity of the reported activities. A major limitation of the PDPAR however, is that because only one activity is indicated per 30-minute block, PA levels are likely to be overestimated.

Recent advancements in mobile and sensor technologies allow for PA data to be collected in real time, across contexts (e.g., mode, type, and location). Ecological momentary assessment (EMA) collects momentary self-reports in situ via electronic diaries on mobile devices (i.e., smartphones or tablets; Robbins & Kubiak, 2014), but can also be collected using traditional pencil and paper format (Kanning & Schlicht, 2010; Rouse & Biddle, 2010). EMA has the potential to reduce recall errors and bias because it collects self-reports in real-time rather than retrospectively (Schwarz, 2007). Non-compliant behaviour, including backfilling and completing diaries in bulk, can also be overcome by deactivating prompt access to the electronic diary following a specific time window (Wen et al., 2017). EMA has been used in child (Dunton, Intille et al., 2012; 2014; Wen et al., 2017) and adult populations (Dunton, Liao et al., 2012; Liao, Intille, & Dunton, 2015; Pickering et al., 2016). Recently, Knell and colleagues (2017) found that EMA data collected using mobile phones showed better correlation and agreement to accelerometer assessed PA estimates than traditional self-report methods. However, there are some challenges and drawbacks to EMA such as battery drainage, software failure, reactivity, and participant burden which can limit the quality and quantity of data collected and complicate the data analysis process (Dunton, 2017).

In summary, despite their low administrative and processing costs, recall-based PA measures have several limitations. Most notably, they are attributable to social desirability bias and frequently over- and underestimate time spent engaged in activity compared to objective measures (Adamo et al., 2009; Troiano et al., 2008). A further limitation of many self-report measures is that they are sensitive to changes in PA behaviour during interventions and are instead more suitable for assessing PA prevalence in the population (Sallis, 2010; Taber et al., 2009). However, presently they are the only field measure able to capture the mode and the context of PA. These attributes can offset the limitations described above.

Chapter summary

- PA researchers have a wide range of measurement tools at their disposal but this degree of choice can present challenges when trying to select the most appropriate method
- Researchers' decision making should be driven by the characteristics of the project design (e.g., population [e.g., pre-schoolers, adults], planned PA outcomes [e.g., volume of PA undertaken, time spent in MVPA during school hours], study type [e.g., surveillance, intervention], and available resources [e.g., available funding, staffing]), as well as an understanding of the strengths and weaknesses of each method

- Accuracy of the chosen method should be balanced against its ease of use in the context of the target population and the available resources
- Researcher expertise in the preparation, administration, and data processing is essential, irrespective of the measurement method and only trained individuals should undertake these tasks
- Combining methods may be appropriate in some studies, particularly where there are multiple planned PA outcomes

References

Adamo, K.B., Prince, S.A., Tricco, A.C., Connor-Gorber, S., & Tremblay, M. (2009). A comparison of indirect versus direct measures for assessing physical activity in the pediatric population: a systematic review. *International Journal of Pediatric Obesity, 4*, 2–27.

Ainsworth, B.E., Caspersen, C.J., Matthews, C.E., Mâsse, L.C., Baranowski, T., & Zhu, W. (2012). Recommendations to improve the accuracy of estimates of physical activity derived from self report. *Journal of Physical Activity and Health, 9*(01), S76–S84.

Ainsworth, B.E., Haskell, W.L., Whitt, M.C., Irwin, M.L., Swartz, A.M., Strath, S.J., . . . Leon, A.S. (2000). Compendium of physical activities: an update of activity codes and MET intensities. *Medicine and Science in Sports and Exercise, 32*(9), S498–S516.

Anderson, C.B., Hagströmer, M., & Yngve, A. (2005). Validation of the PDPAR as an adolescent diary: effect of accelerometer cut points. *Medicine and Science in Sports and Exercise, 37*(7), 1224–1230.

Angelopoulos, P.D., Milionis, H.J., Grammatikaki, E., Moschonis, G., & Manios, Y. (2009). Changes in BMI and blood pressure after a school based intervention: the CHILDREN study. *European Journal of Public Health, 19*(3), 319–325.

Armstrong, N. (1998). Young people's physical activity patterns as assessed by heart rate monitoring. *Journal of Sports Sciences, 16*, S9–S16.

Bai, Y., Chen, S., Laurson, K.R., Kim, Y., Saint-Maurice, P.F., & Welk, G.J. (2016). The Associations of Youth Physical Activity and Screen Time with Fatness and Fitness: The 2012 NHANES National Youth Fitness Survey. *PLoS ONE, 11*(1): e0148038.

Bain, T.M., Frierson, G.M., Trudelle-Jackson, E., & Morrow, J.R. Jr., (2010). Internet reporting of weekly physical activity behaviors: The WIN Study. *Journal of Physical Activity and Health, 7*, 527–532.

Baquet, G., Stratton, G., Van Praagh, E., & Berthoin, S. (2007). Improving physical activity assessment in prepubertal childen with high-frequency accelerometry monitoring: a methodological issue. *Preventive Medicine, 44*, 143–147.

Bassett, D.R., & Strath, S.J. (2002). Use of pedometers to assess physical activity. In G. Welk (Ed.), *Physical Activity Assessments for Health-Related Research* (pp. 163–177). Champaign, IL: Human Kinetics.

Beets, M.W., Morgan, C.F., Banda, J.A., Bornstein, D., Byun, W., Mitchell, J., . . . Erwin, H. (2011). Convergent validity of pedometer and accelerometer estimates of moderate-to-vigorous physical activity of youth. *Journal of Physical Activity and Health, 8 Suppl 2*, S295–S305.

Bergier, J., Kapka-Skrzypczak, L., Biliński, P., Paprzycki, P., & Wojtyła, A. (2012). Physical activity of Polish adolescents and young adults according to IPAQ: a population based study. *Annals of Agricultural and Environmental Medicine, 19*(1), 109–115.

Biddle, S.J.H., Gorely, T., Pearson, N., & Bull, F.C. (2011). An assessment of self-reported physical activity instruments in young people for population surveillance: Project ALPHA. *International Journal of Behavioral Nutrition and Physical Activity, 8*, 1.

Boon, R.M., Hamlin, M.J., Steel, G.D., & Ross, J.J. (2010). Validation of the New Zealand Physical Activity Questionnaire (NZPAQ-LF) and the International Physical Activity Questionnaire (IPAQ-LF) with accelerometry. *British Journal of Sports Medicine, 44*, 741–746.

Bouchard, C., Tremblay, A., Leblanc, C., Lortie, G., Savard, R., & Thériault, G. (1983). A method to assess energy expenditure in children and adults. *American Journal of Clinical Nutrition, 37*(3), 461–467.

Brage, S., Brage, N., Franks, P.W., Ekelund, U., Wong, M.-Y., Andersen, L.B., . . . Wareham, N.J. (2004). Branched equation modelling of simultaneous accelerometry and heart rate monitoring improves estimate of directly measured physical activity energy expenditure. *Journal of Applied Physiology, 96*, 343–351.

Brage, S., Westgate, K., Franks, P.W., Stegle, O., Wright, A., Ekelund, U., & Wareham, N.J. (2015) Estimation of free-living energy expenditure by heart rate and movement sensing: a doubly-labelled water study. *PLoS ONE*. https://doi.org/10.1371/journal.pone.0137206.

Bravata, D.M., Smith-Spangler, C., Sundaram, V., Gienger, A.L., Lin, N., Lewis, R., . . . Sirard, J.R. (2007). Using pedometers to increase physical activity and improve health: a systematic review. *JAMA, 298*(19), 2296–2304. doi:10.1001/jama.298.19.2296.

Bull, F.C., Maslin, T.S., & Armstrong, T. (2009). Global physical activity questionnaire (GPAQ): nine country reliability and validity study. *Journal of Physical Activity and Health, 6*(6), 790–804.

Butte, N., Wong, W. Adolph, A., Puyau, M., Vohra, F. & Zakeri, I. (2010). Validation of cross-sectional time series and multivariate adaptive regression splines models for the prediction of energy expenditure in children and adolescents using doubly labeled water. *J. Nutr., 140*, 1516–1523.

Byrom, B., Stratton, G., McCarthy, M., & Muehlhausen, W. (2016). Objective measurement of sedentary behaviour using accelerometers. *International Journal of Obesity*. doi:10.1038/ijo.2016.136.

Calabró, M.A., Stewart, J.M., & Welk, G.J. (2013). Validation of pattern-recognition monitors in children using doubly labeled water. *Med Sci Sports Exerc, 45*(7), 1313–1322. doi: 10.1249/MSS. 0b013e31828579c3.

Calabró, M.A., Welk, G.J., & Eisenmann, J.C. (2009). Validation of the SenseWear Pro Armband algorithms in children. *Medicine and Science in Sports and Exercise, 41*(9), 1714–1720.

Casiraghi, F., Lertwattanarak, R., Luzi, L., Chavez, A.O., Davalli, A.M., Naegelin, T., . . . Folli, F. (2013). Energy expenditure evaluation in humans and non-human primates by SenseWear Armband. Validation of energy expenditure evaluation by SenseWear Armband by direct comparison with indirect calorimetry. *PLoS ONE, 8*(9), e73651. doi:10.1371/journal.pone.0073651.

Casperson, C.J., Powell, K.E., & Christenson, G.M. (1985). Physical activity, exercise, and physical fitness: definitions and distinctions for health-related research. *Public Health Reports, 100*, 126–131.

Celis-Morales, C.A., Perez-Bravo, F., Ibañez, L., Salas, C., Bailey, M.E.S., & Gill, J.M.R. (2012). Objective vs. self-reported physical activity and sedentary time: effects of measurement method on relationships with risk biomarkers. *PLoS ONE, 7*(5), e36345.

Chillón, P., Ortega, F.B., Ruiz, J.R., De Bourdeaudhuij, I., Martínez-Gómez, D., Vicente-Rodriguez, G., . . . HELENA study group. (2011). Active commuting and physical activity in adolescents from Europe: results from the HELENA study. *Pediatric Exercise Science, 23*(2), 207–217.

Chinapaw, M.J.M., Mokkink, L.B., van Poppel, M.N.M., van Mechelen, W., & Terwee, C.B. (2010). Physical activity questionnaires for youth: a systematic review of measurement properties. *Sports Medicine, 40*(7), 539–563.

Chowdhury, E.A., Western, M.J., Nightingale, T.E., Peacock, O.J., & Thompson, D. (2017). Assessment of laboratory and daily energy expenditure estimates from consumer multi-sensor physical activity monitors. *PLoS ONE, 12*(2), e0171720. doi:10.1371/journal.pone.0171720.

Chu, A.H.Y., Ng, S.H.X., Koh, D., & Müller-Riemenschneider, F. (2015). Reliability and validity of the self- and interviewer-administered versions of the Global Physical Activity Questionnaire (GPAQ). *PLoS ONE, 10*(9), e0136944.

Clark, C.C.T., Barnes, C.M., Stratton, G., McNarry, M.A., Mackintosh, K.A., & Summers, H.D. (2016). A review of emerging analytical techniques for objective physical activity measurement in humans. *Sports Medicine*, 1–9. doi:10.1007/s40279-016-0585-y.

Cleland, C.L., Hunter, R.F., Kee, F., Cupples, M.E., Sallis, J.F., & Tully, M.A. (2014). Validity of the Global Physical Activity Questionnaire (GPAQ) in assessing levels and change in moderate-vigorous physical activity and sedentary behaviour. *BMC Public Health,* 14:1255.

Clemes, S.A., & Deans, N.K. (2012). Presence and duration of reactivity to pedometers in adults. *Medicine and Science in Sports and Exercise, 44*(6), 1097–1101.

Cooper, A., Page, A., Wheeler, B., Hillsdon, M., Griew, P., & Jago, R. (2010). Patterns of GPS measured time outdoors after school and objective physical activity in English children: the PEACH project. *International Journal of Behavioral Nutrition and Physical Activity, 7*, 31.

Cooper, J.A., Watras, A.C., O'Brien, M.J., Luke, A., Dobratz, J.R., Earthman, C.P., & Schoeller, D.A. (2009). Assessing validity and reliability of resting metabolic rate in six gas analysis systems. *J Am Diet Assoc, 109*(1), 128–132. doi:10.1016/j.jada.2008.10.004.

Costa, S., Barber, S.E., Griffiths, P.L., Cameron, N., & Clemes, S.A. (2013). Qualitative feasibility of using three accelerometers with 2–3-year-old children and both parents. *Research Quarterly for Exercise and Sport, 84*(3), 295–304.

Craig, C.L., Marshall, A.L., Sjöström M., Bauman, A.E., Booth, M.L., Ainsworth, B.E., . . . Oja, P. (2003). International Physical Activity Questionnaire: 12-country reliability and validity. *Medicine and Science in Sports and Exercise, 35*, 1381–1395.

Dac Minh Tuan, N., Lecoultre, V., Sunami, Y., & Schutz, Y. (2013). Assessment of physical activity and energy expenditure by GPS combined with accelerometry in real-life conditions. *Journal of Physical Activity and Health, 10*(6), 880–888.

Dai, S., Carroll, D.D., Watson, K.B., Paul, P., Carlson, S.A., & Fulton, J.E. (2015). Participation in types of physical activities among US Adults—National Health and Nutrition Examination Survey 1999–2006. *Journal of Physical Activity and Health, 12*(1), S128–S140.

De Vries, S.I., Garre, F.G., Engbers, L.H., Hildebrandt, V.H., & Van Buuren, S. (2011). Evaluation of neural networks to identify types of activity using accelerometers. *Medicine and Science in Sports and Exercise, 43*(1), 101–107.

Doherty, A.R., Hodges, S.E., King, A.C., Smeaton, A.F., Berry, E., Moulin, C.J.A., . . . Foster, C. (2013). Wearable cameras in health: the state of the art and future possibilities. *American Journal of Preventive Medicine, 44*(3), 320–323.

Doherty, A.R., Jackson, D., Hammerla, N., Plötz, T., Olivier, P., Granat, M.H., . . . Wareham, N.J. (2017). Large scale population assessment of physical activity using wrist worn accelerometers: the UK Biobank Study. *PLoS ONE, 12*(2), e0169649. doi:10.1371/journal.pone.0169649.

Doherty, A.R., Kelly, P., Kerr, J., Marshall, S., Oliver, M., Badland, H., . . . Foster, C. (2013). Using wearable cameras to categorise type and context of accelerometer-identified episodes of physical activity. *International Journal of Behavioral Nutrition and Physical Activity, 10*(1), 22.

Dollman, J., Okely, A.D., Hardy, L., Timperio, A., Salmon, J., & Hills, A.P. (2009). A hitchhiker's guide to assessing young people's physical activity: deciding what method to use. *Journal of Science and Medicine in Sport, 12*(5), 518–525.

Dunton, G.F. (2017). Ecological momentary assessment in physical activity research. *Exercise and Sport Sciences Reviews, 45*(1), 48–54.

Dunton, G.F., Huh, J., Leventhal, A., Riggs, N., Spruijt-Metz, D., Pentz, M.A., & Hedeker, D. (2014). Momentary assessment of affect, physical feeling states, and physical activity in children. *Health Psychology, 33*(3), 255–263.

Dunton, G.F., Intille, S.S., Wolch, J., & Pentz, M.A. (2012). Children's perceptions of physical activity environments captured through ecological momentary assessment: a validation study. *Preventive Medicine, 55*, 119–121.

Dunton, G.F., Liao, Y., Kawabata, K., & Intille, S. (2012). Momentary assessment of adults' physical activity and sedentary behavior: feasibility and validity. *Frontiers in Psychology, 3*:260.

Dwyer-Lindgren, L., Freedman, G., Engell, R.E., Fleming, T.D., Lim, S.S., Murray, C.J.L., & Mokdad, A.H. (2013). Prevalence of physical activity and obesity in US counties, 2001–2011: a road map for action. *Population Health Metrics, 11*:7.

Ekelund, U., Sepp, H., Brage, S., Becker, W., Jakes, R., Hennings, M., & Wareham, N.J. (2006). Criterion-related validity of the last 7-day, short form of the International Physical Activity Questionnaire in Swedish adults. *Public Health Nutrition, 9*, 258–265.

Ekelund, U., Sjöström, M., Yngve, A., Poortviet, E., Nilsson, A., Froberg, K., Wedderkopp, N., & Westerterp, K.R. (2001). Physical activity assessed by activity monitor and doubly labeled water in children. *Medicine and Science in Sports and Exercise, 33*(2), 275–281.

Evenson, K., Goto, M., & Furberg, R. (2015). Systematic review of the validity and reliability of consumer-wearable activity trackers. *International Journal of Behavioral Nutrition and Physical Activity, 12*(1), 159.

Fairclough, S.J., Noonan, R., Rowlands, A.V., Van Hees, V., Knowles, Z., & Boddy, L.M. (2016). Wear compliance and activity in children wearing wrist- and hip-mounted accelerometers. *Medicine and Science in Sports and Exercise, 48*(2), 245–253.

Freedson, P.S., Bowles, H.R., Troiano, R., & Haskell, W. (2012). Assessment of physical activity using wearable monitors: recommendations for monitor calibration and use in the field. *Med Sci Sports Exerc, 44*(1 Suppl 1), S1–S4.

Freedson, P.S., Melanson, E., & Sirard, J. (1998). Calibration of the Computer Science and Applications, Inc. accelerometer. *Medicine and Science in Sports and Exercise, 30*(5), 777–781.

Gomersall, S.R., Ng, N., Burton, N.W., Pavey, T.G., Gilson, N.D., & Brown, W.J. (2016). Estimating physical activity and sedentary behavior in a free-living context: a pragmatic comparison of consumer-based activity trackers and ActiGraph accelerometry. *Journal of Medical Internet Research, 18*(9), e239. doi:10.2196/jmir.5531.

Gore, C. (Ed.) (2000). *Quality Assurance in Exercise Physiology Laboratories: Physiological Testing for Elite Athletes.* Champaign, IL: Human Kinetics.

Green, J. (2009). 'Walk this way': public health and the social organization of walking, *Social Theory & Health, 7*, 20–38.

Gurrin, C., Qiu, Z., Hughes, M., Caprani, N., Doherty, A.R., Hodges, S.E., & Smeaton, A.F. (2013). The smartphone as a platform for wearable cameras in health research. *American Journal of Preventive Medicine, 44*(3), 308–313.

Hagströmer, M., Ainsworth, B.E., Oja, P., & Sjöström, M. (2010). Comparison of a subjective and an objective measure of physical activity in a population sample. *Journal of Physical Activity and Health, 7*, 541–550.

Hagströmer, M., von Berlepsch, J., Phillipp, K., Ortega, F.B., Sjöström, M., Ruiz, J.R., . . . HELENA study group. (2008). Concurrent validity of a modified version of the International Physical Activity Questionnaire (IPAQ-A) in European adolescents: the HELENA study. *International Journal of Obesity, 32*(Suppl 5), S42–S48.

Ham, S.A., Kruger, J., & Tudor-Locke, C. (2009). Participation by US adults in sports, exercise, and recreational physical activities. *Journal of Physical Activity and Health, 6*, 6–14.

Hansen, A.W., Grønbæk, M., Helge, J.W., Severin, M., Curtis, T., & Tolstrup, J.S. (2012). Effect of a web-based intervention to promote physical activity and improve health among physically inactive adults: a population-based randomized controlled trial. *Journal of Medical Internet Research, 14*(5):e145.

Harrell, J.S., McMurray, R.G., Baggett, C.D., Pennell, M.L., Pearce, P.F., & Bangdiwala, S.I. (2005). Energy costs of physical activities in children and adolescents. *Medicine and Science in Sports and Exercise, 37*(2), 329–336.

Harrison, F., Atkin, A.J., van Sluijs, E.M.F., & Jones, A.P. (2017). Seasonality in swimming and cycling: exploring a limitation of accelerometer based studies. *Preventive Medicine Reports, 7*, 16–19.

Haskell, W.L. (2012). Physical activity by self-report: a brief history and future issues. *Journal of Physical Activity and Health, 9*(Suppl1), S5–S10.

Helmerhorst, H.J.F., Brage, S., Warren, J., Besson, H., & Ekelund, U. (2012). A systematic review of reliability and objective criterion-related validity of physical activity questionnaires. *International Journal of Behavioral Nutrition and Physical Activity, 9*, 103.

Herrmann, S.D., Heumann, K.J., Der Ananian, C.A., & Ainsworth, B.E. (2014). Validity and reliability of the Global Physical Activity Questionnaire (GPAQ). *Measurement in Physical Education and Exercise Science, 17*(3), 221–235.

Hesketh, K., McMinn, A., Ekelund, U., Sharp, S., Collings, P., Harvey, N., . . . van Sluijs, E. (2014). Objectively measured physical activity in four-year-old British children: a cross-sectional analysis of activity patterns segmented across the day. *International Journal of Behavioral Nutrition and Physical Activity, 11*(1), 1.

Hills, A.P., Mokhtar, N., & Byrne, N.M. (2014). Assessment of physical activity and energy expenditure: an overview of objective measures. *Frontiers in Nutrition, 1.* doi:10.3389/fnut.2014.00005.

Hollis, J.L., Williams, A.J., Sutherland, R., Campbell, E., Nathan, N., Wolfenden, L., . . . Wiggers, J. (2016). A systematic review and meta-analysis of moderate-to-vigorous physical activity levels in elementary school physical education lessons. *Preventive Medicine, 86*, 34–54.

Hoos, M.B., Plasqui, G., Gerver, W.J., & Westerterp, K.R. (2003). Physical activity level measured by doubly labeled water and accelerometry in children. *Eur J Appl Physiol., 89*(6), 624–626.

Hoos, T., Espinoza, N., Marshall, S., & Arredondo, E.M. (2012). Validity of the Global Physical Activity Questionnaire (GPAQ) in adult Latinas. *Journal of Physical Activity and Health, 9*(5), 698–705.

Hurtig-Wennlof, A., Hagströmer, M., & Olsson, L.A. (2010). The International Physical Activity Questionnaire modified for the elderly: aspects of validity and feasibility. *Public Health Nutrition, 13*(11), 1847–1854.

Jakovljevic, D.G., Nunan, D., Donovan, G., Hodges, L.D., Sandercock, G.R.H., & Brodie, D.A. (2008). Lack of agreement between gas exchange variables measured by two metabolic systems. *Journal of Sports Science and Medicine, 7*, 15–22.

Janz, K.F. (2002). Use of heart rate monitors to assess physical activity. In G.J. Welk (Ed.), *Physical Activity Assessments for Health-Related Research* (pp. 143–162). Champaign, IL: Human Kinetics.

Jørgensen, M.E., Sørensen, M.R., Ekholm, O., & Rasmussen, N.K. (2013). Importance of questionnaire context for a physical activity question. *Scandinavian Journal of Medicine & Science in Sports, 23*(5), 651–656.

Kang, M., & Rowe, D.A. (2015). Issues and challenges in sedentary behavior measurement. *Measurement in Physical Education and Exercise Science, 19*(3), 105–115.

Kanning, M., & Schlicht, W.J. (2010). Be active and become happy: an ecological momentary assessment of physical activity and mood. *Journal of Sport and Exercise Psychology, 32*(2), 253–261.

Karvonen, J., & Vuorimaa, T. (1988). Heart rate and exercise intensity during sports activities. *Sports Medicine, 5*, 303–312.

Karvonen, M., Kentela, E., & Mustala, O. (1957). The effects of training heart rate: a longitudinal study. *Annales Medicinae Experimentalis et Biologiae Fennae, 35*, 307–315.

Kelly, P., Marshall, S.J., Badland, H., Kerr, J., Oliver, M., Doherty, A.R., & Foster, C. (2013). An ethical framework for automated, wearable cameras in health behavior research. *American Journal of Preventive Medicine, 44*(3), 314–319.

Kerr, J., Marshall, S.J., Godbole, S., Chen, J., Legge, A., Doherty, A.R., . . . Foster, C. (2013). Using the SenseCam to improve classifications of sedentary behavior in free-living settings. *American Journal of Preventive Medicine, 44*(3), 290–296.

Kim, Y., Hibbing, P., Saint-Maurice, P.F., Ellingson, L.D., Hennessy, E., Wolff-Hughes, D.L., . . . Welk, G.J. (2017). Surveillance of youth physical activity and sedentary behavior with wrist accelerometry. *American Journal of Preventive Medicine, 52*(6), 872–879.

Knaeps, S., Bourgois, J.G., Charlier, R., Mertens, E., Lefevre, J., & Wijndaele, K., (2016). Ten-year change in sedentary behaviour, moderate-to-vigorous physical activity, cardiorespiratory fitness and cardiometabolic risk: independent associations and mediation analysis. *British Journal of Sports Medicine*, doi: 10.1136/bjsports-2016-096083.

Knell, G., Gabriel, K.P., Businelle, M.S., Shuval, K., Wetter, D.W., & Kendzor, D.E. (2017). Ecological momentary assessment of physical activity: validation study. *Journal of Medical Internet Research, 19*, 7, e253.

Kooiman, T.J.M., Dontje, M.L., Sprenger, S.R., Krijnen, W.P., van der Schans, C.P., & de Groot, M. (2015). Reliability and validity of ten consumer activity trackers. *BMC Sports Science, Medicine and Rehabilitation, 7*, 24.

Kowalski, K.C., Crocker, P.R.E., & Donen, R.M. (2004). *The Physical Activity Questionnaire for Older Children (PAQ-C) and Adolescents (PAQ-A) Manual*. Saskatoon, SK, Canada: University of Saskatchewan.

Lacey, B., Golledge, J., Yeap, B.B., Lewington, S., Norman, P.E., Flicker, L., . . . Hankey, G.J. (2015). Physical activity and vascular disease in a prospective cohort study of older men: the Health In Men Study (HIMS). *BMC Geriatrics, 15*, 164.

Lee, P.H., Macfarlane, D.J., Lam, T.H., & Stewart, S.M. (2011). Validity of the International Physical Activity Questionnaire Short Form (IPAQ-SF): a systematic review. *International Journal of Behavioral Nutrition and Physical Activity, 8*, 115.

Liao, Y., Intille, S.S., & Dunton, G.F. (2015). Using ecological momentary assessment to understand where and with whom adults' physical and sedentary activity occur. *International Journal of Behavioral Medicine, 22*(1), 51–61.

Loveday, A., Sherar, L.B., Sanders, J.P., Sanderson, P.W., & Esliger, D.W. (2016). Novel technology to help understand the context of physical activity and sedentary behaviour. *Physiological Measurement, 37*(10), 1834–1851.

Macera, C.A., Ham, S.A., Yore, M.M., Jones, D.A., Ainsworth, B.E., Kimsey, C.D., & Kohl, H.W. 3rd. (2005). Prevalence of physical activity in the United States: Behavioral Risk Factor Surveillance System, 2001. *Preventing Chronic Disease, 2*(2), A17.

Macfarlane, D.J., & Wong, P. (2012). Validity, reliability and stability of the portable Cortex Metamax 3B gas analysis system. *Eur J Appl Physiol, 112*(7), 2539–2547. doi: 10.1007/s00421-011-2230-7.

Mackintosh, K.A., Fairclough, S.J., Stratton, G., & Ridgers, N.D. (2012). A calibration protocol for population-specific accelerometer cut-points in children. *PLoS ONE, 7*(5), e36919.

Martínez-Gómez, D., Puertollano, M.A., Wärnberg, J., Calabró, M.A., Welk, G.J., Sjöström, M., Veiga, O.L., & Marcos, A. (2009). Comparison of the ActiGraph accelerometer and Bouchard diary to estimate energy expenditure in Spanish adolescents. *Nutricion Hospitalaria, 24*(6), 701–710.

Martínez-Gómez, D., Wärnberg, J., Welk, G.J., Sjöström, M, Veiga, O.L., & Marcos, A. (2010). Validity of the Bouchard activity diary in Spanish adolescents. *Public Health Nutrition, 13*(2), 261–268.

Mathew, M., Morrow J.R. Jr., Frierson, G.M., & Bain, T.M. (2011). Assessing digital literacy in web-based physical activity surveillance: The WIN Study. *American Journal of Health Promotion, 26*(2), 90–95.

Matthews, C.E., Keadle, S.K., Sampson, J., Lyden, K., Bowles, H.R., Moore, S.C., . . . Fowke, J.H. (2013). Validation of a previous-day recall measure of active and sedentary behaviors. *Medicine and Science in Sports and Exercise, 45*(8), 1629–1638.

Matton, L., Wijndaele, K., Duvigneaud, N., Duquet, W., Philippaerts, R., Thomis, M., & Lefevre, J. (2007). Reliability and validity of the Flemish Physical Activity Computerized Questionnaire in adults. *Research Quarterly for Exercise and Sport, 78*(4), 293–306.

McBrearty, D., McCrorie, P., Granat, M., Duncan, E., & Stansfield, B. (2014). Objective assessment of intensity categorization of the previous day physical activity recall questionnaire in 11–13 year old children. *Physiological Measurement, 35*(11), 2329–2342.

McKenzie, T.L. (2002). Use of direct observation to assess physical activity. In G.J. Welk (Ed.), *Physical Activity Assessments for Health-Related Research* (pp. 179–195). Champaign, IL: Human Kinetics.

McKenzie, T.L. (2010). 2009 C.H. McCloy Lecture. Seeing is believing: observing physical activity and its contexts. *Research Quarterly for Exercise and Sport, 81*(2), 113–122.

McKenzie, T.L., Cohen, D.A., Sehgal, A., Williamson, S., & Golinelli, D. (2006). System for Observing Play and Recreation in Communities (SOPARC): reliability and feasibility measures. *Journal of Physical Activity and Health, 3 Suppl 1*, S208–S222.

McKenzie, T.L., Marshall, S., Sallis, J.F., & Conway, T.L. (2000). Leisure-time physical activity in school environments: an observational study using SOPLAY. *Preventive Medicine, 30*, 70–77.

McKenzie, T.L., Sallis, J.F., & Nader, P.R. (1991). SOFIT: System for Observing Fitness Instruction Time. *Journal of Teaching in Physical Education, 11*, 195–205.

McKenzie, T.L., & van der Mars, H. (2015). Top 10 research questions related to assessing physical activity and its contexts using systematic observation. *Research Quarterly for Exercise and Sport, 86*(1), 13–29.

McNeil, D.A., Wilson, B.N., Siever, J.E., Ronca, M., & Mah, J.K. (2009). Connecting children to recreational activities: results of a cluster randomized trial. *American Journal of Health Promotion, 23*(6), 376–387.

Migueles, J.H., Cadenas-Sanchez, C., Ekelund, U., Delisle Nyström, C., Mora-Gonzalez, J., Löf, M., . . . Ortega, F.B. (2017). Accelerometer data collection and processing criteria to assess physical activity and other outcomes: a systematic review and practical considerations. *Sports Medicine,* 1–25. doi:10.1007/s40279-017-0716-0.

Mindell, J., Biddulph, J.P., Hirani, V., Stamatakis, E., Craig, R., Nunn, S., & Shelton, N. (2012). Cohort profile: The Health Survey for England. *International Journal of Epidemiology, 41*(6), 1585–1593.

Murakami, H., Kawakami, R., Nakae, S., . . . Miyachi, M. (2016). Accuracy of wearable devices for estimating total energy expenditure: comparison with metabolic chamber and doubly labeled water method. *JAMA Internal Medicine, 176*(5), 702–703.

Nelson, M.B., Kaminsky, L.A., Dickin, D.C., & Montoye, A.H.K. (2016). Validity of consumer-based physical activity monitors for specific activity types. *Medicine and Science in Sports and Exercise, 48*(8), 1619–1628.

Ottevaere, C., Huybrechts, I., De Meester, F., De Bourdeaudhuij, I., Cuenca-Garcia, M., & De Henauw, S. (2011). The use of accelerometry in adolescents and its implementation with non-wear time activity diaries in free-living conditions. *Journal of Sports Sciences, 29*, 103–113.

Phillips, L.R., Parfitt, G., & Rowlands, A.V. (2013). Calibration of the GENEA accelerometer for assessment of physical activity intensity in children. *Journal of Science and Medicine in Sport, 16*(2), 124–128.

Pickering, T.A., Huh, J., Intille, S., Liao, Y., Pentz, M.A., & Dunton, G.F. (2016). Physical activity and variation in momentary behavioral cognitions: an ecological momentary assessment study. *Journal of Physical Activity and Health, 13*(3), 344–351.

Plasqui, G., Bonomi, A.G., & Westerterp, K.R. (2013). Daily physical activity assessment with accelerometers: new insights and validation studies. *Obesity Reviews, 14*(6), 451–462.

Raask, T., Maestu, J., Latt, E., Jurimae, J., Jurimae, T., Vainik, U., & Konstabel, K. (2017). Comparison of IPAQ-SF and two other physical activity questionnaires with accelerometer in adolescent boys. *PLoS ONE, 12*(1), e0169527.

Reece, J.D., Barry, V., Fuller, D.K., & Caputo, J. (2015). Validation of the SenseWear Armband as a measure of sedentary behavior and light activity. *Journal of Physical Activity and Health, 12*(9), 1229–1237.

Ridgers, N.D., McNarry, A.M., & Mackintosh, A.K. (2016). Feasibility and effectiveness of using wearable activity trackers in youth: a systematic review. *JMIR Mhealth Uhealth, 4*(4), e129. doi:10.2196/mhealth.6540

Ridgers, N.D., Stratton, G., & McKenzie, T.L. (2010). Reliability and validity of the System for Observing Children's Activity and Relationships During Play (SOCARP). *Journal of Physical Activity and Health, 7*(1), 17–25.

Rivièrea, F., Widad, F.Z., Speyer, E. Erpelding, M.L., Escalon, H. & Vuillemin, A. (2016). Reliability and validity of the French version of the global physical activity questionnaire. *Journal of Sport and Health Science,* doi.org/10.1016/j.jshs.2016.08.004.

Robbins, M.L., & Kubiak, T. (2014). Ecological momentary assessment in behavioral medicine. In D.I. Mostovsky (Ed.), *The Handbook of Behavioral Medicine, I* (pp. 429–446). Hoboken, NJ: John Wiley & Sons.

Rothney, M.P., Schaefer, E.V., Neumann, M.M., Choi, L., & Chen, K.Y. (2008). Validity of physical activity intensity predictions by ActiGraph, Actical, and RT3 accelerometers. *Obesity* (Silver Spring), 16(8), 1946–1952. doi: 10.1038/oby.2008.279.

Rouse, P.C., & Biddle, S.J.H. (2010). An ecological momentary assessment of the physical activity and sedentary behaviour patterns of university students. *Health Education Journal, 69*(1), 116–125.

Rowe, D.A., & Kang, M. (2015). "Don't just sit there – do something!" – the measurement of sedentary behavior. *Measurement in Physical Education and Exercise Science, 19*(3), 103–104.

Rowlands, A.V., Fraysse, F., Catt, M., Stiles, V.H., Stanley, R.M., Eston, R.G., & Olds, T.S. (2015). Comparability of measured acceleration from accelerometry-based activity monitors. *Medicine and Science in Sports and Exercise, 47*, 201–210.

Rzewnicki, R., Vanden Auweele, Y., & De Bourdeaudhuij, I. (2003). Addressing overreporting on the International Physical Activity Questionnaire (IPAQ) telephone survey with a population sample. *Public Health Nutrition, 6*(3), 299–305.

Saint-Maurice, P.F., Kim, Y., Hibbing, P., Oh, Y., Perna, F.M., Welk, G.J. (2017). Calibration and validation of the youth activity profile: The FLASHE Study. *American Journal of Preventive Medicine, 52*(6), 880–887.

Saint-Maurice, P.F., & Welk, G.J. (2014). Web-based assessments of physical activity in youth: considerations for design and scale calibration. *Journal of Medical Internet Research, 16*(12), e269.

Saint-Maurice, P.F., & Welk, G.J. (2015). Validity and calibration of the youth activity profile. *PLoS ONE, 10*(12), e0143949.

Saint-Maurice, P.F., Welk, G.J., Beyler, N.K., Bartee, R.T., & Heelan, K.A. (2014). Calibration of self-report tools for physical activity research: the Physical Activity Questionnaire (PAQ). *BMC Public Health, 14*, 461.

Saint-Maurice, P.F., Welk, G., Ihmels, M.A., & Krapfl, J.R. (2011). Validation of the SOPLAY direct observation tool with an accelerometry-based physical activity monitor. *Journal of Physical Activity and Health, 8*(8), 1108–1116.

Sallis, J.F. (2010). Measuring physical activity: practical approaches for program evaluation in Native American communities. *Journal of Public Health Management and Practice, 16*(5), 404–410.

Sasaki, J.E., Howe, C.A., John, D., Hickey, A., Steeves, J., Conger, S., Lyden, K., Kozey-Keadle, S., Burkart, S., Alhassan, S., Bassett Jr, D., & Freedson, P.S. (2016). Energy expenditure for 70 activities in children and adolescents. *Journal of Physical Activity and Health, 13* (Suppl 1), S24–S28 http://dx.doi.org/10.1123/jpah.2015-0712.

Scheers, T., Philippaerts, R., & Lefevre, J. (2012). Assessment of physical activity and inactivity in multiple domains of daily life: a comparison between a computerized questionnaire and the SenseWear Armband complemented with an electronic diary. *International Journal of Behavioral Nutrition and Physical Activity, 9*, 71.

Schrack, J.A., Cooper, R., Koster, A., Shiroma, E.J., Murabito, J.M., Rejeski, W.J., . . . Harris, T.B. (2016). Assessing daily physical activity in older adults: unraveling the complexity of monitors, measures, and methods. *The Journals of Gerontology: Series A, 71*(8), 1039–1048.

Schutz, Y., Weinsier, R.L., & Hunter, G.R. (2001). Assessment of free-living physical activity in humans: an overview of currently available and proposed new measures. *Obesity Research, 9*(6), 368–379.

Schwarz, N. (2007). Retrospective and concurrent self-reports: the rationale for real time data capture. In A.S. Stone, S.S. Shiffman, A. Atienza, & L. Nebeling (Eds.) *The Science of Real-time Data Capture: Self-report in Health Research.* New York (NY): Oxford University Press.

Sievänen, H., & Kujala, U.M. (2017). Accelerometry—simple, but challenging. *Scandinavian Journal of Medicine & Science in Sports, 27*(6), 574–578.

Silsbury, Z, Goldsmith, R., & Rushton, A. (2015). Systematic review of the measurement properties of self-report physical activity questionnaires in healthy adult populations. *BMJ Open, 5*:e008430.

Sylvia, L.G., Bernstein, E.E., Hubbard, J.L., Keating, L., & Anderson, E.J. (2014). A practical guide to measuring physical activity. *Journal of the Academy of Nutrition and Dietetics, 114*(2), 199–208.

Taber, D.R., Stevens, J., Murray, D.M., Elder, J.P., Webber, L.S., Jobe, J.B., & Lytle, L.A. (2009). The effect of a physical activity intervention on bias in self-reported activity. *Annals of Epidemiology, 19*(5), 316–322.

Thoden J.S. (1991). Testing aerobic power. In: J.D. MacDougall, H.A. Wenger, & H.J. Green (Eds), *Physiological Testing of the High-performance Athlete* (pp. 107–173). Champaign, IL: Human Kinetics.

Thomas, E.L., & Upton, D. (2014). Psychometric properties of the Physical Activity Questionnaire for Older Children (PAQ-C) in the UK. *Psychology of Sport and Exercise, 15*, 280–287.

Tremblay, M.S., Aubert, S., Barnes, J.D., Saunders, T.J., Carson, V., Latimer-Cheung, A.E., . . . Chinapaw, M.J.M. (2017). Sedentary Behavior Research Network (SBRN) – Terminology Consensus Project process and outcome. *International Journal of Behavioral Nutrition and Physical Activity, 14*(1), 75. doi:10.1186/s12966-017-0525-8.

Troiano, R., Berrigan, D., Dodd, K., Masse, L.C., Tilert, T., & McDowell, M. (2008). Physical activity in the United States measured by accelerometer. *Medicine and Science in Sports and Exercise, 40*(1), 181–188.

Troiano, R.P., McClain, J.J., Brychta, R.J., & Chen, K.Y. (2014). Evolution of accelerometer methods for physical activity research. *British Journal of Sports Medicine, 48*(13), 1019–1023.

Troiano, R.P., Pettee Gabriel, K.K., Welk, G.J., Owen, N., & Sternfeld, B. (2012). Reported physical activity and sedentary behavior: why do you ask? *Journal of Physical Activity and Health, 9*(Suppl 1), S68–S75.

Trost, S.G., Drovandi, C.C., & Pfeiffer, K. (2016). Developmental trends in the energy cost of physical activities performed by youth. *Journal of Physical Activity and Health, 13*(6), S35–S40.

Trost, S.G., Wong, W.K., Pfeiffer, K.A., & Zheng, Y. (2012). Artificial neural networks to predict activity type and energy expenditure in youth. *Medicine and Science in Sports and Exercise, 44*(9), 1801–1809.

Tucker, J.M., Welk, G.J., Beyler, N.K., & Kim, Y. (2016). Associations between physical activity and metabolic syndrome: comparison between self-report and accelerometry. *American Journal of Health Promotion, 30*(3), 155–162.

Tudor-Locke, C.E. (2002). Taking steps toward increasing physical activity: using pedometers to measure and motivate. *President's Council of Physical Fitness and Sports Research Digest, 3*(17), 1–8.

Tudor-Locke, C.E., & Myers, A. (2001). Methodological considerations for researchers and practitioners using pedometers to measure physical (ambulatory) activity. *Research Quarterly for Exercise and Sport, 72*(1), 1–12.

Tudor-Locke, C.E., Williams, J., Reis, J., & Pluto, D. (2002). Utility of pedometers for assessing physical activity. Convergent validity. *Sports Medicine, 32*(12), 795–808.

Vandelanotte, C., De Bourdeaudhuij, I., Philippaerts, R., Sjöström, M., & Sallis, J. (2005). Reliability and validity of a computerized and Dutch version of the International Physical Activity Questionnaire (IPAQ). *Journal of Physical Activity and Health, 2*, 63–75.

van der Ploeg, H.P., Tudor-Locke, C., Marshall, A.L., Craig, C., Hagströmer, M., Sjöström, M., & Bauman, A. (2010). Reliability and validity of the international physical activity questionnaire for assessing walking. *Research Quarterly for Exercise and Sport, 81*(1), 97–101.

Vanhelst, J., Mikulovic, J., Fardy, P.S., Bui-Xuan, G., & Béghin, L. (2013). Concurrent validity of the modified International Physical Activity Questionnaire for French obese adolescents. *Perceptual and Motor Skills, 116*(1), 123–131.

Van Kann, D.H.H., de Vries, S.I., Schipperijn, J., de Vries, N.K., Jansen, M.W.J., & Kremers, S.P.J. (2016). Schoolyard characteristics, physical activity, and sedentary behavior: combining GPS and accelerometry. *Journal of School Health, 86*(12), 913–921.

van Poppel, M.N.M., Chinapaw, M.J.M., Mokkink, L.B., van Mechelen, W., & Terwee, C.B. (2010). Physical activity questionnaires for adults: a systematic review of measurement properties. *Sports Medicine, 40*, 565–600.

van Sluijs, E.M.F., & Kriemler, S. (2016). Reflections on physical activity intervention research in young people – dos, don'ts, and critical thoughts. *International Journal of Behavioral Nutrition and Physical Activity, 13*, 25.

Voss, C., Ogunleye, A.A., & Sandercock, G.R.H. (2013). Physical Activity Questionnaire for children and adolescents: English norms and cut-off points. *Pediatrics International, 55*, 498–507.

Wanner, M., Hartmann, C., Pestoni, G., Martin, B.W., Siegrist, M., & Martin-Diener, E. (2017). Validation of the Global Physical Activity Questionnaire for self-administration in a European context. *BMJ Open Sport & Exercise Medicine, 3*:e000206.

Warren, J.M., Ekelund, U., Besson, H., Mezzani, A., Geladas, N., & Vanhees, L. (2010). Assessment of physical activity – a review of methodologies with reference to epidemiological research: a report of the exercise physiology section of the European Association of Cardiovascular Prevention and Rehabilitation. *European Journal of Cardiovascular Prevention & Rehabilitation, 17*(2), 127–139.

Welk, G.J. & Kim, Y. (2015). The context of physical activity in a representative sample of adults. *Medicine and Science in Sports and Exercise, 47*(10), 2102–2110.

Welk, G., Morrow, J.R., Jr., & Saint-Maurice, P.F. (2017). *Measures Registry User Guide: Individual Physical Activity*. Retrieved from: www.nccor.org/downloads/NCCOR_MR_User_Guide_Individual_PA-v7.pdf

Wen, C.K.F., Schneider, S., Stone, A.A., & Spruijt-Metz, D. (2017). Compliance with mobile ecological momentary assessment protocols in children and adolescents: a systematic review and meta-analysis. *Journal of Medical Internet Research, 19*(4), e132.

Westerterp K.R. (2009). Assessment of physical activity: a critical appraisal. *Eur. J. Appl. Physiol, 105*, 823–828.

Westerterp, K.R. (2015). Energy expenditure and energy intake methods. In J.A. Lovegrove, L. Hodson, & S. Sharma et al. (Eds), *Nutrition Research Methodologies* (pp. 186–197). Chichester: Wiley-Blackwell.

Weston, A.T., Petosa, R., & Pate, R.R. (1997). Validation of an instrument of measurement of physical activity in youth. *Med Sci Sports Exerc., 29*(1), 138–143.

Wickel, E.E., Welk, G.J., & Eisenmann, J.C. (2006). Concurrent validation of the Bouchard Diary with an accelerometry-based monitor. *Medicine and Science in Sports and Exercise, 38*(2), 373–339.

Wilms, B., Ernst, B., Thurnheer, M., Weisser, B., & Schultes, B. (2014). Correction factors for the calculation of metabolic equivalents (MET) in overweight to extremely obese subjects. *International Journal of Obesity, 38*(11), 1383–1387.

Wright, S.P., Hall Brown, T.S., Collier, S.R., & Sandberg, K. (2017). How consumer physical activity monitors could transform human physiology research. *American Journal of Physiology – Regulatory, Integrative and Comparative Physiology, 312*(3), R358–R367.

Zhang, K., Pi-Sunyer, F.X., & Boozer, C.N. (2004). Improving energy expenditure estimation for physical activity. *Med Sci Sports Exerc, 36*(5), 883–889.

Zhu, W., & Owen, N. (2017). *Sedentary Behavior and Health. Concepts, Assessments, and Interventions*. Champaign, IL: Human Kinetics.

7   Physical activity prescription

Michael J. Hamlin

Keywords: Exercise, prescription, exercise programming, health, physical activity recommendations

Adult physical activity interventions

Physical activity interventions for adults can be grouped into a number of main areas based around where the interventions take place. While we have not described all of the possible adult interventions we have outlined the major three.

Work-site physical activity interventions

Since most adults spend large amounts of time at work, work-site physical activity interventions have become popular over the years. It seems obvious that if employers take the trouble to put work-site physical activity interventions in place, thereby indicating the care they have for their workers, employees will benefit. The advantage for the employee is greater overall health and fitness (Conn, Hafdahl, Cooper, Brown, & Lusk, 2009), while the benefit for the employer is a reduction in health care costs and absenteeism, a boost in workplace morale and enhanced productivity (Pelletier, 2001; Pronk & Kottke, 2009). Early research by Dishman and co-workers indicated overall such interventions have only a small effect (Dishman, Oldenburg, O'Neal, & Shephard, 1998). But a more ecological approach to physical activity promotion at work (e.g. making work-site environmental changes, public displays of employee's activity or health success, providing on-site physical activity facilities) in conjunction with behaviour change education showed a much bigger effect (Dishman et al., 1998). This research indicates that work-site physical activity interventions need to incorporate individual and environmental strategies if they are to work (Marcus et al., 2006).

Clinical physical activity interventions

Physical activity interventions driven from health care practices and family health clinics are growing in importance. Physical activity interventions driven from clinical-based practices are effective because a large number of people have regular contact with medical professionals at these clinics. Moreover, individual's trust their general practitioner (GP) and respect their advice. Examples of such intervention programmes include the Physical Activity Promotion in PRImary CAre (PAPRICA) programme from Switzerland, the Green Prescription programme from New Zealand and the Exercise Is Medicine (EIM) programme from the USA. While the effectiveness of such interventions is debateable (Eden, Orleans, Mulrow, Pender, & Teutsch, 2002), it seems interventions that reduce the workload of the GP, and introduce physical activity and behaviour modification advice, along with increasing access to community organisations and resources for physical activity from external partners (e.g. leisure centre personnel, exercise professionals) increases the effectiveness considerably (Orrow, Kinmonth, Sanderson, & Sutton, 2012).

Community-wide physical activity interventions

Community-wide physical activity strategies are usually multi-level (can effect different levels of society e.g. pensioners, school children and office workers) and multi-sectorial (could involve the transport sector and the education sector for example). Such interventions can involve site-specific programmes that are part of a larger community action plan to increase physical activity at the population level. Community-wide campaigns have been strongly recommended by the Task Force on Community Preventative Services as a means of changing behaviour (Services, 2001). Such campaigns revolve around community-wide informational approaches which are large scale, highly visible, multicomponent campaigns with direct messages to large audiences using a variety of approaches (TV, radio, newspaper and internet). Community-wide campaigns that are highly recommended also involve behavioural and social approaches (social support in the community setting and individually adapted behaviour change approaches) and environmental and policy approaches (creation of enhanced access for places to be physically active, enhanced environment conducive to activity, promotion of resources such as walking and biking trails, etc.). Examples of community-wide interventions include the 'Agita Mundo' (Shake the World) campaign in Brazil and the 'Push Play' campaign from New Zealand.

Physical activity prescription for adults

This is the process whereby an individual's recommended schedule of physical activity and exercise is planned and designed in a systematic and individualised way. The prescription of physical activity and exercise follows a number of logical steps from the initial goal setting

1. Goal Setting
2. Conduct a Needs Analysis
3. Conduct a Fitness Assessment
4. Construct a Physical Activity Programme
5. Reassess and Adjust Physical Activity Programme

Figure 7.1   Overview of the physical activity prescription process

of the individual where the individual needs to clearly articulate why they are wanting to exercise, through to making decisions about how to exercise and what types of exercise to use, to finally reassessing goals and adjusting the programme after a certain period of time. Be mindful of the saying "Participation is Everything" which highlights the fact that the best laid plans and prescriptions are useless if the individual does not implement the changes and take up the physical activity.

Goal setting

Goal setting is when the individual either alone or with the help of others (GP, fitness instructor, coach, friend), decides on a change in behaviour. Goals help to motivate behaviour change. Individuals that know what they want and how they will get this are the most likely to achieve their goals. A person cannot achieve their goals without changing behaviour, so goals are essential in physical activity prescription. However, goal setting needs to be well thought through and as specific as possible.

SMART goals

It is more likely that a well-considered plan of action will help individuals attain their goals. Using SMART goals will help create plans that will lead to successful goal setting.

1. **S**pecific. Goals need to be specific in order to provide clear objectives. For example, a goal of being more active is not specific enough and will result in a lack of achievement and decreased motivation. However, a goal of "I want to undertake 30 minutes of moderate-intensity physical activity on 5 or more days per week" is very specific and describes what you want to accomplish more precisely. If you are an athlete and planning for a specific competition or event you would need to specify what event, when the event occurs and how long the event is for. This will allow the individual to plan to train the appropriate skills and energy systems in advance of the event. Goals not only need to be specific but they also need to be personal. Goals that are set by the individual are more motivational than those set by others and are therefore more likely to be achieved. When goals involve others, such as a sport team or walking group, individual goals need to be compatible with team or group goals so that all participants' goals are able to be met.
2. **M**easureable. If possible make the goals measureable, as it allows a means of monitoring how the individual is progressing towards achieving their goals. For example "being more active" is not measurable, but "completing 30 minutes of moderate-intensity physical activity on 5 or more days per week" is measureable. If you cannot measure your goal how will you know you have achieved it or not. Measurement of goals also gives feedback to the individual about progress and can assist with motivation.
3. **A**ction-orientated. Goals require an action plan in order for them to be realised. A written action plan helps the individual plan specific actions that will help individuals reach their goals. In most cases there are a number of steps required in the plan. For example the goal of "I want to undertake 30 minutes of moderate-intensity physical activity on 5 or more days per week" may be unachievable to someone that has not exercised for

the last two years. But several small specific action-orientated goals will eventually see them reach their ultimate goal:

a. Exercise for 10 minutes 3 days per week for 1 month
b. Exercise for 20 minutes 3 days per week for 1 month
c. Exercise for 30 minutes 3 days per week for 1 month
d. Exercise for 30 minutes 5 days per week and keep details in a journal

4. <u>R</u>ealistic. Goals need to be attainable and realistic. Setting unrealistic or unachievable goals will only result in failure, discouragement and a loss of enthusiasm and typically individuals will drop out of the physical activity. Goals that are too easy are just as bad as they provide little challenge and motivation and individuals can quickly lose interest and again drop out of the physical activity. While goals need to be realistic and challenging they also need to be malleable. In many circumstances, particularly when thinking about physical activity, difficulties or changes in circumstances arise and if the goal cannot change with the changing circumstances the individual is likely to again drop out. When selecting goals prepare or try to anticipate potential problems that may arise and plan for these eventualities. For example, bad weather stops the individual from exercising on 2–3 days, or a sprained ankle causes a complete stop to weight-bearing physical activity for four weeks. Possible solutions to these problems might involve running in the rain, or going to the gym, or swimming or biking to take the weight off the lower body joints.

5. <u>T</u>imed. Goals need to have a time frame, otherwise the goals may never be realised. For example, "I will improve my endurance fitness so that I can run 10 km in under 1 hour" is not time-specific. This goal does not mention the time frame. A better goal would be "I will improve my endurance fitness so that I can run 10 km in under 1 hour over the next 12 weeks". The time required to achieve the goal needs to be realistic so that physiological and perhaps biomechanical changes can occur to allow the goal to be achieved. On the other hand, the goal should not be too far into the future so that it does not pressure the individual to work at the goal. It seems we like to work to deadlines, so timed goals are important.

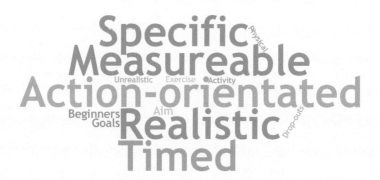

Figure 7.2 Physical activity prescription goals

Conduct a needs analysis

The second stage of the prescription process is to undertake a needs analysis. Remember the specific purposes of physical activity interventions vary with the individual's interest, needs, background and health status. Depending on the aims, the physical activity prescription may be designed to enhance physical fitness, promote health by reducing the risk or re-occurrence of disease, improve body image or increase social interaction. Depending on the individual these common purposes will be given different weighting. For example, an athlete may want to increase physical fitness to improve performance, whereas a non-athlete may want to drop their chances of getting heart disease by losing weight or becoming fitter.

For athletes the needs analysis is mainly focused on the physiological and biomechanical needs of the sport.

For non-athletes the needs analysis should be designed to meet the individual's needs and interests. This might involve asking questions about what types of exercise or physical activity they enjoy, what they want out of the programme and so on.

During the needs analysis the following points need to be addressed:

- Needs and interests of the individual?
- What energy systems are used during the activity or sport the individual is being trained for?
- What muscles, or muscle groups and joints are used during the movements in the activity being trained for?
- What components of fitness are important to the activity being trained for?
- What injuries are likely from the activity being trained for?

(Do not confuse needs with wants, the individual may want to run a marathon but needs to develop cardiorespiratory fitness first.)

Conduct a fitness assessment

If a fitness test is seen to be necessary this would be the time to conduct it and gather the results. But first you must ask yourself "why should I test"?

Why conduct a test?

Functional testing is used to estimate the exercise capacity in a particular component of fitness. For example, a 20-m beep test will give you an estimate of the cardiorespiratory fitness of an individual. The results of such testing provides:

- baseline data for exercise prescription
- feedback for assessing the effectiveness of an individual's training programme
- motivation to ensure exercise compliance
- health status data (this is particularly important for individuals undertaking high-intensity heavy training loads which may create problems in athletes for example, female athlete triad, overtraining or burnout, illness and infection)
- information on clinical status of individuals (e.g. stress testing can give information on heart and cardiovascular health)
- reveals strengths and weaknesses of individuals

- data for elite profiling and talent identification of athletes
- data for coaches to use for team selection (e.g. need to be able to complete a 19 in a Yo-Yo test before being selected for senior team squad)

What testing doesn't do

Fitness testing is not a magical tool that will predict future Olympic champions or supply unequivocal proof that an individual has a health or fitness problem. Remember the human body is a complex set of systems that work together to produce the test performance and parts of the system may fail or work to produce differing results (e.g. psychological, physiological, biomechanical). Use the test results along with your own knowledge to make decisions about the appropriate physical activity prescription.

Effective testing

For fitness and health testing to be relevant and worthwhile ensure the following:

- The variables which are tested are relevant to what the individual wishes to do in terms of physical activity, exercise or sport (for example there is no need to test arm strength if the individual's goal is to complete a half marathon).
- Tests must be *valid*. In other words the test must measure what it claims to measure. A good example of a valid test would be to use the 20-m maximal multistage shuttle test to estimate cardiorespiratory fitness. The 20-m maximal multistage shuttle test is highly correlated to gold standard measures of cardiorespiratory fitness in adults (Palickza, Nichols, & Boreham, 1987) and children (Hamlin et al., 2014).
- Tests must be *reliable*. In other words they must have an appropriate level of sensitivity. If the test is unreliable (in other words it produces wildly fluctuating results for no reason) the tester will not be able to say with certainty that a change in the variable being tested has occurred or not. Therefore the test is of little use. Only use tests that you know are reliable.
- Test administration must be rigidly controlled. Once you have selected a test you must administer this test as per the official instructions and consistently each time. It helps if the tester standardises all procedures so that they are rigidly followed each time a test occurs. Take the simple example of measuring body weight. There is a diurnal change in body weight, body weight also changes with hydration levels, food consumption, clothing and footwear. Therefore, when measuring body weight make sure you do this at the same time of day, at the same time after the last meal, with water intake standardised and in the same footwear and clothing. Also make sure you use the same weighing scales which need to be regularly checked for accuracy.
- The participant's human rights are respected. Testing should be fully explained to the participant and they should be given time to ask questions and withdraw from testing at any time.
- Testing needs to occur at regular intervals. One-off testing has little practical use to the participant as it does not give information on progress and it cannot be used as motivation. It is suggested that testing should occur every 6 to 8 weeks. This allows for adaptations and improvements to occur.
- Results of the test are interpreted correctly. It is all very well to have a valid and reliable test that is conducted appropriately, but it has little value to the individual client if the tester is unable to explain what the result actually means. What does the result of the test mean to the individual?

Minimise any risks

It is important that the tester keeps the testing as safe as possible and minimises any risk to the client. This is especially important in countries where the tester (exercise professional)

The aim of this test is:

To find out your cardiorespiratory fitness which will act as a baseline measure of your stamina (endurance fitness) and will allow us to record changes in this value as you progress through your physical activity programme. Cardiorespiratory fitness has a major influence on health and low levels are associated with a variety of diseases.

Your participation in this test will involve:

Participation in this test is voluntary. Participants can withdraw from the test at any time which includes the withdrawal of their test data. As a test subject you will be asked to exercise on a stationary cycle to a predetermined cadence. The workload will be gradually increased so that you will find it harder and harder to keep up the cadence. Eventually you will find you will not be able to continue at the pre-determined exercise load and you will be forced to stop. The test will normally take 10–12 minutes to complete. During the test you will be asked to indicate how hard you perceive your effort to be. You may also be asked to wear a heart rate monitor or have your heart rate measured from your pulse in your wrist. The testing will occur in a private room at the local gym. You will be asked to abstain from heavy physical exercise and alcohol for 12-h prior to the testing. You will also be instructed not eat a heavy meal and avoid caffeine containing beverages or food for 4-h prior to reporting for testing.

In the performance of the tasks and application of the procedures, there are risks of:

Subjects experiencing fatigue and lethargy for a short period during the later stages of testing. However, these feeling are only temporary and usually subside soon after the test is finished. You will also become warm and may sweat so bring along a towel and a change of clothes. With any exercise there is a danger of illness or even death in a very small proportion of participants, however be assured that all precautions will be taken to avoid any potentially dangerous situations.

Declaration:

I have read and understood the description of the test and what will be required of me as a condition of participation. On this basis I agree to participate in the test with the understanding that confidentiality of my data will be preserved. I understand also that I may at any time withdraw from the test, including withdrawal of any information I have provided.

Name: _____   Signed: _____   Date: _____

Figure 7.3 Example of an informed consent

can be litigated against for any perceived failure to mitigate risks to the client. The following procedures will help in minimising risk:

i. Establish clear emergency procedures. Create a plan of action that can be followed in case of an emergency. Also ensure that exercise professionals have a current first aid certificate.
ii. Ensure privacy and confidentiality of results. Most people object to being tested in front of other people, so be discrete.
iii. Ensure all equipment is clean, in good working condition and calibrated appropriately.
iv. Establish an exercise history.
v. Have an informed consent completed. An example of an informed consent document is shown in Figure 7.3.

Constructing a physical activity programme

Introduction

This is the organisational component of a training session when the instructor, coach or teacher shares with the participants what they are going to do for the activity. This time is typically used for giving advice and encouragement.

Warm up

There is no conclusive evidence for performance increase or a reduction in injury with warming up, although common-sense suggests it's probably worthwhile. Warm up results in:

- Increased temperature of muscles and increased enzymatic activity and thus metabolic reactions associated with the energy systems
- Increased blood flow to muscles which increases their temperature, oxygen delivery and by-product removal
- Decreased reflex time and increased reaction speed

Warm-up exercises should include:

- Gentle activity mimicking that used in your particular activity
- Stretching exercises

Main exercise session

The main exercise session is dedicated to the actual physical activity or sport that the participant is to undertake. The type of activity to be performed in a given day depends on the goals of the participant and in what phase of training they are in (beginner, advanced), along with what equipment or resources are available. For example, for an exercise novice whose goal is to increase cardiorespiratory endurance and lose weight you would choose physical activity that uses a large amount of muscle mass which would not tire the participant too quickly. For this person, swimming, jogging, kayaking, or walking would be suitable.

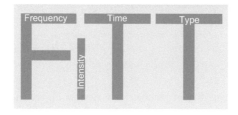

Figure 7.4 The FITT principle

Cool-down

It is suggested a cool-down helps in the following ways:

• Helps to remove metabolic by-products from exercising muscles and re-constitute muscle metabolism
• Maintains the active muscle pump, thereby preventing pooling of blood in the extremities which can reduce blood pressure and lead to dizziness and even syncope
• Stretches during the warm-down also help to bring the muscles back to normal resting length

The physical activity prescription must also take into account the mode (type), intensity, frequency, duration (time) and progression of the physical activity or exercise. These factors can be remembered in a simple principle (FITT).

Frequency

How often will the participant exercise for (e.g. 3 times per week?). This will depend on the underlying health and fitness of the participant and their goals.

Intensity

This refers to how hard the physical activity or exercise is. Probably the hardest part of advising exercise is prescribing the appropriate exercise intensity. Intensity of exercise can be measured in absolute terms (caloric expenditure, absolute oxygen uptake [VO_2]) and METs. A MET (multiple of resting metabolic rate) is an index of energy expenditure. By convention 1 MET is the energy used while sitting at rest doing nothing. Therefore exercising at 3 METs would be using three times as much energy as you would sitting at rest. Absolute intensity measures are not commonly used as they are affected by factors such as body weight, gender and fitness levels. For example, an older person working at 5 METs may be exercising at vigorous intensity which is very difficult for this person, whereas a younger person undertaking the same absolute intensity may be exercising just at moderate intensity due to their superior fitness. This is why it is recommended that a relative measure of exercise intensity is used in exercise prescription (which is the energy cost of the activity relative to their maximal energy capacity). This allows for the differences in the maximum capacity between individuals and with age, sex and so on. There are a number of ways to estimate relative exercise intensity including proportions of heart rate, oxygen consumption and using blood lactate measures. However all of these measures either require sophisticated measurement devices and/or knowledge of exercise physiology.

Table 7.1 Categories of physical activity and exercise intensity using physical descriptors and rating of perceived exertion (RPE) and METs

Intensity	Physical Descriptors	RPE	METs
Sedentary	• Activities that usually involve sitting or lying and have little additional movement and low energy requirement.	< 8	< 2.0
Light	• An aerobic activity that does not cause a noticeable change in breathing rate. • An intensity that can be sustained for at least 60 minutes.	8–10	2.0–2.9
Moderate	• An aerobic activity that is able to be conducted whilst maintaining a conversation uninterrupted. • An activity that causes a small increase in breathing rate. • An intensity that may last between 30 and 60 minutes.	11–13	3.0–5.9
Vigorous	• An aerobic activity in which a conversation generally cannot be maintained uninterrupted. • An activity that causes the participant to huff and puff and start to sweat. • An intensity that may last up to about 30 minutes.	14–16	6.0–8.7
High	• An activity that causes the participant to have a high breathing rate (panting) and high sweating rate. • An intensity that generally cannot be sustained for longer than about 10 minutes.	≥17	≥ 8.8

Physical Descriptors adapted from (Norton et al., 2010). RPE measures from Borg's RPE category scale (Borg, 1998). METs adapted from (Garber et al., 2011).

Table 7.2 Borg scale

Rating of Perceived Exertion	Description of Exertion
6	
7	Very very light
8	
9	Very light
10	
11	Fairly light
12	
13	Somewhat hard
14	
15	Hard
16	
17	Very hard
18	
19	Very very hard
20	

For the average person we suggest using either descriptors of physical change in the exercising person or a rating of perceived exertion (Table 7.1). Ratings of perceived exertion can be used to prescribe and monitor exercise intensity. A common scale used with exercise is the rating scale developed by Borg (Table 7.2) (Borg, 1998).

For those wanting to use new technology much of the worry about working out exercise intensities is taken out of your hands. Wearable technologies like Fitbit, Garmin's Vivosmart, Jawbone's Up, or Polar's Loop-2 activity trackers do all the hard work for you. Even some smartphones have sensors that allow movement to be recorded and tracked which can be put through algorithms supplied with some applications to work out exercise intensities.

Time (duration)

How long will you exercise for? This will depend on goals and fitness levels and time available to exercise. The intensity and duration of exercise are inversely related. In other words, an increase in intensity of an activity normally requires a shorter duration due to increased fatigue with the higher intensity. Alternatively, a lower intensity may allow the participant to exercise for longer. A normal (otherwise healthy) sedentary adult should be able to sustain exercise intensities of 40–60% of relative maximum for 20–30 minutes. Baseline fitness has an effect on physical activity duration. Participants that are fitter can sustain higher intensities for longer. The physical activity specialist is required to prescribe an appropriate combination of exercise intensity and duration to adequately stress the adaptation processes in each individual. Too little stress and no adaptation will occur and the participant will not improve, too much stress the individual may become tired and fatigued, get demotivated and drop-out of the programme.

Type (mode of physical activity)

Once you have the frequency, intensity and time of the activity worked out, you then need to decide on what the activity type will actually be. Again this depends on many things including the goals, experience and motivation of the participants, but also the availability of personal (e.g. bikes, kayaks), and environmental resources (swimming pools, safe bike or running routes). Different types of activities are suited to different goals (Table 7.3).

Table 7.3   Examples of exercise modality to match physical activity goals

Physical Activity Goal	Typical modes of exercise
Cardiorespiratory Fitness (cardiorespiratory endurance or stamina)	Activity involving large muscle groups involving rhythmic movement (e.g. walking, jogging, running, swimming, cycling, kayaking, skiing).
Muscular Strength	Resistance exercises typically using moderate to heavy loads and moderate to low repetitions (resistance can be own body weight, free or fixed weights in a gym or recreation centre).
Muscular Endurance	Resistance exercises typically using light to moderate loads and moderate to high repetitions (resistance can be own body weight, free or fixed weights in a gym or recreation centre).

The American College of Sports Medicine (ACSM) recommends that all adults should partake in regular physical activity that includes cardiorespiratory, resistance, flexibility and neuromotor (balance) exercise training over and above that which occurs during daily living (Garber et al., 2011). More specifically the recommendation suggests most adults should engage in:

> Moderate-intensity cardiorespiratory exercise for 30 minutes or more per day on 5 or more days per week, (for a total of at least 150 minutes per week), vigorous-intensity cardiorespiratory exercise for 20 minutes or more per day on 3 or more days per week (for a total of at least 75 minutes per week), or a combination of moderate and vigorous-intensity exercise to achieve a total energy expenditure of between 500 and 1000 MET-minutes per week (a MET-minute is simply a way of quantifying the total physical activity completed in a standardised way, e.g. walking [at an intensity of 3 METs] for 30 minutes on 4 days per week would equal 360 METs-minutes per week). On 2–3 day per week adults should also perform resistance exercise for the major muscle groups and neuromotor physical activity involving balance, agility and co-ordination exercises. Finally, flexibility exercises are recommended (1 minute per exercise on at least 2 days per week), for each of the major muscle groups to maintain adequate joint range of movement.
>
> (Garber et al., 2011)

Recent research also suggests that health can be improved by becoming less sedentary. In other words, sitting for long periods of time, should be avoided. Therefore, ACSM have recommended the following to go with their physical activity recommendations: to reduce total time engaged in sedentary behaviour and to insert frequent, short bouts of standing and physical activity between periods of sedentary activity, even in already physically active adults (Garber et al., 2011).

The ACSM now include resistance, neuromotor and flexibility in their physical activity recommendations. These components of fitness are particularly important as the individual ages and is susceptible to sarcopenia, osteoporosis and joint problems.

- F   5 or more days per week
- I   moderate-to-vigorous intensity
- T   at least 30 minutes
- T   Cardiorespiratory physical activity that uses
       large muscle mass (e.g. walking, swimming, running)

In addition
- Resistance exercise for 2–3 days per week on major muscle groups
- Flexibility exercises 2 days per week on major muscle groups
- Neuromotor activities 2–3 days per week for older adults

Figure 7.5   Adult physical activity recommendations from ACSM

Resistance exercise

Resistance exercises can take the form of movements against almost any resistance including one's own body weight, or using specific equipment including free or machine weights, hydraulic and pulley devices and rubber bands. The use of resistance exercise can help improve all components of muscular fitness including power, strength and endurance. Improper technique during resistance training can result in injury, therefore good technique should be encouraged throughout any resistance training programme. Individuals should be encouraged to complete the full range of motion (concentric and eccentric movement) for each exercise in a controlled manner with each repetition, while holding the body in a suitably controlled position and breathing normally (not holding your breath). In general (those that are not involved in sports training), two sessions per week of resistance exercise is recommended. These sessions should involve resistance exercises targeting the major muscles groups (chest, shoulders, upper and lower back, abdomen, pelvic area and legs). It is important that at least two days separates the resistance training on the same muscle groups to aid with recovery. The resistance exercises should be multi-joint (effect two or more joints and all the muscles around those joints) in nature (e.g. bench press, less press, shoulder press, triceps dips). Depending on the aims of the resistance programme, but in general for normal healthy adults to improve muscular strength or endurance, the individual would complete resistance training described in Table 7.4.

It can be seen from Table 7.4 that to improve muscular strength a resistance should be selected that allows the individual to complete 8–12 repetitions (reps – individual muscle movements without rest). Such a resistance would be equivalent to approximately 60–80% of the individual's maximal resistance load (otherwise known as 1-repetition maximum [1-RM], or the greatest amount of weight that could be lifted just once). The individual would complete the same 8–12 reps after a rest of about 2–3 minutes a further 2–4 times (sets). While this is the recommended resistance programme for normal healthy adults, even one set of resistance training will give strength improvements. If the objective of the programme is to improve muscular endurance the resistance can be lowered (there is an inverse relationship between number of reps and weight lifted) but the reps increased. For older, or very unfit adults, ACSM recommends one or more sets of 10–15 reps of moderate resistance (60–70% 1-RM). As individuals adapt and get stronger to the resistance training, individuals should continue to increase the resistance being lifted (overload) to continue to increase muscle strength and mass. To do this, participants can increase the load being lifted (resistance weight), the number of reps per set (Reps) or the number of sets per exercise (Sets). A common procedure for introducing more overload is that when the participants can lift the required resistance more than the required number of times in the set (e.g. can easily lift the resistance more than 12 times when the reps are set at 8–12) an additional amount of resistance is added (2–5%).

Table 7.4 Resistance training regimes

Fitness Component to be Trained	Weight (% 1-RM)	RPE	Reps	Sets	Rest
Strength	60–80%	13–16	8–12	2–4	2–3 min
Endurance	< 50%	< 10	15–25	1–2	1–2 min

Flexibility

Similar to resistance training, flexibility is also recommended in any physical activity programme for adults. Improving flexibility may not prevent injury but it does have a beneficial effect on range of motion and physical function, both of which decrease with age. The benefit of stretching before or after sporting activities remains controversial (American College of Sports Medicine, 1998), however, there is no definite evidence to cease the practice of stretching before exercise, except in sports that require muscular strength, power and endurance, where stretching is recommended post-game rather than pre-game (Thacker, Gilchrist, Stroup, & Kimsey Jr, 2004). The ACSM recommends that a stretching programme of at least 10 minutes be incorporated 2–3 days per week. The stretches should involve all the major muscle groups and should be held for 15–60 seconds for static stretches. Stretching can also be performed using dynamic (ballistic) movements or assisted muscle stretching through proprioceptive neuromuscular facilitation stretching. Stretching exercises should be held to the point of discomfort within the range of motion but no further as injury may result.

Neuromotor exercise

Finally some form of neuromotor (neuromuscular) exercise is recommended, particularly for older adults with a higher risk of falling. While such exercise has not been proven to be required for younger people, older adults who have increased risk of falling and have functional or mobility impairments will benefit from such exercise. Any movements that involve balance, coordination and increased proprioceptive feedback such as Tai Chi, Yoga, Pilates and some forms of gym work are recommended to be completed 2–3 days per week for these older adults.

Rate of progression

It is important to understand that individuals will progress towards their physical activity goals at different rates depending on a number of factors including their underlying fitness levels and health status, age, gender and exercise goals. For cardiorespiratory fitness there are generally three stages of progression.

1 Early training stage (4–6 weeks)

Progression may be slow, especially if fitness is low. Individuals with health problems may remain in this stage for longer. Exercise professionals should be wary of exercises that

1. Early Training Stage (4–6 weeks)
2. Improvement Training Stage (12–20 weeks)
3. Maintenance Training Stage (> 6 months)

Figure 7.6   Rate of progression

may cause muscle soreness in this stage as this may increase drop-out rates. It is important that exercise intensity is towards the lower range in this stage (11–13 RPE or 3–6 METs), which may require frequent adjustment as the individual becomes more comfortable with the activity. As with intensity, the duration at this stage may be very low (especially if the participant has a health issue), but should target at least 10–15 minutes per session. The frequency of physical activity at this stage depends on the initial level of fitness. A person with a higher level of initial fitness will recover faster and be able to exercise again sooner than someone with a lower level of fitness. The aim should be at least 3 days per week or more at this stage.

2 Improvement training stage (12–20 weeks)

The individual usually progresses at a faster rate in this stage. The individual can usually cope with more work and adapts to that work faster. Exercise intensity in this stage is usually increased to the target level (11–16 RPE or 3–8.7 METs). The duration of activity increases to match the desired duration of the prescription (i.e. 30 minutes per day). The rate of progression and increase in the frequency and size of work increments in this stage is dictated by how the individual recovers and adapts. Some authors suggest that the duration should increase in small bouts (5–10 minutes per session) to approximately 20–30 minutes before increasing the exercise intensity.

3 Maintenance training stage (> 6 months)

During this stage the individual reaches a satisfactory level of cardiorespiratory fitness. If adequate cardiorespiratory fitness is achieved, the individual can maintain this fitness without increasing exercise load further. Normally this is an important period for re-evaluation of goals and aims of the physical activity intervention.

Note that these stages are only indications and some individuals will reach fitness milestones quicker than others due to individual variation in training adaptation. These stages describe typical changes in cardiorespiratory fitness training and may not represent the typical changes that occur with other types of training (i.e. strength training). In addition, adjustments in the exercise prescription (in all the components of FITT) may be required occasionally if individuals either have adverse effects due to too much exercise, or for other reasons like contracting a cold, increased stress from other sources and so on.

Reassess and adjust physical activity programme

Once the individual arrives at the maintenance training stage the programme should be reassessed for fitness level changes and whether goals were met. Exercise professionals need to be aware of the "Law of Diminishing Returns" here. That is, the magnitude and time it takes for changes to occur will gradually diminish as fitness levels increase. So large and quick changes that occur at the start of the programme are much harder to sustain as the individual improves their fitness. At this time point the objectives of the physical activity intervention should be reviewed and realistic goals set again. It is common to introduce some alterations to physical activity intervention at this stage to keep it fresh and enjoyable. Individuals may also require motivation and encouragement to maintain their activity programmes. Be mindful that "participation is everything" – the best physical activity prescription in the world is worthless unless the individual actually implements the plan.

Risks associated with physical activity

To some extent there is risk in almost all physical activity whether it be a pulled muscle, twisted ankle, or a heart attack (myocardial infarction). Therefore one must decide whether the benefits of exercise outweigh the risks of having an unwanted medical event. The risk of a heart attack is very low in healthy individuals performing low-intensity activities, but increases as you move into vigorous-intensity activities, especially for individuals who are already diagnosed with cardiovascular disease (Giri et al., 1999; Willich et al., 1993). Other risk factors include diabetes, smoking and obesity. For this reason, it is advisable to have individuals complete a medical history questionnaire (Balady, 1998) and undergo a risk stratification prior to exercise. At the very least a Physical Activity Readiness Questionnaire (PAR-Q) (Figure 7.7) should be completed to help distinguish those with elevated risk to seek further medical advice prior to undertaking exercise. While this chapter does not deal with health screening and stratification of risk, we encourage those individuals that will be prescribing physical activity programmes to familiarise themselves with the ACSM procedures and protocols in this area. These individuals are encouraged to gather more information on this important area from American College of Sports Medicine (2013) prior to prescribing exercise.

Children physical activity interventions

It is suggested that establishing positive habits early in life helps to cement those habits over the rest of the lifespan. Eating a healthy diet, taking regular exercise, managing stress, and positively connecting with others, are behaviours that can be impressed on children during their early development by the influence of parents and society in general. So do physically active and athletically competent parents have physically active and athletic children? Although this is a controversial topic, some evidence suggests that having two active parents increases the child's odds of being physically active 4–9 fold compared with having inactive parents (Eriksson, Nordqvist, & Rasmussen, 2008), which corroborated earlier evidence indicating active fathers tended to have active children (Yang, Ielamo, & Laakso, 1996). In another study that used objective measures of physical activity (accelerometers), and followed children for approximately six years, physical activity behaviour tended to track moderately from childhood to adulthood (Kristensen et al., 2008). It seems that if good physical activity behaviours in young children can be developed, they are likely to carry these behaviours on to adolescence and adulthood.

Thirty years ago children and adolescents were physically active in different ways than children of today. Many either walked or cycled to school, and may have had jobs before or after school. Given the fact that children are more sedentary and less physically active today than their peers in the past, what are our options for increasing physical activity in children moving forward? There are a number of strategies that have been suggested to increase physical activity in children. In many cases these interventions have been school-based due to the fact that large numbers of children can be affected at once in a relatively inexpensive way. Because of the importance of the family environment on physical activity behaviour, interventions within

This questionnaire has been designed for screening out individuals who are at risk when exercising due to cardiovascular or metabolic disease.

Are you ready and able to participate in exercise? Complete the following questionnaire.

Name: _____ Signed: _____ Date: _____

Many health benefits are associated with regular exercise, and the completion of the PAR-Q is a sensible first step to take if you are planning to increase the amount of physical activity in your life. For most people, physical activity should not pose any problem or hazard. PAR-Q has been designed to identify the small number of adults for whom physical activity might be inappropriate, or those who should have medical advice concerning the type of activity most suitable for them. Common sense is your best guide in answering these few questions. Please read them carefully and check YES or NO opposite the question if it applies to you.

YES   NO

☐   ☐   1. Has your doctor ever said you have a heart condition <u>and</u> that you should only do physical activity recommended by a doctor?

☐   ☐   2. Do you feel pain in your chest when you do physical activity?

☐   ☐   3. In the past month, have you had chest pain when you were doing physical activity?

☐   ☐   4. Do you lose balance because of dizziness or do you ever lose consciousness?

☐   ☐   5. Do you have a bone or joint problem that could be made worse by a change in your activity?

☐   ☐   6. Is your doctor currently prescribing drugs (for example, water pills) for your blood pressure or heart condition?

☐   ☐   7. Do you know of <u>any other reason</u> why you should not do physical activity?

If you have answered **NO** honestly to <u>all</u> PAR-Q questions, you can be reasonably sure that you can:

        1. Start a graduated exercise program

        2. Take part in a fitness appraisal

However, if you have a minor illness (e.g. cold), you should postpone activity until well.

If you answered **YES** to one or more PAR-Q questions, you should consult your physician if you have not done so recently before starting an exercise program and/or having a fitness appraisal.

Figure 7.7 Example of the Physical Activity Readiness Questionnaire (PAR-Q)

the family are now getting more support (Sallis et al., 2000). Similarly, because much of children's and adolescents' physical activity is undertaken in the community within sports and leisure groups, or through community-owned and serviced facilities, community-led interventions are also becoming more popular.

School-based interventions

Most of these interventions are based around improving or increasing physical activity within the Physical Education (PE) programme at schools. A review (Almond & Harris, 1998) found that school-based interventions that indicated positive results were mainly due to increased PE time, something that is unlikely to occur due to other curriculum pressures. While undertaking PE at school is important for children's development, it probably does not provide enough physical activity for students to meet physical activity recommendations by itself. It also seems that school-based programmes have little effect on out-of-school physical activity levels (Stone, McKenzie, Welk, & Booth, 1998), indicating the difficulty school-based interventions have at affecting overall behaviour change. Other school-based interventions outside of PE classes have focused on changing the environment to change behaviour. For example, altering playground markings can have a beneficial effect on physical activity levels during breaks (Stratton, 2000), although other factors such as availability of equipment was also involved. A recent study (Pilot Primary Schools Physical Activity Project) investigated a more unified approach to increasing the quality and quantity of PE and physical activity over the whole school (Cowley, Grimley, Hamlin, Hargreaves, & Price, 2005). This unique approach employed physical activity co-ordinators (one for every 4 schools), and lead teachers who underwent additional professional development to drive the PE and physical activity development at the schools. A major objective was to link opportunities within the community to the school's programme. The key success factors identified were the leadership skills of the lead teachers, the support of the physical activity co-ordinator, and the support of the principal and the school community. The results suggested the intervention had a significant impact upon children's awareness and opportunities to be physically active and their attitudes and perceptions about physical activity and physical education. Time devoted to timetabled physical activity subjects increased significantly post-intervention. The physical activity co-ordinator was instrumental in raising the awareness of physical activity and providing opportunities for the children to be physically active.

This research suggests that school-based interventions may be more successful if arranged in a more holistic fashion where there are unified messages from teachers and administrators and specialists are recruited to help teachers drive the programme. Using the information gathered from the Pilot Primary Schools Physical Activity Project a new through-school nutrition and physical activity programme called 'Project Energize' was set-up in a large number of schools in New Zealand. The aim of the programme, that was introduced in 2005 and continues today, was to increase primary school (5–13 year-olds) children's physical activity levels, reduce sedentary time, and optimise nutritional intake through changes in the school environment and culture (Graham et al., 2008). For each school, a group of people (Team Energize) were specifically recruited to support the delivery and development of the project Energize programme which was individualised for each school. Team Energize staff met with school administrators, senior teaching staff, school board and parents and conducted a needs assessment and goal-setting exercise to set the general direction of the activities at the school (see Graham et al., 2008 for more information). The success of this holistic approach was demonstrated by a lowering in the prevalence of obesity, reduction in BMI and increased physical fitness levels in the children attending the Project Energize schools (Rush, McLennan, Obolonkin, Cooper, & Hamlin, 2015). In addition, such a model is cost effective (Rush et al., 2014).

Family-based interventions

No matter how much education and behaviour change you may be able to achieve with young people at school, if it is not reinforced and practiced in the home environment it is unlikely to change. Take for example nutritional advice, where many schools educate students about a healthy diet and the importance of the food pyramid and reducing excess consumption of unhealthy snacks and drinks. If the child's family do not adhere to the same messages, it's unlikely the child will change. Coming home to fast food meals, easy and frequent access to calorie-dense snacks and high-sugar drinks will not encourage the child to take up the recommended behaviour. The family is an important avenue for role modelling, social support and encouragement. Research suggests that the effectiveness of home-based interventions are low for already healthy children and slightly more effective for unfit or obese children (Sallis, 1998). Previous attempts at incorporating family-based interventions within other multi-level interventions have been underwhelming. In many cases these family-based interventions have a positive effect on attitudes but little effect on actual behaviour change (Nader et al., 1996), or behaviour change reverts quickly back to normal without continued intervention.

Our research group recently looked at a family-based intervention for obese children. The aim of intervention (Active Families Canterbury) was to make more children and their families more active, more often. The intervention consisted of a 6-month activity plan developed for the family which focused on the obese child which included monthly one-on-one family meetings with an Active Families Advisor and fortnightly phone support provided by the Practice Nurse. Participants were also encouraged to attend the Active Families Club weekly for activity sessions and nutrition education. Medical Practices were randomly assigned to control or intervention groups with Practice Nurses receiving motivational and behaviour change training. Inactive obese children aged 2–12 years old were referred to the programme which is detailed below (Table 7.5).

As with many other weight control interventions the outcome variable in our study was a positive change in children's BMI. The BMI data was standardised to the U.S. reference data from the Centres for Disease Control (McDowell, Fryar, Hirsch, & Ogden, 2005), and we found a significant decrease in the standardised BMI in the intervention children at 12 months post-intervention compared to baseline. Approximately 60% of the intervention children showed an improvement in their standardised BMI score at 12 months post-intervention. While overall the intervention children put on an average of about 5.8 kg in the 12 months post-intervention approximately 5.5 kg of this mass was new muscle or bone and only 0.4 kg was fat mass. This suggests that the increased physical activity during the intervention slowed down the build-up of adipose tissue and increased the laying down of healthier non-adipose tissue. The Paediatric Quality of Life data demonstrated that after only six months the intervention compared to the control group substantially increased their total Quality of Life score indicating an improved self-esteem in these children. It has been suggested that a significant behavioural change is unlikely to occur unless some psychological change has occurred first. However as with previous research, children soon reverted back to their old habits as soon as the intervention ceased. Most of the positive physical activity behaviours showed an

Table 7.5   Timetable of the follow-up and support procedures for the Active Families patients in this study

Timeframe	Support and follow-up details
Day 1	Patient visits their GP or practice nurse and an Active Family's script is administered. With the patient's consent a copy of the prescription is forwarded to the Regional Sports Trust acting as the Active Family Advisor (AFA).
First week	A telephone call from an AFA is made to arrange a meeting with the family, practice nurse and AFA. This initial meeting takes places in the general practice and the questionnaires, physical tests and health measures are taken. An initial activity plan is agreed.
1–6 months	Practice nurse calls child and family fortnightly. AFA calls family once per month and meets family monthly to both motivate and support the family providing progression and assistance to overcome barriers to physical activity. Families are encouraged to attend the weekly Active Families Club where families get together to be active and socialise.
6 months	A consultation with the practice nurse and AFA takes place in the general practice and the questionnaires, physical tests and health measures are repeated. No further support is provided to the family.

improvement after six months but after 12 months the children had dropped activity levels back to baseline values. Parents have a significant influence on their children's behaviours and decision making, which is why this particular intervention focused its efforts on the family rather than on the child.

Future interventions for children should involve the whole family as much as possible, incorporating not only physical and leisure activity change but also nutritional, budgeting and psychological change advice. Such interventions should concentrate on providing physical activities that suit children including less formal, unstructured play and activities like swimming; use schools, parents and friends as motivators for children; but probably the most important factor would be the ongoing support of such families and children. A programme that was able to build a self-sufficient and self-managing resource for such families would be ideal.

Community interventions

Traditionally physical activity interventions for children have been structured around the home or school environment, however recently the influence of the community at encouraging young people to be active has emerged. Even the two interventions described above (Project Energize and Active Families Canterbury) that were situated in the school or home environment recognise the influence of the community on physical activity levels and encouraged community relationships as much as possible. Individual children live in communities, they play and discover in communities, so it seems logical that communities will influence behaviours in these children. Again it seems pointless giving messages of the importance of regular physical activity and exercise if these messages are not adopted and supported by the community. Although the research indicates contradictory results (Pate et al., 2000; Stone et al., 1998) it is well understood that for the sustainability of any physical activity intervention, the community, family and school need to be involved. It has been suggested the large drop-off in physical activity that occurs with young adults after secondary school (years 9–13) is due to the disconnection between community-linked resources for physical activity and the young adults moving out of school into the community. Because the students have been catered for so well in the school system in terms of active leisure, sport and recreation opportunities, when left to fend for themselves the connection between the community that provides these resources and the students is lost resulting in less activity being undertaken.

Physical activity prescription for children

Formal physical activity or exercise prescription for children is difficult because children prefer being active through play and games and engage in sporadic rather than continuous activities. Encouraging children and adolescents to be active in as many ways as possible is desirable whether that be through active transport, during school, or while at home or in the community. Additionally being less sedentary is also a major goal for health and some authorities have incorporated recommendations on television viewing time to try and reduce sedentariness and the negative influence of advertising on children. For example, the American Academy of Pediatrics (2001) and the Australian Physical Activity Recommendations (Salmon & Shilton, 2004) recommend that children spend no more than two hours watching television and using electronic entertainment devices per day (outside of the school environment). Figure 7.8 shows the formalised ACSM children and adolescents exercise prescription guidelines using the FITT analogy (American College of Sports Medicine, 2013).

Frequency
At least 3–5 days per week but preferably daily.

Intensity
Moderate (noticeably increases breathing, sweating and heart rate) to vigorous (substantially increases breathing, sweating and heart rate) intensity activity.

Time
30 minutes a day of moderate and 30 minutes a day of vigorous intensity to total 60 minutes per day of accumulated physical activity.

- **F**   3–5 days per week but preferably daily
- **I**   Moderate-to-vigorous intensity
- **T**   60 minutes per day (at least 30 minutes of moderate and 30 of vigorous)
- **T**   A variety of activities that are enjoyable and developmentally appropriate

Figure 7.8   Child physical activity recommendations from ACSM

Type

A variety of activities that are enjoyable and developmentally appropriate for the child or adolescent.

Special considerations for children and adolescents

- Provided proper and safe supervision is given, children and adolescents can safely undertake strength training. It is recommended that sets be 8–15 reps and should be undertaken to the point of mild fatigue but with good posture and proper lifting technique at all times.
- It is recommended that children and adolescents should exercise in thermo-neutral environments because thermo-regulatory systems may still be underdeveloped in this age group.
- Overweight or physically inactive children/adolescents may not be able to achieve 60 minutes of activity per day, therefore the time should be reduced and slowly increased as the individual gets fitter and healthier.
- Children with health issues like asthma, cystic fibrosis, diabetes mellitus, and cerebral palsy should have their physical activity prescription tailored to their specific needs by an exercise professional.

Summary and practical applications

Recent health trends including an increase in obesity and non-communicable diseases along with an accompanying, ever-escalating, health cost, has not only increased the awareness of the problem to the general society, but it has also increased emphasis on possible solutions. Physical activity in adults as well as children and adolescents, is becoming increasingly important in the fight against these chronic diseases. For years physical activity and exercise has been systematically squeezed out of our lives as the race to mechanise jobs, increase profits, reduce time and manual labour marches on. Passive transportation and inactive leisure pursuits are slowly eating into our daily physical activity levels. And yet, it is exactly this (i.e. physical activity) that is the solution to many of these health problems. There is overwhelming evidence that regular physical activity and exercise is beneficial for health, can reduce stress and improve life expectancy as well as life enjoyment. However, once lost, regular physical activity can be challenging to find again. In this chapter we have investigated some of the ways in which individuals and societies can incorporate physical activity back into their lives. Ultimately it is a personal decision on whether to be physically active or not, and although we have not discussed the decision-making process, reading this chapter will help those individuals who have made the decision to make physical activity part of their life. This chapter outlines proven approaches required for physical activity implementation at a number of levels as well as six practical steps required to start and maintain a physical activity programme.

Steps to start and maintain a physical activity programme

1. Before prescribing physical activity, think about the needs and wants of the individual and how these can be satisfied
2. Follow the FITT principle when putting together physical activity programmes
3. Make sure any physical activity is safe for the participant

4. Successful long-term exercise adherers make physical activity part of their daily routine
5. Bad habits can be ingrained in children at an early age, so take all opportunities to be active with your children
6. Enjoyment and variety are most important for continued regular physical activity

Chapter summary

- Being physically active and taking part in regular exercise is fundamental to the normal development of the human being
- Programmes and approaches to exercise prescription should differ for children and adults
- Using SMART goals will help to create plans that will lead to successful goal setting
- Using the FITT principle will help with prescription for adults and children
- ACSM recommend that adults take part in 30 min of moderate-intensity exercise on five or more days per week
- ACSM recommend that children and adolescents take part in 30 min moderate and 30 min vigorous physical activity each day.
- Interventions with children should involve the whole family as much as possible

References

Almond, L., & Harris, J. (1998). Interventions to promote health-related physical education. In S. Biddle, N. Cavill, & J. Sallis (Eds.), *Young and Active? Young People and Health-enhancing Physical Activity: Evidence and Implications* (pp. 133–149). London: Health Education Authority.

American Academy of Pediatrics. (2001). Children, adolescents, and television (RE0043). *Pediatrics, 107*, 423–426.

American College of Sports Medicine. (1998). Position Stand: The recommended quantity and quality of exercise for developing and maintaining cardiorespiratory and muscular fitness, and flexibility in healthy adults. *Medicine and Science in Sports and Exercise, 30*(6), 975–991.

American College of Sports Medicine. (2013). *ACSM's Guidelines for Exercise Testing and Prescription* (9th ed.). Baltimore, MD: Lippincott Williams & Wilkins.

Balady, G. (1998). American College of Sports Medicine and American Heart Association Joint Position Statement: Recommendations for cardiovascular screening, staffing, and emergency policies at health/fitness facilities. *Medicine and Science in Sports and Exercise, 30*(6), 1009–1018.

Borg, G. (1998). *Borg's Perceived Exertion and Pain Scales*. Champaign, IL: Human Kinetics.

Conn, V.S., Hafdahl, A.R., Cooper, P.S., Brown, L.M., & Lusk, S.L. (2009). Meta-analysis of workplace physical activity interventions. *American Journal of Preventive Medicine, 37*(4), 330–339.

Cowley, V., Grimley, M., Hamlin, M., Hargreaves, J., & Price, C. (2005). *Evaluation of the Pilot Primary Schools Physical Activity Project*. Retrieved from Christchurch: College of Education, Christchurch, New Zealand.

Dishman, R.K., Oldenburg, B., O'Neal, H., & Shephard, R.J. (1998). Worksite physical activity interventions. *American Journal of Preventive Medicine, 15*(4), 344–361.

Eden, K.B., Orleans, C.T., Mulrow, C.D., Pender, N.J., & Teutsch, S.M. (2002). Does counseling by clinicians improve physical activity? A summary of the evidence for the US Preventive Services Task Force. *Annals of Internal Medicine, 137*(3), 208–215.

Eriksson, M., Nordqvist, T., & Rasmussen, F. (2008). Associations between parents' and 12-year-old children's sport and vigorous activity: The role of self-esteem and athletic competence. *Journal of Physical Activity and Health, 5*(3), 359.

Garber, C.E., Blissmer, B., Deschenes, M.R., Franklin, B.A., Lamonte, M.J., Lee, I.-M., . . . Swain, D.P. (2011). American College of Sports Medicine position stand. Quantity and quality of exercise for developing and maintaining cardiorespiratory, musculoskeletal, and neuromotor fitness in apparently healthy adults: Guidance for prescribing exercise. *Medicine and Science in Sports and Exercise, 43*(7), 1334–1359.

Giri, S., Thompson, P.D., Kiernan, F.J., Clive, J., Fram, D.B., Mitchel, J.F., . . . Waters, D.D. (1999). Clinical and angiographic characteristics of exertion-related acute myocardial infarction. *Journal of American Medical Association, 282*(18), 1731–1736.

Graham, D., Appleton, S., Rush, E., McLennan, S., Reed, P., & Simmons, D. (2008). Increasing activity and improving nutrition through a schools-based programme: Project Energize. 1. Design, programme, randomisation and evaluation methodology. *Public Health Nutrition, 11*(10), 1076–1084.

Hamlin, M.J., Fraser, M., Lizamore, C.A., Draper, N., Shearman, J.P., & Kimber, N.E. (2014). Measurement of cardiorespiratory fitness in children from two commonly used field tests after accounting for body fatness and maturity. *Journal of Human Kinetics, 40*(1), 83–92.

Kristensen, P.L., Møller, N., Korsholm, L., Wedderkopp, N., Andersen, L.B., & Froberg, K. (2008). Tracking of objectively measured physical activity from childhood to adolescence: The European youth heart study. *Scandinavian Journal of Medicine & Science in Sports, 18*(2), 171–178.

Marcus, B.H., Williams, D.M., Dubbert, P.M., Sallis, J.F., King, A.C., Yancey, A.K., Claytor, R.P. (2006). Physical activity intervention studies what we know and what we need to know: A scientific statement from the American Heart Association Council on Nutrition, physical activity, and metabolism (Subcommittee on Physical Activity); Council on Cardiovascular Disease in the Young; and the Interdisciplinary Working Group on Quality of Care and Outcomes Research. *Circulation, 114*(24), 2739–2752.

McDowell, M.A., Fryar, C.D., Hirsch, R., & Ogden, C.L. (2005). *Anthropometric Reference Data for Children and Adults: U.S. Population, 1999–2002.* Retrieved from Hyattsville, MD: National Center for Health Statistics, 2005.

Nader, P.R., Sellers, D.E., Johnson, C.C., Perry, C.L., Stone, E.J., Cook, K.C., . . . Luepker, R.V. (1996). The effect of adult participation in a school-based family intervention to improve children's diet and physical activity: The Child and Adolescent Trial for Cardiovascular Health. *Preventive Medicine, 25*(4), 455–464.

Norton, K., Norton, L., and Sadgrove, D. (2010). Position statement on physical activity and exercise intensity terminology. *Journal of Science and Medicine in Sport, 13*, 496–502.

Orrow, G., Kinmonth, A.-L., Sanderson, S., & Sutton, S. (2012). Effectiveness of physical activity promotion based in primary care: Systematic review and meta-analysis of randomised controlled trials. *British Medical Journal, 344*. doi:10.1136/bmj.e1389

Palickza, V., Nichols, A., & Boreham, C.A. (1987). Multistage shuttle run as a predictor of running performance and maximal oxygen uptake in adults. *British Journal of Sports Medicine, 21*(4), 163–165.

Pate, R.R., Trost, S.G., Mullis, R., Sallis, J.F., Wechsler, H., & Brown, D.R. (2000). Community interventions to promote proper nutrition and physical activity among youth. *Preventive Medicine, 31*(2), S138–S149.

Pelletier, K.R. (2001). A review and analysis of the clinical- and cost-effectiveness studies of comprehensive health promotion and disease management programs at the worksite: 1998–2000 update. *American Journal of Health Promotion, 16*(2), 107–116.

Pronk, N.P., & Kottke, T.E. (2009). Physical activity promotion as a strategic corporate priority to improve worker health and business performance. *Preventive Medicine, 49*(4), 316–321.

Rush, E., McLennan, S., Obolonkin, V., Cooper, R., & Hamlin, M. (2015). Beyond the randomised controlled trial and BMI – evaluation of effectiveness of through-school nutrition and physical activity programmes. *Public Health Nutrition*, 1–4.

Rush, E., Obolonkin, V., McLennan, S., Graham, D., Harris, J., Mernagh, J.P., & Weston, J.A. (2014). Lifetime cost effectiveness of a through-school nutrition and physical programme: Project Energize. *Obesity Research & Clinical Practice, 8*(2), e115–e122.

Sallis, J. (1998). Family and community interventions to promote physical activity in young people. In S. Biddle, N. Cavill, & J. Sallis (Eds.), *Young and Active? Young People and Health-enhancing Physical Activity: Evidence and Implications* (pp. 150–161). London: Health Education Authority.

Sallis, J.F., Patrick, K., Frank, E., Pratt, M., Wechsler, H., & Galuska, D.A. (2000). Interventions in health care settings to promote healthful eating and physical activity in children and adolescents. *Preventive Medicine, 31*(2), S112–S120.

Salmon, J., & Shilton, T. (2004). Endorsement of physical activity recommendations for children and youth in Australia. *Journal of Science and Medicine in Sport, 7*(3), 405–406.

Services, T. F. o. C. P. (2001). Increasing physical activity: A report on recommendations of the Task Force on Community Preventive Services: Morbidity and Mortality Weekly Reports Recommendations and Reports. *Centers for Disease Control, 50.*

Stone, E.J., McKenzie, T.L., Welk, G.J., & Booth, M.L. (1998). Effects of physical activity interventions in youth: Review and synthesis. *American Journal of Preventive Medicine, 15*(4), 298–315.

Stratton, G. (2000). Promoting children's physical activity in primary school: An intervention study using playground markings. *Ergonomics, 43*(10), 1538–1546.

Thacker, S.B., Gilchrist, J., Stroup, D.F., & Kimsey Jr, C.D. (2004). The impact of stretching on sports injury risk: A systematic review of the literature. *Medicine and Science in Sports and Exercise, 36*(3), 371–378.

Willich, S.N., Lewis, M., Lowel, H., Arntz, H.-R., Schubert, F., & Schroder, R. (1993). Physical exertion as a trigger of acute myocardial infarction. *New England Journal of Medicine, 329*(23), 1684–1690.

Yang, X., Telamo, R., & Laakso, L. (1996). Parents' physical activity, socioeconomic status and education as predictors of physical activity and sport among children and youths – a 12 year follow up study. *International Review of Sociology of Sport, 31*(3), 273–294.

Part II

Sport science disciplines and physical activity

8   Growth and development and physical activity

Lynne Boddy and Gareth Stratton

Keywords: Growth and development, body composition, musculoskeletal health, children and adolescents, older adults

Introduction

The pathway from birth to adulthood involves many processes that ebb and flow and influence participation in and are influenced by physical activity (PA). Terms such as growth, development and maturation are often used interchangeably yet they have different definitions. Growth is a biological process that can be defined as 'the increase in the size of the body as a whole and of its parts' (Malina, 2014, p. 157). Development "is a broader concept, encompassing growth, maturation, learning and experience" (Beunen, 2009, p. 74). Maturation can be considered as the process of becoming mature or progress towards the adult state (Baxter-Jones, Eisenmann, & Sherar, 2005), and there are several different aspects of maturation that are often considered, including sexual, skeletal and morphological.

PA influences a range of systems by providing a 'load' on the body and through its influence on energy expenditure. As a result, PA has a direct influence on the growth and development of children and young people, but also helps to prevent losses associated with ageing. Therefore PA has an important role throughout the life course. The following chapter highlights some key areas related to PA, growth and development and provides a snapshot of some research for each area.

Physical activity during the growing years

PA contributes to the healthy development of the musculoskeletal system, healthy body composition, and the maintenance and promotion of fitness. The contribution of PA to these key areas varies across the individual's 'growing years'.

Body size and adiposity

Early childhood is an important period for promoting PA, although the amount of PA needed to optimise growth and development remains unclear (Timmons et al., 2012). In comparison to older children and adolescents, the pre-school group has received far less attention from researchers. During early childhood children grow very quickly, becoming taller and leaner.

Young children's body mass index (BMI) reduces until the age of 4–6 years and then rapidly increases, which is often termed the obesity rebound (Butte et al., 2016) (see Figure 8.1 for BMI growth charts from 2–20 years). Earlier onset of adiposity rebound is associated with increased weight gain, adiposity during childhood and an increased BMI during childhood, adolescence and young adulthood (Malina, 2014). This stage of growth is therefore viewed as a period in which PA could play a key role.

A growing body of evidence has described an inverse association between PA and adiposity and/or body size within the preschool age group. The study by Butte and colleagues (2016) examined the associations between moderate to vigorous-intensity PA (MVPA) and body size and composition in pre-schoolers. Authors concluded that MVPA and total PA were associated with reduced adiposity. Prospective analyses described positive associations between MVPA and total PA with BMI and fat free mass, but not with fat mass, suggesting that MVPA promotes healthy development of fat free mass. Collings et al. (2013) examined the associations between objectively assessed PA and body composition in 4-year-old children. Their results showed that vigorous PA (VPA) exhibited a strong, inverse association with total and abdominal adiposity. Moderate PA (MPA) was not related to fatness, and there were no associations observed between sedentary time and body composition, thus suggesting VPA should be promoted within this age group (Collings et al., 2013). Other evidence suggests that the effects of early childhood MVPA on adiposity may persist throughout childhood, therefore the benefits of MVPA during this period may be sustained over time (Janz et al., 2009).

Many studies have examined the relationships between PA and body size or composition within children aged ~5–12 years, mainly due to the large increases in obesity prevalence observed over the past two decades within this age group. Evidence from the European Youth Heart Study (Ekelund et al., 2004) demonstrated significant yet modest associations between objectively assessed MVPA and VPA with body fatness. The study showed that children who accumulated <60 minutes/day of MVPA were significantly fatter than those who accumulated >120 minutes/day. There is, however, contradictory evidence regarding the associations between PA and body size and/or composition, which has mainly been attributed to inadequate measures of PA and poor study designs undermining study results. A review of the research that used objective methods to estimate PA in children and adolescents described consistent evidence of negative associations between PA and adiposity, supporting the view that higher levels of PA protect against childhood obesity (Jiménez-Pavón, Kelly, & Reilly, 2010). However the dose-response relationship is yet to be fully elucidated.

Adolescence is a period that is characterised by rapid growth and changes in body composition (Rogol, Roemmich, & Clark, 2002). During adolescence changes in body composition differ between boys and girls, where boys exhibit an increase in fat free mass and decrease in percentage fat mass, and girls increase in percent body fat and increase fat free mass to a lesser degree than boys. These periods of rapid growth correspond with a well-documented decline in PA. Therefore the promotion of PA during this age group is important. Recent evidence from the Pelotas birth cohort study provides support for regular participation in MVPA and the development of favourable body composition. The study found that the consistent practice of MPA and VPA during adolescence was directly related to lean mass index (lean mass relative to height) in boys and girls. VPA was also shown to be inversely related to fat mass index (fat mass relative to height) in boys (Ramires et al., 2016). Thus suggesting consistent or maintained PA had beneficial effects on body composition.

Early studies examined whether PA, training and sport participation had detrimental effects on adolescent growth, particularly when considering stature. Malina (1994) reviewed some of this earlier evidence, which looked at stature, age at peak height velocity and growth velocity in boys classified as active vs. inactive. The study also looked at boys and girls who regularly took part in sport vs. those who took part in lower volumes of sport. The results of Malina's study found that regular PA, sport participation and training had no effect on stature, timing of peak height velocity or timing of peak height velocity in boys. At the time of Malina's review, longitudinal data documenting girls' PA was not available, however the paper found that regular training had no adverse effects on structural growth, therefore suggesting that PA, regular sport participation and/or training does not negatively influence the growth of adolescents (Malina, 1994). This paper effectively de-bunked theories regarding PA and sport being detrimental to growth in children and adolescents. Subsequently, the field has moved towards examining the potential benefits of regular PA, sport participation and/or training on growth and body composition rather than focusing on the potential risks.

PA represents the voluntary component of energy expenditure, with the involuntary component often termed resting energy expenditure (REE). Resting energy expenditure has historically been closely associated with changes in body mass, and absolute REE increases through adolescence during puberty. Recent evidence from the longitudinal EarlyBird Study has challenged this theory (Mostazir et al., 2016). This study described small reductions in absolute REE in adolescents around the period of peak height velocity. When REE relative to size was modelled and body composition and other confounding variables were controlled for within analyses a decline in REE of approximately 450 kcal/24 hrs was observed during the period of peak height velocity. This represents a substantial decline in REE, which although potentially advantageous from an evolutionary perspective, in today's society where energy sources are plentiful this may represent a key time at which individuals are at risk of developing obesity and overweight (Mostazir et al., 2016). Therefore, this emerging evidence highlights a potentially greater role for PA and may spur additional research into the benefits of PA within this age group.

Maturation

Maturation is a continuous process throughout the child and adolescent years (Baxter-Jones et al., 2005). Children grow and mature at different rates. Sexual maturation during the pubertal years occurs under the influence of hormones and substantial individual variation exists with regards to the timing of the onset of puberty and associated physiological changes, therefore individuals of a similar chronological age can differ substantially in terms of their biological age (Baxter-Jones et al., 2005). During puberty, PA declines, which has potentially important consequences for adult health and health behaviours. It is commonly reported that boys are more active than during childhood and adolescence, however these differences are attenuated in adolescents when maturation is accounted for within analysis (Rodrigues et al., 2010).

The longitudinal EarlyBird Study examined the potential biological and environmental factors that may influence PA patterns from childhood through adolescence (Metcalf, Hosking, Jeffery, Henley, & Wilkin, 2015). The study described declines in PA between 9 to 15 years of age of ~30% and ~20% in girls and boys, respectively. Half of the decline was due to falls in LPA with a quarter attributed to declining MVPA. The decline in PA was similarly related to biological and chronological age, and pubertal stage accelerated the decline in girls. Interestingly the declines were consistent across different environmental settings (e.g. areas of low vs. high deprivation), suggesting that the declines in PA observed during the pubertal/adolescent period may be to some extent under biological control (Metcalf et al., 2015).

Research has often focused on the effect of exercise training on timing of maturation and pubertal growth, rather than the influence of 'usual' free-living PA. Sports such as artistic gymnastics, where competitors tend to be of short stature and exhibit delayed maturation, have been one focus of attention for this type of research. For example, Malina et al., (2013) reported the outcomes of an expert committee convened to review the role of intensive training in the growth and maturation of artistic gymnasts. The committee concluded that gymnastics training does not: (1) compromise adult or near adult height, (2) attenuate the growth of the upper (sitting height) or lower body (legs) segment lengths, or (3) attenuate pubertal growth and maturation. Finally the committee concluded that the data available were inadequate to examine any changes in the endocrine system and that although gymnasts tend to be shorter and lighter than average, they have appropriate weight-for-height (Malina et al., 2013). Therefore, the characteristics of gymnasts may be due to a selection bias within the sport, i.e. favouring those who are shorter, rather than any negative effects of training on growth and maturation.

Skeletal development and health

The growing years are the most important when considering bone strength, as individuals reach peak bone mass by the end of the second or early in the third decade of life (Baxter-Jones, Faulkner, Forwood, Mirwald, & Bailey, 2011). It is important that individuals maximise their peak bone mass during the growing years to protect against osteoporosis in later life. Peak bone mass is achieved via an interaction between genetic and environmental variables. The environmental variables include the influence of hormones, nutrition and mechanical loading (Klentrou, 2016). PA produces the mechanical load that can stimulate an increase in bone mass and improved bone strength. High impact, load-bearing activities such as jumping, gymnastics and bounding have been associated with the largest benefits in bone mineral development and accrual. Muscle forces and lean mass mediate the loads placed on bones during PA (Janz et al., 2007), therefore lean mass has a close association with bone mineral content.

Several researchers have examined the relationships between PA and skeletal health across various stages of childhood and adolescence. Harvey et al. (2012) examined the cross-sectional relationships between daily MVPA, dietary calcium intake and bone size and density in 4-year-old children. The study found that time spent in MVPA was positively associated with femoral size and density but not height or weight. Other evidence from the IDEFICS study (Herrmann et al., 2015) examined the combined effects of PA and weight-bearing exercise on bone stiffness, an indicator of bone health in young children. Results showed that for every additional 10 minutes/day of MPA or VPA bone stiffness increased by 1 or 2%, respectively. The study also found that participation in weight-bearing exercise was associated with 2% higher bone stiffness in pre-schoolers. The results demonstrate the positive relationship between PA and bone health, however the authors emphasised the need for researchers to use objective methods to quantify PA to better examine dose-response relationships (Herrmann et al., 2015).

The pre- and early pubertal periods are key times to attempt to maximise bone mass and strength (Janz et al., 2014; Tan et al., 2014) as the skeleton has increased responsiveness to loading (Duckham et al., 2014). In the 2016 review, Klentrou highlights two longitudinal bone health studies: The Saskatechewan Pediatric Bone Mineral Accrual Study (Bailey, McKay,

Mirwald, Crocker, & Faulkner, 1999; Baxter-Jones, Eisenmann, Mirwald, Faulkner, & Bailey, 2008) and the Iowa Bone Development Study (Janz et al., 2007). The Saskatechwan Pediatric Bone Mineral Accrual Study examined the relationship between PA and peak bone mineral accrual in children passing through adolescence. The longitudinal design allowed researchers to control for maturational differences between children of equivalent chronological ages, which meant participants could be compared at a common maturational time or landmark. Evidence from the study described significant main effects for PA on peak bone mineral accrual and total accrual. An increase of 9% and 17% in total body bone mineral content was observed for active boys and girls, respectively, in comparison to inactive participants (Bailey et al., 1999). The Saskatchewan study also described the beneficial effects of PA in adolescence on markers of tibial bone strength in young adulthood (Duckham et al., 2014), suggesting long-term benefits of PA in adolescence. The Iowa Bone Development Study examined PA and bone health, specifically hip geometry, in a cohort of 4- to 12-year-old healthy children (Janz et al., 2007). The study found that MVPA was a positive predictor of femoral neck cross-sectional area (an index of axial strength) and section modulus (an index of bending strength). On average, children who participated in 40 minutes of MVPA/day would have a 3–5% greater femoral neck cross-sectional area and section modulus at aged 8 years than those who accrued 10 minutes of MVPA/day. The Iowa study also found that girls and boys with persistently high levels of MVPA during childhood had greater bone mass and geometry at 17 years of age (Janz et al., 2014), thus highlighting the beneficial effects of PA throughout childhood.

It is worth noting that although measures of bone strength and mineralisation have been explored, the effect of high volumes of PA on bone turnover in children and adolescents are relatively unexplored and contradictory evidence exists (Klentrou, 2016). More research into bone turnover is required to establish whether a threshold exists for the beneficial effects of PA on bone health, and whether when exceeded through excessive loading detrimental effects could occur.

Fitness

Fitness is made up of a number of health- and skill-related components and "the components of fitness change as a function of growth, maturation development and the interactions between these processes" (Malina, 2014, p. 165). Much of the current evidence related to fitness in children and young people has focused on cardiorespiratory fitness (CRF), mainly because of the reported associations with cardiometabolic risk and other health markers (Ortega, Ruiz, Castillo, & Sjöström, 2008). When observing maturational changes in peak oxygen uptake (VO_2 peak, see Figure 8.2), the optimum assessment of CRF in children, increases are observed in girls and boys from age ~8 years through to around 16 years, with some evidence to suggest that absolute VO_2 peak (L/min) plateaus in girls at around age 14 years (Armstrong, Tomkinson, & Ekelund, 2011). The sex differences observed in absolute VO_2 peak (L/min) strengthen over time, with girls exhibiting approximately 10% lower VO_2 peak values during childhood, rising to approximately 35% at age 16 (Armstrong et al., 2011). If VO_2 peak is scaled differently, for example by expressing relative VO_2 peak in ml/kg/min, boys' VO_2 peak remains stable from ~8 years to 18 years, at around 48 ml/kg/min whereas girls' relative VO_2 peak declines from around 45 ml/kg/min to 35 ml/kg/min over the same age range (Armstrong et al., 2011).

One issue to consider when examining fitness and performance, is the influence of relative age. Many sports and fitness assessments are organised according to chronological age. For a given chronological age, children can vary substantially. In addition to this, when we consider children within their school year groups, children can also vary considerably in terms of their actual chronological age. For example, in England a child born on the 1 September falls within the same school year as a child born on the 31 August 364 days later, thus children's chronological age can vary by almost a full year. This provides the older children with an advantage both in the short and long term. This grouping system is common in competitive sport contexts and the 'relative age effect' has been documented in several competitive sports. For example one meta-analysis highlighted the presence of relative age effects across

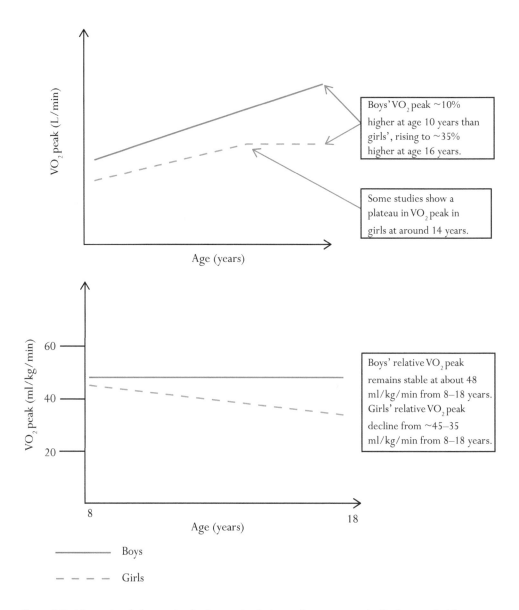

Boys' VO$_2$ peak ~10% higher at age 10 years than girls', rising to ~35% higher at age 16 years.

Some studies show a plateau in VO$_2$ peak in girls at around 14 years.

Boys' relative VO$_2$ peak remains stable at about 48 ml/kg/min from 8–18 years. Girls' relative VO$_2$ peak decline from ~45–35 ml/kg/min from 8–18 years.

————— Boys

– – – – Girls

Figure 8.2 Maturational changes in absolute and relative peak oxygen uptake for boys and girls

a range of sports and also described a strengthening of the effect at representative levels (e.g. national, regional) in highly popular sports (Cobley, Baker, Wattie, & McKenna, 2009). Relative age effects also influence fitness. Differences in field-assessed CRF have been described between children born in quarters of the school calendar, with children born in quarter 1 (September–November) performing significantly better on the 20m multi-stage shuttle runs test than those born in quarter 4 (June–August) after controlling for somatic maturation (Roberts, Boddy, Fairclough, & Stratton, 2012). It is important therefore, that in addition to the complications associated with biological age, that an appreciation of how children are grouped during the growing years can also have an effect and this is especially important where fitness testing is used as a tool for health screening or talent identification.

Fitness is often viewed as the product of recent PA, but evidence to support this in children and adolescents is weaker than may be expected, with relatively low associations reported depending on the component of fitness examined and measurement methods utilised (Andersen, Riddoch, Kriemler, & Hills, 2011; Armstrong et al., 2011). Despite this, some studies have reported significant differences in fitness in active versus inactive children (Boddy et al., 2014), and adolescents (Ortega, Ruiz, Hurtig-Wennlof, & Sjöström, 2008) and positive changes in fitness as a result of lifestyle changes, for example cycling to school (Andersen et al., 2011). The relationship between fitness and PA is likely to differ depending on the intensity of the PA stimulus and the measurement methods used, which may account for the weak relationships observed within some studies.

Historically, controversy existed regarding the trainability of children, mainly due to theories suggesting that a maturational threshold, usually viewed as the onset of puberty, existed before which training would be ineffective. The period immediately following the maturational threshold was viewed as a time in which adolescents may be more receptive to training and thus exhibit significant gains. In more recent years, researchers have addressed this issue. A 2014 BASES expert statement summarised the key issues regarding the trainability of children and adolescents and concluded that CRF gains are inversely related to baseline fitness, changes in some of the parameters of aerobic function are independent of maturity and appropriately designed training can result in improvements in VO_2 peak of around 7.7% in children aged <11 years and 8.6% in children aged >11 years (McNarry et al., 2014). When considering strength training, gains increase with increasing maturity and age, where larger gains in speed were evident in pre- and post-pubertal groups rather than mid-pubertal groups. The expert statement therefore concluded that no thresholds for gains or windows of opportunity were evident (McNarry et al., 2014). The balance of evidence therefore suggests that appropriately designed training programmes can stimulate changes in various components of fitness in children and adolescents, irrespective of their stage of maturation. As methods are better able to capture PA behaviours and classify intensities of PA, the relationships between habitual PA, exercise training and fitness will become clearer.

PA During adulthood

Physical activity during adulthood is health protective, playing an important role in disease prevention, reducing age related decline, and a therapeutic role for existing conditions. It is important to consider the effect of PA across the lifespan, especially in the context of an ageing society.

All-cause mortality and non communicable diseases

A well-established negative association exists between PA and all-cause mortality, though it has been suggested that the complex relationships between PA and body composition may mediate this. Ekelund et al. (2015) examined whether total and abdominal adiposity modified the association between PA and all-cause mortality. Participants were classified into groups based on BMI, waist circumference and PA (active, moderately active, moderately inactive and inactive). PA was inversely associated with all-cause mortality at all levels of adiposity, and the greatest reductions in mortality risk were observed between the inactive and moderately inactive groups, suggesting that small increases in PA in inactive people may have substantial public health benefits. The analysis found that if all the inactive individuals became moderately inactive, the number of deaths would reduce by 7.35% (Ekelund et al., 2015), therefore high-lighting the important, independent effect of PA on all-cause mortality.

The ACSM position statement on PA in older adults (Nelson et al., 2007) concisely sum-marises a range of benefits of PA, both in terms of prevention of diseases such as cardio-vascular disease, hypertension, osteoporosis, obesity, cancer, anxiety and depression and the prevention of age-related issues such as fall risk and functional limitations (Nelson et al., 2007). The statement also highlights the therapeutic effect of PA in the management of a wide range of conditions including heart disease, hypertension, osteoporosis, dementia, pain, stroke, and depression (Nelson et al., 2007). The statement recommends that adults aged 65+ (or those aged 50–64 years with existing conditions/functional limitations) should participate in 30 minutes of MPA on five days every week or 20 minutes of VPA on three days per week, or a combination of both intensities. An important difference between the recommendations presented for older adults and the general adult population is the acknowledgement that lev-els of fitness vary considerably within this age group, therefore the intensity of activity should be modified accordingly and individualised. Strengthening activities should be performed on a minimum of two days per week and flexibility exercises should be incorporated on two days per week for at least 10 minutes. Finally balance exercises should be included to help prevent falls. ACSM also recommend older adults use a PA plan that integrates the preventive and therapeutic PA recommendations.

Despite the widely discussed health benefits of PA across the lifespan, systematic reviews have highlighted the lack of longitudinal studies available to fully examine the long-term effects of PA on the risk of non-communicable and age-related diseases (Reiner, Niermann, Jekauc, & Woll, 2013). In the 2013 review, Reiner et al. (2013) described that most studies included found negative relationships between PA and weight gain/obesity over time, coronary heart disease, risk of type 2 diabetes mellitus, Alzheimer's disease and dementia, thus suggesting a protective effect of PA. However, the lack of longitudinal studies and the use of self-reported PA within most studies limited the conclusions drawn from the review, especially related to dose-response relationships and clear guidance on the frequency, intensity and type of activity required to minimise the risk of non-communicable and age-related disease.

Age-related declines

It has been theorised that PA could help to prevent reduced mobility in older adults, which is a risk factor for disability, morbidity, hospitalisation and mortality. Stenholm et al. (2015) examined whether PA in early adulthood, late midlife and old age as well as cumulative PA history were associated with changes in physical functioning and mortality in old age. The researchers asked participants aged 65+ to recall PA levels across two age periods (20–40 years and 40–60 years) and over the past year. Participants were classified as inactive, moderately active and physically active and assessed physical performance, mobility related disability and mortality in three-year intervals from 2001–2003 through to 2007–2008. Those who were inactive at baseline exhibited a greater decline in physical performance, mobility disability and mortality in comparison to active participants. Being active throughout adulthood was associated with a lower risk of premature death, smaller declines in physical performance and a lower risk of mobility disability in comparison to those who had been less active throughout their adult years (Stenholm et al., 2016). This study therefore presents further evidence of the protective effect of PA across the adult years.

Intervention studies have shown promise in terms of promoting PA and reducing age-related declines. For example, Pahor et al. (2014) conducted a randomised clinical trial to examine whether a long-term structured PA programme was more effective than a health education programme in reducing the risk of major mobility disability in 70- to 89-year-old adults. Half of the group were assigned to a structured PA programme which involved two centre visits per week and home based activity 3–4 times a week. The other half of the cohort were assigned to a health education programme that focused on 'successful aging'. At two years follow-up the PA intervention group had maintained a 40 min/week difference in MPA in comparison to the health education group (Pahor et al., 2014). The study also found significant differences in the incidence of major mobility disability between groups, with disability evident in 30.1% of the PA programme participants and 35.5% of the health education group. In addition, significantly more participants in the education group experienced persistent mobility disability, and major mobility disability or death in comparison to the PA group (Pahor et al., 2014). The study therefore highlights the potential benefits of PA promoting interventions within older adults.

Physical activity across the life course and specifically in older age has protective effects upon the maintenance of muscle and bone mass, which in turn helps to protect function and reduces the risk of falls. The loss of muscle mass and function, or sarcopenia, has received a lot of attention from researchers in recent years. This is because sarcopenia is associated with a range of negative outcomes including disability, poor quality of life and mortality (Cruz-Jentoft et al., 2010). The MRC National Survey of Health and Development birth cohort study examined PA levels across adult life and grip strength in early old age (ages 60–64 years) (Dodds, Kuh, Aihie Sayer, & Cooper, 2013). Previous analyses from the study described no associations between grip strength and PA in adults at age 53 years, but the authors hypothesised that the associations may not become apparent until later in life. The study looked at leisure time PA at ages 36, 43, 53 and 60–64 and found evidence of a cumulative effect of leisure time PA across mid-life on grip strength at age 60–64 (Dodds et al., 2013). These results are pertinent as reduced grip strength has been associated with increased fall risk in older adults and is commonly used in the assessment of sarcopenia.

The importance of PA during the growing years for the accrual of peak bone mass and strength is well established. Physical activity is important in the subsequent years for the maintenance of bone, especially in postmenopausal women where bone reabsorption accelerates, increasing the risk of osteoporosis. Positive associations between exercise (a sub-component of PA) and bone mass and geometry in postmenopausal women have been described (Hamilton, Swan, & Jamal, 2010). Findings from another review reported that MVPA was associated with a 45% and 38% risk reduction in hip fracture in men and women, respectively (Moayyeri, 2008). Further research is required to determine the required dose of PA to maximise gains in mass and geometry and to fully examine the magnitude of any benefits in bone mineral density and quality, but the benefits of PA for skeletal health are widely acknowledged.

Another area where age-related declines are evident is in cognitive function. For example Dregan and Gulliford (2013) examined the association between leisure time PA from age 11 to 50 years and cognitive function in late mid-adulthood. Participants self-reported leisure-time PA at ages 11, 16, 33, 42, 46 and 50 years of age. Executive, cognitive and memory functioning were also assessed at age 50 years (Dregan & Gulliford, 2013). PA was scored in terms of frequency and intensity of activity using cumulative scores from the repeated surveys. A positive association between PA frequency and cognitive index, memory and executive functioning was observed in men and women. Strong evidence for improvements in cognitive scores with increasing intensity of PA were also reported in men and women, and a consistent dose-response relationship was observed between cumulative PA and cognitive function outcomes at age 50 years (Dregan & Gulliford, 2013). Therefore, in addition to the physical benefits of PA, regular participation in PA during adulthood may help to prevent the cognitive declines that are also associated with the aging process.

Chapter summary

- Growth and development involves many processes that ebb and flow throughout life.
- PA can positively impact upon a range of systems and health variables throughout the life course.
- Physical activity positively influences body composition, musculoskeletal health, fitness and physical functioning across the lifespan.
- Our understanding of the relationships between PA and growth and development is improving as studies utilise better measurement methods and robust designs, however more longitudinal studies are required.

References

Andersen, L.B., Riddoch, C., Kriemler, S., & Hills, A.P. (2011). Physical activity and cardiovascular risk factors in children. *Br J Sports Med, 45*(11), 871–876. doi:10.1136/bjsports-2011-090333

Armstrong, N., Tomkinson, G., & Ekelund, U. (2011). Aerobic fitness and its relationship to sport, exercise training and habitual physical activity during youth. *Br J Sports Med, 45*(11), 849–858. doi:10.1136/bjsports-2011-090200

Bailey, D.A., McKay, H.A., Mirwald, R.L., Crocker, P.R.E., & Faulkner, R.A. (1999). A six-year longitudinal study of the relationship of physical activity to bone mineral accrual in growing children: The University of Saskatchewan Bone Mineral Accrual Study. *Journal of Bone and Mineral Research, 14*(10), 1672–1679.

Baxter-Jones, A.D., Eisenmann, J.C., Mirwald, R.L., Faulkner, R.A., & Bailey, D.A. (2008). The influence of physical activity on lean mass accrual during adolescence: a longitudinal analysis. *J Appl Physiol (1985), 105*(2), 734–741. doi:10.1152/japplphysiol.00869.2007

Baxter-Jones, A.D., Eisenmann, J.C., & Sherar, L.B. (2005). Controlling for maturation in pediatric exercise science. *Pediatric Exercise Science, 17*, 18–30.

Baxter-Jones, A.D., Faulkner, R.A., Forwood, M.R., Mirwald, R.L., & Bailey, D.A. (2011). Bone mineral accrual from 8 to 30 years of age: an estimation of peak bone mass. *J Bone Miner Res, 26*(8), 1729–1739. doi:10.1002/jbmr.412

Beunen, G. (2009). Physical growth, maturation and performance. In R. G. Eston & T. Reilly (Eds.), *Kinanthropometry and exercise physiology laboratory manual: Tests, procedures and data* (3rd ed., Vol. 1 *Anthropometry*, pp. 73–100). Abingdon: Routledge.

Boddy, L.M., Murphy, M.H., Cunningham, C., Breslin, G., Foweather, L., Gobbi, R., . . . Stratton, G. (2014). Physical activity, cardiorespiratory fitness, and clustered cardiometabolic risk in 10- to 12-year-old school children: the REACH Y6 study. *Am J Hum Biol, 26*(4), 446–451. doi:10.1002/ajhb.22537

Butte, N.F., Puyau, M.R., Wilson, T.A., Liu, Y., Wong, W.W., Adolph, A.L., & Zakeri, I.F. (2016). Role of physical activity and sleep duration in growth and body composition of preschool-aged children. *Obesity* (Silver Spring), *24*(6), 1328–1335. doi:10.1002/oby.21489

Cobley, S., Baker, J., Wattie, N., & McKenna, J. (2009). Annual age-grouping and athlete development: a meta-analytical review of relative age effects in sport. *Sports Med, 39*(3), 235–256. doi:10.2165/00007256-200939030-00005

Collings, P.J., Brage, S., Ridgway, C.L., Harvey, N.C., Godfrey, K.M., Inskip, H.M., . . . Ekelund, U. (2013). Physical activity intensity, sedentary time, and body composition in preschoolers. *Am J Clin Nutr, 97*(5), 1020–1028. doi:10.3945/ajcn.112.045088

Cruz-Jentoft, A.J., Baeyens, J.P., Bauer, J.M., Boirie, Y., Cederholm, T., Landi, F., . . . European Working Group on Sarcopenia in Older People. (2010). Sarcopenia: European consensus on definition and diagnosis: Report of the European Working Group on Sarcopenia in Older People. *Age Ageing, 39*(4), 412–423. doi:10.1093/ageing/afq034

Dodds, R., Kuh, D., Aihie Sayer, A., & Cooper, R. (2013). Physical activity levels across adult life and grip strength in early old age: updating findings from a British birth cohort. *Age Ageing, 42*(6), 794–798. doi:10.1093/ageing/aft124

Dregan, A., & Gulliford, M.C. (2013). Leisure-time physical activity over the life course and cognitive functioning in late mid-adult years: a cohort-based investigation. *Psychol Med, 43*(11), 2447–2458. doi:10.1017/S0033291713000305

Duckham, R.L., Baxter-Jones, A.D., Johnston, J.D., Vatanparast, H., Cooper, D., & Kontulainen, S. (2014). Does physical activity in adolescence have site-specific and sex-specific benefits on young adult bone size, content, and estimated strength? *Journal of Bone and Mineral Research, 29*(2), 479–486.

Ekelund, U., Sardinha, L.B., Anderssen, S.A., Harro, M., Franks, P.W., Brage, S., . . . Froberg, K. (2004). Associations between objectively assessed physical activity and indicators of body fatness in 9- to 10-y-old European children: a population-based study from 4 distinct regions in Europe (the European Youth Heart Study). *Am J Clin Nutr, 80*(3), 584–590.

Ekelund, U., Ward, H.A., Norat, T., Luan, J., May, A.M., Weiderpass, E., . . . Riboli, E. (2015). Physical activity and all-cause mortality across levels of overall and abdominal adiposity in European men and women: the European Prospective Investigation into Cancer and Nutrition Study (EPIC). *Am J Clin Nutr, 101*(3), 613–621. doi:10.3945/ajcn.114.100065

Hamilton, C.J., Swan, V.J., & Jamal, S.A. (2010). The effects of exercise and physical activity participation on bone mass and geometry in postmenopausal women: a systematic review of pQCT studies. *Osteoporos Int, 21*(1), 11–23. doi:10.1007/s00198-009-0967-1

Harvey, N.C., Cole, A., Crozier, S.R., Kim, M., Ntani, G., Goodfellow, L., Robinson, S.M., Inskip, H.M., Godfrey, K.M., Dennison, E.M., Wareham, N., Ekelund, U., & Cooper, C. (2012). Physical activity, calcium intake and childhood bone mineral: a population-based cross-sectional study. *Osteoporosis, 23*, 121–130.

Herrmann, D., Buck, C., Sioen, I., Kouride, Y., Marild, S., Molnár, D., . . . consortium, I. (2015). Impact of physical activity, sedentary behaviour and muscle strength on bone stiffness in 2–10-year-old children-cross-sectional results from the IDEFICS study. *Int J Behav Nutr Phys Act, 12*, 112. doi:10.1186/s12966-015-0273-6

Janz, K.F., Gilmore, J.M., Levy, S.M., Letuchy, E.M., Burns, T.L., & Beck, T.J. (2007). Physical activity and femoral neck bone strength during childhood: the Iowa Bone Development Study. *Bone, 41*(2), 216–222. doi:10.1016/j.bone.2007.05.001

Janz, K.F., Kwon, S., Letuchy, E.M., Eichenberger Gilmore, J.M., Burns, T.L., Torner, J.C., . . . Levy, S.M. (2009). Sustained effect of early physical activity on body fat mass in older children. *Am J Prev Med, 37*(1), 35–40. doi:10.1016/j.amepre.2009.03.012

Janz, K.F., Letuchy, E.M., Burns, T.L., Gilmore, J.M.E., Torner, J.C., & Levy, S.M. (2014). Objectively measured physical activity trajectories predict adolescent bone strength: Iowa Bone Development Study. *British Journal of Sports Medicine, 48*, 1032–1036.

Jiménez-Pavón, D., Kelly, J., & Reilly, J.J. (2010). Associations between objectively measured habitual physical activity and adiposity in children and adolescents: systematic review. *Int J Pediatr Obes, 5*(1), 3–18. doi:912756490 [pii] 10.3109/17477160903067601

Klentrou, P. (2016). Influence of exercise and training on critical stages of bone growth and development. *Pediatr Exerc Sci, 28*(2), 178–186. doi:10.1123/pes.2015-265

Malina, R.M. (1994). Physical activity and training: effects on stature and the adolescent growth spurt. *Med Sci Sports Exerc, 26*(6), 759–766.

Malina, R.M. (2014). Top 10 research questions related to growth and maturation of relevance to physical activity, performance, and fitness. *Res Q Exerc Sport, 85*(2), 157–173. doi:10.1080/02701 367.2014.897592

Malina, R.M., Baxter-Jones, A.D., Armstrong, N., Beunen, G.P., Caine, D., Daly, R.M., . . . Russell, K. (2013). Role of intensive training in the growth and maturation of artistic gymnasts. *Sports Med, 43*(9), 783–802. doi:10.1007/s40279-013-0058-5

McNarry, M., Barker, A., Lloyd, R.S., Buchheit, M., Williams, C., & Oliver, J. (2014). The BASES expert statement on trainability during childhood and adolescence. *The Sport and Exercise Scientist, 41*, 22–23.

Metcalf, B.S., Hosking, J., Jeffery, A.N., Henley, W.E., & Wilkin, T.J. (2015). Exploring the adolescent fall in physical activity: a 10-yr cohort study (EarlyBird 41). *Med Sci Sports Exerc, 47*(10), 2084–2092. doi:10.1249/MSS.0000000000000644

Moayyeri, A. (2008). The association between physical activity and osteoporotic fractures: a review of the evidence and implications for future research. *Ann Epidemiol, 18*, 827–835.

Mostazir, M., Jeffery, A., Hosking, J., Metcalf, B., Voss, L., & Wilkin, T. (2016). Evidence for energy conservation during pubertal growth: a 10-year longitudinal study (EarlyBird 71). *Int J Obes.* doi:10.1038/ijo.2016.158

Nelson, M.E., Rejeski, W.J., Blair, S.N., Duncan, P.W., Judge, J.O., King, A.C., . . . Castaneda-Sceppa, C. (2007). Physical activity and public health in older adults: recommendation from the American College of Sports Medicine and the American Heart Association. *Med Sci Sports Exerc, 39*(8), 1435–1445. doi:10.1249/mss.0b013e3180616aa2

Ortega, F.B., Ruiz, J.R., Castillo, M.J., & Sjöström, M. (2008). Physical fitness in childhood and adolescence: a powerful marker of health. *Int J Obes* (Lond), *32*(1), 1–11. doi:10.1038/sj.ijo.0803774

Ortega, F.B., Ruiz, J.R., Hurtig-Wennlof, A., & Sjöström, M. (2008). [Physically active adolescents are more likely to have a healthier cardiovascular fitness level independently of their adiposity status. The European youth heart study]. *Rev Esp Cardiol, 61*(2), 123–129.

Pahor, M., Guralnik, J.M., Ambrosius, W.T., Blair, S., Bonds, D.E., Church, T.S., . . . Life Study Investigators. (2014). Effect of structured physical activity on prevention of major mobility disability in older adults: the LIFE study randomized clinical trial. *JAMA, 311*(23), 2387–2396. doi:10.1001/jama.2014.5616

Ramires, V.V., Dumith, S.C., Wehrmeister, F.C., Hallal, P.C., Menezes, A.M., & Goncalves, H. (2016). Physical activity throughout adolescence and body composition at 18 years: 1993 Pelotas (Brazil) birth cohort study. *Int J Behav Nutr Phys Act, 13*(1), 105. doi:10.1186/s12966-016-0430-6

Reiner, M., Niermann, C., Jekauc, D., & Woll, A. (2013). Long-term health benefits of physical activity –a systematic review of longitudinal studies. *BMC Public Health, 13*, 813. doi:10.1186/1471-2458-13-813

Roberts, S.J., Boddy, L.M., Fairclough, S.J., & Stratton, G. (2012). The influence of relative age effects on the cardiorespiratory fitness levels of children age 9 to 10 and 11 to 12 years of age. *Pediatr Exerc Sci, 24*(1), 72–83.

Rodrigues, A.M.M., Silva, M., Mota, J., Cumming, S.P., Sherar, L.B., Neville, H., & Malina, R.M. (2010). Confounding effect of biologic maturation on sex differences in physical activity and sedentary behaviour in adolescents. *Pediatric Exercise Science, 22*(3), 442–453.

Rogol, A.D., Roemmich, J.N., & Clark, P.A. (2002). Growth at puberty. *Journal of Adolescent Health, 31*, 192–200.

Stenholm, S., Koster, A., Valkeinen, H., Patel, K.V., Bandinelli, S., Guralnik, J.M., & Ferrucci, L. (2016). Association of physical activity history with physical function and mortality in old age. *J Gerontol A Biol Sci Med Sci, 71*(4), 496–501. doi:10.1093/gerona/glv111

Tan, V.P.S., Macdonald, H.M., Kim, S., Nettlefold, L., Gabel, L., Ashe, M.C., & McKay, H.A. (2014). Influence of physical activity on bone strength in children and adolescents: a systematic reivew and narrative synthesis. *Journal of Bone and Mineral Research, 29*(10), 2161–2181.

Timmons, B.W., Leblanc, A.G., Carson, V., Gorber, S.C., Dillman, C., Janssen, I., . . . Trembley, M.S. (2012). Systematic review of physical activity and health in the early years (aged 0–4 years). *Applied Physiology, Nutrition, and Metabolism, 37*, 773–792.

9 Motor skill development and physical activity

Jenny Clarke

Keywords: Motor skill development, gross motor skills, locomotor, object control, fundamental movement skills

Motor skill development refers to the acquisition and evolution of movement skills through an individual's lifespan. Fundamental Movement Skills (FMS) are distinct movement patterns that involve various body parts and provide the basis for the more advanced movements, such as those required for day-to-day living and sport-specific skills. Children acquire fundamental movement skills from their first kick and grasping movement through to running, jumping and throwing, to competently putting on clothes, feeding themselves and writing. Acquisition of increasingly sophisticated gross and fine motor skills occurs through repeated participation in physical activity and sports, and in turn these skills encourage continued participation and enjoyment of active lives.

The health-related benefits of physical activity at various stages of the lifespan are well documented (Janssen & LeBlanc, 2010; Strong et al., 2005; Warburton, Nicol, & Bredin, 2006). Benefits include reduced risk of premature death from non-communicable diseases, such as several types of cancer, diabetes, hypertension, and bone and joint diseases. Conversely, the risks and effects of a sedentary childhood have also been explored in some depth, identifying unfavourable body composition, low self-esteem, decreased fitness, and decreased academic achievement (Tremblay et al., 2011).

There is plenty of evidence that successful fundamental motor skill development in early years paves the way for a physically active life. While proficiency at motor skill tests has repeatedly been shown to be positively correlated to the amount of physical activity an individual undertakes, particularly in studies involving young children, causality has yet to be firmly established. However, the health benefits of physical activity are well established; as are the positive outcomes associated with success in motor skill performance, and the relationship between the two certainly warrants better understanding.

This chapter will present evidence in relation to the positive and negative effects of physical activity and inactivity on motor skill development across the lifespan. This includes a brief review of key motor skill acquisition milestones in a child's early years and tools for assessing motor development. The efficacy of physical activity related interventions on motor skill development will be explored, as well as the effect of lifelong physical activity on motor skill development through adolescence to late adulthood. The neurological basis of motor skill development, whereby myelin is laid down over neuronal axons to provide speed and accuracy of impulse propagation, is explored in Chapter 13. Exploration of the relationship between motor and cognitive development is beyond the scope of this chapter.

Motor skill development and fundamental movement skills

Motor skill development refers to the acquisition and changes in motor skills of an individual throughout their life. Motor learning by contrast is a change in the ability for a skilled performance resulting from new experiences and from practice. Motor learning can take the form of the development of new or refined skills, or the re-acquisition of previously mastered skills following serious illness, injury or long-term non-participation in a specific activity.

Fundamental movement skills are developed in most children's pre-school years through play and practice. FMS generally refer to *gross motor skills*, movements created by involving large muscle groups as well as core stabilisation provided by the body to support movement. Gross motor skills can be divided into: *locomotor skills*, moving the body about by running, jumping, hopping, etc.; *object control*, which involves manipulating objects for example throwing and catching balls and striking objects with bats; and, *balance/body management skills*, which develop core stability and posture control (Centers for Disease Control and Prevention, 2013). Developing children acquire and refine gross motor skills as they progress through the 'toddler' years towards becoming accomplished walkers, runners and stair climbers. Alongside this development comes the acquisition and refinement of *fine motor skills*, typically involving the small muscles in the hands and the production of finely controlled movements such as manipulation of small objects, tying shoe laces, writing and art (Centers for Disease Control and Prevention, 2013).

In addition to FMS being a precursor to successful performance of sport-specific skills, Seefeldt and colleagues have suggested that the acquisition of fundamental motor skills must reach a certain level of competency, which they have termed the "proficiency barrier", to progress to performing sporting skills and participating successfully in motor tasks later in life (Seefeldt & Nadeau, 1980; Stodden, True, Langendorfer, & Gao, 2013).

Assessment and checkpoints for motor skill development

Motor skill development milestones

At various stages, normally developing children will meet key FMS milestones, with pre-school age particularly significant for FMS development (Gallahue, Ozmun, & Goodway, 2012). New skills start from infants raising their heads and pointing at pictures in books to toddlers walking stiff-legged before developing a normal walking gait. Three-year-old toddlers will often be walking and begin to run, jump and hop, as well as starting to kick, throw and catch balls and gain fine motor skills to support feeding themselves. Around this age children will also start to develop a preference for a dominant hand. Normally developing pre-schoolers will ride tricycles, walk up and down steps using alternate feet, and start to draw simple stick figures. Once children reach school age (5–7 years) they begin to demonstrate clear adult-like skills, replicating sport-specific actions with smoother, more controlled movements. These include faster running and swimming, riding a bicycle without training wheels, and playing organised sports. Fine motor skills continue to develop with children learning to write letters and numbers, and create artwork. With improvements comes competence at dressing and undressing and the ability of children to feed and groom themselves.

While FMS development milestones can be used as reference points to track normal development, it is important to remember that there are great differences in the motor skills of children of the same age range. The indicators above provide an approximate set of ages at which development will occur, though individual differences, particularly between locomotor, object control and fine motor skill development are not necessarily signs of problems (Centers for Disease Control and Prevention, 2013).

Motor skill development assessment

Assessment of motor skill development involves testing children across a battery of skills using validated measurement instruments. In order to accurately assess skilled performance, participants must first be briefed on the tasks, with demonstrations and the opportunity to attempt the tasks prior to testing. This ensures it is the performance being tested, rather than simple understanding of the task. As several skills are typically tested in one session, it is important to create a motivating and fun environment where children feel encouraged and positively challenged (Stratton, Foweather, Rotchell, English, & Hughes, 2015; Theeboom, De Knop, & Weiss, 1995).

The *Test of Gross Motor Development* 2nd edition (TGMD-2) was designed to test 12 gross motor skills in children aged from 3–10 years (Ulrich, 2000). The skills assessed are separated into locomotor skills (run, hop, gallop, leap, horizontal jump, and slide) and object control skills (ball skills such as hitting a stationary ball, stationary dribble, catching, kicking, overhand throw, and underhand roll). Many similar tools have been developed (see for example, Cools, De Martelaer, Samaey, & Andries, 2009). More recently, Sport Wales (Stratton et al., 2015) introduced the Dragon Challenge assessment tool. This tool uses a game-like iPad interface to increase student motivation as they select skills to perform and complete each 'challenge'.

The majority of tools have been developed assuming equality of motor skill development and performance between boys and girls under 11 years of age (Cools et al., 2009). It is important to note, however, that some studies have identified differences in task performance between male and female children in specific tasks (Cliff, Okely, Smith, & McKeen, 2009; Goodway, Robinson, & Crowe, 2010; Pedersen, Sigmundsson, Whiting, & Ingvaldsen, 2003; Sääkslahti et al., 1999; Sport New Zealand, 2012). The New Zealand study which found differences between males and females in some tasks also identified a challenge with using ageing metrics for motor skill development. Comparing around 450 students aged 8–9 and 12–13 in 2002 with a further 240 students of the same ages four years later, significant increases in performance were found between the two groups in the majority of skills assessed (Sport New Zealand, 2012).

Observation involves one or two assessors scoring children on predetermined and prevalidated measures of motor skill performance, with a cross-check providing a test for inter-rater reliability where multiple assessors are used. The tasks need to be short with assessment carried out at the time of testing, rather than by reviewing recordings after the fact, as multiple tasks are assessed in a given session and many children are assessed in each session.

The relationship between physical activity and motor skill development

The health benefits of regular physical activity have been extensively studied (Janssen & LeBlanc, 2010; Strong et al., 2005; Warburton et al., 2006). In addition, there is evidence that physical activity intensity has an inverse relationship to mortality (Lee & Skerrett, 2001), with Janssen & LeBlanc and Strong et al. recommending at least 60 minutes of daily moderate physical activity for children and young people. As well as supporting longevity and overall health, there is growing evidence supporting the positive interrelationship between physical activity and motor skill development. Physical activity, in particular moderate to vigorous physical activity (MVPA) supports the development of motor skills (Fisher et al., 2005), while children with well-developed motor skills participate more frequently in physical activity and report greater self-efficacy (Lopes, Rodrigues, Maia, & Malina, 2011).

Causality between on-time motor skill development in young children and physical activity at young and older ages is difficult to establish. Cross-sectional studies are able only to demonstrate correlations between physical activity in very young children and the development of fundamental motor skills, as well as between measured motor skills in school-aged children and measured or self-reported amount of physical activity. Longitudinal studies are expensive and challenging to conduct, however there is some evidence from the few that have been conducted in this area that successful development of movement skills in childhood may play a causal role in determining future physical activity engagement (Barnett, van Beurden, Morgan, Brooks, & Beard, 2009).

Table 9.1 summarises the relationship between motor skills and physical activity from the literature. The general findings are a low positive relationship between physical activity and play and motor skill performance. A few studies suggest a difference in motor skill performance between sexes, though the evidence is weak, and only observed by some researchers for the performance of some locomotor skills. The results in Table 9.1 show a stronger relationship was found between more vigorous physical activity and motor skill acquisition.

Fisher and colleagues (2005) reported a low correlation between gross motor skills and physical activity in a study involving 4-year-old children ($n = 394$). This correlation was significant between total time spent in MVPA and motor skill score ($r = 0.18$, $p < 0.001$), but not for time spent in light-intensity physical activity ($r = 0.02$, $p > 0.05$). In a longitudinal study which tested motor control of a group of over 1,000 students aged 8–12, and re-tested 294 of the original sample six years later, Barnett et al., (2009) found that object control proficiency (kick, catch, overhand throw) was a significant predictor of adolescents' physical activity levels. This supports the need for attention to object control development and potential interventions to support object control development to enhance time spent in physical activity during the lifespan.

Motivation, physical activity and motor skill acquisition

Theeboom et al. (1995) explored the relationship between motivational climate and motor skill development in teaching the Chinese martial art of Wushu to a group of 8–10-year-old children ($n = 119$). The children were randomly assigned to one of two groups for three weeks of Wushu lessons during a larger organised sports programme. The children in the control group were taught using traditional instruction in a performance climate where successful performances were acknowledged publicly, supporting an environment where students compared their performance to the norms of their peer group. The study group involved mastery oriented instruction, using athlete-centred approaches to give students more ownership of their learning and encouraging incremental improvements in personal performance. In addition to reporting higher levels of perceived competence and intrinsic motivation, students in the mastery group sought increasingly difficult challenges and reported greater enjoyment of

Table 9.1 Relationship between motor skills and physical activity in published literature

Author	Age (N participants)	Relationship	Motor Skill tests	Correlation/significance of some results
Williams et al. (2008)	3–4 (N=198)	Significant relationship between total motor skills and MVPA and VPA for children in top motor skill tertile	CMSP (CHAMPS motor skill protocol)	MVPA: $r=0.2$ $p<0.01$ VPA: $r=0.26$, $p<0.001$
Butcher and Eaton (1989)	5	Low positive correlation between indoor free play and motor skills	Running speed and agility assessed	
Sääkslahti et al. (1999)	3–4 (N=105)	Low positive correlation between sports participation and motor skill proficiency	APM-Inventory (Finland)	E.g. very active indoor play and throwing at a target: $r=0.24$, $p=0.014$)
Raudsepp and Pall (2006)	7–8	Participation in jumping-related activities related to skill in jumping	Observations	$r=0.55$
Okely, Booth, and Patterson (2001)	12–16 (N=1844)	Significant relationship between FMS and self-reported participation in physical activity in adolescents	New South Wales Schools Fitness and Physical Activity Survey 1997	
Theeboom et al. (1995)	8–10	Higher performance between mastery learning group in Wushu class than traditionally coached group	Expert assessment of Wushu forward jump kick	Effect size = 0.50
Fisher et al. (2005)	3–5 (N=394)	Significant positive relationship between MVPA and movement performance, no significant correlation with light-intensity physical activity (PA)	Movement Assessment Battery (15 skills)	MVPA: $r=0.18$ $p<0.001$ light PA: $r=0.02$, $p>0.05$
B. D. Ulrich (1987)	5–10 (N=250)	Children in organised sport programmes performed selected gross motor tasks better than nonparticipants	The Perceived Competence Scale for Children	
Barnett et al. (2009)	8–12 (N=294)	Adolescent time in MVPA and organised physical activity was positively associated with childhood object control proficiency	"Get Skilled, Get Active" movement battery	
Cliff et al. (2009)	3–5 (N=46)	Object-control skills associated with physical activity. Gender differences in locomotor skills	TGMD-II	Object control, boys MVPA: $r=0.48$, $p=0.015$

the sessions. Motor skill proficiency of the children was assessed through the performance of a 'forward jump kick'. Children in the mastery group scored higher on the jump kick performance than those in the traditional group (effect size = 0.50).

The finding of Theeboom et al. (1995) suggests children may benefit from a supportive and motivational environment where they have some control over their activities. It also suggests a relationship may exist between participation in skill-specific physical activity and development of specific motor skills. This has also been observed by Raudsepp and Pall (2006), who implemented a training intervention which focused on jumping-related activities, and demonstrated a significant improvement in jumping-related skills among the participants.

The relationship between a child's self-perception of their motor skill proficiency and participation in physical activity as an adolescent was also examined in the longitudinal study of Barnett, Morgan, van Beurden, and Beard (2008). These results suggest a need to not only assist children to develop fundamental motor skills, but to also ensure that children develop efficacy in their own skills.

The results described in this section support the use of games-based approaches to encourage physical activity participation. Popular research-supported games-based approaches include Teaching Games for Understanding (Bunker & Thorpe, 1982), Game Sense (den Duyn, 1997), and Positive Pedagogy (Light, 2016). The latter provides applications to individual and technique-dominated sports. In these approaches modified versions of games are used to progressively develop game-related skills along with tactical understanding. Modified games can be used to vary the intensity as well as the skill focus of games, with questioning used to encourage active learning and engagement.

Influence of inactivity on motor skill development

Self-efficacy and task confidence are closely related with motivation to participate in specific activities (Lopes et al., 2011; Theeboom et al., 1995; Williams et al., 2008).

Williams et al. (2008) observed 198 pre-school children, also finding significantly lower physical activity participation from children with poor motor skill performance, although the relationship was found to only be significant with regard to the quality of locomotor skills. They also discovered that children with higher locomotor skills spent significantly more time in MVPA than those with lower skills. This latter finding is particularly significant with regard to participation in lifelong physical activity, and argues for attention to the promotion and development of fundamental movement skills in the developing child.

In addition to the positive findings of motivation, participation, and motor skill development discussed in the previous section, children with gross motor difficulties commonly display disinterest and avoidance of physical tasks (Lopes et al., 2011). Such children will commonly choose tasks that are either too easy, or too difficult. This avoids the risk of failure in suitably challenging tasks. Lopes' study is particularly interesting, consisting of longitudinal study of 285 boys and girls from ages 6 to 10. They found that physical activity of the group declined significantly across the five years of the study, although the decrease among children who initially scored high in motor skills was very small compared to the much sharper drop from the middle tertile and particularly those who recorded low motor skill scores.

These results highlight the importance of on-time development of fundamental motor skills in children to support lifelong engagement in physical activity. In the following section, the efficacy of interventions to enhance motor skill performance where deficits have been identified are explored.

Physical activity interventions to enhance motor skill development

Earlier sections have identified a link between physical activity at pre-school ages and the development of fundamental motor skills, and have further discussed the influence of motor skill acquisition on physical activity in childhood and adolescence. Many of the tests of motor skill development are aimed at identifying developmental delays or abnormalities. With the implementation of targeted support, through MVPA in modified games, for example, it is possible to support motor skill development. This section discusses interventions which have been used and the findings from those studies.

Goodway and Branta (2003) implemented a 12-week motor skill intervention with disadvantaged pre-school children ($n = 59$) using the earlier version of the TGMD tool to evaluate performance. Students had been identified as having delayed motor skill development, and scored low on both locomotor skills and object control. In this context, students may be considered disadvantaged due to a lack of support to engage in physical activity in their upbringing. Examples where support or encouragement may be lacking include: poverty, single parent, incarcerated or drug dependent parent. These disadvantages have been shown to lead to developmental FMS delays in many children (Hamilton, Goodway, & Haubenstricker, 1999). The pre-test showed that most of the students were significantly delayed in development of both locomotor and object control skills. The intervention featured direct instruction to purposefully develop selected motor skills, and was seen to produce significant gains, which exceeded the modest gains of the control group who engaged in free play as part of their programme. In a further study, Goodway and Branta (2003) tested fundamental skills of disadvantaged (primarily through poverty) African-American ($n = 275$) and Hispanic ($n = 194$) pre-school children. They also found students were behind expectation in FMS development, and that boys outperformed girls in most of the TGMD-2 items. Differences in motor skill performance in girls and boys may well represent different socialisation into different activities, and further investigation in this area is warranted.

In addition to assessing the efficacy of a motor skill development intervention, Ishee and Hoffman (2003) concluded that normal development is supported if "physical educators and pre-school teachers engage their students in activities necessary to facilitate positive motor skill development". This supports Goodway and Branta's finding (2003) that purposeful attention to developing motor skills produces significantly greater motor skill gains.

Physical activity, motor performance and ageing

Much of the discussion in this chapter has addressed the development and needs of pre-school and school-aged children. Even later in life, as motor development moves from gaining new skills toward maintenance and some loss of proficiency, the interplay between physical activity, motor development and health is important to understand.

Motor skill development continues into adolescence, when specialised movement skills are enhanced through deliberate practice. The 'ten thousand hours' theory of expert performance for example posits that, on average, an athlete needs to spend 10,000 hours in deliberate practice to become world class in their pursuit (Baker, 2003; Gladwell, 2008). While this theory is the subject of some debate, the fact remains that practice does indeed lead to the development and enhancement of motor skills at all ages. Motor skill acquisition is also specialised, in that the learner may become highly proficient at one set of skills, for example become a talented soccer player, but may be weak at throwing and catching a ball. This specialisation demonstrates the importance of providing opportunities for motor skill development across a wide range of activities (Schmidt & Wrisberg, 2004).

As we age, the performance and functioning of the body's physiological systems begin to decline. Vision, hearing, muscular strength and nervous system functions are less efficient, among other established changes in the older adult (Huang & Tang, 2010; Klein et al., 1991). Age-related changes differ markedly between individuals, with some systems retaining their functioning through the lifespan, while others compensate for declining systems. Various underlying mechanisms have been proposed to explain the observed changes, from a general 'wearing out' of body systems – which is contradicted by the improved performance seen in physically active older people – to the damaging effects at cellular level of free radicals, changes in body composition and posture affecting internal organ functioning and a general decline in the ability of the body to respond quickly to changing environmental factors to maintain homeostasis (Gallahue et al., 2012). Significant changes have been observed in older adults with regard to visual acuity (Klein et al., 1991) and auditory performance (Huang & Tang, 2010), which can contribute to reduced reaction times and poorer motor performance in tasks performed in dimly lit environments, or where task requirements are explained verbally and might not be accurately and fully heard. Other changes associated with reaction time may be due to differing priorities in the young and old – with older people choosing to complete tasks with more care, prioritising accuracy, while younger performers seek speed. Choice and motivation can therefore potentially account for changes in performance timing, rather than physical decline. With this in mind, it is interesting to review what has been observed of the interaction of physical activity and age-related changes that have been observed in motor performance.

Christensen et al. (2003) examined the reaction time performance of 45 men aged between 60 and 70 and found that those in the top tertile of physical activity exhibited both faster reactions, and lower error in the tests conducted, while those in the lowest tertile performed the worst. This finding supports several earlier studies that also found that physical activity is associated with a lesser decline in motor function. Further, regular physical activity, and indeed physical activity interventions in older adults, has been shown to also contribute to enhanced joint flexibility, muscular strength, and improved posture (see, for example, Warburton et al. (2006) for an extensive review of the field). These are all important factors in maintaining balance and avoiding injury from falls, a major concern in the elderly. There is a wealth of evidence that age-related declines in motor performance can be reduced significantly by continued, and specific physical activity. This can be seen in the performance athletes competing at 'masters' level, many to a much higher skill level than accomplished younger athletes.

Concluding remarks

A clear body of evidence demonstrates the relationship between physical activity and the development of FMS in pre-school children. While milestones have been laid down with which to assess development of children and adolescents, and a battery of tools developed to study motor skill acquisition, it is important to be cognisant of individual differences and timings in skill acquisition.

Equally important is the link, across the lifespan, between motor skill proficiency and the volume and intensity of physical activity which people engage in. While there is only a weak link established to support early motor skill proficiency as the driver for future amount of physical activity, rather than the latter driving the former, it is clear that engaging developing children in play and movement activities supports habits of lifelong physical activity and positive motor skill development. There is also evidence of a positive link between the specificity of physical activity, as well as participant motivation, and motor skill acquisition. This provides support for the delivery of modified games-based approaches to teaching and coaching to improve motor learning outcomes.

The efficacy of physical activity interventions has been demonstrated in improving motor skill development in disadvantaged populations, providing opportunities to address deficits. This is particularly important when assessing the needs of the developing child from the earliest years through into adolescence. Finally, the amount of physical activity in which people engage in later years has been shown to be related to a reduced loss of motor skill performance.

Chapter summary

- Physical activity, through play and purposeful activity, is critical to supporting development of fundamental movement skills in the early years of children's lives.
- Fundamental motor skills are the building blocks for the performance of sport-specific skills.
- Fundamental motor skill development deficiencies are correlated with reduced child participation in physical activity and feelings of low self-efficacy.
- The causal relationship between motor skill development and physical activity is not clearly understood, however correlations between movement skills and physical activity are clearly established across the lifespan.
- Short, intense but specific, motor skill training interventions provide measurable gains in motor skill performance.
- Maintenance of physical activity through the lifespan is associated with lesser decline in motor performance in late adulthood.

References

Baker, J. (2003). Early specialization in youth sport: A requirement for adult expertise? *High Ability Studies, 14*(1), 85–94.

Barnett, L.M., Morgan, P.J., van Beurden, E., & Beard, J.R. (2008). Perceived sports competence mediates the relationship between childhood motor skill proficiency and adolescent physical activity and fitness: A longitudinal assessment. *International Journal of Behavioral Nutrition and Physical Activity, 5*(1), 1.

Barnett, L.M., van Beurden, E., Morgan, P.J., Brooks, L.O., & Beard, J.R. (2009). Childhood motor skill proficiency as a predictor of adolescent physical activity. *Journal of Adolescent Health, 44*(3), 252–259.

Bunker, D., & Thorpe, R. (1982). A model for the teaching of games in secondary schools. *Bulletin of Physical Education, 18*(1), 5–8.

Butcher, J.E., & Eaton, W.O. (1989). Gross and fine motor proficiency in preschoolers – relationships with free play behavior and activity level. *Journal of Human Movement Studies, 16*(1), 27–36.

Centers for Disease Control and Prevention. (2013). *Developmental Milestones*.

Christensen, C.L., Payne, V.G., Wughalter, E.H., Van, J.H., Henehan, M., & Jones, R. (2003). Physical activity, physiological, and psychomotor performance: A study of variously active older adult men. *Research Quarterly for Exercise and Sport, 74*(2), 136–142.

Cliff, D.P., Okely, A.D., Smith, L.M., & McKeen, K. (2009). Relationships between fundamental movement skills and objectively measured physical activity in preschool children. *Pediatric Exercise Science, 21*(4), 436–449.

Cools, W., De Martelaer, K., Samaey, C., & Andries, C. (2009). Movement skill assessment of typically developing preschool children: A review of seven movement skill assessment tools. *Journal of Sports Science and Medicine, 8*(2), 154–168.

den Duyn, N. (1997). Coaching children: Game Sense – it's time to play! *Sports Coach, 19*, 9–11.

Fisher, A., Reilly, J.J., Kelly, L.A., Montgomery, C., Williamson, A., Paton, J.Y., & Grant, S. (2005). Fundamental movement skills and habitual physical activity in young children. *Med Sci Sports Exerc, 37*(4), 684–688.

Gallahue, D.L., Ozmun, J.C., & Goodway, J. (2012). *Understanding Motor Development: Infants, children, adolescents, adults*: McGraw-Hill.

Gladwell, M. (2008). *Outliers: The story of success*: Hachette UK.

Goodway, J.D., & Branta, C.F. (2003). Influence of a motor skill intervention on fundamental motor skill development of disadvantaged preschool children. *Research Quarterly for Exercise and Sport, 74*(1), 36–46.

Goodway, J.D., Robinson, L.E., & Crowe, H. (2010). Gender differences in fundamental motor skill development in disadvantaged preschoolers from two geographical regions. *Research Quarterly for Exercise and Sport, 81*(1), 17–24.

Hamilton, M., Goodway, J., & Haubenstricker, J. (1999). Parent-assisted instruction in a motor skill program for at-risk preschool children. *Adapted Physical Activity Quarterly, 16*, 415–426.

Huang, Q., & Tang, J. (2010). Age-related hearing loss or presbycusis. *European Archives of Oto-Rhino-Laryngology, 267*(8), 1179–1191. doi:10.1007/s00405-010-1270-7

Ishee, J.H., & Hoffman, J. (2003). The influence of motor skill interventions on disadvantaged children. *Journal of Physical Education, Recreation & Dance, 74*(8), 14–14.

Janssen, I., & LeBlanc, A.G. (2010). Systematic review of the health benefits of physical activity and fitness in school-aged children and youth. *International Journal of Behavioral Nutrition and Physical Activity, 7*(1), 1.

Klein, R., Klein, B.E., Linton, K.L., & De Mets, D.L. (1991). The Beaver Dam eye study: Visual acuity. *Ophthalmology, 98*(8), 1310–1315.

Lee, I.-M., & Skerrett, P.J. (2001). Physical activity and all-cause mortality: What is the dose-response relation? *Medicine and Science in Sports and Exercise, 33*(6; SUPP), S459–S471.

Light, R. (2016). *Positive Pedagogy for Sport Coaching: Athlete-centred coaching for individual sports*: Routledge.

Lopes, V.P., Rodrigues, L.P., Maia, J.A., & Malina, R.M. (2011). Motor coordination as predictor of physical activity in childhood. *Scandinavian Journal of Medicine & Science in Sports, 21*(5), 663–669.

Okely, A.D, Booth, M.L., & Patterson, J.W. (2001). Relationship of physical activity to fundamental movement skills among adolescents. *Medicine and Science in Sports and Exercise, 33*(11), 1899–1904. http://dx.doi.org/10.1097/00005768-200111000-00015.

Pedersen, A., Sigmundsson, H., Whiting, H., & Ingvaldsen, R. (2003). Sex differences in lateralisation of fine manual skills in children. *Experimental Brain Research, 149*(2), 249–251.

Raudsepp, L., & Pall, P. (2006). The relationship between fundamental motor skills and outside-school physical activity of elementary school children. *Pediatric Exercise Science, 18*(4), 426.

Sääkslahti, A., Numminen, P., Niinikoski, H., Rask-Nissilä, L., Viikari, J., Tuominen, J., & Välimäki, I. (1999). Is physical activity related to body size, fundamental motor skills, and CHD risk factors in early childhood? *Pediatric Exercise Science, 11*, 327–340.

Schmidt, R.A., & Wrisberg, C.A. (2004). *Motor Learning and Performance*. Champaign: Human Kinetics.

Seefeldt, V., & Nadeau, C. (1980). Developmental motor patterns: Implications for elementary school physical education. *Psychology of Motor Behavior and Sport*, 314–323.

Sport New Zealand. (2012). *Fundamental Movement Skills among children in New Zealand*. Wellington: Sport New Zealand.

Stodden, D.F., True, L.K., Langendorfer, S.J., & Gao, Z. (2013). Associations among selected motor skills and health-related fitness: Indirect evidence for Seefeldt's proficiency barrier in young adults? *Research Quarterly for Exercise and Sport, 84*(3), 397–403.

Stratton, G., Foweather, L., Rotchell, J., English, J., & Hughes, H. (2015). *Dragon Challenge V1.0 Manual*. Cardiff: Sport Wales.

Strong, W.B., Malina, R.M., Blimkie, C.J., Daniels, S.R., Dishman, R.K., Gutin, B., . . . Pivarnik, J.M. (2005). Evidence based physical activity for school-age youth. *The Journal of Pediatrics, 146*(6), 732–737.

Theeboom, M., De Knop, P., & Weiss, M.R. (1995). Motivational climate, psychological responses, and motor skill development in children's sport: A field-based intervention study. *Journal of Sport and Exercise Psychology, 17*, 294–311.

Tremblay, M.S., LeBlanc, A.G., Kho, M.E., Saunders, T.J., Larouche, R., Colley, R.C., . . . Gorber, S.C. (2011). Systematic review of sedentary behaviour and health indicators in school-aged children and youth. *International Journal of Behavioral Nutrition and Physical Activity, 8*(1), 1.

Ulrich, B.D. (1987). Perceptions of physical competence, motor competence, and participation in organized sport: Their interrelationships in young children. *Research Quarterly for Exercise and Sport, 58*(1), 57–67.

Ulrich, D.A. (2000). *Test of Gross Motor Development – 2*. Austin: Prod-Ed.

Warburton, D.E., Nicol, C.W., & Bredin, S.S. (2006). Health benefits of physical activity: The evidence. *Canadian Medical Association Journal, 174*(6), 801–809.

Williams, H.G., Pfeiffer, K.A., O'Neill, J.R., Dowda, M., McIver, K.L., Brown, W.H., & Pate, R.R. (2008). Motor skill performance and physical activity in preschool children. *Obesity, 16*(6), 1421–1426

10 Exercise physiology and physical activity

Michael J. Duncan

Keywords: Energy balance, Non-Exercise Activity Thermogenesis, NEAT, EPOC, inactivity

Introduction

This chapter provides an overview of the physiology of physical activity (and inactivity). The chapter outlines the concept of energy balance, followed by an overview of what occurs when an individual engages in a sustained bout of physical activity (acute) and then if physical activity is engaged in with regularity (chronic). In such cases nearly all of the systems and organs in the human body are engaged in some form or another, and as such, understanding the physiology of physical activity is a key component for effective research and practice in sport, exercise and health sciences. Then, if undertaken regularly the physiological changes we typically see as a result of physical activity change as the body adapts to an increased demand on the body to undertake exercise. The second half of this chapter will then present information relating to the physiological changes that occur as a consequence of prolonged inactivity and the concept of Non-Exercise Activity Thermogenesis (NEAT)

Energy balance

Before beginning to understand the physiology of physical activity (or inactivity) an overview of energy balance is relevant. In its most basic sense energy balance is a simple concept where:

Energy balance = Energy intake − Energy expenditure

Where energy intake and expenditure are different we experience an energy imbalance. In cases where energy intake is greater than energy expenditure humans will tend to experience an increase in body mass and where energy intake is less than energy expenditure humans will tend to experience a decrease in body mass. Such changes do not tend to occur in response to acute periods (e.g. days) or energy imbalance but rather happen over a longer period of times, usually months to years. In the context of the current chapter, low levels of energy expenditure (as a result of inactivity) will result in increased body mass, comprised of adipose tissue, if not matched with low levels of energy intake. If this imbalance is sustained, over time an individual will become overweight, then obese and will have increased mortality and morbidity as a consequence.

When considering the physiology of physical activity energy balance and the determinants of energy expenditure are important. The major component of energy expenditure is Basal Metabolic Rate (BMR) (Levine, 2004). BMR is considered as the daily amount of energy expenditure required to maintain basic physiological functions including breathing and circulation of blood. BMR typically reflects the energy expended when an individual is supine at complete rest, in the morning, after sleep (Levine, 2004). For individuals with sedentary occupations, BMR accounts for approximately 60% of total daily energy expenditure (Levine, 2004). However, as a component of overall energy expenditure, BMR can become less significant when an individual engages in high levels of physical activity. Body mass is another key variable which influences BMR, and subsequently the impact of physical activity on human physiology, but size has a contrasting effect depending on what type of mass is involved. Body composition is therefore important when considering the effect of physical activity on physiology as adipose tissue has a lower metabolic demand compared to other tissues, particularly muscle. As increasing energy expenditure, relative to intake, is associated with increased muscle mass and decreased fat mass and decreasing energy expenditure is associated with decreased muscle mass and increased fat mass, considering body composition of the individual is important in estimating and understanding the physiological changes expected from changing physical activity habits.

BMR is however only one of the principal components of human energy balance, the other two being the thermic effect of feeding and activity thermogenesis. The thermic effect of feeding accounts for around 10–15% of total daily energy expenditure (Levine, 2004) and will not be explained in great detail as part of this chapter. Activity thermogenesis is the key focus of the current chapter and can be separated into two subcomponents, exercise related activity thermogenesis and Non-Exercise Activity Thermogenesis (NEAT) (Levine, 2004). Both are important when describing the physiological effects of physical activity.

Physiological responses to acute bouts of different types of physical activity

An acute bout of physical activity will elicit some form of physiological response and that response may differ depending on the type of physical activity engaged in and depending which physiological system we examine.

As energy derived from oxygen consumption accounts for the majority of energy used in any physical activity, examining the changes in the volume of oxygen consumed (VO_2) that occur when moving from rest and then undertaking an acute bout of exercise is important in understanding how the cardiovascular and respiratory systems change in order to meet the increased oxygen demand placed on the body as a result of whatever activity the body is engaged in. An individual's VO_2 max, or the maximal amount of oxygen that can be taken and used by the body is key in this response and will influence the response to an acute bout of physical activity.

In basic terms, when an individual moves from rest to exercise there is a shift in the oxygen demand placed on the body. When the bout of physical activity or exercise that is undertaken is constant (e.g., walking/running on a treadmill at a consistent, unchanging speed), the body has an increased O_2 requirement in comparison to its resting O_2 requirement. This is demonstrated in Figure 10.1 which presents the VO_2 values for a 9-year-old child engaging moving from supine to light to moderate PA.

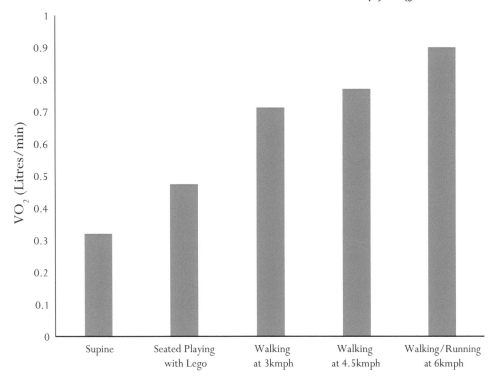

Figure 10.1 VO$_2$ values (litres/min) for a 9-year-old engaged in sedentary activity, light and moderate
intensity physical activity

The human body cannot instantaneously meet the increased O$_2$ demand for the bout of
physical activity using aerobic energy sources and instead has to meet this demand using other
(anaerobic) sources of energy. This is often termed 'oxygen deficit' as other energy sources,
phosphocreatine and glycolysis provide the energy to meet the required O$_2$ cost during the first
minutes of a bout of physical activity. The greater the exercise intensity, the greater the oxygen deficit. Over time, the body is then able to meet the required O$_2$ demand using oxidative
(aerobic) metabolism. Once the bout of physical activity finishes, the VO$_2$ does not however return back to resting O$_2$ requirement instantaneously either. Instead there is a gradual
reduction in VO$_2$ consumed from the O$_2$ requirement for physical activity to the resting O$_2$
requirement. This has variously been referred to as oxygen debt or excess post-exercise oxygen
consumption (EPOC). EPOC is characterised by a rapid reduction in VO$_2$ consumed in the 2–3
minutes immediately after physical activity/exercise cessation and then a slower reduction of
VO$_2$ back to the resting O$_2$ requirement. This takes place to replenish phosphocreatine and oxygen stores in muscle and then to resynthesise lactic acid to glucose (Gaesser & Brooks, 1984).
A typical exercise and EPOC response, demonstrated during a bout of submaximal arm crank
ergometry is shown in Figure 10.2. On this figure, the increase in O$_2$ consumption at the onset
of exercise is clearly shown, followed by steady state O$_2$ consumption to meet the demands
of the exercise bout. This is then followed by a slower decline in O$_2$ consumption on exercise
cessation representing EPOC.

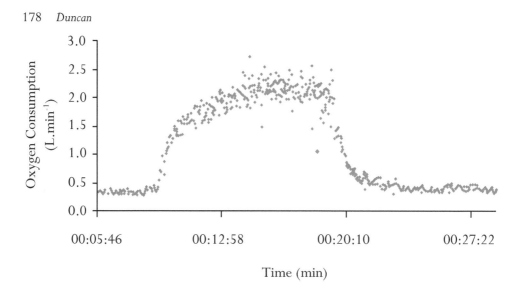

Figure 10.2 Typical oxygen consumption and EPOC pattern demonstrated as a consequence of submaximal arm crank ergometry in an adult male (data courtesy of Dr Mike Price)

The response shown in Figure 10.2 occurs in any instance where an individual moves
from rest to undertaking any form of physical activity, however the magnitude of the O_2
deficit and EPOC is dependent on the intensity and duration of the activity undertaken with
physical activity of higher intensity or longer duration resulting in increased oxygen debt
and longer EPOC.

The heart rate and ventilatory response to physical activity follows a similar pattern to that
of the VO_2 consumed. This results in a lag in the delivery of O_2 to the working muscles resulting in the initial oxygen debt at the commencement of a bout of physical activity.

Blood pressure responses during acute bouts of physical activity are also intensity dependant. Typically, systolic blood pressure increases with exercise intensity whereas diastolic blood
pressure remains the same or slightly decreases. In combination this results in a slight increase
in mean arterial blood pressure. On cessation of the physical activity bout there is a reduction
in blood pressure, termed postexercise hypotension, which has been documented to last for
several hours post exercise (Keese, Farinatti, Pescatello, & Monteiro, 2011). Similarly, with
physical activity there is an increased demand from the working muscles to extract oxygen
from arterial blood. In order to bring more O_2 into the body, and blood via gas exchange,
pulmonary ventilation increases. Ventilation increases in a linear fashion from rest to light to
moderate intensity physical activity. After this point, when physical activity becomes more
vigorous in intensity, ventilation rate is shown to increase dramatically. This point is often
referred to as the ventilatory threshold and has been more commonly used in sports science
type research as a non-invasive estimate of the lactate threshold.

Acute bouts of physical activity also have potential to produce different responses in the
endocrine system. Again, such changes are intensity and mode dependant. Key hormones, testosterone, cortisol, growth hormone and insulin-like growth factor-1 are impacted by acute
bouts of physical activity and are important as they initiate various physiological cascades that
contribute to increased capillary density, muscle hypertrophy and mitochondrial biogenesis

(Kraemer & Ratamess, 2005; Andersen & Henriksson, 1977; Goffart & Wiesner, 2003), in addition to maintaining homeostasis. Typically, testosterone will increase as a result of an acute bout of exercise or physical activity. Heavy resistance exercise exhibits the largest post-exercise increase in testosterone (Kraemer & Ratamess, 2005). Responses of a smaller magnitude of change seen for aerobically based exercise or submaximal resistance exercise (Tremblay, Copeland & Van Helder, 2005; Vuorimaa et al., 1999; Linnamo, Pakarinen, Komi, Kraemer, & Häkkinen, 2005) including reduced testosterone following submaximal resistance exercise (Linnamo et al., 2005). With aerobically based activity that is longer in duration (2 hours+) testosterone levels decrease and cortisol levels increase (Tremblay et al., 2005). Growth hormone concentrations typically increase as a consequence of aerobically or resistance-based exercise, which in turn stimulates insulin-like growth factor-1 production. This is important in the context of physical activity as insulin-like growth factor-1 has been associated with a number of parameters representing 'good health' including body fatness and aerobic fitness (Nindl, Santtila, Vaara, Häkkinen, & Kyröläinen, 2011).

Physiological adaptations to physical activity

Acute bouts of physical activity elicit acute physiological responses both during and immediately post exercise. Engagement in habitual and regular physical activity results in physiological adaptations that, in some instances are a consequence of repeated acute physiological responses, as may be the case with blood pressure (Keese et al., 2011), or occur as a result of the overload principle (Gunter, Almstedt, & Janz, 2012) in the case of muscle or bone.

In respect to cardiovascular and respiratory changes seen as a result of habitual and regular physical activity, these are intensity dependent with a greater magnitude of response being seen with higher intensity exercise programmes. The magnitude of adaptation is also dependent on the length of engagement in the physical activity programme and mode of exercise.

Broadly, regular, aerobically based physical activity results in several changes that collectively contribute to increasing the capability of the body to take in and use oxygen for movement. Cardiac output at rest and during submaximal exercise remains relatively unchanged but can be increased following regular physical activity if the intensity of the activity programme is sufficiently intense (e.g., endurance training). There are also changes in stroke volume at rest and during submaximal and maximal exercise as well as decreased resting and submaximal exercise heart rates. Again, if the intensity of the activity programme is sufficiently intense there are longer term cardiac changes including hypertrophy of the left ventricle resulting in more forceful emptying of the left ventricle per heart beat and thus more blood (and oxygen) being distributed around the body. In normotensive individuals, longer term engagement results in a small reduction in resting and submaximal exercise blood pressure. Reduction in resting and submaximal exercise blood pressure of a greater magnitude is seen in hypertensive individuals.

There is also potential for the respiratory system to change as a consequence of physical activity. Again, adaptations to the respiratory system are intensity dependent with endurance exercise training resulting in increases in the maximal rate of pulmonary ventilation and an increase in the pulmonary diffusion at maximal rates of exercise.

When an individual undertakes a sustained and regular programme of physical activity, skeletal muscle will adapt over time. The nature of the adaptation depends on the type of physical activity that the individual engages in. Low to moderate intensity, aerobically based physical activity (e.g., brisk walking) results in a small increase in the cross-sectional area of slow twitch muscle fibres (Abernethy, Thayer, & Taylor, 1990) and endurance exercise can result in a change of fast twitch fibres from type b to a, which have a higher oxidative capability (Abernethy et al., 1990). For more vigorous intensity, aerobically based physical activity, there is also an increase in the capilliarisation of the skeletal muscle (Terjung, 1995). This is useful in terms of exercise performance as it allows for increased blood flow in the active muscles during activity. If the mode of physical activity is more resistance based, over time there is increased hypertrophy (increased muscle size) and also increased muscle fibre recruitment. In addition to changes in the skeletal muscle, there are other related physiological adaptations to physical activity that enable the musculoskeletal system to effectively function. There is some evidence, particularly with higher intensity exercise, that ligaments and tendons become stronger (Tipton & Vailas, 1990).

In addition to adaptations seen in the cardiovascular, respiratory and muscular systems, long-term engagement in physical activity also prompts a number of metabolic changes. As with any form of exercise training, engaging in physical activity over a prolonged period can result in increases in the size and number of mitochondria with a concomitant increase in the activity of oxidative enzymes in the muscle. These changes, coupled with the increase in muscle capillaries and blood flow work to enhance the overall oxidative capacity of the trained muscle. In addition to this, a period of regular and habitual exercise/physical activity can also increase muscle glycogen storage and the ability of the muscle to use fat as an energy source (Kenny, Wilmore, & Costill, 2015). It has been suggested that the increased ability to use fat as an energy source following exercise training is a consequence of improved ability of the body to mobilise free fatty acids from fat depots and better capacity of oxidised fat (Kenny et al., 2015). Typically such changes have been demonstrated following a period of endurance type training rather than lower levels of physical activity. However, meta-regression analysis has demonstrated that improved ability to oxidise fat occurs with an average physical activity duration of 135 minutes per week at a moderate intensity (Romain et al., 2012) and mitochondrial adaptations have been shown with as little as 90 minutes per week at moderate intensity (Sahlin, Mogensen, Bagger, Fernström, & Pedersen, 2007).

Physiological changes as a consequence of prolonged inactivity/bed rest studies

Just as there are physiological adaptations which occur as a consequence of engaging in physical activity, if an individual who is highly physically active then ceases to be so, any physiological adaptations will be reversed. This is akin to the detraining effect seen when athletes stop undertaking endurance or resistance exercise training. The majority of research that has investigated the physiological effects of prolonged inactivity has done so employing bed rest studies. In these instances apparently healthy individuals have been placed in bed for up to three weeks following a control period, where baseline physiological measurements have been assessed. This should not be confused with sedentary behaviour, rather scientists have sought to examine the physiological changes that occur if an individual simply stops being active. The effects of bed rest on physiological function are similar to the effect of reduced gravitational forces attained during space flight and are particularly marked compared to detraining type studies where only exercise is discontinued. In the case of the latter, individuals continue their daily routine and remain upright during the day.

The results of bed rest studies show marked decrements in physiological function, particularly cardiovascular and respiratory function where the reduction in function is proportional to the duration of bed rest (Saltin et al., 1968; Shephard, 1994). The changes in physiological function are seen within days of bed rest with the reduced daily energy expenditure contributing to changes in metabolism such as glucose intolerance and changes in insulin resistance (Lipman et al., 1972). The body also goes into negative nitrogen and calcium balance, signalling loss of muscle protein and bone, respectively (Bloomfield & Coyle, 1993).

Aerobic exercise performance is also severely reduced following a period of total inactivity. Bloomfield and Coyle (1993) reported a reduction of 15% in VO_2 max after 10 days bed rest and a 27% reduction after 21 days bed rest (equivalent to 0.8% reduction per day). This decrease in VO_2 max is a result of decreased maximal cardiac output, which, in turn is a result of reduced stroke volume and decreased cardiac contractility (Bloomfield & Coyle, 1993). Although maximal heart rate does not change markedly as a consequence of bed rest, because stroke volume decreases, submaximal heart rate during exercise tends to be increased.

Skeletal muscle is also profoundly influenced following a period of bed rest. Muscle mass decreases, as does strength. There is also a reduction in bone mineral density that is proportional to the duration of inactivity (Bloomfield & Coyle, 1993). However, muscle atrophies faster than bone loses density with Bloomfield and Coyle (1993) reporting a 21% decrease in peak isokinetic knee extensor torque but only a 0.3–3% decrease in bone density at the lumbar spine following one month of bed rest. Of key importance, once normal physical activity is resumed, the decrements in cardiorespiratory, metabolic and muscle function can be reversed relatively quickly, within days and weeks (Bloomfield & Coyle, 1993). Likewise, Hortobágyi et al. (2000) reported an overall 47% decrease in eccentric, concentric and isometric strength following three weeks of limb immobilisation but after two weeks spontaneous recovery, muscle strength was only 11% lower than pre immobilisation values.

Lifespan physical activity

Although different methods of analysis have been used across studies, PA has protective effects on multiple facets of health in humans across the age spectrum. Importantly, it appears that physical activity tracks at low to moderate levels during adolescence, from adolescence into adulthood, and across various ages in adulthood (Malina, 1996). There has been considerable research attention devoted to understanding how PA impacts various aspects of human physiology in children and older adults particularly. This is understandable given a focus in children in developing PA habits that will persist into adulthood and in older adults given the link between PA and independent living and physical function for tasks of daily living. For older adults particularly there is a reported year on year decrease in moderate to vigorous PA at a rate of 1 minute/day between the ages of 65 and 85 (Hansen, Kolle, Dyrstad, Holme, & Anderssen, 2012). As an example, we also see, using data from our laboratory, distinct dose-response curves for PA on parameters related to health physiology and physical function in adults aged 50–80, where PA levels of less than 7,500 steps/day (Low PA) are associated with high levels of body fatness and there is a graded response where increased PA is associated with lower levels of body fatness (see Figure 10.3).

Recent research by Matthews et al. (2016) has also demonstrated dose response relations between PA and mortality in a sample of 4,840 US adults. Their work evidenced lower mortality risk for individuals with greater levels of accelerometer assessed PA and suggested that in less-active adults, replacing 1 h of sedentary time with either light- or moderate- to vigorous-intensity activity was associated with 18% and 42% lower mortality. The effect of lifespan PA on physiology can be evidenced in multiple ways, including mortality, as demonstrated above.

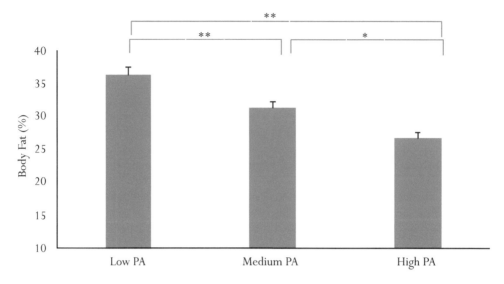

Figure 10.3 Mean SE of body fat percentage, determined by BIA, in 201 independently living adults aged 50–80 years (*P = .002, **P = .001)

However, the concept of lifespan PA is not the primary focus of the current chapter and is picked up more comprehensively in Chapters 3 and 10.

Non-Exercise Activity Thermogenesis (NEAT)

As mentioned earlier in this chapter, NEAT represents one of the subcomponents of activity thermogenesis which contribute to human energy expenditure. In relative terms the contribution of exercise-related activity thermogenesis is much less than NEAT. NEAT comprises the energy expenditure of occupations, leisure, sitting, standing, walking, dancing, shopping and a multitude of other activities such as playing musical instruments, toe-tapping, fidgeting and even chewing gum (Levine, 2004). As a consequence our understanding of the effects of exercise-related activity thermogenesis has been more widely studied due to ease of doing so. Studying the physiological (and other) effects of an acute bout of treadmill running or cycling or a sustained training programme engaged in structured exercise does help our understanding of the effect of physical activity on obesity. However, physical activity as a behaviour is multifaceted, comprising many different modes of movement and energy expenditure. A better awareness of NEAT is therefore important in understanding the impact of physical activity on physiological variables. The enormous variety of components within NEAT has made it a more difficult area to study but, arguably, it is of more importance in understanding physical activity behaviour as NEAT comprises activities such as walking, gardening and stair climbing, all of which have been key modes of physical activity intervention for health benefit (Levine, 2004). As NEAT comprises such a variety of activities it is also the most variable component of energy expenditure, representing from 15% of total energy expenditure in very sedentary individuals to 50% or greater in highly active individuals (Dauncey, 1990; Livingstone et al., 1991).

Influences on NEAT

NEAT is influenced by a number of different factors including occupation, built environment, gender and education. Individuals employed in different occupations can have different levels of NEAT, for example a sedentary worker, mostly sat at a desk each day, compared to a builder, where there will be considerably more movement and muscular load per day. This distinction also holds where an individual may undertake greater or lesser amounts of housework (Leibel, Rosenbaum, & Hirsch, 1995). Likewise, NEAT tends to be lower in more urbanised and industrialised environments as labour and time-saving facets of the built environment (e.g., drive through restaurants, lifts) contribute to lower physical activity, and lower NEAT as a consequence (Hill & Peters, 1998). Gender, although biologically determined, does impact NEAT as there are differences in physical activity levels between males and females and boys and girls (Levine et al., 2001) which contribute to different NEAT. Society and culture also contribute to differences in the level of NEAT undertaken by males and females (Levine et al., 2001). In more developed countries a higher level of education is also associated with higher NEAT, whereas the opposite is true in developing countries.

There are also biological factors which influence NEAT that also need to be considered in the context of understanding how physical activity might influence physiology. Even trivial movement can increase energy expenditure above resting levels which can potentially have a cumulative effect on physiological responses to physical activity (Levine, 2004). For example, chewing can increase energy expenditure by up to 20% greater than resting levels and low level movements such as fidgeting can increase energy expenditure by 20–40% (Levine, Baukol, & Pavlidis, 1999; Levine, Schleusner, & Jensen, 2000). Walking at very slow speeds (1 mph) doubles and walking at 3 mph triples energy expenditure (Bouten, Verboeket-van de Venne, Westerterp, Verduin, & Janssen, 1996).

NEAT presents a concept which is clearly important to understand if trying to interpret the effect of physical activity on physiology as the activities within NEAT comprise some of the activities prescribed to individuals who want to start a structured physical activity programme such as gardening or walking. The activities within NEAT are also distinct from structured modes of exercise such as running or cycling, where much of our understanding of the effect of physical activity on physiology is derived. However, while the mechanisms by which exercise effects physiology is relatively well understood, the mechanism for NEAT and the extent to which it will effect human physiology is currently less well understood. Further research is needed to fully elucidate this due to the paucity of data on how NEAT and its components are modulated in physiology. However, given the application of NEAT in energy balance, current levels of overweight and obesity worldwide and a move towards getting more people more physically active for health benefit, it will remain a key concept for scientists and practitioners wanting to understand how physical activity can influence physiology.

Chapter summary

- Where energy intake and expenditure are different we experience an energy imbalance. Where energy intake is greater than energy expenditure humans will tend to experience an increase in body mass and where energy intake is less than energy expenditure humans will tend to experience a decrease in body mass.
- When an individual moves from rest to exercise there is a shift in the oxygen demand placed on the body. When the bout of physical activity or exercise that is undertaken is

constant (e.g., walking/running on a treadmill at a consistent, unchanging speed), the body has an increased O_2 requirement in comparison to its resting O_2 requirement.

- The term 'oxygen deficit' describes a state where other energy sources, phosphocreatine and glycolysis provide the energy to meet the required O_2 cost during the first minutes of a bout of physical activity, as the body cannot instantaneously meet the increased O_2 demand of exercise.

- Regular physical activity results in several changes that collectively contribute to increasing the capability of the cardiovascular, muscle, skeletal, respiratory and endocrine systems. Cessation of physical activity results in a gradual reversal of these effects.

- Non-Exercise Activity Thermogenesis (NEAT) represents one of the subcomponents of activity thermogenesis which contribute to human energy expenditure. NEAT comprises activities such as walking, gardening, stair climbing, standing and fidgeting. It is the most variable component of energy expenditure, representing from 15–50% of total energy expenditure in sedentary to highly active individuals, respectively.

References

Abernethy, P.J., Thayer, R., & Taylor, A.W. (1990). Acute and chronic responses of skeletal muscle to endurance and sprint exercise: a review. *Sports Medicine, 10*, 365–389.

Andersen, P., & Henriksson, J. (1977). Capillary supply of the quadriceps femoris muscle of man: adaptive response to exercise. *The Journal of Physiology, 270*, 677–690.

Bloomfield, S.A., & Coyle, E.F. (1993). Bed rest, detraining, and retention of training-induced adaptation. In: Durstine, J.L., King, A.C., Painter, P.L., Roitman, J.L., & Zwiren, L.D., (Eds.) *ACSM's resource manual for guidelines for exercise testing and prescription* (2nd ed.) (pp. 115–128). Philadelphia: Lea and Febiger.

Bouten, C.V., Verboeket-van de Venne, W.P., Westerterp, K.R., Verduin, M., & Janssen, J.D. (1996). Daily physical activity assessment: comparison between movement registration and doubly labeled water. *Journal of Applied Physiology, 81*, 1019–1026.

Dauncey, M.J. (1990). Activity and energy expenditure. *Canadian Journal of Physiology and Pharmacology, 68*, 17–27.

Gaesser, G.A., & Brooks, G.A., (1984). Metabolic basis of excess post-exercise oxygen consumption: a review. *Medicine and Science in Sports and Exercise, 16*, 29–43.

Goffart, S., & Wiesner, R. (2003). Regulation and co-ordination of nuclear gene expression during mitochondrial biogenesis. *Experimental Physiology, 88*, 33–40.

Gunter, K.B., Almstedt, H.C., & Janz, K.F. (2012). Physical activity in childhood may be the key to optimizing lifespan skeletal health. *Exercise and Sports Science Reviews, 40*, 13–21.

Hansen, B.M., Kolle, E., Dyrstad, S.M., Holme, I., & Anderssen, S.A. (2012). Accelerometer-determined physical activity in adults and older people. *Medicine and Science in Sports and Exercise, 44*, 266–272.

Hill, J.O., & Peters, J.C. (1998). Environmental contributions to the obesity epidemic. *Science, 280*, 1371–1374.

Hortobágyi, T., Dempsey, L., Fraser, D., Zheng, D., Hamilton, G., Lambert, J., & Dohm, L. (2000). Changes in muscle strength, muscle fibre size and myofibrillar gene expression after immobilization and retraining in humans. *Journal of Physiology, 524*, 293–304.

Keese, F., Farinatti, P., Pescatello, L., & Monteiro, W.A. (2011). Comparison of the immediate effects of resistance, aerobic, and concurrent exercise on postexercise hypotension. *Journal of Strength Conditioning Research, 25*, 1429–1436.

Kenny, W.L., Wilmore, J.H., & Costill, D.L. (2015). *Physiology of sport and exercise.* Champaign, IL: Human Kinetics.

Kraemer, W.J., & Ratamess, N.A. (2005). Hormonal responses and adaptations to resistance exercise and training. *Sports Medicine, 35*, 339–361.

Leibel, R.L., Rosenbaum, M., & Hirsch, J. (1995). Changes in energy expenditure resulting from altered body weight. *New England Journal of Medicine, 332*, 621–628.

Levine, J.A. (2004). Nonexercise activity thermogenesis: environment and biology. *American Journal of Physiology Endocrinology and Metabolism, 286*, E675–E685.

Levine, J.A., Baukol, P.A., & Pavlidis, Y. (1999). The energy expended chewing gum. *New England Journal of Medicine, 341*, 2100.

Levine, J.A., Schleusner, S.J., & Jensen, M.D. (2000). Energy expenditure of nonexercise activity. *American Journal of Clinical Nutrition, 72*, 1451–1454.

Levine, J.A., Weisell, R., Chevassus, S., Martinez, C.D., Burlingame, B., & Coward, W.A. (2001). The work burden of women. *Science, 294*, 812.

Linnamo, V., Pakarinen, A., Komi, P.V., Kraemer, W.J., & Häkkinen, K. (2005). Acute hormonal responses to submaximal and maximal heavy resistance and explosive exercises in men and women. *Journal of Strength and Conditioning Research, 19*, 566–571.

Lipman, R.L., Raskin, P., Love, T., Triebwasser, J., Lecocq, F.R., & Schnure, J.J. (1972). Glucose intolerance during decreased physical activity in man. *Diabetes, 21*, 101–107.

Livingstone, M.B., Strain, J.J., Prentice, A.M., Coward, W.A., Nevin, G.B., Barker, M.E., Hickey, R.J., McKenna, P.G., & Whitehead, R.G. (1991) Potential contribution of leisure activity to the energy expenditure patterns of sedentary populations. *British Journal of Nutrition, 65*, 145–155.

Malina, R.M. (1996) Tracking of physical activity and physical fitness across the lifespan. *Research Quarterly for Exercise and Sport, 67*, S48–S57.

Matthews, C.E., Keadle, S.K., Troiano, R.P., Kahle, L., Koster, A., Brychta, R., Van Domelen, D., Caserotti, P., Chen, K.Y., Harris, T.B., & Berrigan, D. (2016). Accelerometer-measured dose-response for physical activity, sedentary time, and mortality in US adults. *American Journal of Clinical Nutrition, 104*, 1424–1432.

Nindl, B.C., Santtila, M., Vaara, J., Häkkinen, K., & Kyröläinen, H. (2011). Circulating IGF-I is associated with fitness and health outcomes in a population of 846 young healthy men. *Growth Hormone & IGF Research, 21*, 124–128.

Romain, A.J., Carayol, M., Desplan, M., Fedou, C., Ninot, G., Mercier, J., Avignon, A., & Brun, J.F. (2012). Physical activity targeted at maximal lipid oxidation: a meta-analysis. *Nutrition and Metabolism, 2012*, 285395.

Sahlin, K., Mogensen, M., Bagger, M., Fernström, M., & Pedersen, P.K. (2007). The potential for mitochondrial fat oxidation in human skeletal muscle influences whole body fat oxidation during low-intensity exercise. *American Journal of Physiology, 292*, E223–E230.

Saltin, B., Blomqvist, G., Mitchell, J.H., Johnson, R.L., Wildenthal, K., & Chapman, C.B. (1968). Response to exercise after bed rest and after training: a longitudinal study of adaptive changes in oxygen transport and body composition. *Circulation, 38*, 1–78.

Shephard, R.J. (1994). *Aerobic fitness and health*. Champaign, IL: Human Kinetics.

Terjung, R.L. (1995). Muscle adaptations to aerobic training. *Sports Science Exchange, 8*, 1–4.

Tipton, C.M., & Vailas, A.C. (1990). Bone and connective tissue adaptations to physical activity. In: Bouchard, C., Shephard, R.J., Stephens, T., Sutton, J.R., & McPherson, B.D., (Eds.) *Exercise, fitness, and health: a consensus of current knowledge* (pp. 331–344). Champaign, IL: Human Kinetics.

Tremblay, M.S., Copeland, J.L., & Van Helder, W. (2005). Influence of exercise duration on post-exercise steroid hormone responses in trained males. *European Journal of Applied Physiology, 94*, 505–513.

Vuorimaa, T., Vasankari, T., Mattila, K., Heinonen, O., & Häkkinen, K., & Rusko (1999). Serum hormone and myocellular protein recovery after intermittent runs at the velocity associated with $\dot{V}O_{2max}$. *European Journal of Applied Physiology and Occupational Physiology, 80*, 575–581.

11 Paediatric physical activity and aerobic fitness

Neil Armstrong

Keywords: Children, health, peak oxygen uptake, physical activity, time trends

Physical activity (PA), exercise and physical fitness are associated with a plethora of health-related benefits in children and adolescents (Janssen & LeBlanc, 2010). The terms PA, exercise and physical fitness are, however, frequently used interchangeably even though they are not synonymous. This practice has clouded understanding of youth health-related research where it is important to clearly define, differentiate and justify the study of behaviours and physiological variables. This is particularly important if the intention is to use them in subsequent statistical analyses with health-related variables.

This chapter will clarify the development of PA and aerobic fitness during childhood and adolescence, analyse the PA and aerobic fitness of today's young people in relation to previous generations and interrogate the relationship between PA and aerobic fitness. It is recognised that both PA and aerobic fitness have heritable characteristics but genetics are outside the scope of the chapter and interested readers are referred to Schutte and colleagues (2017) for a comprehensive discussion.

Physical activity

Youth PA consists of a complex set of behaviours which can be divided into dimensions such as frequency, intensity and duration. It can be expressed in terms of mode/type of PA being performed (e.g. cycling, walking, running) or as a domain of PA describing the context in which PA takes place (e.g. school-time PA, sports-time PA, leisure-time PA). Exercise is a sub-component of PA that is planned, structured and repetitive. Normally in PA research sedentary behaviour (i.e. time spent engaging in very low energy expenditure behaviours such as sitting and lying during waking hours) is differentiated from physical inactivity (i.e. not meeting the recommended dose of PA according to public health recommendations). The focus here will be on PA in relation to young people's health and well-being where the PA behaviour of primary interest is habitual PA (HPA) which is 'the usual PA carried out in normal daily life in every domain and in any dimension' (Hildebrand & Ekelund, 2017).

Assessment of habitual physical activity

Numerous techniques have been developed to estimate dimensions of PA and to classify HPA into PA categories such as moderate (MPA), moderate-to-vigorous (MVPA) or vigorous

(VPA) but all methods have limitations which are often amplified in youth. Young people are characterised by intermittent bouts of a few seconds of variable intensity PA (Bailey et al., 1995) which has substantial implications for the measurement, processing and interpretation of data. Both subjective and objective techniques have been developed but estimations of PA from different methodologies should be compared cautiously as correlations between methods are, at best, low to moderate (Adamo, Prince, Tricco, Connor-Gorbor & Tremblay, 2009). Herein methods of assessment of young people's PA will only be outlined to provide a framework for later sections and interested readers are referred to Hildebrand and Ekelund (2017) for a detailed critique of methodology

Subjective assessment

Subjective methods of estimating PA are founded on self-recall (or proxy-recall by parents or teachers) of previous events over a specified time period and include questionnaires, interviews and activity diaries. Children are less time conscious than adults and to recall details of dimensions of PA from specific events in the past places considerable demands on their cognitive abilities. During childhood and adolescence potential for errors in recall is augmented by sociocultural variations in lifestyle and the timing and tempo of maturation. Errors may be substantial in estimating an individual's HPA but several large, well-designed, multinational surveys have provided valuable descriptions of young people's HPA at population level (e.g. Roberts, Tynaka & Komkov, 2004).

Objective assessment

Objective assessment techniques involving external monitors must be socially acceptable, should not burden the young person with cumbersome equipment and should not (or only minimally) influence normal PA. Some account should be taken of day-to-day variation and ideally monitors worn for at least 10 h per day for 3–7 continuous days, including both weekdays and weekends (Hildebrand & Ekelund, 2017).

Simple motion sensors such as pedometers which record the number of steps taken over a period of time have been used to estimate PA since the 1920s, although Leonardo da Vinci is reputed to have designed a pedometer to measure distance by counting steps somewhat earlier. Pedometers are unable to distinguish dimensions of PA and with body size differences data are not directly comparable across ages during growth and maturation. There is no consensus on number of steps equivalent to youth PA guidelines and recommendations for adults (e.g. 10,000 steps per day) should not be extrapolated for use with young people. Nevertheless, pedometry continues to be used and has provided informative comparative data in large studies (e.g. Raustorp, Pangrazi & Stahle, 2004).

Physiological sensors do not directly measure PA but they can provide clinically relevant data with which to evaluate relationships between PA and health-related behaviour. For example, heart rate (HR) monitoring provides an indication of the stress placed upon the cardiovascular system rather than a direct measure of PA. During low-intensity PA, HR data are difficult to interpret but with appropriate calibration HR monitoring lends itself to the application of threshold values of MPA and VPA with which to interpret PA guidelines. By the 1970s HR monitors had been introduced to the study of youth PA. As HR monitors became less cumbersome they were used extensively in the 1980s and 1990s and provided new insights into youth PA (Armstrong, 1998a).

Over the last two decades HR monitors have generally been replaced by or used in combination with sophisticated motion sensors such as accelerometers which measure the acceleration of the body or parts of the body for specific, pre-determined time periods (epochs). Accelerometry data are expressed as activity counts per minute (cpm) and translated into estimates of PA via laboratory calibration studies. There is currently a lively debate on interpretation of data with a lack of consensus on the best model of accelerometer, appropriate monitor placement, optimum epoch length and the cpm cut-off points to align with PA intensity thresholds. In particular, the variable use of cpm in relation to PA intensity thresholds is a major challenge to accurate quantification of the number of young people who are sufficiently active and there is an urgent need to establish agreed alignment between cpm and PA intensity thresholds in relation to age. Ekelund, Tomkinson and Armstrong (2011) have advocated the reporting of data from multiple cut-off points (~2000–3500 cpm) in order to interpret youth PA across studies. Nevertheless, despite the need for a consensual, evidence-based approach to data interpretation the development and application of accelerometry has provided significant advances in understanding youth PA and it is currently viewed as the reference method (Guinhouya, Samouda & de Beaufort, 2013).

Interpretation of habitual physical activity

Having quantified the dimensions of HPA it is necessary to put it into the context of health and well-being. Proposals for health-related PA guidelines for young people have evolved over the last 30 years. The earliest youth PA guidelines were proposed by the American College of Sports Medicine (ACSM, 1988) who based their proposals on the ACSM guidelines for adults. ACSM recommended that, for 'optimal functional capacity and health' children and adolescents should achieve 20–30 min of VPA each day.

Five years later an invited group of experts convened an International Consensus Conference (ICC) and systematically reviewed the scientific literature relating HPA to health-related outcomes (e.g. Alpert & Wilmore, 1994; Armstrong & Simons-Morton, 1994; Bailey & Martin, 1994; Bar-Or & Baranowski, 1994). Founded on the extant evidence the ICC proposed that young people should, i) be physically active daily or nearly every day and, ii) engage in three or more sessions per week of activities that last 20 min or more at a time and that require moderate-to-vigorous levels of exertion. MVPA was defined as requiring at least as much effort as brisk walking (Sallis, Patrick & Long, 1994). As the first evidence-informed guidelines specifically developed for youth the ICC guidelines informed most studies of young people's habitual PA in the 1990s.

In 1998 the UK Health Education Authority (UKHEA) commissioned a similar series of systematic reviews. Following a consensus conference drawing from the same evidence-base as the ICC the primary recommendation of the UKHEA was that all young people should participate in PA of at least moderate intensity for 60 min per day (Biddle, Cavill & Sallis, 1998). This recommendation shifted the emphasis from MVPA to MPA and from sustained periods of PA to PA accumulated over a day. Subsequent PA guidelines from numerous national and international organisations and agencies have been generally consistent with the UKHEA proposal although more recent guidelines (see Janssen, 2007 for a tabulated summary of youth PA guidelines) have emphasised the importance of daily MVPA. It has also been suggested that VPA may provide more health benefits than MVPA and that sporadic (accumulated) PA may not be as beneficial as sustained 5–10 min bouts of PA (Janssen & LeBlanc, 2010). The World Health Organization [WHO] (2010) promotes the inclusion of three sessions of VPA per week and a recent study has proposed that current guidelines should be updated to increase the amount of MVPA and a daily amount of VPA should be prescribed (Fussenich et al., 2016).

In truth there is no compelling evidence to support a single dose-response relationship between PA and health in children and adolescents. The minimal and optimal doses of PA required to promote most aspects of health during growth and maturation remain unclear and more rigorously conducted dose-response studies in relation to gender, age and maturation are warranted. The need for young people to engage in *daily* PA to maintain good health remains to be proven. It is unknown whether a child or adolescent who accumulates a daily 60 min of MVPA over a week would have greater health benefits than one who accumulates 7 h of MVPA in a week with different amounts being performed each day and some days with no MVPA (Janssen & LeBlanc, 2010).

It therefore seems that, as elegantly argued by Twisk (2001) current youth PA guidelines are, at best, evidence-informed rather than evidence-based. Nevertheless, evidence-informed PA guidelines provide a framework for evaluating population levels of HPA in youth. The most widely utilised health-related PA guideline is that 5–18 year-olds participate daily in 60 min or more of MVPA. This guideline stems from a systematic review of the literature (Strong et al., 2005) and, where possible, it will be adopted herein as the criterion guideline of health-related PA.

Are young people physically active?

Young people's HPA is extensively documented but space precludes a systematic review of the literature. Representative studies using different methodologies will therefore be used to overview the prevalence of health-related PA in youth. Readers seeking more detail are referred to comprehensive reviews which have tabulated study synopses (e.g. Armstrong & Welsman, 2006; Ekelund et al., 2011; Guinhouya et al., 2013, van Hecke et al., 2016).

Subjective assessment

Several multinational surveys have been sponsored by the WHO and generally a wide variation across countries of young people meeting PA guidelines has been noted. One of the most comprehensive studies involved 31 European countries, Canada, Israel and the United States (US) and included the self-reported HPA of 162,036 young people aged 11, 13 and 15 years (Roberts et al., 2004). Participants were asked to recall the time spent in 'any activity that increases your heart rate and makes you out of breath some of your time' and to calculate the number of days they experienced this level of PA for at least 60 min in a typical week. On average, 40% of boys and 27% of girls reported meeting this guideline on at least five days. A strong trend of HPA decreasing with age was noted. Similarly, data from 16,410 US adolescents indicated that 46% of boys and 28% of girls met a similar PA guideline (Eaton et al., 2010). In contrast a WHO sponsored survey of 72,845 13–15 year-olds from 34 developing countries reported only 24% of boys and 15% of girls met a guideline of a daily 60 min of MVPA (Guthold, Cowan, Autenrieth, Kann & Riley, 2010).

Variation in questionnaire design, sample characteristics and data collection periods demands that comparisons across studies be carried out cautiously. The findings that HPA declines with age and that girls are less likely to meet PA guidelines than boys are generally consistent but quantifying the prevalence of young people meeting PA guidelines is challenging. An International Olympic Committee (IOC) sponsored expert group analysed the extant evidence and concluded that on the basis of self-report ~30–40% of youth meet current health-related PA guidelines (Mountjoy, Andersen, Armstrong, et al., 2011).

Objective assessment

Studies using pedometers have been reviewed and tabulated elsewhere but they provide limited insights into the prevalence of young people meeting PA guidelines. They are, however, consistent in reporting boys' HPA to be higher than girls at all ages from 7 to 18 years with HPA declining in both sexes with age (Armstrong & Welsman, 2006).

Bradfield and colleagues (1971) appear to have been the first to monitor boys' HR in the context of PA (actually energy expenditure) but the most extensive series of HR monitoring studies with youth was performed by Armstrong and his colleagues from 1985 to 2000. They monitored the HR of 1,227 5–16 year-olds for at least 10 hours on each of three weekdays. In a subsequent review the data were merged and re-analysed in accord with school attended; i) first school (mean age 7.2 years) ii) middle school (11.0 years); and iii) high school (13.3 years). Boys in each category were reported to spend significantly more time in both MPA and VPA than girls. The mean percentage of time spent in at least MPA was 11.9% and 8.6% for boys and girls, respectively, in first school with corresponding figures in middle school of 9.2% and 7.7%, and in high school of 6.3% and 4.7%. Ten and 20 min sustained periods of at least MPA were sparse but among the younger children 93% of boys and 78% of girls experienced a daily 5 min sustained period of MPA. The corresponding figures for the older children were 82% and 34% for boys and girls, respectively (Armstrong & Welsman, 2006).

Investigations of PA using HR monitoring consistently report more boys than girls to meet PA guidelines and HPA to decline with age. In addition, a longitudinal study of ~200 11–13 year-olds demonstrated that with age controlled using multilevel regression modelling stage of biological maturity exerts a significant, independent, negative effect on PA in both sexes (Armstrong, Welsman & Kirby, 2000).

Inconsistency in the interpretation of cpm cut-off points (and to a lesser extent epoch length) has resulted in studies reporting sufficient PA in from 0–100% of young people. For example, two UK studies of 10-year-olds (n=1862 and n=2071) used 2000 cpm as their threshold of MPA and reported 76–82% of boys and 53–59% of girls to meet PA guidelines (Steele, van Sluijs, Cassidy, Griffin & Ekelund, 2009; Owen et al., 2009). In contrast another UK study of 5,595 11–12 year-olds used 3600 cpm as the criterion of MVPA and reported ~5% of boys and <1% of girls to meet PA guidelines (Riddoch et al., 2007).

Guinhouya et al.'s (2013) extensive review concluded that the percentage of European children and adolescents who meet PA guidelines varies from 20–87% with a cut-off of 2000 cpm, through less than 10% with a cut-off of 3000 cpm to ~1% with a cut-off of 4,000 cpm. In the studies reviewed boys met the PA guideline between 1.1 and 12.8 times more frequently than girls but unlike data from other methodologies the association between age and PA was unclear. The IOC consensus statement based on Ekelund et al.'s (2011) review of international data concluded that, on balance, studies using PA intensity thresholds above 3000 cpm (broadly equivalent to brisk walking or MPA) indicate that less than 25% of young people meet current PA guidelines (Mountjoy et al., 2011). On the basis of an accelerometry database of 24,025 participants, it appears that VPA reduces with each year of age (5–18 years) at a faster rate than MPA (6.9% vs. 6.0%). The gender difference in the decline of VPA is particularly marked with girls' VPA decreasing at a rate of 10.7% per year of age compared with boys' VPA declining at a rate of 2.9% per year of age (Corder, Sharp, Atkin et al., 2016).

Are today's young people less physically active than previous generations?

Reliable data collected prior to 1990 are sparse but several subjective and objective studies have reported time trends in HPA over the last two to three decades. The first indication that youth HPA had stabilised emerged from HR monitoring studies in the South West of England. The HPA of secondary school students (11–16 years) over 10 hours on each of 3 days was first estimated in 1989–90 (Armstrong, Balding, Gentle & Kirby, 1990a) and the study was repeated 10 years later using the same methodology in the same schools (Welsman & Armstrong, 2000a). The percentage of time spent by girls in at least MPA increased from 4% to 6% over the decade whereas the boys' values were stable at 6% on each measurement occasion. Analyses of 5, 10 and 20 min of sustained periods of MPA revealed a strikingly similar pattern a decade apart and the authors concluded, controversially at the time, that youth HPA levels had remained stable in the 1990s.

These findings have been subsequently substantiated by a number of studies from different parts of the world. In a comprehensive analysis of seven published studies of data from the Youth Risk and Behaviour Surveillance Survey, Li, Treuth, and Wang (2010) demonstrated that there was no clear evidence of US youth becoming less active over the period 1991–2007. Similarly a WHO study of seven European countries (n = 47,201 11–15 year-olds) reported stability or a small increase in PA from the mid-1980s to the early 2000s (Samdal, Tynjala, Roberts, Sallis, Villberg & Wold, 2006). The Pan-European data were supported by an Icelandic survey of 27,426 14 and 15 year-olds, which reported an overall increase in VPA in both sexes from 1992 to 2006 (Eiosdottir, Kristjansson, Sigfusdottir & Allegrante, 2008). In Australia, Okely et al., (2008) analysed data on 12–15 year-olds surveyed in 1985 (n = 1055) and 2004 (n = 1226) and reported that youth PA, particularly MVPA, had considerably increased in all age and sex groups studied over the 19-year period.

There are few studies of time trends in PA using objective methodology but extant data are consistent. Two Swedish studies recorded daily step counts over four days using pedometers and reported that 7–9 year-olds significantly increased their daily step counts from 2000 to 2006, girls by 10% and boys by 6% (Raustrop & Ludvigsson, 2007) and 13–14 year-olds reported no change in daily step counts from 2000 to 2008 (Raustrop & Ekroth, 2010). Another study used accelerometers to compare the PA of cohorts of 6–10 year-olds 18 months apart and confirmed the stability of Swedish youth PA over this period of time (Nyberg, Ekelund & Marcus, 2009). The Swedish data have been supported by a Danish study which used accelerometers to compare the percentage of time 8–10 year-olds spent in MPA in 1997/98 with 2003/04 and noted no significant changes in HPA over the 6-year period (Moller, Kristensen, Wedderkopp, Andersen & Froberg, 2009).

In summary, studies across methodologies strongly indicate that i) HPA decreases from childhood through adolescence; ii) VPA declines at a faster rate with age than MPA and the decrease is more marked in girls than boys; iii) more boys than girls meet PA guidelines; iv) precise quantification of how many young people can be classified as experiencing sufficient PA is clouded by methodological inconsistencies and the need for more dose-response evidence; v) evidence indicates that, on balance, ~60–75% of children and adolescents do not meet current PA guidelines although there are wide cross-country variances; and vi) empirical evidence supports stability in youth PA, at least over the last 25 years.

Physical fitness

Physical fitness has both health-related and skill-related components. Health-related fitness is not a unitary concept but consists of several discrete physical and physiological attributes including aerobic fitness, muscular fitness, metabolic fitness and morphological fitness. All of these attributes are relevant to health but it is aerobic fitness (i.e. the ability to deliver oxygen to the muscles and to utilise it to generate energy to support muscle activity during exercise) which is most frequently associated with health and well-being in youth (Ferreira & Twisk, 2017). In one chapter it is not possible to discuss adequately all postulated indicators of aerobic fitness so, in accord with the vast majority of studies in the field of youth health, the present chapter will adopt peak oxygen uptake (peak $\dot{V}O_2$) as the criterion measure of youth aerobic fitness. Interested readers are referred to Armstrong and McManus (2017) for a critical review of the assessment and interpretation of components of youth aerobic fitness.

Assessment of aerobic fitness

Maximal $\dot{V}O_2$ is internationally recognised as the best single measure of adults' aerobic fitness. However, only a minority of young people exhibit in a single test the $\dot{V}O_2$ plateau which conventionally confirms maximal $\dot{V}O_2$ in adults (Åstrand, 1952) and it has become more common in paediatric exercise science to label the highest rate at which oxygen can be consumed during an exercise test to exhaustion as peak $\dot{V}O_2$. It has been demonstrated that rigorously determined peak $\dot{V}O_2$ from an incremental exercise test to exhaustion can be accepted as a maximal variable (Armstrong, Welsman & Winsley, 1996). However, the method of choice for the confident determination of peak $\dot{V}O_2$ as a maximal index of young people's aerobic fitness is probably a short duration ramp test to exhaustion followed by a 'supramaximal' test as described by Barker and colleagues (2011). Young people's ability to recover quickly from exhaustive exercise (Ratel & Williams, 2017) allows the use of a follow-up 'supramaximal' effort after ~15 min of active/passive recovery to verify whether a maximal effort was elicited in the initial test. The 'supramaximal' test normally consists of 2 min pedalling at 10 W followed by a step transition to 105% of the peak power achieved during the initial ramp test and exercise to exhaustion. This methodology has been used successfully with children of varying aerobic fitness (e.g. Robben, Poole & Harms, 2013). For a review of the assessment and interpretation of peak $\dot{V}O_2$ across health conditions see McManus and Armstrong (2017).

The laboratory determination of young people's peak $\dot{V}O_2$ is expensive, time consuming, dependent on sophisticated apparatus and reliant on skilled technical assistance. This has encouraged some researchers to predict peak $\dot{V}O_2$ from field tests of performance. The 20 metre shuttle run test (20mSRT) has emerged as the most popular test of youth maximal performance but the number of completed shuttle runs (laps or stages) is not a physiological measure of aerobic fitness. Shuttle run performance is influenced by a network of social, behavioural, physical, biomechanical and psychosocial factors as well as physiological variables (Tomkinson & Olds, 2007). There are at least 17 different published equations to predict young people's peak $\dot{V}O_2$ from 20mSRT performance, equations that differ in validity and result in substantially different estimates of peak $\dot{V}O_2$ (Tomkinson et al., 2017). A meta-analysis of young people's 20mSRT performance in relation to peak $\dot{V}O_2$ reported that of studies which met eligibility criteria for inclusion, over 50% of correlation coefficients explained less than 50% of the variance in peak $\dot{V}O_2$ (Mayorga-Vega, Aguiler-Soto & Viciana, 2015). In addition, shuttle run performance can be improved by practice and various training methods without a concomitant increase in peak $\dot{V}O_2$ (Harrison et al., 2015). It is therefore clearly evident that the use of performance scores from the 20mSRT as surrogates or predictors of peak $\dot{V}O_2$ not only misrepresents youth aerobic fitness but also confounds putative relationships with health-related variables.

Interpretation of aerobic fitness

Physiological data on peak $\dot{V}O_2$ (L·min^{-1}) in youth are well-documented and consistent but spurious interpretation of the data in relation to age, sex, body size and maturation has clouded understanding of aerobic fitness in childhood and adolescence.

Boys' peak $\dot{V}O_2$ (in L·min^{-1}) increases in a near-linear manner by ~150% from 8 to 16 years. Girls' data show a similar trend with peak $\dot{V}O_2$ increasing by ~80% over the same age range. Longitudinal data from boys generally concur with cross-sectional data although some studies have reported that the greatest annual increase in peak $\dot{V}O_2$ accompanies the attainment of peak height velocity. Longitudinal peak $\dot{V}O_2$ data from girls are sparse but indicate a near-linear rise from 8 to 13 years before beginning to plateau from ~14 years in accord with some cross-sectional studies. Boys' peak $\dot{V}O_2$ values are higher than those of girls from an early age and from 10 to 16 years the sex difference increases from ~10–35%, illustrating the futility of reporting descriptive statistics of aerobic fitness from mixed sex groups (Armstrong & Welsman, 1994).

Boys' increase in skeletal muscle mass accounts for most of the progressive sexual divergence in peak $\dot{V}O_2$ in puberty and it is supplemented by a sex-specific increase in haemoglobin concentration in the late teens. The explanation for pre-pubertal sex differences in peak $\dot{V}O_2$ has been attributed to boys' greater stroke index, boys' higher maximal arteriovenous oxygen difference and sexual dimorphism in the balance between oxygen delivery and utilisation in the muscles (Armstrong & McManus, 2017).

Muscle mass, which facilitates oxygen utilisation and augments venous return and therefore oxygen delivery, is the dominant influence in the increase in youth peak $\dot{V}O_2$ with age. Both lean body mass (LBM) and the muscle mass used in the peak $\dot{V}O_2$ determination (e.g. the muscle mass of the legs) are therefore highly correlated with peak $\dot{V}O_2$ and in some circumstances are the scaling factors of choice (Graves, Batterham & Foweather et al., 2013). However, as the accurate assessment of LBM and muscle mass of the legs is complex, body size differences are typically 'controlled' (or scaled) by dividing peak $\dot{V}O_2$ by total body mass and expressing it as a ratio (mL·kg^{-1}·min^{-1}). Peak $\dot{V}O_2$ reported in ratio with body mass is, however, strongly influenced by largely metabolically inert body fat content as well as muscle mass. When peak $\dot{V}O_2$ is expressed in mL·kg^{-1}·min^{-1} a different picture emerges from that apparent when absolute values (L·min^{-1}) are presented. Boys' peak $\dot{V}O_2$ decreases slightly or remains essentially unchanged from 8 to 18 years while girls' values progressively decline through adolescence (Armstrong & McManus, 2017).

The fallacy of expressing peak $\dot{V}O_2$ in ratio with body mass has been documented for almost 70 years (Tanner, 1949) yet despite periodic critical reviews of the methodology over several decades (e.g. Katch & Katch, 1974; Armstrong & Welsman, 1994; Welsman & Armstrong, 2000b; Loftin, Sothern, Abe & Bonis, 2016) it is still widely used in health-related studies. It has been frequently demonstrated that ratio-scaled peak $\dot{V}O_2$ (mL·kg^{-1}·min^{-1}) is negatively and significantly correlated with body mass (kg) thus illustrating the inability of ratio scaling to remove the influence of body mass (Armstrong & McManus, 2017).

Ratio scaling 'over-scales', favours lighter individuals and penalises heavier and more mature young people. When body mass is controlled for appropriately using allometry or multilevel modelling male peak $\dot{V}O_2$ values, in direct contrast to ratio scaling, increase from childhood, through adolescence and into young adulthood. In females, peak $\dot{V}O_2$ increases up to ~13 years and subsequently stabilises with no decline into young adulthood (Welsman, Armstrong, Kirby, Nevill & Winter, 1996). Ratio scaling has also obscured the true relationship between aerobic fitness and biological maturity. Peak $\dot{V}O_2$ expressed in mL·kg^{-1}·min^{-1} has persistently been reported as being unrelated to biological maturity status but both cross-sectional and longitudinal studies have unequivocally demonstrated that with age and body mass appropriately controlled using either allometry or multilevel modelling there are significant, additional effects of biological maturity status on peak $\dot{V}O_2$ (Armstrong, Welsman & Kirby, 1998a, Armstrong & Welsman, 2001).

Detailed analysis of the interpretation of physiological variables and exercise performance in relation to body size is beyond the scope of this chapter and interested readers are referred to Welsman and Armstrong (2008) where the theoretical and statistical principles of allometry and multilevel modelling are explained and applied to paediatric data sets. Nevertheless, the importance of clarifying the meaning of youth aerobic fitness and its interpretation in health-related studies can be simply illustrated by considering a lean boy who becomes progressively obese. His 20mSRT performance will decline with extra body fat being transported. Peak $\dot{V}O_2$ expressed in ratio with body mass will decrease as body fat content increases. Peak $\dot{V}O_2$ expressed relative to LBM will remain stable. But, because of the concomitant increase in muscle tissue which occurs with obesity his actual peak $\dot{V}O_2$ (L·min^{-1}) will increase. Therefore depending on how it is normalised for body size this boy's peak $\dot{V}O_2$ can be interpreted as decreasing or not changing as he becomes more obese. His absolute aerobic fitness (peak $\dot{V}O_2$) will, however, increase (Rowland, 2017). A recent review provides several examples where inappropriate scaling of body mass has not only confounded understanding of the aerobic fitness of obese and overweight young people but also misrepresented relationships between aerobic fitness and cardiovascular risk factors where a statistical relationship is likely to reflect obesity or overweight status to a greater extent than aerobic fitness (Loftin et al., 2016).

Are young people fit?

Health-related thresholds of peak $\dot{V}O_2$ based on, for example, expert opinion (Bell, Macek, Rutenfranz, & Saris, 1986), extrapolations from adult cut-off points (The Cooper Institute, 2004) or statistical links with cardiometabolic risk factors (Adegboye, Andersen, Froberg, et al., 2011) have been advocated in the literature. Proposed threshold values are similar across publications but evidence of their credibility is unconvincing. The proposals are not founded on direct determinations of young people's peak $\dot{V}O_2$, they are compromised by ignoring the significant effect of biological maturity status and, in particular, by expressing peak $\dot{V}O_2$ recommendations in ratio with body mass. Nevertheless, working on the dubious assumption that aerobic fitness thresholds are meaningful, very few UK children and adolescents appear to present 'unhealthy' values of peak $\dot{V}O_2$. Normally it is not possible to calculate the number of young people who meet threshold values from published studies but a re-analysis of data from two large UK studies of untrained volunteer participants show the thresholds recommended by Bell et al. (1986) to be met by >95% of 307 (140 girls) 13–15 year-olds and 100% of 164

(53 girls) pre-pubertal, 11-year-olds (Armstrong, Balding, Gentle, Williams & Kirby, 1990b: Armstrong, Kirby, McManus & Welsman, 1995).

Credible international standards or norms for aerobic fitness in childhood and adolescence are not available. As would be expected with age-related comparisons peak $\dot{V}O_2$ varies within studies of healthy young volunteers with typical coefficients of variation of ~15% and elite young athletes present values ~40–50% higher than healthy, non-athletic peers. There is, however, no compelling evidence to suggest that the current generation of children and adolescents have low or unhealthy levels of aerobic fitness (Armstrong, Tomkinson & Ekelund, 2011; Mountjoy et al., 2011; Rowland, 2007).

Are today's young people less fit than previous generations?

Scrutiny of published studies since Robinson's (1938) seminal investigation 80 years ago reveals a remarkable consistency in young people's peak $\dot{V}O_2$ over time. Individual studies only provide local snapshots of the aerobic fitness of volunteer participants who might not reflect the population from which they are drawn. But, taken collectively compilations of data, at least from Europe and North America, reinforce the view that aerobic fitness has remained remarkably stable over several decades (Freedson & Goodman, 1993; Eisenmann & Malina, 2002; Armstrong et al., 2011). In the Children's Health and Exercise Research Centre ~3,000 young people, aged 8–18 years, from the same Exeter schools have had their peak $\dot{V}O_2$ determined with no discernible change in values noted over a 30-year period (N. Armstrong, unpublished data).

In contrast to peak $\dot{V}O_2$, young people's 20mSRT performance has been reported to deteriorate over the last 40 years (Armstrong et al., 2011) and this has often been wrongly attributed to a reduction in youth aerobic fitness rather than an increase in body fatness (Olds, Ridley & Tomkinson, 2007). As most health-related PA involves transporting body mass a decrease in young people's maximal performance is a cause for concern and the underlying mechanisms worthy of further investigation. But, in rigorous scientific studies of the health of children and adolescents the use of shuttle run performance as a proxy for aerobic fitness is untenable (Armstrong, 2017).

In summary, youth aerobic fitness (peak $\dot{V}O_2$) increases with age and biological maturity and there is no convincing evidence to suggest that the current generation of young people have low levels of aerobic fitness or that aerobic fitness is deteriorating over time. However, it is readily apparent that the use of ratio scaling and/or 20mSRT data i) have clouded understanding of aerobic fitness during growth and maturation; ii) have obscured the true aerobic fitness of young people; iii) have misrepresented current levels and time trends in young people's aerobic fitness; and iv) have generated spurious associations when these data are incorporated into subsequent statistical analyses with health-related variables.

What is the relationship between physical activity and aerobic fitness in youth?

To elucidate the association between PA and aerobic fitness it is necessary to define and distinguish between aspects of PA, in particular exercise training and HPA. Exercise training consists of a structured exercise programme that is sustained for a sufficient length of time, with sufficient intensity and frequency to induce improvements in components of physical fitness (Armstrong & Barker, 2011). In contrast, HPA consists of usual PA carried out in normal daily life in every domain and any dimension (Hildebrand & Ekelund, 2017).

Exercise training and peak oxygen uptake

The concept of children's responses to exercise training being reliant on a 'maturation threshold' is embedded in the paediatric literature. A persuasive theoretical argument can be made (Rowland, 1997) but there is no convincing empirical evidence to support the case for a maturation effect on the response of peak $\dot{V}O_2$ to exercise training (McNarry & Armstrong, 2017). Studies which have directly compared the trainability of children and adults have reported comparable increases in peak $\dot{V}O_2$ irrespective of age (Eisenmann & Golding, 1975; Savage et al., 1986).

The vast majority of training intervention programmes that have reported increases in young people's peak $\dot{V}O_2$ has involved sustained periods of constant-intensity exercise training (CIET). It is, however, surprising that high-intensity interval training (HIIT) protocols have not been more popular in paediatric exercise training studies (Armstrong & McNarry, 2016). It was demonstrated over 20 years ago that pre-pubertal girls could improve their peak $\dot{V}O_2$ through either CIET or HIIT (McManus, Armstrong & Williams, 1997) but it is only recently that a concerted research effort has focused on HIIT as a means of enhancing aerobic fitness (Costigan, Eather, Plotnikoff, Taaffe & Lubans, 2015).

An IOC-sponsored systematic review of the literature located 69 published studies and scrutinised 21 investigations which had rigorously examined the effect of exercise training on young people's peak $\dot{V}O_2$ (Mountjoy, Armstrong, Bizzini et al., 2008). There was insufficient evidence to confidently recommend an optimal HIIT programme. It was concluded that a 12-week training programme involving a mixture of continuous and interval exercise at 85–90% of HR max will induce, on average, an 8–9% increase in peak $\dot{V}O_2$ which is independent of age, biological maturity and sex. The review noted that there is a small but significant inverse relationship between baseline peak $\dot{V}O_2$ and training-induced changes but no significant relationship between pre-training HPA and peak $\dot{V}O_2$ responses to training (Armstrong & Barker, 2011).

Habitual physical activity and peak oxygen uptake

Seliger and colleagues (1974) were the first to objectively estimate HPA and compare the data with directly determined peak $\dot{V}O_2$. They estimated the HPA of 11–12 year-old boys from one day HR monitoring and found no significant relationships with peak $\dot{V}O_2$. These findings have been extended and confirmed in subsequent studies which have consistently observed either no relationship or, at best, a very weak association between peak $\dot{V}O_2$ and HPA. Table 11.1 summarises studies which have objectively monitored PA for at least three days and directly determined peak $\dot{V}O_2$. Based on empirical evidence periodic reviews of the literature have consistently concluded that there is no meaningful relationship between peak $\dot{V}O_2$ and objectively monitored HPA (Morrow & Freedson, 1994; Armstrong, 1998b; Armstrong et al., 2011).

Cross-sectional data are strongly supported by longitudinal investigations. A three-year study of $\sim$200 ($\sim$100 girls) British children used multilevel modelling to examine age, biological maturity state and body mass influences on VPA and MPA from the ages of 11–13 years. With the primary variables controlled peak $\dot{V}O_2$ was introduced to the model as an additional variable and a non-significant parameter estimate demonstrated no relationship between peak $\dot{V}O_2$ and HPA. An analysis of accumulated time spent in at least MPA over three 10-hour periods of monitoring in relation to peak $\dot{V}O_2$ clearly showed that HPA decreased with age

Table 11.1 Habitual physical activity and peak oxygen uptake in youth

Citations	Participants	Means of physical activity estimation	Mode of exercise in peak $\dot{V}O_2$ determination	Outcomes
Armstrong, Balding, Gentle, Williams & Kirby (1990c)	111 girls, 85 boys; aged 11–16 years	3-day HR monitoring	Cycle ergometer or treadmill	No significant relationships. Non-significant correlation coefficients ranged from r=0.01 to −0.26
Armstrong, McManus, Welsman & Kirby (1996)	63 girls, 60 boys; aged 12.2 years	3-day HR monitoring	Treadmill	No significant relationships. Non-significant correlation coefficients ranged from r=0.13 to 0.16 in boys and from r=−0.02 to 0.04 in girls
Armstrong, Welsman & Kirby (1998b)	43 girls, 86 boys; aged 10–11 years	3-day HR monitoring	Treadmill	No significant relationships. Non-significant correlation coefficients ranged from r=−0.15 to 0.09
Armstrong, Welsman & Kirby (2000)	98/70/79 girls, 104/73/81 boys: longitudinal study from 11–13 years	3-day HR monitoring	Treadmill	In a multilevel regression model, peak $\dot{V}O_2$ was a non-significant parameter estimate of PA
Ekelund, Poortvleit, Nilsson, Yngve, Holmberg & Sjöström (2001)	40 girls, 42 boys; aged 14–15 years	3-day HR monitoring	Treadmill	No significant relationship between MVPA and peak $\dot{V}O_2$ (r=−0.04); AEE explained 14% of the variance in peak $\dot{V}O_2$
Eiberg, Hasselstrom, Gronfeldt, Froberg, Svensson & Andersen (2005)	309 boys, 283 girls; aged 6–7 years	3-day accelerometry	Treadmill	Sustained periods of PA explained 9% of the variance in peak $\dot{V}O_2$
Dencker, Thorsson, Karlsson, Linden, Svensson, Wollmer & Andersen (2006)	101 girls, 127 boys; aged 8–11 years	3–4 day accelerometry	Cycle ergometer	In a multiple forward regression analysis VPA and MDPA together explained 10% of the variance in peak $\dot{V}O_2$ (VPA 9%, and MDPA 1%)
Butte, Puyau, Adolph, Vohra & Zakeri (2007)	424 non-overweight and 473 overweight 4–19 year-olds	3-day accelerometry	Treadmill	PA explained 1–3% of the variance in peak $\dot{V}O_2$
Dencker, Bugge, Hermansen & Andersen (2010)	222 girls, 246 boys; aged 6–7 years	4-day accelerometry	Treadmill	PA explained 0–8% and 0–2% of the variance in peak $\dot{V}O_2$ in boys and girls, respectively

PA is physical activity; TDEE is total daily energy expenditure; MPA is moderate physical activity; MVPA is moderate to vigorous physical activity; VPA is vigorous physical activity; MDPA is mean daily physical activity; AEE is activity-related energy expenditure; HR is heart rate. Table adapted and updated from Armstrong and Fawkner (2007).

whereas peak $\dot{V}O_2$ in both L·min^{-1} and appropriately normalised for body mass increased from 11 to 13 years in both sexes (Armstrong, Welsman, Nevill & Kirby, 1999; Armstrong, Welsman & Kirby 2000). Similarly, Kemper and Koppes (2004) analysed longitudinal data collected from participants in the Amsterdam Growth and Health Longitudinal Study over 23 years and concluded that no clear association could be proved between HPA and maximal $\dot{V}O_2$ in free-living males and females.

In summary, exercise training can enhance aerobic fitness but the lack of a meaningful positive relationship between HPA and peak $\dot{V}O_2$ is not surprising as i) young people rarely experience the intensity and duration of PA necessary to increase their peak $\dot{V}O_2$ and ii) youth HPA typically decreases from childhood through adolescence whereas peak $\dot{V}O_2$, even when appropriately normalised for body mass, increases over the same period.

Concluding remarks

Lack of clarity in experimental studies and the paucity of empirical evidence-based debate have confused understanding of PA and aerobic fitness in youth. The emergence of sophisticated motion sensors has the potential to revolutionise youth PA data collection and analysis but more research is warranted on the application of movement data (e.g. accelerometer cpm) to the monitoring of free-ranging PA. Rigorously determined dose-response evidence is required before health-related PA guidelines can be confidently prescribed for young people. The assessment and interpretation of peak $\dot{V}O_2$ in youth have sound scientific foundations but ubiquitous data from maximal performance tests such as 20 m shuttle running and inappropriate scaling of body mass have clouded the conceptual bases of youth aerobic fitness. Exercise training has been demonstrated to enhance the peak $\dot{V}O_2$ of both children and adolescents but a meaningful relationship between HPA and peak $\dot{V}O_2$ remains to be proven.

Peak $\dot{V}O_2$ is not the only indicator of aerobic fitness and further insights into youth aerobic fitness and how it relates to dimensions of PA are likely to rest in the transient responses to forcing exercise regimens. More research in this area is required and interested readers are referred to Armstrong (2017) for discussion of potential areas of future research.

Much remains to be learned about paediatric PA and aerobic fitness in relation to health and well-being but effective progress requires investigators to clearly define, differentiate and justify the inclusion of behaviours and physiological variables in future studies. This is crucial if the intention is to use them in subsequent statistical analyses with health-related morphological or cardio-metabolic variables leading to recommendations or policy statements impacting on young people's health and well-being.

Chapter summary

- In the context of youth health and well-being physical activity (PA) and aerobic fitness (peak $\dot{V}O_2$) should not be used interchangeably.
- Youth health-related PA guidelines are evidence-informed not evidence-based. The physiological assessment and interpretation of peak $\dot{V}O_2$ have a sound scientific foundation but the use of 20mSRT performance scores and ratio-scaling of data have confounded understanding of youth aerobic fitness.
- Boys tend to be more active than similarly aged girls and PA declines in both sexes through the teen years, particularly girls' vigorous PA. Aerobic fitness increases with chronological age and biological maturation.

- Only ~25–40% of young people meet PA guidelines. In contrast the view that the current generation of children and adolescents have low or unhealthy levels of peak $\dot{V}O_2$ cannot be substantiated with empirical evidence.
- There is no compelling evidence to support a temporal decline in either youth PA or aerobic fitness, at least over recent decades.
- Appropriate exercise training enhances the aerobic fitness of both children and adolescents but a meaningful relationship between habitual PA and peak $\dot{V}O_2$ has not been verified.

References

Adamo, K.B., Prince, S.A., Tricco, A.C., Connor-Gorbor, S. & Tremblay, M.A. (2009). Comparison of indirect versus direct measures for accessing physical activity in the pediatric population: a systematic review. *International Journal of Pediatric Obesity, 4*, 2–27.

Adegboye, A.R., Andersen, S.A., Froberg, K., Sardinha, L.B., Heitmann, B.L., Steene-Johannessen, J., Kolle, E. & Andersen, L.B. (2011). Recommended aerobic fitness level for metabolic health in children and adolescents: a study of diagnostic accuracy. *British Journal of Sports Medicine, 45*, 722–728.

Alpert, B.S. & Wilmore, J.H. (1994). Physical activity and blood pressure in adolescents. *Pediatric Exercise Science, 6*, 361–380.

American College of Sports Medicine. (1988). Physical fitness in children and youth. *Medicine and Science in Sports and Exercise, 20*, 422–423.

Armstrong, N. (1998a). Young people's physical activity patterns as assessed by heart rate monitoring. *Journal of Sport Sciences, 16(Suppl)*, S9–S16.

Armstrong, N. (1998b). Physical fitness and physical activity during childhood and adolescence. In K.M. Chan, & L. Micheli (Eds.), *Sports and children* (pp. 50–75). Hong Kong: Williams & Wilkins.

Armstrong, N. (2017). Top 10 research questions related to youth aerobic fitness. *Research Quarterly for Exercise and Sport, 88*, 130–148.

Armstrong, N., Balding, J., Gentle, P. & Kirby, B.J. (1990a). Patterns of physical activity amongst 11 to 16 year old British children. *British Medical Journal, 301*, 203–205.

Armstrong, N., Balding, J., Gentle, P., Williams, J. & Kirby B.J. (1990b). Peak oxygen uptake of British children with reference to age, sex and sexual maturity. *European Journal of Applied Physiology, 62*, 369–375.

Armstrong, N., Balding, J., Gentle, P., Williams, J. & Kirby, B.J. (1990c). Peak oxygen uptake and physical activity in 11 to 16 year olds. *Pediatric Exercise Science, 2*, 349–358.

Armstrong, N. & Barker, A.R. (2011). Endurance training and elite young athletes. *Medicine and Sport Science, 56*, 84–96.

Armstrong, N. & Fawkner, S.G. (2007). Aerobic fitness. In N. Armstrong (Ed.), *Paediatric exercise physiology* (pp. 161–187). Edinburgh: Churchill Livingstone.

Armstrong, N., Kirby, B.J., McManus, A.M. & Welsman, J.R. (1995). Aerobic fitness of pre-pubescent children. *Annals of Human Biology, 22*, 427–441.

Armstrong, N. & McManus, A.M. (2017). Aerobic fitness. In N. Armstrong & W. van Mechelen (Eds.), *Oxford textbook of children's sport and exercise medicine* (pp. 161–180). Oxford: Oxford University Press.

Armstrong, N., McManus, A., Welsman, J. & Kirby, B. (1996). Physical activity patterns and aerobic fitness among pre-pubescents. *European Physical Education Review, 2*, 7–18.

Armstrong, N. & McNarry, M. (2016). Aerobic fitness and trainability in healthy youth. Gaps in our knowledge. *Pediatric Exercise Science, 28*, 171–177.

Armstrong, N. & Simons-Morton, B. (1994). Physical activity and blood lipids in adolescents. *Pediatric Exercise Science, 6*, 381–405.

Armstrong, N., Tomkinson, G.R. & Ekelund, U. (2011). Aerobic fitness and its relationship to sport, exercise training and habitual physical activity during youth. *British Journal of Sports Medicine, 45*, 849–858.

Armstrong, N. & Welsman, J.R. (1994) Assessment and interpretation of aerobic fitness in children and adolescents. *Exercise and Sport Sciences Reviews, 22*, 435–476.

Armstrong, N. & Welsman, J.R. (2001). Peak oxygen uptake in relation to growth and maturation in 11–17-year-old humans. *European Journal of Applied Physiology, 85*, 546–551.

Armstrong, N. & Welsman, J.R. (2006). The physical activity patterns of European youth with reference to methods of assessment. *Sports Medicine, 36*, 1067–1086.

Armstrong, N., Welsman, J.R. & Kirby, B.J. (1998a). Peak oxygen uptake and maturation in 12-year-olds. *Medicine and Science in Sports and Exercise, 30*, 165–169.

Armstrong, N., Welsman, J. & Kirby, B.J. (1998b). Physical activity, peak oxygen uptake and performance on the Wingate anaerobic test in 12-year-olds. *Acta Kinesiologie Universitatis Tartu, 3*, 7–21.

Armstrong, N., Welsman, J.R. & Kirby, B.J. (2000). Longitudinal changes in 11–13-year-olds' physical activity. *Acta Paediatrica, 89*, 775–780.

Armstrong, N., Welsman, J.R., Nevill, A.M. & Kirby, B.J. (1999). Modeling growth and maturation changes in peak oxygen uptake in 11–13-yr olds. *Journal of Applied Physiology, 87*, 2230–2236.

Armstrong, N., Welsman, J.R. & Winsley, R.J. (1996). Is peak $\dot{V}O_2$ a maximal index of children's aerobic fitness? *International Journal of Sports Medicine, 17*, 356–359.

Åstrand, P.O. (1952). *Experimental studies of physical working capacity in relation to sex and age.* Copenhagen: Munksgaard.

Bailey D.A. & Martin, A.D. (1994). Physical activity and skeletal health in adolescents. *Pediatric Exercise Science, 6*, 330–347.

Bailey, R.C., Olsen, J., Pepper, S.L., Porszasc, J., Barstow, T.J. & Cooper, D.M. (1995). The level and tempo of children's physical activities: an observational study. *Medicine and Science in Sports and Exercise, 27*, 1033–1041.

Barker, A.R., Williams, C.A., Jones, A.M. & Armstrong, N. (2011). Establishing maximal oxygen uptake in young people during a ramp test to exhaustion. *British Journal of Sports Medicine, 45*, 498–503.

Bar-Or, O. & Baranowski, T. (1994). Physical activity, adiposity and obesity among adolescents. *Pediatric Exercise Science, 6*, 348–360.

Bell, R.D., Macek, M., Rutenfranz, J. & Saris, W.H.M. (1986). Health indicators and risk factors of cardiovascular diseases during childhood and adolescence. In J. Rutenfranz, R. Mocellin & F. Klimt (Eds.), *Children and exercise XII* (pp. 19–27). Champaign, IL: Human Kinetics.

Biddle, S., Cavill, N. & Sallis, J. (1998). Policy framework for young people and health-enhancing physical activity. In S. Biddle, J. Sallis & N. Cavill (Eds.), *Young and active?* (pp. 3–16). London: Health Education Authority.

Bradfield, R.B., Chan, H., Bradfield, N.E. & Payne, R.R. (1971). Energy expenditures and heart rates of Cambridge boys at school. *American Journal of Clinical Nutrition, 24*, 439–446.

Butte, N.F., Puyau, M.R., Adolph, A.L., Vohra, F.A. & Zakeri, I. (2007). Physical activity in non-overweight and overweight Hispanic children and adolescents. *Medicine and Science in Sports and Exercise, 39*, 1257–1266.

Corder, K., Sharp, S.J., Atkin, A.J., Andersen, L.B., Cardon, G., Page, A., Davey, R., Grontved, A., Hallal, P.C., Janz, K.J., Kordas, K., Kriemler, S., Puder, J.J., Sardinha, L.B., Ekelund, U. & van Sluijs E.M.F. (2016). Age-related patterns of vigorous-intensity physical activity in youth: The International Children's Accelerometry Database. *Preventive Medicine Reports, 4*, 17–22.

Costigan, S.A., Eather, N., Plotnikoff, R.C., Taaffe, D.R. & Lubans, D.R. (2015). High-intensity interval training for improving health-related fitness in adolescents: a systematic review and meta-analysis. *British Journal of Sports Medicine, 49*, 1253–1261.

Dencker, M., Bugge, A., Hermansen, B. & Andersen, L.B. (2010). Objectively measured daily physical activity related to aerobic fitness in young children. *Journal of Sports Sciences, 28*, 139–145.

Dencker, M., Thorsson, O., Karlsson, M.K., Linden, C., Svensson, J., Wollmer. P. & Andersen, L.B. (2006). Daily physical activity and its relation to aerobic fitness in children aged 8–11 years. *European Journal of Applied Physiology, 96*, 587–592.

Eaton, D.K, Kann, L., Kinchen, S., Shanklin, S., Ross, J. & Hawkins, J. (2010). Youth risk behavior surveillance – United States, 2009, *MMWR Surveillance Summit, 59*, 1–142.

Eiberg, S., Hasselstrom, H., Gronfeldt, V., Froberg, K., Svensson, J. & Andersen, L.B. (2005). Maximum oxygen uptake and objectively measured physical activity in Danish children 6–7 years of age: the Copenhagen school child intervention study. *British Journal of Sports Medicine, 39*, 725–730.

Eiosdottir, S., Kristjansson, A.L., Sigfusdottir, I.D. & Allegrante, J.P. (2008). Trends in physical activity and participation in sports clubs among Icelandic adolescents. *European Journal of Public Health, 18*, 289–293.

Eisenmann, J.C. & Malina, R.M. (2002). Secular trend in peak oxygen consumption among United States youth in the 20th century. *American Journal of Human Biology, 14*, 699–706.

Eisenmann, P.A. & Golding, L.A. (1975). Comparison of effects of training on VO_2 max in girls and young women. *Medicine and Science in Sports and Exercise, 7*, 136–138.

Ekelund, U., Poortvleit, E., Nilsson, A., Yngve, A., Holmberg, A. & Sjöström, M. (2001). Physical activity in relation to aerobic fitness and body fat in 14- to 15-year-old boys and girls. *European Journal of Applied Physiology, 85*, 195–201.

Ekelund, U., Tomkinson, G.R. & Armstrong, N. (2011). What proportion of youth are physically active? Measurement issues, levels and recent time trends. *British Journal of Sports Medicine, 45*, 859–866.

Ferreira, I. & Twisk, J.W.R. (2017). Physical activity, physical fitness, and cardiovascular health. In N. Armstrong & W. van Mechelen (Eds.), *Oxford textbook of children's sport and exercise medicine* (pp. 239–254). Oxford: Oxford University Press.

Freedson, P.S. & Goodman, T.L. (1993). Measurement of oxygen consumption. In T.W. Rowland (Ed.), *Pediatric laboratory exercise testing* (pp. 91–114). Champaign, IL: Human Kinetics.

Fussenich, L.M., Boddy, L.M., Green, D.J., Graves, L.E.F., Foweather, L., Dagger, R.M., McWhannell, N., Henaghan, J., Ridgers, N.D., Stratton, G. & Hopkins, N.D. (2016). Physical activity guidelines and cardiovascular risk in children: a cross-sectional analysis to determine whether 60 minutes is enough. *BMC Public Health, 16*, 67.

Graves L.E.F., Batterham, A.M., Foweather L., McWannell, N., Hopkins N.D., Boddy, L.M., Gobbi, R., Stratton, G. (2013). Scaling of peak oxygen uptake in children. A comparison of body size index models. *Medicine and Science in Sports and Exercise, 45*, 2341–2345.

Guinhouya, B.C., Samouda, H. & de Beaufort, C. (2013). Level of physical activity among children and adolescents in Europe. A review of physical activity assessed by accelerometry. *Public Health, 127*, 301–311.

Guthold, R., Cowan, M.J., Autenrieth, C.S., Kann, L. & Riley, L.M. (2010). Physical activity and sedentary behavior among schoolchildren: a 34-country comparison. *Journal of Pediatrics, 157*, 43–49.

Harrison, C.B., Gill, N.D., Kinugasa, T. & Kilding, A.E. (2015). Development of aerobic fitness in young team sport athletes. *Sports Medicine, 45*, 969–983.

Hildebrand, M. & Ekelund, U. (2017). Assessment of physical activity. In N. Armstrong & W. van Mechelen (Eds.), *Oxford textbook of children's sport and exercise medicine* (pp. 303–314). Oxford: Oxford University Press.

Janssen, I. (2007). Physical activity guidelines for children and youth. *Applied Physiology, Nutrition and Metabolism, 32*, S109–S121.

Janssen, I. & LeBlanc, A.G. (2010). Systematic review of the health benefits of physical activity and fitness in school-aged children and youth. *International Journal of Behaviour, Nutrition and Physical Activity, 7*, 40.

Katch, V.L. & Katch, F.I. (1974). Use of weight-adjusted oxygen uptake scores that avoid spurious correlation. *Research Quarterly, 45*, 447–451.

Kemper, H.C.G. & Koppes, L.L.J. (2004). Is physical activity important for aerobic power in young males and females? *Medicine and Sport Science, 47*, 153–166.

Li, S., Treuth, M.S. & Wang, Y. (2010). How active are American adolescents and have they become less active? *Obesity Reviews, 11*, 847–862.

Loftin, M., Sothern, M., Abe, T. & Bonis, M. (2016). Expression of $\dot{V}O_{2peak}$ in children and youth with special reference to allometric scaling. *Sports Medicine, 46*, 1451–1460.

Mayorga-Vega, D., Aguiler-Soto, P. & Viciana, J. (2015). Criterion-related validity of the 20-m shuttle run test for estimating cardiorespiratory fitness: a meta-analysis. *Journal of Sports Science and Medicine, 14*, 536–547.

McManus, A.M. & Armstrong, N. (2017). Maximal oxygen uptake. In: T.W. Rowland (Ed), *Cardiopulmonary exercise testing in children and adolescents* (pp. 79–93). Champaign, IL: Human Kinetics.

McManus, A.M., Armstrong, N. & Williams, C.A. (1997). Effect of training on the aerobic power and anaerobic performance of prepubertal girls. *Acta Paediatrica, 86*, 456–459.

McNarry, M.A. & Armstrong, N. (2017). Aerobic trainability. In N. Armstrong & W. van Mechelen (Eds.), *Oxford textbook of children's sport and exercise medicine* (pp. 465–476). Oxford: Oxford University Press.

Moller, N.C., Kristensen, P.L., Wedderkopp, N., Andersen, L.B. & Froberg, K. (2009). Objectively measured habitual physical activity in 1997/1998 vs 2003/2004 in Danish children: the European youth heart study. *Scandinavian Journal of Medicine & Science in Sports, 19*, 19–29.

Morrow, J.R. & Freedson, P.S. (1994). The relationship between habitual physical activity and aerobic fitness in adolescents. *Pediatric Exercise Science, 6*, 315–329.

Mountjoy, M., Andersen, L.B, Armstrong, N., Biddle, S., Boreham, C., Bedenbeck, H-P.B., Ekelund, U., Engebretsen, L., Hardman, K., Hills, A., Kahlmeier, S., Kriemler, S., Lambert, E., Ljungqvist, A., Matsudo, V., McKay, H., Micheli, L., Pate, R., Riddoch, C., Schamasch, P., Sundberg, C.J., Tomkinson, G., van Sluis, E. & van Mechelen, W. (2011). International Olympic Committee consensus statement on health and fitness of young people through physical activity and sport. *British Journal of Sports Medicine, 45*, 839–848.

Mountjoy, M., Armstrong, N., Bizzini, L., Blimkie, C., Evans, J., Gerrard, D., Hangen, J., Knoll, K., Micheli, L., Sangenis, P. & van Mechelen, W. (2008). International Olympic Committee consensus statement on training the elite athlete. *Clinical Journal of Sports Medicine, 18*, 122–123.

Nyberg, G., Ekelund, U. & Marcus, C. (2009). Physical activity in children measured by accelerometry: stability over time. *Scandinavian Journal of Medicine & Science in Sports, 19*, 30–35.

Okely, A. D., Booth, M.L., Hardy, L., Dobbins, T. & Denney-Wilson, E. (2008). Changes in physical activity participation from 1985–2004 in a state-wide survey of Australian adolescents. *Archives of Pediatric and Adolescent Medicine, 162*, 176–180.

Olds, T.S, Ridley, K. & Tomkinson, G.R. (2007). Declines in aerobic fitness: are they only due to increasing fatness? *Medicine and Sport Science, 50*, 226–240.

Owen, C.G., Nightingdale, C.M., Rudnicka, A.R., Cook, D.G., Ekelund, U. & Whincup, P.H. (2009). Ethnic and gender differences in physical activity levels among 9–10 year-old children of white European, South Asian and African-Caribbean origin: the Child Heart Health Study in England (CHASE Study). *International Journal of Epidemiology, 38*, 1082–1089.

Ratel, S. & Williams, C.A. (2017). Neuromuscular fatigue. In N. Armstrong & W. van Mechelen (Eds), *Oxford textbook of children's sport and exercise medicine* (pp. 121–130). Oxford: Oxford University Press.

Raustrop, A. & Ekroth, Y. (2010). Eight year secular trends of pedometer determined physical activity in Swedish adolescents. *Journal of Physical Activity and Health, 7*, 368–374.

Raustrop, A. & Ludvigsson, J. (2007). Secular trends of pedometer-determined physical activity in Swedish schoolchildren. *Acta Paediatrica, 96*, 1824–1828.

Raustorp, A., Pangrazi, R.P. & Stahle, A. (2004). Physical activity level and body mass index among schoolchildren in south eastern Sweden. *Acta Paediatrica, 93*, 400–404.

Riddoch, C.J., Mattocks, C., Deere, K., Saunders, J., Kirkby, J. & Tilling, K. (2007). Objective measurement of level and patterns of physical activity. *Archives of Disease in Childhood, 92*, 963–969.

Robben, K.E., Poole, D.C. & Harms, C.A. (2013). Maximal oxygen uptake validation in children with expiratory flow limitation. *Pediatric Exercise Science, 25*, 84–100.

Roberts, C., Tynaka, J. & Komkov, A. (2004). Physical activity. In C. Currie, C. Roberts, A. Morgan, R. Smith, W. Setertsbulte & D. Sandal (Eds.). *Young people's health in context* (pp. 90–97). Copenhagen: World Health Organization.

Robinson, S. (1938). Experimental studies of physical fitness in relation to age. *Arbeitsphysiologie, 10*, 251–323.

Rowland, T.W. (1997). The 'trigger hypothesis' for aerobic trainability: a 14-year follow-up. *Pediatric Exercise Science, 9*, 1–9.

Rowland, T.W. (2007). Evolution of maximal oxygen uptake in children. *Medicine and Sport Science, 50*, 200–209.

Rowland, T.W. (2017). Cardiovascular function. In N. Armstrong & W. van Mechelen (Eds.), *Oxford textbook of children's sport and exercise medicine* (pp. 147–160). Oxford: Oxford University Press.

Sallis, J.F., Patrick, K. & Long, B.J. (1994). Overview of the international consensus conference on physical guidelines for adolescents. *Pediatric Exercise Science, 6*, 299–302.

Samdal, O., Tynjala, J., Roberts, C., Sallis, J.F., Villberg, J. & Wold, B. (2006). Trends in vigorous physical activity and TV watching of adolescents from 1986 to 2002 in seven European countries. *European Journal of Public Health, 17*, 242–248.

Savage, M.P., Petratis, M.M., Thomson, W.H., Berg, K., Smith, J.L. & Sady, S.P. (1986). Exercise training effects on serum lipids in prepubescent boys and adult men. *Medicine and Science in Sports and Exercise, 18*, 197–204.

Schutte, N.M., Bartels, M. & de Gues, E.J.C. (2017). Genetics of physical activity and physical fitness. In N. Armstrong & W. van Mechelen (Eds.), *Oxford textbook of children's sport and exercise medicine* (pp. 293–302). Oxford: Oxford University Press.

Seliger, V., Trefny, S., Bartenkova, S. & Pauer, M. (1974). The habitual physical activity and fitness of 12 year old boys. *Acta Paediatrica Belgica, 28*, 54–59.

Steele, R.M., van Sluijs, E.M., Cassidy, A., Griffin, S.J. & Ekelund, U. (2009). Targeting sedentary time or moderate and vigorous intensity activity: independent relations with adiposity in a population-based study of 10 yr-old British children. *American Journal of Clinical Nutrition, 90*, 1185–1192.

Strong, W.B., Malina, R.M., Blimkie, C.J.R., Daniels, S.R., Dishman, R.K., Gutin, B., Hergenroeder, A.C., Must, A., Nixon, P.A., Pivarnik, J.M., Rowland, T.W., Trost, S, & Trudeau, F. (2005). Evidence-based physical activity for school-age youth. *Journal of Pediatrics, 146*, 732–737.

Tanner, J.M. (1949). Fallacy of per-weight and per-surface area standards and their relation to spurious correlation. *Journal of Applied Physiology, 2*, 1–15.

The Cooper Institute for Aerobics Research. (2004). *Fitnessgram test administration manual.* (3rd edition). Champaign, IL: Human Kinetics.

Tomkinson, G.R., Lang, J.J., Tremblay, M., Dale, M., LeBlanc, A.G., Belanger, K., Ortega, F.B. & Léger, L. (2017). International normative 20 m shuttle run values from 1,142,026 children and youth representing 50 countries. *British Journal of Sports Medicine, 51*, 1545–1554.

Tomkinson, G.R. & Olds, T.S. (2007). Secular changes in aerobic fitness test performance of Australasian children and adolescents. *Medicine and Sport Science, 50*, 168–182.

Twisk, J.W. (2001). Physical activity guidelines for children and adolescents: a critical review. *Sports Medicine, 31*, 617–627.

van Hecke, L., Loyen, A., Verloigne, M., van der Ploeg, H.P., Lakerveld, J., Brug, J., de Bourdeahdhuij, I., Ekelund, U., Donnelly, A., Hendriksen, I. & Deforche, B. (2016). Variation in population levels of physical activity in European children and adolescents according to cross-European studies: a systematic literature review within DEDIPAC. *International Journal of Behavioral Nutrition and Physical Activity, 13*, 70.

Welsman, J.R. & Armstrong, N. (2000a). Physical activity patterns in secondary schoolchildren. *European Journal of Physical Education, 5*, 147–157.

Welsman, J.R. & Armstrong, N. (2000b). Statistical techniques for interpreting body size-related exercise performance during growth. *Pediatric Exercise Science, 12*, 112–127.

Welsman, J.R. & Armstrong, N. (2008). Interpreting exercise performance data in relation to body size. In N. Armstrong & W. van Mechelen (Eds.), *Paediatric exercise science and medicine* (2nd ed.). (pp. 13–28). Oxford: Oxford University Press.

Welsman, J.R., Armstrong, N., Kirby, B.J., Nevill, A.M. & Winter, E.M. (1996). Scaling peak $\dot{V}O_2$ for differences in body size. *Medicine and Science in Sports and Exercise, 28*, 259–265.

World Health Organization. (2010). *Global recommendations on physical activity for health.* Geneva: World Health Organization.

12   Nutrition and physical activity

Daniel Bailey, Julia Zakrzewski-Fruer and Faye Powell

Keywords: Nutrient intake, dietary assessment, appetite control, energy balance, eating disorders

Nutrition for the physically active person

Optimal nutrition

An optimal diet supplies adequate amounts of energy and all of the essential nutrients that the body requires for tissue maintenance, repair and growth. These essential nutrients are divided into two categories:

1. Macronutrients: carbohydrates, fats and protein. These nutrients serve as dietary sources of energy and are required in relatively large quantities.
2. Micronutrients: vitamins and minerals. These nutrients do not serve as dietary sources of energy and are required in relatively small quantities.

When considering physically active men and women who engage in recreational physical activity or perform at the elite level, optimal nutrition will (a) provide sufficient energy for the demands of physical activity, (b) facilitate repair and recovery from intense physical exercise, (c) optimise physical conditioning during training and athletic performance in competition, (d) help to avoid injury, and (e) promote overall health and well-being (American College of Sports Medicine, 2009). Optimal nutrition may be achieved by following relevant dietary recommendations, but will also depend on individual characteristics, such as age, sex and body composition. In particular, it is essential that dietary recommendations for physically active individuals take into account the energy demands of training and competition and the requirement of all essential nutrients to maintain health (American College of Sports Medicine, 2009).

Dietary guidelines

The current UK dietary guidelines were developed by the Committee on Medical Aspects of Food Policy (COMA) for the general population with the aim of promoting well-being and reducing morbidity and mortality from inadequate nutrient intake (COMA, 1991). Dietary Reference Values (DRVs) specify the recommended daily intake of energy and the essential nutrients for the whole population and for population subgroups based on age, sex, physiological status and physical activity level.

For physically active individuals, one of the key dietary considerations is energy balance, which becomes particularly important during periods of intense training with high energy expenditures. A person's daily energy requirement is determined by their basal metabolic rate, the thermic effect of digesting food, and the thermic effect of physical activity. When daily energy intake is equal to daily energy expenditure (i.e., energy balance), body mass will remain relatively constant. If the amount of daily calories consumed exceeds energy expenditure, the body will store this excess energy as fat in subcutaneous adipose tissue, around organs, or within muscle, causing increased body weight. When energy expenditure exceeds the amount of calories consumed, energy demands will be met by storage sites within the body leading to reduced body fat, lean mass and total body weight; prolonged negative energy balance may lead to potential disruptions in endocrine function, such as menstrual cycle disturbances (Williams, Helmreich, Parfitt, Caston-Balderrama, & Cameron, 2001). Individuals who expend a high amount of energy during physical activity, therefore, need to ensure they replenish their energy reserves to meet the continued demands of training.

To estimate an individual's daily energy requirements, basal metabolic rate (BMR) and physical activity energy expenditure must be calculated. There are a number of different equations to estimate BMR, such as the Harris and Benedict (Frankenfield, Muth, & Rowe, 1998) and Schofield equations (Schofield, 1985). The commonly used Schofield (1985) equations are as follows:

Men	18–29 years	$BMR (kcal/d) = (0.063W + 2.896) \times 239$
	30–59 years	$BMR (kcal/d) = (0.048W + 3.653) \times 239$
Women	18–29 years	$BMR (kcal/d) = (0.062W + 2.036) \times 239$
	30–59 years	$BMR (kcal/d) = (0.034W + 3.538) \times 239$

W = body mass (kg)

Daily energy expenditure is then estimated by multiplying the BMR value by a physical activity level factor that corresponds to the person's normal activity levels: 1.2 corresponds to bed rest, 1.4 to sedentary activity, 1.6 to light activity, 1.8 to moderate activity, 2.0 to heavy activity, and 2.2 to vigorous activity. Subsequently, the estimated daily energy expenditure can be used in diet planning to ensure the adequate consumption of macronutrients (carbohydrate, fat, protein) to meet individual energy demands for the maintenance of body weight. Alternatively, energy intake can be reduced or increased appropriately to meet specific goals related to weight loss or weight gain, respectively.

The UK Eatwell Guide (Public Health England, 2016a) is a visual aid showing the proportions of different food types that are needed for a well-balanced and healthy diet (Figure 12.1). The guide can be used in combination with the macronutrient and energy intake recommendations outlined above for meal planning with physically active individuals and can be applied to most population groups. It recommends the consumption of nutrient-rich foods in place of energy-dense and nutrient-poor foods, which are commonly consumed in the UK diet. This pattern of dietary intake increases the risk of obesity, cardio-metabolic abnormalities (e.g. increased cholesterol and blood sugar levels) and reduced micronutrient intake. The largest segments of the Eatwell Guide occupy about 30% each consisting of (i) starchy

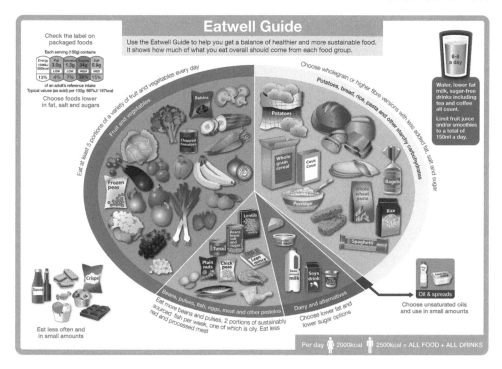

Figure 12.1 The Eatwell Guide
Source: Public Health England in association with the Welsh Government, Food Standards Scotland and the Food Standards Agency in Northern Ireland © Crown copyright 2016

foods (potatoes, bread, rice and pasta, which should be wholegrain or high fibre varieties) and (ii) fruit and vegetables (a variety of at least five portions each day). Moderate amounts of foods in the diet should come from the beans, pulses, fish, eggs, meat and other proteins group and the dairy and alternatives group. Limited amounts of oil and spreads should be consumed (these should be the unsaturated varieties) and foods and drinks high in fat, salt or sugar should be consumed less often and in small amounts. A total of 6 to 8 cups/glasses of fluid are recommended each day, but daily fruit juice and smoothie consumption should be limited to 150 ml. There are also energy requirement guidelines for the general population, although the Schofield equations described above would permit a more accurate estimate for an individual (Schofield, 1985).

Substrate oxidation and macronutrient recommendations for physical activity

Carbohydrate and fat are the main substrates that contribute to exercise energy expenditure. Carbohydrate exists in the body as blood glucose (i.e. exogenous carbohydrate) and as glycogen stored in the muscle and liver (i.e. endogenous carbohydrate). Although substrate oxidation during exercise depends on various factors related to the exercise characteristics (e.g. mode, duration and intensity) and the individual (e.g. nutritional status, body composition and training status), exercise intensity is known to be a particularly influential factor. As exercise intensity increases, there is a progressive increase in the relative contribution of carbohydrate oxidation and decrease in the relative contribution of fat oxidation to energy expenditure (Brooks & Mercier, 1994). In absolute terms, carbohydrate oxidation increases proportionally with exercise intensity, whereas fat oxidation increases from low to moderate intensities and then declines at higher intensities (Achten, Gleeson, & Jeukendrup, 2002; Romijn et al., 1993). This is because the body can metabolise carbohydrate for energy more rapidly than fat, thus allowing a higher intensity level to be achieved. Accordingly, insufficient glucose availability to skeletal muscle and the central nervous system will limit performance during prolonged sub-maximal or intermittent high-intensity physical activity.

Carbohydrate intake before, during and after exercise is considered important to ensure sufficient availability of glycogen pre-exercise and replenishment post exercise. For the general adult population, 50% of daily energy intake should come from carbohydrate (COMA, 1991). A daily intake of 6–10 g·kg^{-1} body weight·day^{-1} carbohydrate is recommended for highly active adults and 5–7 g·kg^{-1} body weight·day^{-1} for moderately active adults (American College of Sports Medicine, 2009; Burke, Hawley, Wong, & Jeukendrup, 2011). There is evidence that a high-carbohydrate diet that elevates muscle glycogen content prior to exercise can postpone fatigue by approximately 20% in endurance events lasting more than 90 minutes and can improve endurance performance by 2–3% where a pre-determined distance is covered as quickly as possible (Hawley, Schabort, Noakes, & Dennis, 1997). In contrast, adequate quantities of glycogen remain in the working muscles at the end of a single exhaustive bout of high-intensity exercise lasting less than 5 minutes or for moderate-intensity running or cycling lasting 60 to 90 minutes; thus elevating pre-exercise muscle glycogen content has little effect on performance (Hawley et al., 1997). In the 1- to 4-hour period before physical activity lasting >60 min, it is recommended that the meal should be relatively high in carbohydrate (1–4 g·kg^{-1} body weight) to maximise the maintenance of blood glucose (Burke et al., 2011). During prolonged continuous physical activity (≥60 min), approximately 30–60 g·h^{-1} carbohydrate intake is recommended to maintain blood glucose (American College of Sports Medicine, 2009). Following exercise, it is important to replenish muscle glycogen to ensure sufficient energy stores are available for the next physical activity bout and to avoid injury and fatigue. A carbohydrate intake of 1.0–1.5 g·kg^{-1} body weight 30 min after physical activity and again every 2 h for 4–6 h is recommended (American College of Sports Medicine, 2009).

Fat (lipids) serves as a major energy source at rest and during light to moderate-intensity physical activity. Total fat intake for the general population to promote good health should not be more than 35% of total energy intake (COMA, 1991). Of this, no more than 11% of total energy should come from saturated fatty acids (COMA, 1991). There are no clear recommendations on optimal fat intake for physically active individuals. However, consuming ≤20% of energy from fat appears to be detrimental to endurance performance in males and females (Horvath, Eagen, Fisher, Leddy, & Pendergast, 2000) and can lead to reductions in testosterone levels in response to resistance training in men, which may compromise muscle tissue anabolism (Volek, 2004). Low-fat diets are, thus, not recommended for physically active individuals (American College of Sports Medicine, 2009). High-fat diets (>40% fat) cause a shift in substrate metabolism to greater fat oxidation and it is proposed that this could spare glycogen stores during intense aerobic physical activity (Burke et al., 2002). However, the research is controversial with some studies reporting improvements in endurance performance (Vogt et al., 2003) and others reporting no benefits (Burke et al., 2002) or reduced training capacity and increased fatigue (Helge, 2002; Helge, Richter, & Kiens, 1996). When considering the evidence as a whole, high-fat diets are generally not recommended for physically active individuals (American College of Sports Medicine, 2009).

The contribution of protein to energy during physical activity is relatively small (approximately 2–8% depending on the exercise intensity). It is, however, important for protein to be consumed after physical activity to provide essential amino acids required for synthesis and repair of muscle tissue. Protein recommendations for males and females are 55.5 g·day^{-1} and 45.0 g·day^{-1}, respectively (Public Health England, 2016b), and this recommendation also applies to highly active individuals. For endurance and strength trained individuals, recommendations for protein intake ranges from 1.2 to 1.7 g·kg^{-1} body weight·day^{-1} (American College of Sports Medicine, 2009). It is important to note that for optimal protein use, energy balance is important so that amino acids are spared for protein synthesis and not oxidised to contribute to energy demands.

Child–adult differences in substrate oxidation during physical activity

When compared with adults, boys and girls exhibit lower respiratory exchange ratio values during submaximal exercise performed at similar absolute (Montoye, 1982) and relative (Foricher, Ville, Gratas-Delamarche, & Delamarche, 2003; Martinez & Haymes, 1992) exercise intensities. This indicates a higher reliance on fat and lower reliance on carbohydrate oxidation in children, an effect that appears to be attributed to puberty rather than chronological age (Timmons, Bar-Or, & Riddell, 2007a, 2007b). The mechanisms explaining these child–adult differences in substrate oxidation were first thought to be related to an 'underdeveloped glycolytic system' in children, with boys showing a lower muscle glycogen content and activity of the rate limiting enzyme for glycolysis, phosphofructokinase, when compared with untrained men (Eriksson, Gollnick, & Saltin, 1973). However, more recent evidence using stable isotope techniques has shown that younger, less mature boys rely more on exogenous carbohydrate oxidation during exercise and that exogenous carbohydrate is preferable over fat as a fuel when provided at a sufficient rate (Timmons et al., 2007b). Therefore, it appears that children do not have an underdeveloped glycolytic flux and that glycogen stores may limit carbohydrate oxidation. Due to their limited capacity to utilise endogenous carbohydrate (Timmons et al., 2007b), it is possible that the reported benefits of pre-exercise carbohydrate consumption for endurance performance (via elevated glycogen stores) in adults do not apply to children. However, the effects of high-carbohydrate diets on muscle glycogen stores and exercise performance have not been studied in children. Nevertheless, children may benefit from consuming adequate carbohydrate immediately before or during exercise due to their preference for exogenous carbohydrate as a fuel (Timmons, Bar-Or, & Riddell, 2003; Timmons et al., 2007b).

Assessing dietary intake

Assessing an individual's dietary intake is a fundamental step in monitoring their nutritional status. This could be important for physically active individuals to determine whether their diet is nutritionally adequate, identify potential risk behaviours, and promote optimal training adaptations and performance. There are a number of methods available for dietary assessment that vary with respect to precision and practicality. The method of choice will depend on the type of information required and the resources available.

24-hour recall

This is a retrospective method where the individual is asked to recollect all food and drinks consumed over the previous 24 hours. To obtain important details such as food preparation methods and snacking to produce accurate estimates of energy and nutrient intake, it is recommended that the recall is conducted by a trained interviewer who will ask probing questions (F.E. Thompson & Byers, 1994). Usual household measures are often used to record portion sizes (e.g. cups, spoons), although photographs of various portions are also sometimes used. The recalled information can then be translated into energy and nutrient intakes using food composition tables (see below, p. 212). The main strength of the 24-hour recall is that it is quick and simple taking around 15–20 minutes to complete. As this is a retrospective method, the individual is unlikely to change their dietary behaviour in response to the monitoring.

This approach may be useful to identify patterns of eating behaviour or aspects of the diet that require further investigation, however, due to a number of measurement errors the 24-hour recall should not be used to characterise an individual's usual diet. The ability of individuals to quantify portion sizes varies substantially and may therefore be incorrect, even with the use of portion size aids (Poslusna, Ruprich, de Vries, Jakubikova, & van't Veer, 2009). Research suggests that energy intake may be underreported by 22–67% using this method, which is likely a result of individual's forgetting some of the items they have consumed (Poslusna et al., 2009). Furthermore, the day that is selected for recall may need to be carefully chosen when working with athletes as their dietary intake may vary according to their regime. A single 24-hour recall may not be sufficient and several recalls conducted across different training, competition and rest days may be needed to obtain adequate information (Magkos & Yannakoulia, 2003).

Food frequency questionnaires

The food frequency questionnaire (FFQ) is a retrospective method comprising of a short or long list of foods and drinks from which the individual indicates how often each item is consumed within a specified period of time. This may vary from frequency of consumption in a single day to several months with responses available for selection ranging from 'never' through 'once per month' to 'more than once a day'. Many FFQs also include portion size questions to permit estimation of energy and nutrient intakes, some of which have been validated for this purpose (Bohlscheid-Thomas, Hoting, Boeing, & Wahrendorf, 1997). A major strength of using this method over the 24-hour recall is that foods consumed infrequently (e.g. less than daily) can be identified. Furthermore, most FFQs are self-administered and therefore less time consuming for the observer and are often less burdensome for the responder compared with other dietary assessment methods.

The FFQ is a good tool for identifying general patterns of dietary intake; however, quantification of food intake is less accurate compared with recalls or food diaries. This is due to questionnaires not comprising of all possible food items in the diet, errors in individuals' estimations of consumption frequency, and errors in portion size estimation. A major limitation of FFQs is that they are population-specific and thus include only the most common foods consumed by the target population. If the questionnaire is not appropriate for the population group being assessed it may lead to underestimation of food intake. There are currently a very limited number of FFQs that have been developed for use in athletes (Braakhuis, Hopkins,

Lowe, & Rush, 2011; Fogelholm et al., 1992). Due to these limitations, FFQs are better suited for ranking individuals according to their frequency of consumption of particular foods as opposed to estimating levels of intake (F.E. Thompson & Byers, 1994).

Food diaries

Food diaries (also called food records) are widely considered to be the most accurate approach to dietary assessment. This prospective method requires the individual to record all food and drink consumed usually over a period of three to seven days. The amounts of each item consumed are either estimated using household measures or weighing the items (weighed food diary); the latter being the more accurate and considered the 'gold-standard' method of dietary assessment (Black, 2001). Individuals completing a food diary should provide as much detail as possible, including cooking methods used, brand names of items consumed, and details of any leftovers. The observer must then determine nutrient intake using food composition tables (see below, p. 212). Prospective dietary evaluations are advantageous as they are less susceptible to memory errors, less likely to omit foods being consumed, and should provide greater accuracy of portion sizes compared with recalling portions of foods previously consumed. The foods consumed are also likely to be described in greater detail. However, this approach is much more burdensome for the responder and observer compared with retrospective methods and requires motivation and literacy from the responder for accurate and complete recording. The requirement to weigh and record each item at the time of consumption may also be impractical for the responder. This may be particularly problematic for individuals who consume their food whilst engaging in physical activity or those who eat frequently throughout the day to maintain their high energy requirements (Benardot & Thompson, 1999).

A food diary should be completed over a minimum of three days including both weekday and weekend days to account for an individual's daily variation in dietary intake (Magkos & Yannakoulia, 2003). However, the number of incomplete records becomes higher as more days of records are kept, which may decrease the validity of the food diary in the later days (F.E. Thompson & Byers, 1994). For individuals who are physically active, a monitoring period of three to seven days is suggested to provide reasonably accurate estimations of habitual energy and nutrient intake (Black, 2001). As with other dietary assessment methods, though, estimated and weighed food diaries can result in misreporting of energy intake. A review of studies reported that energy intake may be underestimated by 7–22% when using estimated food diaries and underestimated by 10–20% with weighed diaries (Poslusna et al., 2009). Each of these methods of dietary assessment should therefore be used with consideration of their advantages and limitations.

Analysis of dietary intake

Once a dietary assessment has been completed the next step is to analyse the information provided. If the energy and nutrient intake within the diet is of interest, it will be necessary to carry out calculations to determine their values. How this analysis is conducted will depend on the resources available to the observer but will involve either manual work with food composition tables or nutrient analysis software. Whichever approach is taken, the quality of the analysis will depend on the quality of the dietary information collected. If the dietary record provided is vague and has missing information then the subsequent outcome of the dietary analysis will be flawed and not suitable for drawing conclusions about that person's diet. When conducting the dietary analysis it is important to use food composition data that is relevant to the country in which the dietary record has been conducted as nutrient content of similar foods can vary between different countries.

Food composition tables

Food composition tables contain lists of thousands of commonly consumed foods and the amount of each nutrient per 100 g. These tables provide the majority of information for analysis of nutrient intake. The UK Nutrient Databank is maintained by the Food Standards Agency and a range of books have been produced containing the nutrient composition data; the McCance and Widdowson's *The Composition of Foods* series. The dataset can also be accessed online and downloaded as a Microsoft Excel file at www.gov.uk/government/publications/composition-of-foods-integrated-dataset-cofid. Analysing nutrient intake using these tables requires calculation of the amount of each nutrient in each portion of food consumed until the total consumption within the dietary record is determined. This process is therefore often tedious and time consuming.

Nutrient analysis software

The data contained within published food composition tables is available in a range of dietary analysis software packages. The software will typically include a description of each food item, a code for the food, and the nutrient composition per 100 g of the food. The observer is required to input each food and beverage consumed and the portion size and the software will then calculate nutrient intakes from this information. In addition to inputting food weights, the software will also convert common household measures into estimated weights. This emphasises the importance of gathering detailed and accurate information within the food record to enable a precise calculation of nutrient intake. Once nutrient intake is determined, it is usually most appropriate to compare these against dietary standards (see above, p. 205).

Physical activity, energy balance and appetite

Energy balance describes a state where energy intake equals energy expenditure. Energy intake consists of all energy-containing ingested foods and beverages, i.e. those that contain carbohydrate, fat, protein and/or alcohol. Energy expenditure consists of resting metabolic rate, the thermic effect of food and physical activity. Exercise not only influences energy balance through increased physical activity energy expenditure, it can also influence appetite and energy intake. An understanding of the impact of physical activity on appetite is fundamental for overweight and obesity management, where weight gain results from an extended period of energy intake exceeding energy expenditure. This topic also has implications for athletes to optimise performance and maintain long-term health, and for those who are exposed to extreme environments, e.g. mountaineers at high altitudes.

Appetite regulation

Appetite regulation is a complex process involving communication between the hypothalamus within the brain, various gastrointestinal organs (including the stomach, pancreas and intestines) and adipose (fat) tissue. Hunger refers to the drive to eat, whereas satiation describes the process that leads to the termination of eating and satiety describes the feeling of fullness after eating. Following food intake, satiety is induced via neural signals of gastric distension from the stomach to the brain. Subsequently, various appetite-regulating hormones that sense the digestion and absorption of nutrients are released from the gastrointestinal tract. Episodic hormonal signals occur in unison with episodes of eating and thus control hunger and satiety on a meal-to-meal basis. These hormones include acylated ghrelin, peptide tyrosine tyrosine (PYY), glucagon-like peptide-1 (GLP-1) and pancreatic polypeptide, which signal hunger or satiety either via the vagus nerve (which connects the gut to the brain) or via blood perfusing the hypothalamus. In contrast, the tonic hormones insulin (released from the pancreas) and leptin (released from adipose tissue) regulate long-term changes in energy balance and body fat (Murphy & Bloom, 2006).

Research on physical activity and appetite has predominantly focused on the episodic hormones ghrelin, PYY and GLP-1. Ghrelin is unique in that it is the only known orexigenic (appetite-stimulating) peptide hormone (M. Kojima et al., 1999). It is produced primarily by cells in the oxyntic glands of the stomach and circulates in two forms: acylated and unacylated. The acylation of ghrelin is thought to be essential for appetite regulation, as only the acylated form of the hormone can cross the blood-brain barrier (Murphy & Bloom, 2006). Importantly, acylated ghrelin accounts for only 10–20% of total circulating ghrelin (Ghigo et al., 2005; Hosoda et al., 2004); thus, measuring total ghrelin concentrations may mask changes in the acylated form. Temporal fluctuations indicate that that circulating ghrelin is involved in coordinating meal initiation, with concentrations peaking preprandially and being suppressed postprandially (Cummings et al., 2001). Acting in opposition to acylated ghrelin, various anorexigenic gastrointestinal hormones signal satiety to terminate eating. PYY is predominately synthesised and secreted in the intestinal L-cells and exists in two forms in the circulation: PYY_{3-36} and PYY_{1-36}. Despite PYY_{3-36} being the most abundant and biologically active form, with peripheral infusions reducing energy intake (Batterham et al., 2002), concentrations of total PYY are sensitive to manipulations in food intake, being low in the fasted state and increasing rapidly after food to signal satiety (Degen et al., 2005). Similarly, GLP-1 is secreted from the intestinal L-cells in response to nutrient intake and contributes to meal termination and satiety (Flint, Raben, Astrup, & Holst, 1998).

Acute physical activity (1 to 2 days)

A large body of evidence has shown that acute aerobic exercise does not lead to an increase in appetite or energy intake to restore energy balance (Donnelly et al., 2014) and that high-intensity exercise (≥70% maximal oxygen uptake [$\dot{V}O_{2max}$]) may actually induce transient declines in appetite (Broom, Batterham, King, & Stensel, 2009). This temporary suppression of appetite has been termed 'exercise-induced anorexia'. Even when the exercise energy expenditure is as high as 5324 kJ (1272 kcal), there is no increase in energy intake for the subsequent 22.5 hours (J.A. King, Miyashita, Wasse, & Stensel, 2010). Furthermore, two consecutive days of high-dose exercise (7566 kJ [1808 kcal] across two days) still did not increase energy intake and thus resulted in a large energy deficit (negative energy balance) (Douglas et al., 2015).

Changes in appetite-regulating hormones have been identified as a possible mechanism explaining exercise-induced declines in hunger (Broom et al., 2009). Acute exercise has a small to moderate effect on appetite-regulating hormones, transiently suppressing acylated ghrelin and increasing circulating concentrations of PYY, GLP-1 and pancreatic polypeptide (Schubert, Sabapathy, Leveritt, & Desbrow, 2014). While this observation is mainly based on aerobic exercise ranging from 50 to 75% $\dot{V}O_{2max}$ and lasting approximately 30 to 60 minutes (J.A. King et al., 2010; Shorten, Wallman, & Guelfi, 2009; Ueda et al., 2009), resistance exercise (90-min free weight lifting session) also suppressed appetite with no change in energy intake (Broom et al., 2009). This appetite-suppressing effect of resistance exercise coincided with reduced acylated ghrelin, but no change in PYY (Broom et al., 2009). Similarly, low volume sprint interval training appears to induce reductions in appetite that coincide with reduced acylated ghrelin and increased PYY concentrations (Deighton, Barry, Connon, & Stensel, 2013). Furthermore, acylated ghrelin is suppressed to the same extent when comparing running and cycling exercise performed at 70% of mode-specific $\dot{V}O_{2max}$ (Wasse, Sunderland, King, Miyashita, & Stensel, 2013). Despite anecdotal reports of acute swimming exercise often making people feel like eating more, appetite and acylated ghrelin were suppressed during swimming with no change in subsequent energy intake (J.A. King, Wasse, & Stensel, 2011). Therefore, the exercise-induced suppression in appetite and the lack of compensatory increase in energy intake appears to apply to a range of exercise modes.

The finding that swimming suppresses appetite, akin to land-based exercise, is somewhat in contrast to anecdotal and scientific reports indicating that colder environmental temperatures can stimulate appetite. Indeed, energy intake was lower after exercise in a hot (30°C) environment compared with a thermoneutral (20°C) environment, and higher in cold (8–10°C) compared with a thermoneutral (20°C) environment (Crabtree & Blannin, 2015; Wasse, King, Stensel, & Sunderland, 2013). However, there is no consensus on whether appetite-regulating hormones mediate the suppression of energy intake in hotter environments (Crabtree & Blannin, 2015; C. Kojima, Sasaki, Tsuchiya, & Goto, 2015; Shorten et al., 2009; Wasse, King, et al., 2013). Altitude is another important environmental determinant of appetite. As part of the 1981 American Medical Research Expedition to Everest, Boyer and Blume (1984) observed reductions in energy intake, fat absorption and body weight in Caucasians ascending to high altitude. However, body weight remained stable in the Sherpa guides who habitually reside in these environmental conditions. This loss of appetite in lowlanders acutely exposed to high altitude has been termed 'high altitude anorexia'. Although the mechanisms linking altitude and appetite are not well understood, there is some evidence of reductions in acylated ghrelin and a tendency for reduced total PYY concentrations during acute exposure to hypoxia (12.7% oxygen; ~4000 m) with or without exercise (Wasse, Sunderland, King, Batterham, & Stensel, 2012). Furthermore, the reduced food intake and body weight after one week of exposure to hypoxia was accompanied by an increase in the tonic hormone leptin in obese males (Lippl et al., 2010). Overall, the influence of environmental conditions and appetite is not yet well-understood, but the current evidence suggests that individuals exercising in hot environments or at high altitudes may be prone to large energy deficits, which could exacerbate weight loss in the long term.

As appetite is multi-faceted, perceived appetite is typically assessed using multiple subjective visual analogue scales for feelings of hunger, fullness, satisfaction and prospective food consumption in the studies discussed within this chapter section. However, perceived appetite is not consistently associated with changes in appetite-regulating hormones and energy intake (Gibbons et al., 2013). Other factors that may be involved in the exercise-induced suppression of appetite include reduced neuronal responses in brain regions involved in food reward when subjects are shown images of food (Evero, Hackett, Clark, Phelan, & Hagobian, 2012).

In addition, carbohydrate oxidation accounted for 37% of the variance in post-exercise energy intake in overweight and obese women, indicating that substrate oxidation may be another mechanism explaining the link between exercise and appetite (Hopkins, Blundell, & King, 2014).

Finally, it should be highlighted that the findings on acute exercise and appetite are predominantly based on samples of healthy young men and cannot necessarily be translated to women who may possess more effective mechanisms to maintain body fat (Hagobian & Braun, 2010). When comparing overweight/obese men and women, four days of exercise altered appetite-regulating hormones in a direction expected to stimulate energy intake (e.g. increased acylated ghrelin) in women regardless of whether they were in energy balance or deficit, whereas energy balance abolished this response in men (Hagobian, Sharoff et al., 2009). Similarly, 12 weeks of exercise training lowered leptin concentrations, indicating less satiety and low energy stores, in women but not in men (Hickey et al., 1997). In contrast, acute exercise resulted in equal reductions in relative energy intake (i.e. energy intake minus the energy cost of exercise) and no observable changes in acylated ghrelin and PYY_{3-36} concentrations in men and women (Hagobian, Yamashiro et al., 2013). With respect to individual differences, a meta-analysis showed that weight status did not explain the variation in appetite responses between studies (Schubert et al., 2014). This is despite differences in postprandial ghrelin (English, Ghatei, Malik, Bloom, & Wilding, 2002), PYY (Batterham et al., 2003) and GLP-1 (Madsbad, 2014) responses in obese and non-obese individuals. Nevertheless, further research is required to assess the impact of individual differences (e.g. sex, age, ethnicity, weight status, health status) on interactions between acute exercise and appetite so that exercise can be prescribed to the needs of specific individuals.

Regular physical activity (≥ two days)

Since a single exercise session appears to be effective in eliciting an immediate energy deficit that lasts for at least one to two days, it is somewhat paradoxical that longer term exercise interventions often produce weight loss that is less than theoretically expected (Thomas et al., 2012). With this in mind, compensatory mechanisms including increased energy intake or decreased 'non-exercise energy expenditure' (i.e. the energy expended outside of prescribed exercise, including rest and all other physical activities) may oppose the 'exercise energy expenditure' (i.e. the energy expended during prescribed exercise only) at some point after one to two days of beginning an exercise regimen. Indeed, it seems logical that the cumulative impact of continued daily exercise sessions on energy balance would be different to those of a single acute bout.

Cross-sectional data on differences in energy intake between physically active and physically inactive individuals has been available for many decades. Around 60 years ago, studies on army cadets showed no meaningful association between measures of energy expenditure in daily activities and energy consumed in meals and snacks within a single day, but there was a clear association over two weeks (Edholm, Fletcher, Widdowson, & McCance, 1955). At this time, Edholm et al. (1955) argued that 'the differences between the intakes of food must originate in the differences in energy expenditure'. In a subsequent study on Bengali jute mill workers whose daily occupations ranged from 'sedentary' to 'very heavy', Mayer, Roy and Mitra (1956) proposed a J-shaped relationship between daily energy expenditure and daily energy intake, which were closely matched at higher levels of daily physical activity. Conversely, this coupling was lost at low levels of daily physical activity, with daily energy intake exceeding expenditure in those performing 'sedentary' or 'light' work (Mayer et al., 1956). Since then, evidence has accumulated that suggests habitual physical activity may improve appetite control via enhancing satiety signalling. For example, regular exercisers are better at detecting the difference in energy content between low- and high-energy preloads compared with their sedentary counterparts and adjust their subsequent energy intake accordingly (Long, Hart, & Morgan, 2002). In line with these findings, a recent systematic review (Beaulieu, Hopkins, Blundell, & Finlayson, 2016) reported that habitually active individuals show more accurate compensation for the energy density of foods and supported the J-shaped relationship between physical activity level and energy intake originally reported by Mayer et al. (1956).

Although cross-sectional studies indicate that appetite and energy intake are both related to physical activity level, experimental interventions are required to determine the causal nature of these relationships. As modest weight loss is typically seen with exercise interventions lasting three to 12 months, compensatory behaviours are likely to oppose the exercise-induced energy deficit and thus negate weight loss. Although evidence has shown no change in hunger or energy intake when exercise is performed over periods of two weeks to 18 months, the exercise is often unsupervised and energy intake is typically measured via participant self-report (Donnelly et al., 2014). Nevertheless, some well-controlled studies using sensitive measures of energy balance have shown partial compensation during five to 16 days of daily exercise. For example, initial compensatory behaviours have been detected during five to seven days of exercise, where women appear to compensate through energy intake by ~33% of the exercise-induced energy deficit and men compensate through a reduction in non-exercise energy expenditure (Stubbs et al., 2002a; Stubbs et al., 2002b). Another study showed that exercise for 16 days increased average daily energy expenditure by 3.5 MJ and resulted in 30% compensation in energy intake (Whybrow et al., 2008). Importantly, interventions conducted over 12 to 32 weeks show a large degree of inter-individual variability in compensatory responses to increased physical activity levels (Church, Earnest, Skinner, & Blair, 2007; Church et al., 2009; N.A. King, Hopkins, Caudwell, Stubbs, & Blundell, 2008). Part of this individual variability may be explained by between-sex differences, with women often showing less and more variable weight loss and men showing more consistent weight loss in response to exercise training (Donnelly et al., 2003; Donnelly, Jacobsen, Heelan, Seip, & Smith, 2000).

Possible reasons for the compensatory responses to long-term exercise in individuals who do not achieve predicted weight loss may be related to increases in fasting hunger, which is also highly variable between individuals (N.A. King et al., 2008). Somewhat in contrast, long-term exercise can enhance postprandial satiety signalling from meals (Martins, Kulseng, King, Holst, & Blundell, 2010). Therefore, it has been proposed that the effect of long-term exercise on appetite comprises two components: first, a tonic stimulation of (fasting) appetite and, second, a meal-related episodic inhibition that may be related to changes in the sensitivity to appetite-regulating hormones (Martins et al., 2010). On the other side of the energy balance equation, prescribed exercise does not appear to decrease non-exercise energy expenditure in healthy adults, although, again, this finding requires confirmation in larger studies that employ accurate measures of energy balance (Washburn et al., 2014).

Overall, individuals involved in physical activity should acknowledge the relationship with energy balance and may need to make conscious efforts to increase or reduce their energy intakes depending on their individual goals. In overweight and obese individuals, exercise is recommended to promote negative energy balance for weight loss through increased energy expenditure and may have the added benefit of inducing acute reductions in appetite. However, this negative energy balance must be maintained in the long term for weight loss to occur and be maintained. On the other hand, athletes expending large amounts of energy on a daily basis should be aware of the acute appetite-suppressing effects of exercise and may need to increase their energy intakes to maintain optimal performance and health. This may be of particular relevance for individuals exercising in hot temperatures or at high altitudes, as these environments can induce further suppressions in appetite.

Physical activity and eating behaviour

Lifestyle behaviours such as physical activity and a healthy diet often coexist. Individuals who are physically active also tend to smoke less, consume less alcohol and have a healthier diet and body weight (Maier & Barry, 2015; Poortinga, 2007). Therefore, understanding the association between health-related behaviours is important for both health promotion and disease prevention, particularly as risk behaviours often occur in combination (Poortinga, 2007). Whilst physical activity is often associated with an array of health benefits, it can also involve health risks such as low energy availability, disordered eating behaviour and eating disorders (Torstveit, Rosenvinge, & Sundgot-Borgen, 2008). This section seeks to explore the relationship between physical activity, dietary intake, eating behaviour and disordered eating.

Physical activity and dietary intake

Associations between physical activity and diet are reported in youths, adolescents and adults (Gillman et al., 2001; Lytle, Seifert, Greenstein, & McGovern, 2000). Some evidence suggests that exercise promotes a preference for high-fat, sweet foods among some individuals (Finlayson, Bryant, Blundell, & King, 2009) and can lead to an increase in snack intake (Werle, Wansink, & Payne, 2011). However, also well documented is the association between physical activity and healthy eating, such as higher levels of fruit and vegetable intake (Maier & Barry, 2015). Longitudinal research tracking children across adolescence into early adulthood found that physical activity was positively associated with diet quality indicators as early as 12 years of age, with the strength of the relationship increasing with age (Maier & Barry, 2015). Similarly, research involving middle-aged men and women in the UK observed a weak but significant relationship between leisure-time physical activity and fruit and vegetable intake (Sodergren, McNaughton, Salmon, Ball, & Crawford, 2012).

However, the nature of the relationship between physical activity and diet remains unclear (Sodergren et al., 2012). It is often difficult to determine whether physical activity leads to an increase in healthful behaviours, such as increased fruit and vegetable intake, or whether these healthful behaviours lead to increases in physical activity. Untargeted increases in physical activity have been reported in interventions to promote fruit and vegetable consumption (Berrigan, Dodd, Troiano, Krebs-Smith, & Barbash, 2003). Regardless of the direction of this relationship, overall, evidence seems to suggest that these health behaviours facilitate rather than hinder each other, which may be explained through psychological constructs (Fleig, Kuper, Lippke, Schwarzer, & Wiedemann, 2015). For example, research exploring health behaviour change suggests that individuals who are more confident in their ability to be physically active also hold more positive beliefs about their ability to develop healthy eating habits (Annesi & Marti, 2011). Similarly, motivation to change physical activity has been associated with intention to change dietary intake (Kremers,

De Bruijn, Schaalma, & Brug, 2004). This has implications for weight management interventions as physical activity may affect weight loss through these psychological pathways associated with eating changes.

Physical activity and disordered eating

Whilst physical activity is often associated with an array of health benefits, it can also involve health risks such as low energy availability, disordered eating behaviour and eating disorders (Byrne & McLean, 2001). Particularly amongst elite athletes, disordered eating can be common, with up to 20% of female and 8% of male elite athletes meeting the criteria for an eating disorder (Sundgot-Borgen, & Torstveit, 2004). Within weight-sensitive sports that emphasise a low weight and lean body shape (such as endurance, track and field and aesthetic sports), features of disordered eating may be present in up to 50% of athletes (Torstveit et al., 2008). On the contrary, competing in sport at a non-elite level may have a protective effect against eating disorders with lower levels of eating psychopathology reported in this group compared with elite athletes (Smolak, Murnen, & Ruble, 2000). As the most common onset of eating disorders is during adolescence, age is considered a risk factor within sport and coaches and athletes should therefore attempt to identify indicators of these disorders from a young age (Byrne & McLean, 2001).

Eating disorders increase an athlete's risk of injury, often due to reduced energy availability and reduced bone density (Pollock et al., 2010). They can also impact upon an athlete's quality of life (Mond, Hay, Rodgers, & Owen, 2006) and psychological well-being (Meyer, Taranis, Goodwin, & Haycraft, 2011). For female athletes, disordered eating is a particular concern as it increases the risk of female athlete triad, which is a syndrome characterised by inadequate energy availability, decreased bone mineral density and menstrual disorders (Nattiv et al., 2007). Lack of menstruation (amenorrhea) can be perceived as relatively normal among athletes and as such may not be recognised as a potential sign of disordered eating. Identification of eating disorders can be particularly difficult given that these symptoms can be hidden or difficult to identify and athletes may attempt to deny the issue (Sherman, Thompson, DeHass, & Wilfert, 2005).

There are a range of psychosocial and personality factors that may impact upon an athlete's risk of developing an eating disorder or maladaptive attitudes towards food. Psychological indicators such as self-efficacy, self-esteem and body image have been associated with eating disorder risk (Stice & Agras, 1998). Amongst athletes, a positive outlook on life and high self-efficacy may serve as protective factors against disordered eating (Fulkerson, Keel, Leon, & Dorr, 1999), whereas low self-esteem is most often viewed as a risk factor (Johnson et al., 2004). Similarly, personality traits such as perfectionism have been associated with eating disorder risk within both athletes (Haase, Prapavessis & Glynn Owens, 2002) and non-athletes (Halmi et al., 2000). Whilst high levels of perfectionism can be viewed as an adaptive and necessary trait to help athletes to achieve elite performance (Gould, Dieffenbach, & Moffett, 2002), the combination of exceedingly high standards accompanied with overly critical evaluations of behaviour can increase the likelihood of an athlete developing an eating disorder (Forsberg & Lock, 2006). The athlete's socio-cultural environment is also important, particularly amongst younger athletes, whereby family dysfunction and poor parent–child relationships can impact upon eating disorder symptomology (Kluck, 2008). Societal and peer group influences, particularly comments from peers relating to body shape and weight, represent another risk factor (Wade, Bergin, Martin, Gillespie, & Fairburn, 2006). It is important that professionals working within sport understand the broad range of risk factors for disordered eating that may impact upon both athlete performance and their health and well-being.

Coaches have been identified as important figures in the emergence and development of disordered eating (Papathomas & Lavallee, 2010) and also in the prevention and identification of eating disorders in their athletes (Plateau, McDermott, Arcelus, & Meyer, 2014). Thus, it is important to explore how coach actions may contribute towards, or reduce features of, the sporting environment that may foster disordered eating. Coaches' attitudes, behaviours and remarks may be implicated in the emergence of eating problems in athletes. For example, track and field coaches have reported that they place a high level of importance on body weight for performance and an 'ideal' female athlete body (Plateau, McDermott, et al., 2014). Similarly, coaches may expect certain athletes, such as gymnasts or distance runners, to be slim and may not notice when weight loss is occurring (R.A. Thompson & Trattner Sherman, 1999). Whilst some experienced coaches working in high risk sports understand the impact of disordered eating on health and performance, many lack knowledge and confidence in identifying early signs of disordered eating among their athletes. Research involving track and field coaches in the UK suggests that coaches require additional information, advice and guidance in order to improve knowledge and confidence in identifying disordered eating among athletes (Plateau, McDermott, et al., 2014).

Physical activity is predominantly viewed as a positive health behaviour that provides individuals with a range of physical and psychological benefits. However, some individuals can develop compulsive exercise (also termed excessive exercise or exercise dependence), where they feel compelled to exercise, often pushing themselves to physical injury and exhaustion (Meyer et al., 2011). Compulsive exercise does not simply refer to excess volumes of exercise but includes an emotional and cognitive aspect as well (Steffen & Brehm, 1999). Features include routine-like patterns of exercise which are continued despite negative consequences and feelings of anxiety and distress if exercise cannot be completed (Meyer et al., 2011). The motivation to exercise in compulsive exercisers is commonly related to eating, weight and shape concerns and exists in athletes, the general population, and patients with a clinical eating disorder (Lipsey, Barton, Hulley, & Hill, 2006; Plateau, Shanmugam, et al., 2014; Taranis, Touyz, & Meyer, 2011). The challenge amongst athlete populations is deciphering whether an individual is demonstrating high commitment to training or engaging in potentially harmful exercise behaviours that could be indicative of an eating disorder (R.A. Thompson & Trattner Sherman, 1999). In athletes, a definition of problematic exercise focusing on the frequency, intensity and duration of exercise may not be relevant (Plateau, Shanmugam, et al., 2014). Instead, there is a need to consider a multidimensional model incorporating body weight and shape control (Fairburn, Cooper, & Shafran, 2003) and cognitive behavioural maintenance factors such as exercise as a mood regulatory strategy to avoid negative emotions (Plateau, Shanmugam, et al., 2014) and intense feelings of guilt if exercise sessions cannot be completed (Meyer et al., 2011). As elite athletes will engage in high volume and frequency of exercise that is likely to be repetitive, routine and performance oriented, it is important that coaches look out for these specific features of 'compulsive exercise' that may be relevant and problematic.

Chapter summary

This chapter has highlighted the interdisciplinary nature of nutrition and physical activity. In order to maximise physical activity performance and health in the general public and athletic populations, nutrient intake is an important consideration and dietary guidelines have been provided for use in practice. There are a variety of methods available to assess dietary intake that vary in terms of accuracy and practicality. Practitioners are guided on how to utilise these methods and conduct a dietary analysis for the client they may be working with. Physical activity and exercise training have the potential to promote negative energy balance through increased energy expenditure and acute reductions in appetite. However, regular exercise may result in compensatory responses that negate weight loss and this issue is complicated by the large degree of inter-individual variability in the compensatory responses to exercise. Lastly, this chapter has highlighted that although physical activity is often associated with an array of healthful behaviours, there are also health risks associated with being physically active. Some athletes can develop maladaptive eating and exercise behaviours that impact upon health, psychological well-being and performance. Practitioners need to be aware of risk factors and early symptoms of disordered eating and compulsive exercise in order to prevent and treat them.

- Optimal nutrition is essential for individuals to promote performance and overall health and well-being.
- Energy balance and macronutrient composition of the diet are key considerations for optimal nutrition.
- Dietary assessment is important in monitoring nutritional status and can help refine nutritional practices of individuals.
- Exercise can suppress appetite and energy intake acutely, but in the long-term there may be a compensatory effect in which active individuals achieve a state of energy balance.
- Although physical activity is often associated with healthful behaviours such as a healthy diet and lower alcohol consumption, it can also be accompanied by health risks.
- Maladaptive practices, such as compulsive exercise and disordered eating, can impact upon exercise performance, health and psychological well-being.

References

Achten, J., Gleeson, M., & Jeukendrup, A.E. (2002). Determination of the exercise intensity that elicits maximal fat oxidation. *Med Sci Sports Exerc, 34*(1), 92–97.

American College of Sports Medicine. (2009). American College of Sports Medicine position stand. Nutrition and athletic performance. *Med Sci Sports Exerc, 41*(3), 709–731. doi: 10.1249/MSS.0b013e31890eb86

Annesi, J.J., & Marti, C.N. (2011). Path analysis of exercise treatment-induced changes in psychological factors leading to weight loss. *Psychol Health, 26*(8), 1081–1098. doi: 10.1080/08870446.2010.534167

Batterham, R.L., Cohen, M.A., Ellis, S.M., Le Roux, C.W., Withers, D.J., Frost, G.S., . . . Bloom, S.R. (2003). Inhibition of food intake in obese subjects by peptide YY3–36. *N Engl J Med, 349*(10), 941–948. doi: 10.1056/NEJMoa030204

Batterham, R.L., Cowley, M.A., Small, C.J., Herzog, H., Cohen, M.A., Dakin, C.L., . . . Bloom, S.R. (2002). Gut hormone PYY(3–36) physiologically inhibits food intake. *Nature, 418*(6898), 650–654. doi: 10.1038/nature02666

Beaulieu, K., Hopkins, M., Blundell, J., & Finlayson, G. (2016). Does habitual physical activity increase the sensitivity of the appetite control system? A systematic review. *Sports Med, 46*(12), 1897–1919. doi: 10.1007/s40279-016-0518-9

Benardot, D., & Thompson, W. (1999). Energy from food for physical activity: enough and on time. *ACSM Health Fit J, 3*, 14–18.

Berrigan, D., Dodd, K., Troiano, R.P., Krebs-Smith, S.M., & Barbash, R.B. (2003). Patterns of health behavior in U.S. adults. *Prev Med, 36*(5), 615–623.

Black, A. (2001). Dietary assessment for sports dietetics. *Nutr Bull, 26*, 26–42.

Bohlscheid-Thomas, S., Hoting, I., Boeing, H., & Wahrendorf, J. (1997). Reproducibility and relative validity of energy and macronutrient intake of a food frequency questionnaire developed for the German part of the EPIC project. European Prospective Investigation into Cancer and Nutrition. *Int J Epidemiol, 26 Suppl 1*, S71–81.

Boyer, S.J., & Blume, F.D. (1984). Weight loss and changes in body composition at high altitude. *J Appl Physiol Respir Environ Exerc Physiol, 57*(5), 1580–1585.

Braakhuis, A.J., Hopkins, W.G., Lowe, T.E., & Rush, E.C. (2011). Development and validation of a food-frequency questionnaire to assess short-term antioxidant intake in athletes. *Int J Sport Nutr Exerc Metab, 21*(2), 105–112.

Brooks, G.A., & Mercier, J. (1994). Balance of carbohydrate and lipid utilization during exercise: the 'crossover' concept. *J Appl Physiol (1985), 76*(6), 2253–2261.

Broom, D.R., Batterham, R.L., King, J.A., & Stensel, D.J. (2009). Influence of resistance and aerobic exercise on hunger, circulating levels of acylated ghrelin, and peptide YY in healthy males. *Am J Physiol Regul Integr Comp Physiol, 296*(1), R29–35. doi: 90706.2008 [pii]10.1152/ajpregu.90706.2008

Burke, L.M., Hawley, J.A., Angus, D.J., Cox, G.R., Clark, S.A., Cummings, N.K., . . . Hargreaves, M. (2002). Adaptations to short-term high-fat diet persist during exercise despite high carbohydrate availability. *Med Sci Sports Exerc, 34*(1), 83–91.

Burke, L.M., Hawley, J.A., Wong, S.H., & Jeukendrup, A.E. (2011). Carbohydrates for training and competition. *J Sports Sci, 29 Suppl 1*, S17–27. doi: 10.1080/02640414.2011.585473

Byrne, S., & McLean, N. (2001). Eating disorders in athletes: a review of the literature. *J Sci Med Sport, 4*(2), 145–159.

Church, T.S., Earnest, C.P., Skinner, J.S., & Blair, S.N. (2007). Effects of different doses of physical activity on cardiorespiratory fitness among sedentary, overweight or obese postmenopausal women with elevated blood pressure: a randomized controlled trial. *JAMA, 297*(19), 2081–2091. doi: 10.1001/jama.297.19.2081

Church, T.S., Martin, C.K., Thompson, A.M., Earnest, C.P., Mikus, C.R., & Blair, S.N. (2009). Changes in weight, waist circumference and compensatory responses with different doses of exercise among sedentary, overweight postmenopausal women. *PLoS ONE, 4*(2), e4515. doi: 10.1371/journal.pone.0004515

COMA. (1991). *Report on Health and Social Subjects no. 41. Dietary Reference Values for Food Energy and Nutrients for the United Kingdom*. London: HMSO.

Crabtree, D.R., & Blannin, A.K. (2015). Effects of exercise in the cold on ghrelin, PYY, and food intake in overweight adults. *Med Sci Sports Exerc, 47*(1), 19–57. doi: 10.1249/MSS.0000000000000391

Cummings, D.E., Purnell, J.Q., Frayo, R.S., Schmidova, K., Wisse, B.E., & Weigle, D.S. (2001). A preprandial rise in plasma ghrelin levels suggests a role in meal initiation in humans. *Diabetes, 50*(8), 1714–1719.

Degen, L., Oesch, S., Casanova, M., Graf, S., Ketterer, S., Drewe, J., & Beglinger, C. (2005). Effect of peptide YY3–36 on food intake in humans. *Gastroenterology, 129*(5), 1430–1436. doi: 10.1053/j.gastro.2005.09.001

Deighton, K., Barry, R., Connon, C.E., & Stensel, D.J. (2013). Appetite, gut hormone and energy intake responses to low volume sprint interval and traditional endurance exercise. *Eur J Appl Physiol, 113*(5), 1147–1156. doi: 10.1007/s00421-012-2535-1

Donnelly, J.E., Herrmann, S.D., Lambourne, K., Szabo, A.N., Honas, J.J., & Washburn, R.A. (2014). Does increased exercise or physical activity alter ad-libitum daily energy intake or macronutrient composition in healthy adults? A systematic review. *PLoS ONE, 9*(1), e83498. doi: 10.1371/journal.pone.0083498

Donnelly, J.E., Hill, J.O., Jacobsen, D.J., Potteiger, J., Sullivan, D.K., Johnson, S.L., . . . Washburn, R.A. (2003). Effects of a 16-month randomized controlled exercise trial on body weight and composition in young, overweight men and women: the Midwest Exercise Trial. *Arch Intern Med, 163*(11), 1343–1350. doi: 10.1001/archinte.163.11.1343

Donnelly, J.E., Jacobsen, D.J., Heelan, K.S., Seip, R., & Smith, S. (2000). The effects of 18 months of intermittent vs. continuous exercise on aerobic capacity, body weight and composition, and metabolic fitness in previously sedentary, moderately obese females. *Int J Obes Relat Metab Disord, 24*(5), 566–572.

Douglas, J.A., King, J.A., McFarlane, E., Baker, L., Bradley, C., Crouch, N., . . . Stensel, D.J. (2015). Appetite, appetite hormone and energy intake responses to two consecutive days of aerobic exercise in healthy young men. *Appetite, 92*, 57–65. doi: 10.1016/j.appet.2015.05.006

Edholm, O.G., Fletcher, J.G., Widdowson, E.M., & McCance, R.A. (1955). The energy expenditure and food intake of individual men. *Br J Nutr, 9*(3), 286–300.

English, P.J., Ghatei, M.A., Malik, I.A., Bloom, S.R., & Wilding, J.P. (2002). Food fails to suppress ghrelin levels in obese humans. *J Clin Endocrinol Metab, 87*(6), 2984. doi: 10.1210/jcem.87.6.8738

Eriksson, B.O., Gollnick, P.D., & Saltin, B. (1973). Muscle metabolism and enzyme activities after training in boys 11–13 years old. *Acta Physiol Scand, 87*(4), 485–497. doi: 10.1111/j.1748–1716.1973.tb05415.x

Evero, N., Hackett, L.C., Clark, R.D., Phelan, S., & Hagobian, T.A. (2012). Aerobic exercise reduces neuronal responses in food reward brain regions. *J Appl Physiol (1985), 112*(9), 1612–1619. doi: 10.1152/japplphysiol.01365.2011

Fairburn, C.G., Cooper, Z., & Shafran, R. (2003). Cognitive behaviour therapy for eating disorders: a 'transdiagnostic' theory and treatment. *Behav Res Ther, 41*(5), 509–528.

Finlayson, G., Bryant, E., Blundell, J.E., & King, N.A. (2009). Acute compensatory eating following exercise is associated with implicit hedonic wanting for food. *Physiol Behav, 97*(1), 62–67. doi: 10.1016/j.physbeh.2009.02.002

Fleig, L., Kuper, C., Lippke, S., Schwarzer, R., & Wiedemann, A.U. (2015). Cross-behavior associations and multiple health behavior change: a longitudinal study on physical activity and fruit and vegetable intake. *J Health Psychol, 20*(5), 525–534. doi: 10.1177/1359105315574951

Flint, A., Raben, A., Astrup, A., & Holst, J.J. (1998). Glucagon-like peptide 1 promotes satiety and suppresses energy intake in humans. *J Clin Invest, 101*(3), 515–520. doi: 10.1172/JCI990

Fogelholm, G.M., Himberg, J.J., Alopaeus, K., Gref, C.G., Laakso, J.T., Lehto, J.J., & Mussalo-Rauhamaa, H. (1992). Dietary and biochemical indices of nutritional status in male athletes and controls. *J Am Coll Nutr, 11*(2), 181–191.

Foricher, J.M., Ville, N., Gratas-Delamarche, A., & Delamarche, P. (2003). Effects of submaximal intensity cycle ergometry for one hour on substrate utilisation in trained prepubertal boys versus trained adults. *J Sports Med Phys Fitness, 43*(1), 36–43.

Forsberg, S., & Lock, J. (2006). The relationship between perfectionism, eating disorders and athletes: a review. *Minerva Pediatr, 58*(6), 525–536.

Frankenfield, D.C., Muth, E.R., & Rowe, W.A. (1998). The Harris-Benedict studies of human basal metabolism: history and limitations. *J Am Diet Assoc, 98*(4), 439–445. doi: 10.1016/S0002-8223(98)00100-X

Fulkerson, J.A., Keel, P.K., Leon, G.R., & Dorr, T. (1999). Eating-disordered behaviors and personality characteristics of high school athletes and nonathletes. *Int J Eat Disord, 26*(1), 73–79.

Ghigo, E., Broglio, F., Arvat, E., Maccario, M., Papotti, M., & Muccioli, G. (2005). Ghrelin: more than a natural GH secretagogue and/or an orexigenic factor. *Clin Endocrinol (Oxf), 62*(1), 1–17. doi: 10.1111/j.1365–2265.2004.02160.x

Gibbons, C., Caudwell, P., Finlayson, G., Webb, D.L., Hellstrom, P.M., Naslund, E., & Blundell, J.E. (2013). Comparison of postprandial profiles of ghrelin, active GLP-1, and total PYY to meals varying in fat and carbohydrate and their association with hunger and the phases of satiety. *J Clin Endocrinol Metab, 98*(5), E847-855. doi: 10.1210/jc.2012–3835

Gillman, M.W., Pinto, B.M., Tennstedt, S., Glanz, K., Marcus, B., & Friedman, R.H. (2001). Relationships of physical activity with dietary behaviors among adults. *Prev Med, 32*(3), 295–301. doi: 10.1006/pmed.2000.0812

Gould, D., Dieffenbach, K., & Moffett, A. (2002). Psychological characteristics and their development in Olympic champions. *J Appl Sport Psychol, 14*(3), 172–204. doi: 10.1080/10413200290103482

Haase, A.M., Prapavessis, H., & Glynn Owens, R. (2002). Perfectionism, social physique anxiety and disordered eating: a comparison of male and female elite athletes. *Psychol Sport and Exerc, 3*(3), 209–222. doi: http://dx.doi.org/10.1016/S1469-0292(01)00018-8

Hagobian, T.A., & Braun, B. (2010). Physical activity and hormonal regulation of appetite: sex differences and weight control. *Exerc Sport Sci Rev, 38*(1), 25–30. doi: 10.1097/JES.0b013e3181c5cd98

Hagobian, T.A., Sharoff, C.G., Stephens, B.R., Wade, G.N., Silva, J.E., Chipkin, S.R., & Braun, B. (2009). Effects of exercise on energy-regulating hormones and appetite in men and women. *Am J Physiol Regul Integr Comp Physiol, 296*(2), R233–242. doi: 10.1152/ajpregu.90671.2008

Hagobian, T.A., Yamashiro, M., Hinkel-Lipsker, J., Streder, K., Evero, N., & Hackney, T. (2013). Effects of acute exercise on appetite hormones and ad libitum energy intake in men and women. *Appl Physiol Nutr Metab, 38*(1), 66–72. doi: 10.1139/apnm-2012-0104

Halmi, K.A., Sunday, S.R., Strober, M., Kaplan, A., Woodside, D.B., Fichter, M., . . . Kaye, W.H. (2000). Perfectionism in anorexia nervosa: variation by clinical subtype, obsessionality, and pathological eating behavior. *Am J Psychiatry, 157*(11), 1799–1805. doi: 10.1176/appi.ajp.157.11.1799

Hawley, J.A., Schabort, E.J., Noakes, T.D., & Dennis, S.C. (1997). Carbohydrate-loading and exercise performance. An update. *Sports Med, 24*(2), 73–81.

Helge, J.W. (2002). Long-term fat diet adaptation effects on performance, training capacity, and fat utilization. *Med Sci Sports Exerc, 34*(9), 1499–1504. doi: 10.1249/01.MSS.0000027691.95769.B5

Helge, J.W., Richter, E.A., & Kiens, B. (1996). Interaction of training and diet on metabolism and endurance during exercise in man. *J Physiol, 492 (Pt 1)*, 293–306.

Hickey, M.S., Houmard, J.A., Considine, R.V., Tyndall, G.L., Midgette, J.B., Gavigan, K.E., . . . Caro, J.F. (1997). Gender-dependent effects of exercise training on serum leptin levels in humans. *Am J Physiol, 272*(4 Pt 1), E562–566.

Hopkins, M., Blundell, J.E., & King, N.A. (2014). Individual variability in compensatory eating following acute exercise in overweight and obese women. *Br J Sports Med, 48*(20), 1472–1476. doi: 10.1136/bjsports-2012-091721

Horvath, P.J., Eagen, C.K., Fisher, N.M., Leddy, J.J., & Pendergast, D.R. (2000). The effects of varying dietary fat on performance and metabolism in trained male and female runners. *J Am Coll Nutr, 19*(1), 52–60.

Hosoda, H., Doi, K., Nagaya, N., Okumura, H., Nakagawa, E., Enomoto, M., . . . Kangawa, K. (2004). Optimum collection and storage conditions for ghrelin measurements: octanoyl modification of ghrelin is rapidly hydrolyzed to desacyl ghrelin in blood samples. *Clin Chem, 50*(6), 1077–1080. doi: 10.1373/clinchem.2003.025841

Johnson, C., Crosby, R., Engel, S., Mitchell, J., Powers, P., Wittrock, D., & Wonderlich, S. (2004). Gender, ethnicity, self-esteem and disordered eating among college athletes. *Eat Behav, 5*(2), 147–156. doi: 10.1016/j.eatbeh.2004.01.004

King, J.A., Miyashita, M., Wasse, L.K., & Stensel, D.J. (2010). Influence of prolonged treadmill running on appetite, energy intake and circulating concentrations of acylated ghrelin. *Appetite, 54*(3), 492–498. doi: 10.1016/j.appet.2010.02.002

King, J.A., Wasse, L.K., & Stensel, D.J. (2011). The acute effects of swimming on appetite, food intake, and plasma acylated ghrelin. *J Obes, 2011*. doi: 10.1155/2011/351628

King, N.A., Hopkins, M., Caudwell, P., Stubbs, R.J., & Blundell, J.E. (2008). Individual variability following 12 weeks of supervised exercise: identification and characterization of compensation for exercise-induced weight loss. *Int J Obes* (Lond), *32*(1), 177–184. doi: 10.1038/sj.ijo.0803712

Kluck, A.S. (2008). Family factors in the development of disordered eating: integrating dynamic and behavioral explanations. *Eat Behav, 9*(4), 471–483. doi: 10.1016/j.eatbeh.2008.07.006

Kojima, C., Sasaki, H., Tsuchiya, Y., & Goto, K. (2015). The influence of environmental temperature on appetite-related hormonal responses. *J Physiol Anthropol, 34*(1), 22. doi: 10.1186/s40101-015-0059-1

Kojima, M., Hosoda, H., Date, Y., Nakazato, M., Matsuo, H., & Kangawa, K. (1999). Ghrelin is a growth-hormone-releasing acylated peptide from stomach. *Nature, 402*(6762), 656–660. doi: 10.1038/45230

Kremers, S.P.J., De Bruijn, G.-J., Schaalma, H., & Brug, J. (2004). Clustering of energy balance-related behaviours and their intrapersonal determinants. *Psychol Health, 19*(5), 595–606.

Lippl, F.J., Neubauer, S., Schipfer, S., Lichter, N., Tufman, A., Otto, B., & Fischer, R. (2010). Hypobaric hypoxia causes body weight reduction in obese subjects. *Obesity* (Silver Spring), *18*(4), 675–681. doi: 10.1038/oby.2009.509

Lipsey, Z., Barton, S.B., Hulley, A., & Hill, A.J. (2006). 'After a workout . . .' Beliefs about exercise, eating and appearance in female exercisers with and without eating disorder features. *Psychol Sport and Exerc, 7*(5), 425–436. doi: http://dx.doi.org/10.1016/j.psychsport.2006.01.005

Long, S.J., Hart, K., & Morgan, L.M. (2002). The ability of habitual exercise to influence appetite and food intake in response to high- and low-energy preloads in man. *Br J Nutr, 87*(5), 517–523. doi: 10.1079/BJNBJN2002560

Lytle, L.A., Seifert, S., Greenstein, J., & McGovern, P. (2000). How do children's eating patterns and food choices change over time? Results from a cohort study. *Am J Health Promot, 14*(4), 222–228.

Madsbad, S. (2014). The role of glucagon-like peptide-1 impairment in obesity and potential therapeutic implications. *Diabetes Obes Metab, 16*(1), 9–21. doi: 10.1111/dom.12119

Magkos, F., & Yannakoulia, M. (2003). Methodology of dietary assessment in athletes: concepts and pitfalls. *Curr Opin Clin Nutr Metab Care, 6*(5), 539–549. doi: 10.1097/01.mco.0000087969.83880.97

Maier, J.H., & Barry, R. (2015). Associations among physical activity, diet, and obesity measures change during adolescence. *J Nutr Metab, 2015*, 805065. doi: 10.1155/2015/805065

Martinez, L.R., & Haymes, E.M. (1992). Substrate utilization during treadmill running in prepubertal girls and women. *Med Sci Sports Exerc, 24*(9), 975–983.

Martins, C., Kulseng, B., King, N.A., Holst, J.J., & Blundell, J.E. (2010). The effects of exercise-induced weight loss on appetite-related peptides and motivation to eat. *J Clin Endocrinol Metab, 95*(4), 1609–1616. doi: 10.1210/jc.2009-2082

Mayer, J., Roy, P., & Mitra, K.P. (1956). Relation between caloric intake, body weight, and physical work: studies in an industrial male population in West Bengal. *Am J Clin Nutr, 4*(2), 169–175.

Meyer, C., Taranis, L., Goodwin, H., & Haycraft, E. (2011). Compulsive exercise and eating disorders. *Eur Eat Disord Rev, 19*(3), 174–189. doi: 10.1002/erv.1122

Mond, J.M., Hay, P.J., Rodgers, B., & Owen, C. (2006). Eating Disorder Examination Questionnaire (EDE-Q): norms for young adult women. *Behav Res Ther, 44*(1), 53–62. doi: 10.1016/j.brat.2004.12.003

Montoye, H.J. (1982). Age and oxygen utilization during submaximal treadmill exercise in males. *J Gerontol, 37*(4), 396–402.

Murphy, K.G., & Bloom, S.R. (2006). Gut hormones and the regulation of energy homeostasis. *Nature, 444*(7121), 854–859. doi: nature05484 [pii]10.1038/nature05484

Nattiv, A., Loucks, A.B., Manore, M.M., Sanborn, C.F., Sundgot-Borgen, J., Warren, M.P., & American College of Sports. (2007). American College of Sports Medicine position stand. The female athlete triad. *Med Sci Sports Exerc, 39*(10), 1867–1882. doi: 10.1249/mss.0b013e318149f111

Papathomas, A., & Lavallee, D. (2010). Athlete experiences of disordered eating in sport. *Qualit Res in Sport, Exerc and Health, 2*, 354–370.

Plateau, C.R., McDermott, H.J., Arcelus, J., & Meyer, C. (2014). Identifying and preventing disordered eating among athletes: perceptions of track and field coaches. *Psychol Sport and Exerc, 15*(6), 721–728. doi: http://dx.doi.org/10.1016/j.psychsport.2013.11.004

Plateau, C.R., Shanmugam, V., Duckham, R.L., Goodwin, H., Jowett, S., Brooke-Wavell, K.S.F., . . . Meyer, C. (2014). Use of the compulsive exercise test with athletes: norms and links with eating psychopathology. *J Appl Sport Psychol, 26*(3), 287–301. doi: 10.1080/10413200.2013.867911

Pollock, N., Grogan, C., Perry, M., Pedlar, C., Cooke, K., Morrissey, D., & Dimitriou, L. (2010). Bone-mineral density and other features of the female athlete triad in elite endurance runners: a longitudinal and cross-sectional observational study. *Int J Sport Nutr Exerc Metab, 20*(5), 418–426.

Poortinga, W. (2007). The prevalence and clustering of four major lifestyle risk factors in an English adult population. *Prev Med, 44*(2), 124–128. doi: 10.1016/j.ypmed.2006.10.006

Poslusna, K., Ruprich, J., de Vries, J.H., Jakubikova, M., & van't Veer, P. (2009). Misreporting of energy and micronutrient intake estimated by food records and 24 hour recalls, control and adjustment methods in practice. *Br J Nutr, 101 Suppl 2*, S73–85. doi: 10.1017/S0007114509990602

Public Health England. (2016a). The Eatwell Guide. Available at www.gov.uk/government/publications/the-eatwell-guide (accessed 7 Nov 2016).

Public Health England. (2016b). Government Dietary Recommendations: Government recommendations for food energy and nutrients for males and females aged 1–18 years and 19+ years. Available at: www.gov.uk/government/uploads/system/uploads/attachment_data/file/547050/government__dietary_recommendations.pdf (accessed 9 Nov 2016).

Romijn, J.A., Coyle, E.F., Sidossis, L.S., Gastaldelli, A., Horowitz, J.F., Endert, E., & Wolfe, R.R. (1993). Regulation of endogenous fat and carbohydrate metabolism in relation to exercise intensity and duration. *Am J Physiol, 265*(3 Pt 1), E380–391.

Schofield, W.N. (1985). Predicting basal metabolic rate, new standards and review of previous work. *Hum Nutr Clin Nutr, 39 Suppl 1*, 5–41.

Schubert, M.M., Sabapathy, S., Leveritt, M., & Desbrow, B. (2014). Acute exercise and hormones related to appetite regulation: a meta-analysis. *Sports Med, 44*(3), 387–403. doi: 10.1007/s40279-013-0120-3

Sherman, R.T., Thompson, R.A., DeHass, D., & Wilfert, M. (2005). NCAA coaches survey: the role of the coach in identifying and managing athletes with disordered eating. *Eat Disord, 13*(5), 447–466. doi: 10.1080/10640260500296707

Shorten, A.L., Wallman, K.E., & Guelfi, K.J. (2009). Acute effect of environmental temperature during exercise on subsequent energy intake in active men. *Am J Clin Nutr, 90*(5), 1215–1221. doi: 10.3945/ajcn.2009.28162

Smolak, L., Murnen, S.K., & Ruble, A.E. (2000). Female athletes and eating problems: a meta-analysis. *Int J Eat Disord, 27*(4), 371–380.

Sodergren, M., McNaughton, S.A., Salmon, J., Ball, K., & Crawford, D.A. (2012). Associations between fruit and vegetable intake, leisure-time physical activity, sitting time and self-rated health among older adults: cross-sectional data from the WELL study. *BMC Public Health, 12*, 551. doi: 10.1186/1471-2458-12-551

Steffen, J.J., & Brehm, B.J. (1999). The dimensions of obligatory exercise. *Eating Disorders, 7*(3), 219–226. doi: 10.1080/10640269908249287

Stice, E., & Agras, W.S. (1998). Predicting onset and cessation of bulimic behaviors during adolescence: a longitudinal grouping analysis. *Behavior Therapy, 29*(2), 257–276. doi: http://dx.doi.org/10.1016/S0005-7894(98)80006-3

Stubbs, R.J., Sepp, A., Hughes, D.A., Johnstone, A.M., Horgan, G.W., King, N.A., & Blundell, J.E. (2002a). The effect of graded levels of exercise on energy intake and balance in free-living men, consuming their normal diet. *European Journal of Clinical Nutrition, 56*, 129–140.

Stubbs, R.J., Sepp, A., Hughes, D.A., Johnstone, A.M., King, N., Horgan, G., & Blundell, J.E. (2002b). The effect of graded levels of exercise on energy intake and balance in free-living women. *Int J Obes Relat Metab Disord, 26*(6), 866–869. doi: 10.1038/sj.ijo.0801874

Sundgot-Borgen, J., & Torstveit, M.K. (2004). Prevalence of eating disorders in elite athletes is higher than in the general population. *Clin J Sport Med, 14*(1), 25–32.

Taranis, L., Touyz, S., & Meyer, C. (2011). Disordered eating and exercise: development and preliminary validation of the compulsive exercise test (CET). *Eur Eat Disord Rev, 19*(3), 256–268. doi: 10.1002/erv.1108

Thomas, D.M., Bouchard, C., Church, T., Slentz, C., Kraus, W.E., Redman, L.M., . . . Heymsfield, S.B. (2012). Why do individuals not lose more weight from an exercise intervention at a defined dose? An energy balance analysis. *Obes Rev, 13*(10), 835–847. doi: 10.1111/j.1467-789X.2012.01012.x

Thompson, F.E., & Byers, T. (1994). Dietary assessment resource manual. *J Nutr, 124*(11 Suppl), 2245S–2317S.

Thompson, R.A., & Trattner Sherman, R. (1999). Athletes, athletic performance, and eating disorders: healthier alternatives. *Journal of Social Issues, 55*(2), 317–337. doi: 10.1111/0022-4537.00118

Timmons, B.W., Bar-Or, O., & Riddell, M.C. (2003). Oxidation rate of exogenous carbohydrate during exercise is higher in boys than in men. *J Appl Physiol (1985), 94*(1), 278–284. doi: 10.1152/japplphysiol.00140.2002

Timmons, B.W., Bar-Or, O., & Riddell, M.C. (2007a). Energy substrate utilization during prolonged exercise with and without carbohydrate intake in preadolescent and adolescent girls. *J Appl Physiol (1985), 103*(3), 995–1000. doi: 10.1152/japplphysiol.00018.2007

Timmons, B.W., Bar-Or, O., & Riddell, M.C. (2007b). Influence of age and pubertal status on substrate utilization during exercise with and without carbohydrate intake in healthy boys. *Appl Physiol Nutr Metab, 32*(3), 416–425. doi: 10.1139/H07-004

Torstveit, M.K., Rosenvinge, J.H., & Sundgot-Borgen, J. (2008). Prevalence of eating disorders and the predictive power of risk models in female elite athletes: a controlled study. *Scand J Med Sci Sports, 18*(1), 108–118. doi: 10.1111/j.1600-0838.2007.00657.x

Ueda, S.Y., Yoshikawa, T., Katsura, Y., Usui, T., Nakao, H., & Fujimoto, S. (2009). Changes in gut hormone levels and negative energy balance during aerobic exercise in obese young males. *J Endocrinol, 201*(1), 151–159. doi: JOE-08-0500 [pii]10.1677/JOE-08-0500

Vogt, M., Puntschart, A., Howald, H., Mueller, B., Mannhart, C., Gfeller-Tuescher, L., . . . Hoppeler, H. (2003). Effects of dietary fat on muscle substrates, metabolism, and performance in athletes. *Med Sci Sports Exerc, 35*(6), 952–960. doi: 10.1249/01.MSS.0000069336.30649.BD

Volek, J.S. (2004). Influence of nutrition on responses to resistance training. *Med Sci Sports Exerc, 36*(4), 689–696.

Wade, T.D., Bergin, J.L., Martin, N.G., Gillespie, N.A., & Fairburn, C.G. (2006). A transdiagnostic approach to understanding eating disorders. *J Nerv Ment Dis, 194*(7), 510–517. doi: 10.1097/01.nmd.0000225067.42191.b0

Washburn, R.A., Lambourne, K., Szabo, A.N., Herrmann, S.D., Honas, J.J., & Donnelly, J.E. (2014). Does increased prescribed exercise alter non-exercise physical activity/energy expenditure in healthy adults? A systematic review. *Clin Obes, 4*(1), 1–20. doi: 10.1111/cob.12040

Wasse, L.K., King, J.A., Stensel, D.J., & Sunderland, C. (2013). Effect of ambient temperature during acute aerobic exercise on short-term appetite, energy intake, and plasma acylated ghrelin in recreationally active males. *Appl Physiol Nutr Metab, 38*(8), 905–909. doi: 10.1139/apnm-2013-0008

Wasse, L.K., Sunderland, C., King, J.A., Batterham, R.L., & Stensel, D.J. (2012). Influence of rest and exercise at a simulated altitude of 4,000 m on appetite, energy intake, and plasma concentrations of acylated ghrelin and peptide YY. *J Appl Physiol, 112*(4), 552–559. doi: 10.1152/japplphysiol.00090.2011

Wasse, L.K., Sunderland, C., King, J.A., Miyashita, M., & Stensel, D.J. (2013). The influence of vigorous running and cycling exercise on hunger perceptions and plasma acylated ghrelin concentrations in lean young men. *Appl Physiol Nutr Metab, 38*(1), 1–6. doi: 10.1139/apnm-2012-0154

Werle, C.O., Wansink, B., & Payne, C.R. (2011). Just thinking about exercise makes me serve more food. Physical activity and calorie compensation. *Appetite, 56*(2), 332–335. doi: 10.1016/j.appet.2010.12.016

Whybrow, S., Hughes, D.A., Ritz, P., Johnstone, A.M., Horgan, G.W., King, N., . . . Stubbs, R.J. (2008). The effect of an incremental increase in exercise on appetite, eating behaviour and energy balance in lean men and women feeding ad libitum. *Br J Nutr, 100*(5), 1109–1115. doi: 10.1017/S0007114508968240

Williams, N.I., Helmreich, D.L., Parfitt, D.B., Caston-Balderrama, A., & Cameron, J.L. (2001). Evidence for a causal role of low energy availability in the induction of menstrual cycle disturbances during strenuous exercise training. *The Journal of Clinical Endocrinology & Metabolism, 86*(11), 5184–5193. doi: 10.1210/jcem.86.11.8024.

13 Biochemistry and physical activity

Angus Lindsay and Chris Chamberlain

Keywords: Immune system, metabolism, mitochondria, oxidative stress, signalling

Introduction

Biochemistry is a term given to the study and understanding of chemical properties and processes of biological systems. Physical activity can be described as the utilization of energy that results in the movement of the body. In a symbiotic partnership, physical activity relies on multiple biochemical reactions and pathways at the cellular and molecular level which results in the contraction and relaxation of skeletal and cardiac muscle and the subsequent displacement of the skeleton.

Absolute volume, nature and alterations in a person's physical activity can result in biochemical perturbations that have resonating effects on several physiological pathways. Whether a dramatic or gradual change in activity levels occurs, the downstream effect on protein modifications, metabolism, signaling cascades, immune system function and the hormonal response can directly affect both the acute and long-term health of an individual. Understanding some of these crucial biochemical reactions to physical activity can help monitor and regulate a person's response and ultimately build and develop a suitable approach for sustaining activity and health.

This chapter will focus specifically on the type of physical activity or inactivity on key biochemical processes involved in adaptation with a particular emphasis on selectively chosen cellular and molecular regulatory processes. The reader should develop an understanding for the adaptive changes associated with varying types of physical activity including endurance, high intensity, resistance and inactivity.

Physical activity and immune system function

Immunity is composed of two separate and yet intertwined systems (innate and adaptive/acquired) whose primary objective is to protect the host from a foreign organism. Innate immunity is the non-specific first line of defense against an antigen that becomes activated immediately or within a few hours of detection. Composed primarily of immune cells that are recruited to sites of infection through a complex series of cytokine molecules, it works in tandem with specialized white blood cells, the complement system and interferons to provide a direct barrier of resistance. Adaptive immunity however, becomes activated through a process known as antigen presentation; a process whereby antigen presenting cells display the antigen through a major histocompatibility complex allowing T-cell recognition, destruction and development of a specific immune response. The key players involved in these processes are all susceptible to alterations in physical activity which can lead to either an enhanced or severely compromised immune system, the result of which can cause a person to lose the ability to ward-off, fight or recover from an infection or challenge.

The effect of intensity

Physical activity-induced immune function perturbations were first observed in 1902 by Larrabee (Larrabee, 1902). Since the discovery of leukocytosis in response to a marathon, there has been a dearth of research examining changes in immune system function. It soon became apparent that alterations in immune cells, antibodies and antimicrobial peptides were intensity and duration dependent whilst a lack of physical activity resulted in immune-suppression or compromisation. In response to these observations, Nieman (1994) developed the J-curve; a representation of risk of infection based on exercise intensity (Figure 13.1). It was evident that moderate-intensity workloads provided an individual with a heightened immune system whilst individuals who completed either low or high workloads were more susceptible to infection. In conjunction with this observation, a secondary theory known as the "open-window" was developed (Hoffman-Goetz & Pedersen, 1994; Pedersen & Ullum, 1994); a short-term suppression (3–24 hours (Kakanis et al., 2010; Pereira et al., 2012)) of immune system function following an acute bout of exercise. The theory identifies a window of opportunity to upper respiratory infections where the immune system has become temporarily compromised. An alternative version of this theory is called the S-curve. Developed by Malm (2006), it postulates that those individuals who are of an elite status possess an immune system that is capable of withstanding infections during severe and physiological and psychological stress.

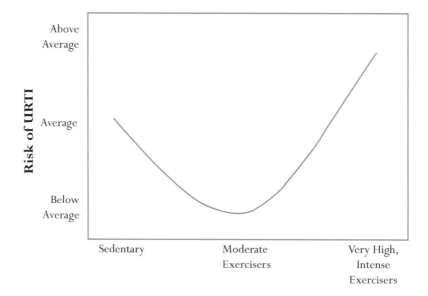

Figure 13.1 J-curve highlighting the risk of infection based on exercise intensity

Table 13.1 The most common immune system components measured in response to physical activity and their response to varying degrees of physical stress

Immune component	Function	Response to physical activity
Neutrophil	The most abundant mammalian leukocyte responsible for phagocytic resolution of a foreign pathogen during the acute stage of inflammation	↓ concentration in obese sedentary women performing regular exercise (Radom-Aizik, Zaldivar, Oliver, Galassetti, & Cooper, 2010) ↑ concentration up to 2 hours post maximum-intensity exercise (Quindry, Stone, King, & Broeder, 2003)
Macrophages	A mononuclear phagocytic leukocyte responsible for destruction of "non-self" debris, microbes and pathogens during both innate and adaptive immunity (M1 – killer). They also play a critical role in anti-inflammatory pathways encouraging tissue repair (M2 – repair)	↓ infiltration in response to regular exercise in severely obese individuals (Bruun, Helge, Richelsen, & Stallknecht, 2006) ↓ anti-inflammatory polarization following 12 weeks of resistance training (Gordon et al., 2012)
Natural Killer cells	A cytotoxic lymphocyte capable of recognizing and destroying "stressed" cells as part of the innate immune response	↓ concentration and cytotoxic activity up to 2 hours following high-intensity exercise (D.C. Nieman et al., 1993) ↑ cell activity in individuals reporting a healthy lifestyle including physical activity (Kusaka, Kondou, & Morimoto, 1992)
Helper T-cells	Lymphocytes ($CD4^+$) that provide immune assistance through rapid division and cytokine secretion following recognition of peptide antigens on the surface of antigen-presenting cells	↑ circulating T-cell function and cytokine production in habitual endurance exercisers (Shinkai et al., 1995) ↓ concentration following an acute intense 5km endurance event (Espersen et al., 1990)
Cytotoxic T-cells	Lymphocytes ($CD8^+$) that destroy virus-infected cells through recognition of major histocompatibility complex I antigen presentation during infection	↑ subset mobilization immediately following 85% intensity exercise (Campbell et al., 2009) ↑ in migration and apoptotic function following resistance exercise (Pereira et al., 2012)
B-cells	Differentiated into plasma and memory cells, B-cells are a type of antibody producing lymphocyte important in adaptive immunity	No change following moderate exercise training in sedentary obese women or long-term intense swimming training (Gleeson et al., 1995; Nehlsen-Cannarella et al., 1991) ↓ concentration during an incremental cycling test in both active and sedentary individuals (Moyna et al., 1996)
Immunoglobulins	Antibodies produced primarily by plasma cells that are utilized for the detection and destruction/neutralization of foreign pathogens	↓ following high-intensity team sport (Lindsay et al., 2015) ↑ following moderate daily physical activity (Shimizu et al., 2007)
Antimicrobial peptides	Small molecular weight proteins with a broad anti-microbial spectrum capable of mediating processes involved in adaptive immunity	↑ serum lactoferrin concentrations following moderate and high-intensity running exercise (Inoue, Sakai, Kaida, & Kaibara, 2004) ↑ salivary lysozyme secretion rate following short high-intensity exercise (Allgrove, Gomes, Hough, & Gleeson, 2008)

Interpretation of these theories needs to consider confounding factors that include previous infections, various stressors other than physical activity, pathogen exposure, diet and sleep among others. Furthermore, program design or implementation of an exercise program for recreational/athletes and sedentary individuals, respectively, should consider the consequence of intensity and the resulting immune-suppression and risk of infection associated.

Effect on immune cell modulation

Humoral (cell-independent) and cell-mediated immunity provide protection against infection which can be directly affected through changes in physical activity. They are comprised of multiple components with specific functions regulating antigen effectiveness; however the immune system and physical activity literature has focused primarily on a select few of these which will be the emphasis of this section. Table 13.1 provides a description of the most commonly measured immune system parameters in response to physical activity and how their concentration and function are affected.

Sedentary individuals or individuals who do not regularly exercise may suffer from a weakened immune system compared to those who complete regular physical activity. This has been established by a number of studies identifying a 29% risk reduction of upper respiratory tract infections (URTI) following two hours of moderate exercise compared to a sedentary lifestyle (Matthews et al., 2002), a reduced risk of self-reported respiratory symptoms when completing moderate-intensity exercise (Kostka, Berthouze, Lacour, & Bonnefoy, 2000; Wong et al., 2008), and a reduced number of days with a URTI in active people compared to sedentary controls (David C. Nieman, Henson, Austin, & Sha, 2011). However, competing in ultra-endurance (high-intensity) based events can cause a 100–500% increase in the risk of infection in the weeks following (D. Nieman, Johanssen, Lee, & Arabatzis, 1990; E. Peters, Goetzsche, Joseph, & Noakes, 1996; E. M. Peters, Goetzsche, Grobbelaar, & Noakes, 1993; E. M. Peters, Shaik, & Kleinveldt, 2010). This can equate to as much as 47% of competitors experiencing a URTI (Robson-Ansley et al., 2012), while intense exercise before or during an infection has been associated with greater morbidity and mortality (Ekblom, Ekblom, & Malm, 2006; Heath et al., 1991).

The change in risk of infection can be attributed in part to alterations in both the concentration and function of the humoral and cell-mediated responses. These responses range from apoptotic and phagocytic ability, sensitivity to chemotaxis and migratory capability, proliferative capacity, response to challenges (PHA and PMA), and generation of cell-specific molecules and proteins for targeted degradation and identification of antigens for host defense. The degree of change is directly associated with the type of physical activity.

Effect of intensity

Physical inactivity and lower exercise workloads have been predominantly associated with a detrimentally affected cell-mediated response including neutrophils, macrophages, natural killer cells (NKCs), T-cells and B-cells. Infiltration is a commonality among the sedentary population (Bruun, Helge, Richelsen, & Stallknecht, 2006; Radom-Aizik, Zaldivar, Oliver, Galassetti, & Cooper, 2010), however absolute concentration, phagocytic function, adherence capacity, chemotaxis and microbicide capacity all increase following exercise of sedentary men and women (Giraldo, Garcia, Hinchado, & Ortega, 2009; LaPerriere et al., 1994; E. Ortega, Barriga, & De la Fuente, 1993; E. Ortega, Collazos, Maynar, Barriga, & De la Fuente,

1993; Rhind, Shek, Shinkai, & Shephard, 1996; Rodriguez, Barriga, & De la Fuente, 1991). Whilst some have identified no difference in the response of monocytes, lymphocytes and NKC cells to exercise between trained and sedentary populations (Brahmi, Thomas, Park, Park, & Dowdeswell, 1985; Moyna et al., 1996), others have observed a decrease in the number of apoptotic lymphocytes based on the training status of an individual (Mooren, Lechtermann, & Lker, 2004). Nonetheless, the ability of a sedentary individual to fight an infection through a cascade of immune and antibody related mechanisms may be diminished compared to someone who engages in regular moderate-intensity exercise (Martin, Pence, & Woods, 2009; Spence et al., 2007). More specifically, animal studies have identified a reduction in mortality of those that complete moderate-intensity exercise compared to sedentary or prolonged protocols when exposed to influenza (Lowder, Padgett, & Woods, 2005).

Since the development of the J-curve and associated theories, moderate-intensity exercise has been the focus of studies monitoring immune system function. Improvement in natural killer cell activity in sedentary women undergoing a moderate endurance training program (D. Nieman, Nehlsen-Cannarella, et al., 1990), un-altered oxidative burst activity of neutrophils and phagocytic function of monocytes and neutrophils (Scharhag et al., 2005), reduced circulating leukocyte senescence (Werner et al., 2009), differentiation of naïve T cells (Drela, Kozdron, & Szczypiorski, 2004; Zhao, Zhou, Davie, & Su, 2012), a reduction in inflammatory biomarkers (Okita et al., 2004) and an un-altered caspase-8–9 activation and DNA fragmentation of lymphocytes compared to a high intensity group (Wang & Huang, 2005) are but a few examples of the beneficial effect of regular moderate-intensity exercise on cell-mediated immunity. Most importantly, this type of exercise can reduce the incidence of URTIs by as much as three-fold in previously sedentary obese women (Chubak et al., 2006).

Of course at the opposite end of sedentary activity is high-intensity exercise. Curiously however, athletes and individuals who complete this type of regular activity are just as likely to suffer from immune-suppression. Lower neutrophil oxidative burst activity in elite swimmers (D. B. Pyne et al., 1995) and following intense up-hill running (D.B. Pyne, Smith, Baker, Telford, & Weidemann, 2000) is in accordance with DNA fragmentation and phosphatidylserine externalization following an ironman (Levada-Pires et al., 2008) and reduced phagocytic capacity following sustained endurance training (Blannin, Chatwin, Cave, & Gleeson, 1996). Total lymphocyte numbers have also been shown to reduce following a 5km run (Espersen et al., 1990) which is corroborated by Nielsen (2003) who identified NKC and B-cell suppression following intense exercise. Most interesting is the observation following 80% VO_2 max exercise in comparison to 60% where the level of apoptotic lymphocytes becomes elevated (Mooren, Blöming, Lechtermann, Lerch, & Völker, 2002) along with granulocyte calcium un-coupling in response to exhaustive exercise (Mooren et al., 2001). In accordance with apoptotic lymphocytes, high-intensity exercise can also diminish the mitochondrial membrane potential of leukocytes which increases their propensity to become apoptotic (Tuan et al., 2008). Resistance training has also been shown to cause an increase in the apoptosis and migration of $CD4^+$ and $CD8^+$ lymphocytes for up to 24 hours (Pereira et al., 2012), alongside a decrease in their circulating concentration (Cardoso et al., 2012).

Like cell-mediated immunity, humoral immunity is also differentially affected by physical activity. With up to 90% of all infections occurring in the mucosae in regard to microbial colonization and entry into the body (Brandtzaeg, 2003), the majority of illnesses associated with physical activity are based around URTIs. It is therefore pertinent to understand the effect of physical activity on changes in mucosae immune system components to establish a link between their perturbations and infection.

Immunoglobulins (Ig) can be separated into five distinct subsets, IgA, IgE, IgG, IgM and IgD. Salivary immunoglobulin A (IgA) is produced by plasma cells (differentiated B lymphocytes) adjacent to ducts and acini of the salivary gland (Korsrud & Brandtzaeg, 1980), whose transport (bound to its secretory component that provides protection against proteolytic degradation (Crottet & Corthésy, 1998)) and function (first line of defense against microbial infection) across the epithelium can occur in three potential ways:

- prevention of pathogen adherence and penetration of the mucosal epithelium
- neutralization of viruses within the epithelial cells during transcytosis
- excretion of locally formed immune complexes across mucosal epithelial cells to the luminal surface (Lamm, 1998).

Modifications in salivary IgA function or capacity to defend can result directly increase susceptibility to clinical and sub-clinical infection.

The effect of exercise on markers of mucosal immunity has been extensively reviewed (Bishop & Gleeson, 2009). In accordance with the aforementioned J-curve, sIgA shows a similar trend with respect to exercise intensity. Salivary immunoglobulin A is unquestionably exercise intensity dependent, with moderate-intensity protocols failing to elicit any significant post-exercise changes (Bratthall & Widerstrom, 1985; McDowell, Chaloa, Housh, Tharp, & Johnson, 1991; Tharp, 1991; N. Walsh, 1999). Similar studies have also identified no change in sIgA following an elite soccer match (Thorpe & Sunderland, 2012), intensive tennis training (Gomes et al., 2013), a collegiate rugby game (Koch et al., 2007), jiu-jitsu matches (Moreira et al., 2012) or resistance exercise (Carlson, Kenefick, & Koch, 2013; Roschel et al., 2011). The sedentary population may also be in an immune-compromised state given that sIgA is lower than moderately trained individuals but similar to those of elite athletes (Saygin et al., 2006).

Meanwhile, there are several studies that have identified immediate post-exercise decreases in sIgA. Ultra-endurance events are considered one of the most physiologically demanding in the world that results in an immediate post-exercise suppression (Gill et al., 2014; Henson et al., 2008; Pedro Tauler, Martinez, Moreno, Martínez, & Aguilo, 2013). Similarly, cycling for two hours at 70% $\dot{V}O_2$ max (N. P. Walsh, Bishop, Blackwell, Wierzbicki, & Montague, 2002), cross country skiing for 50 km (Tomasi, Trudeau, Czerwinski, & Erredge, 1982), supra-maximal cycling (MacKinnon & Jenkins, 1993), competing in a triathlon (Steerenberg et al., 1997) and a professional rugby game (Lindsay et al., 2015) all cause the athlete or subject to become immune-compromised.

Salivary immunoglobulin A monitoring may also be useful in determining the risk of infection (Pedersen & Nieman, 1998; D. Pyne & Gleeson, 1998) and excessive training in athletes (Mackinnon & Hooper, 1994; Shephard & Shek, 1998). Decreased levels of sIgA have been associated with stale, underperforming and over-trained athletes (Budgett, 1998; Foster, 1998; Gleeson et al., 1999). In a swimming study, significant decreases in sIgA during six months of training were observed (Kormanovski, Ibarra, Padilla, & Rodriguez, 2010) which is similar to that previously noted (Gleeson et al., 2000; Gleeson et al., 1999). Elite kayakers have also shown a 27–38% decrease in sIgA secretion rate after each session of training over three weeks (Traeger Mackinnon, Ginn, & Seymour, 1993). While sIgA may provide some insight into potential over-training and reaching and risk of infection, it seems to be biased regarding the type of exercise and the individuals involved.

Another major subset of mucosal compounds include the antimicrobial peptides; lactoferrin, lysozyme, β-defensin-2 and cathelicidin which directly bind free iron resulting in loss of foreign cell membrane potential, hydrolysis of specific linkages of the bacterial cell wall inducing damage, antibiotic properties that are regulated during inflammation, and leukocyte/epithelial cell secretion, respectively. For an extensive review of anti-microbial compounds and the exercise effect, please see West et al. (2006).

In contrast to the majority of research presented, lactoferrin and lysozyme may show a variation in response to physical activity intensity. To begin, it is well established that exercise can cause transient increases and decreases in their salivary concentrations (Gillum et al., 2015; He, Tsai, Ko, Chang, & Fang, 2010; Tsai, Chou, Chang, & Fang, 2011; N. West et al., 2010) with increased and decreased risk of infection and incidence of a URTI (Papacosta & Nassis, 2011); however the concentrations between elite athletes and sedentary controls may not differ (N. West et al., 2010). In fact, concentrations of β-defensin-2 and cathelicidin are higher in sedentary controls than elite marathon runners which correlates with reduced incidence of URTIs (Usui et al., 2012). The same two molecules have also been shown to increase in response to strenuous exercise suggesting an increase in immunity (Usui et al., 2011). It is evident that some salivary antimicrobial compounds may react differently to exercise and training status.

Physical activity and oxidative status

Antioxidants are forever being branded as a beneficial supplement for the sedentary and athlete population. Available both man-made and naturally produced, antioxidants provide cellular protection through an oxidant/radical dependent scavenging action that prevents damage to essential cellular components including DNA, membrane lipids and proteins; the result of which can cause mutation, increased cellular repair (increased metabolic demand), loss of membrane integrity, formation of reactive intermediates and signaling lipids, and loss of enzyme activity, structure and receptor function. Lack of physical activity or acute or chronic exposure can result in maintaining or severely dismantling the balance between molecules that induce oxidative damage and the antioxidants designed for protection. This balance is often referred to as hormesis (Figure 13.2), a dose-response relationship characterized by opposing effects at low and high doses resulting in either a J-shaped or an inverted U-shaped dose-response (Calabrese & Baldwin, 2001, 2002; Kendig, Le, & Belcher, 2010). This has become extended to free radicals and physical exercise with the modulation controlled through exercise and ageing (Radak, Chung, & Goto, 2005, Radak, Chung, Koltai, Taylor, & Goto, 2008). This section will compare the relationship between oxidative stress and the antioxidant defence system and how alterations in physical activity can result in hormesis-dependent changes.

What is oxidative status?

A free-radical is any molecule or atom that is very stable but exceedingly reactive with one or more unpaired electrons. These radicals can be generated as products of homolytic, heterolytic or redox reactions, producing either charged or uncharged radical species (Powers, Ji, Kavazis, & Jackson, 2011) which strive to fill their outer shell with an extra electron by pilfering from a cellular structure. Consequently, this induces both damage and a cascade of detrimental reactions along with the potential generation of another radical. Reactive oxygen species (ROS) and reactive nitrogen species (RNS) also possess the capability of inducing significant cellular damage that requires consistent antioxidant monitoring.

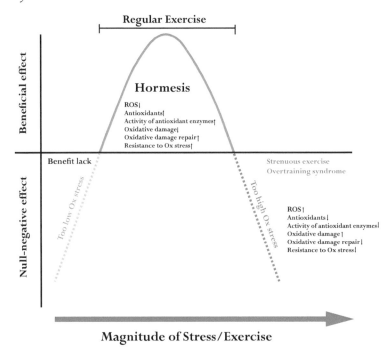

Figure 13.2 The effect of exercise on oxidative status

An antioxidant is a chemical species whose reaction rate with a free radical will out-compete the reaction of the free radical with a bio-molecule. Whether it is the endogenous antioxidant enzymes like catalase or superoxide dismutase, or the endogenous/exogenous antioxidants like urate/uric acid, glutathione and Vitamins A, C and E, antioxidants neutralize free-radical/ROS/RNS as well as repair and replace damaged molecules.

Oxygen dependent metabolism and cell function

An organism relies on oxygen to drive metabolic processes through the ATP generating electron transport chain complexes of the mitochondria and NADPH oxidases. It has been discovered that 0.1% of all the electrons in Complex I and Coenzyme Q are lost as superoxide when electrons leak through side chain reactions onto molecular oxygen (Brand, 2010) in conjunction with hydrogen peroxide generation through complex IV (Grivennikova & Vinogradov, 2006). These reactions are significantly accelerated when exercise increases the metabolic, mechanical and psychological demand for energy through increased skeletal and cardiac muscle contraction and increased respiration. This in turn up-regulates the production of oxygen-centered radicals and ROS which can provide both beneficial and detrimental effects. Whilst the majority of people would consider free radicals as destructive molecules, they are pertinent to several biological reactions including mitochondrial biogenesis (Joseph, Pilegaard, Litvintsev, Leick, & Hood, 2006), antioxidant defense system up-regulation (Leeuwenburgh & Heinecke, 2001), glucose uptake and insulin sensitivity (Henriksen,

Diamond-Stanic, & Marchionne, 2011), regulation of cell differentiation and growth (Rigou-let, Yoboue, & Devin, 2011), skeletal muscle contractility (Reid, Khawli, & Moody, 1993) and gene regulation (Hemmrich, Suschek, Lerzynski, & Kolb-Bachofen, 2003). The production of the metabolically-induced ROS, radicals and immune cell oxidants however, can shift the balance of hormesis resulting in damage to crucial cellular components; one of which can be oxidative damage of the sarcoplasmic ryanodine receptors responsible for calcium release during muscle contraction (Cherednichenko et al., 2004). Similar to the J-curve concept discussed in the previous section, regular exercise maintains a healthy balance between the oxidant and antioxidant systems which allows for adaptive processes to develop; the predom-inant reason for exercise.

Effect of exercise intensity

A sedentary lifestyle can influence two separate oxygen dependent pathways. According to the hormesis theory, lack of physical activity cannot drive the necessary adaptations required for a capable antioxidant defense should the challenge arise. Similarly, physical inactivity is linked to an overwhelming dearth of health-related diseases including atherosclerosis, Alzheimer's, type 2 diabetes, Parkinson's, obesity and certain cancer types (Booth & Lees, 2007; Radak, Chung, & Goto, 2008) that may be associated with an oxidative stress and endothelial dysfunction depen-dent mechanism (Laufs et al., 2005). Furthermore, physical inactivity is related to infiltration and greater abundance of phagocytic immune cells (see above, section 1) that possess a respira-tory burst activity (superoxide and protease generation) capable of inducing secondary damage to surrounding tissues. The magnitude and overwhelming evidence suggests physical inactivity is extremely detrimental to one's health with respect to oxidant/antioxidant hormesis; however what effect does moderate and intense exercise do to the balance of this relationship?

Moderate-intensity exercise has the capacity to up-regulate genes responsible for various antioxidant enzymes (Gomez-Cabrera, Domenech, & Viña, 2008). Specifically, swimming training in children (Gonenc, Acikgoz, Semin, & Ozgonul, 2000), 50% $\dot{V}O_2$ max cycling (Goto et al., 2003) and regular moderate physical exercise in adolescents (Santos-Silva et al., 2001) reduces oxidative stress and potential atherosclerotic tissue generation. Regular physical activity can also reduce type 2 diabetes incidence through antioxidant and anti-inflammatory pathways (Teixeira de Lemos, Oliveira, Páscoa Pinheiro, & Reis, 2012), and induce an anti-atherogenic and anti-hypertensive environment through modulation of nitric oxide bioavailability (Goto et al., 2007; Higashi & Yoshizumi, 2004); however, not all moderate-intensity exercise has the capacity to alter the oxidant-antioxidant status (P. Tauler, Gimeno, Aguilo, Guix, & Pons, 1999; Tiidus, Pushkarenko, & Houston, 1996).

There is also overwhelming murine research indicating exercise of a moderate intensity provides significant adaptations. These include enhancing nuclear erythroid 2 p45-related fac-tor 2 (Nrf2) function (Gounder et al., 2012), extending life duration through a reduction in protein carbonyls, thiobarbituric acid-reactive substances contents of the submitochondrial membranes and increasing antioxidant enzyme activities (Navarro, Gomez, López-Cepero, & Boveris, 2004), and reducing caspase-3 and -8 whilst simultaneously increasing superoxide dismutase activity in diabetic mice (Ghosh et al., 2009).

High-intensity exercise meanwhile can result in equivocal biochemical changes. Com-pleting a cycling stage for example can increase plasma antioxidant activities (Aguiló et al., 2005) and induce cellular lymphocyte adaptations (Cases et al., 2006), whilst high-intensity endurance training can elevate antioxidant enzyme activities in erythrocytes, and decrease neutrophil $O_2^{\cdot-}$ production (Miyazaki et al., 2001). In contrast, acute and chronic high-intensity exercise can overwhelm the antioxidant defence system (J. E. Turner et al., 2013) resulting in substantial oxidative stress (Knez, Coombes, & Jenkins, 2006; Mastaloudis, Leonard, & Traber, 2001; J. Turner, Hodges, Bosch, & Aldred, 2011), DNA damage (Hartmann et al., 1998; Miyata et al., 2008; Niess et al., 1998; Wagner, Reichhold, & Neubauer, 2011), platelet aggregation (Tozzi-Ciancarelli, Penco, & Di Massimo, 2002), increased red blood cell removal associated with premature aging (Santos-Silva et al., 2001), metabolic dysfunction (Fehrenbach & Northoff, 2000) and inducement of autophagy-related and autophagy-regulatory genes (Jamart et al., 2012) that may be gender-specific (Ginsburg, O'Toole, Rimm, Douglas, & Rifai, 2001).

Muscle function is also dramatically affected through oxidative stress hormesis. Altering the mitochondrial antioxidant enzyme profile can reduce calcium-induced muscle myopathies during aging (Umanskaya et al., 2014) whilst the level of free radicals/ROS can have both positive and negative effects on muscle function. These range from alterations in muscle cell signaling, mitochondrial biogenesis genes (PGC1α), fiber type switching, force production and hypertrophy for which the readers are directed to a series of comprehensive reviews (Barbieri & Sestili, 2011; Powers, Duarte, Kavazis, & Talbert, 2010; Powers & Jackson, 2008; Powers et al., 2011; Steinbacher & Eckl, 2015).

Physical activity and metabolism

Carbohydrates and lipids comprise the major fuel source for exercising muscle. The average person with a body composition of 10–30% fat contains enough energy stored in lipids to walk a distance of ~800–2400 km (E. F. Coyle, 1995). However, fat cannot be oxidized at a fast enough rate to accommodate the energy demands of moderate to intensely exercising muscle (E. F. Coyle, Coggan, Hemmert, & Ivy, 1986). Therefore, in order to meet the energy demands of muscle exercising at varying levels of intensity, the human body has adapted a highly regulated, yet highly flexible network of metabolic responses. In this section, we will discuss the metabolic changes associated with muscle exercising at varying levels of intensity and also describe the effects of exercise on mitochondrial function.

There are four major sources of energy for exercising muscle: 1) blood glucose, 2) muscle glycogen, 3) plasma free fatty acids, and 4) intramuscular triglycerides (Flatt, 1995). The relative utilization of each energy source is linked to exercise intensity (Brooks & Mercier, 1994; E. F. Coyle, 1995). During low-intensity exercise (i.e. walking) the vast majority of energy is derived from plasma fatty acids, with a minor contribution from blood glucose (Ahlborg, Felig, Hagenfeldt, Hendler, & Wahren, 1974; Romijn et al., 1993). However, when exercise is increased to moderate intensity (i.e. jogging), the substrate utilization profile shifts dramatically. During moderate exercise, carbohydrate (blood glucose and muscle glycogen) and lipid (plasma fatty acids and intramuscular triglycerides) metabolism each account for ~50% of energy production (Romijn et al., 1993). However, after two hours of moderate-intensity exercise, muscle glycogen stores become depleted and the contribution from blood glucose levels becomes more important. For this reason, carbohydrate ingestion is necessary after ~2 hrs of moderate-intensity exercise in order to maintain blood glucose levels and avoid fatigue (Coggan & Coyle, 1989; E. Coyle et al., 1983). Carbohydrate metabolism is even more important during high-intensity exercise where it accounts for ~2/3 of energy utilization (Katz, Broberg, Sahlin, & Wahren, 1986; Romijn et al., 1993; Wahren, Felig, Ahlborg, & Jorfeldt, 1971).

While lipid metabolism is more prominent during low-intensity exercise, carbohydrate (glucose and glycogen) metabolism becomes increasingly important with greater exercise intensity. To accommodate carbohydrate demand, three critical steps are regulated during exercise: 1) glucose delivery to muscle, 2) glucose transport into muscle, and 3) glucose metabolism within working muscle (Sylow, Kleinert, Richter, & Jensen, 2016). First, glucose delivery is increased during bouts of moderate to intense exercise through a rise in blood flow (Joyner & Casey, 2015). This is accomplished through signaling by molecules that are released by exercising muscle such as nitric oxide. Coupled with increased delivery of glucose to contracting muscle is an increase in muscle permeability to circulating glucose (Jensen & Richter, 2012). This is accomplished by translocation of a highly conserved glucose transporter (GLUT4) into the muscle plasma membrane and T-tubules (Jessen & Goodyear, 2005; Rose & Richter, 2005). GLUT4 mediates transport of circulating glucose into exercising muscle fibers. Lastly, the regulation of glucose and glycogen metabolism in exercising muscle is a tightly regulated process. At the onset of exercise, muscle preferentially utilizes glycogen stores to accommodate energy demand (E. F. Coyle et al., 1986; Romijn et al., 1993). Glycogenolysis is regulated by the enzyme glycogen phosphorylase (Roach, Depaoli-Roach, Hurley, & Tagliabracci, 2012). Breakdown of glycogen increases intracellular concentrations of glucose-6-phosphate, which impairs activity of the enzyme hexokinase (Katz, Sahlin, & Broberg, 1991; Kristiansen, Hargreaves, & Richter, 1997). Since hexokinase is responsible for initiating glucose metabolism, its impairment causes diminished glucose metabolism during the early stages of exercise. Following extended bouts of exercise, muscle glycogen stores become depleted. This results in diminished glucose-6-phosphate levels, re-activation of hexokinase enzyme activity, and stimulates the utilization of circulating glucose (Sylow et al., 2016).

Ultimately, the critical hub of energy production during muscle contraction is the mitochondrion. This organelle houses the protein complexes of the electron transport chain that are required for ATP production, as well as the tricarboxylic acid cycle which is essential for producing the reducing equivalents NADH and $FADH^2$ that feed into the electron transport chain. While the mitochondrion is essential for producing the energy used during muscle contraction, it is also highly regulated by the downstream consequences of muscle activity. Muscle contraction induces several metabolic changes that stimulate mitochondria biogenesis. Increases in AMP/ATP and NAD^+/NADH ratios stimulate key signaling cascades involving AMPK and SIRT1 that then modify factors such as PGCα to stimulate mitochondrial biogenesis (Hawley, Hargreaves, & Zierath, 2006; Hood, Tryon, Carter, Kim, & Chen, 2016). Through this mechanism, exercise training stimulates an increase in muscle mitochondrial content that then increases overall exercise capacity. Mitochondrial function is also impacted as exercise induces an upregulation of the enzymes involved in fatty acid oxidation and the electron transport chain (Lundby & Jacobs, 2016).

In summary, substrate utilization by muscle is dependent upon exercise intensity. Whereas lipids are the predominant fuel for low-intensity exercise, carbohydrate metabolism is more important during moderate to intense exercise. Additionally, the metabolic consequences of muscle contraction including altered AMP/ATP and NAD^+/NADH ratios stimulate an increase in mitochondrial function and biogenesis that ultimately improves overall muscle function.

Physical activity and protein modulation

Seminal work by Holloszy demonstrated that muscles from treadmill-trained rats expressed higher mitochondrial protein content than from untrained rats (Holloszy, 1967).

This and much work since supports the general idea that muscle is adaptive to exercise. At a biochemical level, the mechanism of this adaptive response involves the conversion of electrical, mechanical, and chemical consequences of muscle contraction into cellular signals that impact various cellular processes thus changing the underlying characteristics of muscle.

The signals that stimulate downstream cellular pathways involved in muscle adaptation include increased intracellular Ca^{2+}, reactive oxygen species, AMP, ADP, and fatty acids as well as decreased levels of creatine phosphate and glycogen (Hawley et al., 2006). Altered ratios of NAD^+:NADH and aberrant redox conditions have also been implicated. While this list is certainly not exhaustive, and more signaling molecules will certainly be identified, it is clear that the molecules involved in muscle adaptive signaling are many and varied.

The story becomes even more complex when we begin to dissect the various signaling pathways that become activated in response to the contraction-induced changes (described above). Exercise is known to activate a variety of signaling cascades including Ca^{2+}/calmodulin dependent protein kinase (CamK), calcineurin, mitogen-activated protein kinases (MAPK), AMP-activated protein kinase (AMPK), and mammalian target of rapamycin (mTOR) (Fujii et al., 2000; Rose & Hargreaves, 2003; Widegren et al., 1998; Winder & Hardie, 1996). Activation of these pathways is mediated by direct modulation of proteins within the cascade. Ultimately, these pathways impact regulation of genes involved in various aspects of muscle function (Hawley, Hargreaves, Joyner, & Zierath, 2014).

While a detailed accounting of the varied cellular consequences of exercise-induced signaling cascades is beyond the scope of this chapter, one highly studied factor in this response is peroxisome proliferator-activated receptor γ coactivator 1α (PGC1α), which has emerged as a key regulator of mitochondrial biogenesis in response to repeated bouts of exercise. PGC1α is regulated by both AMPK and p38 MAPK signaling pathways. Importantly, both pathways result in the direct phosphorylation and activation of PGC1α (Jäger, Handschin, Pierre, & Spiegelman, 2007; Puigserver et al., 2001). Additionally, AMPK phosphorylates the transcriptional repressor HDAC5, which relieves inhibition of MEF2, a known transcriptional activator of PGC1α (McGee & Hargreaves, 2010). p38 MAPK phosphorylates ATF-2, which is a transcriptional activator of PGC1α (Akimoto et al., 2005). Therefore, PGC1α protein activity is directly stimulated via phosphorylation by both pathways, and transcription of PGC1α transcript is also activated by both pathways. PGC1α then induces expression of key mitochondria proteins encoded by both nuclear and mitochondrial encoded genes which stimulates mitochondrial biogenesis and increases the total mitochondrial content in exercise trained muscle (Handschin & Spiegelman, 2006).

Recently, the use of mass-spectrometry based approaches has dramatically expanded our ability to monitor the proteomic consequences of exercise. In a recent study, a mass spectrometry-based analysis of global protein phosphorylation was used to compare phosphorylation both before and immediately following a single bout of intense exercise (Hoffman et al., 2015). Importantly, this single-bout of exercise induced phosphorylation of >550 unique proteins, many of which were phosphorylated at multiple sites. While some of these phosphorylated proteins are targets of kinases known to be involved in the muscle adaptive response (i.e. AMPK, MAPK, CamK, etc. . . .), most had not been previously implicated in muscle signaling. This finding illustrates both the complexity of the muscles biochemical response to contraction and also the limits of our current understanding of this physiological system.

Redundancy is also a likely component of the complexity of the biochemical response of muscle contraction. Redundancy here refers to multiple signaling cascades converging on a single physiological outcome. One example is the activation of PGC1α by both AMPK and p38 MAPK pathways. In addition to the redundant pathways activating PGC1α, there are even redundancies within each independent pathway as both activate PGC1α by transcriptional and post-translational mechanisms. Ultimately, activation of both pathways induces an increase in mitochondrial biogenesis through PGC1α (Hawley et al., 2014). Redundancy is useful physiologically as potential defects on one arm of a response may be compensated for by the other pathways involved. However, redundancy makes detailed mechanistic investigations of these pathways difficult. Future work using –omics based approaches will be critical to understanding the biochemical pathways involved in muscle adaptation to exercise. Additionally, new technologies such as CRISPR/Cas9 (Cong et al., 2013; Hsu, Lander, & Zhang, 2014) that allow for easier and more rapid targeting of the multiple genes/proteins involved in regulating these processes will likely prove instrumental in fully elucidating the mechanisms underlying muscle adaptation.

Chapter summary

Exercise and training affect many facets of one's physiology. The goal of this chapter is to introduce the reader to several of the biochemical processes impacted by exercise. We have described how exercise influences immune function, redox homeostasis, metabolism, and mitochondrial function. Additionally, we have described specific changes to various signaling cascades that occur in response to muscle contraction. While an exhaustive description of all the known biochemical consequences of exercise is beyond the scope of any single book chapter, there is a critical idea that underscores all of what was covered here. Ultimately, the varied physiological consequences of exercise and training are dependent on contraction-induced mechanical, electrical, and chemical signals that impact downstream cellular processes. The factors involved in this process form a complex and flexible network that collectively impacts physiology in response to exercise. Developing an understanding of the critical biochemical reactions involved in the body's adaptive response to exercise will help to build and develop a suitable approach for maintaining an active lifestyle.

- Immune system function and compromisation are exercise-intensity dependent. Whilst moderate-intensity workloads generally provide positive adaptation, physical inactivity lifestyles and intense exercise result in increased susceptibility to sub-clinical infection.
- Physical activity can elicit modification and adaptation in the free-radical/oxidant and antioxidant balance (hormesis) which affects mitochondrial biogenesis, muscle contractility, gene regulation and incidence of debilitating health related illnesses and diseases.
- There are four major sources of energy for exercising muscle: 1) blood glucose, 2) muscle glycogen, 3) plasma free fatty acids, and 4) intramuscular triglycerides. Whereas lipids are more important during low-intensity exercise, glucose and glycogen become the primary source of energy during moderate and intense exercise.
- Exercise stimulates mitochondrial biogenesis through the activation of various signaling cascades that act upon PGC1α. PGC1α then stimulates expression of genes involved in mitochondrial function.

- At a biochemical level, electrical, mechanical, and chemical signals associated with muscle contraction are converted into cellular signals that activate downstream signaling cascades including Ca^{2+}/calmodulin dependent protein kinase (CamK), calcineurin, mitogen-activated protein kinases (MAPK), AMP-activated protein kinase (AMPK), and mammalian target of rapamycin (mTOR) thus changing the underlying characteristics of muscle.

References

Aguiló, A., Tauler, P., Fuentespina, E., Tur, J. A., Córdova, A., & Pons, A. (2005). Antioxidant response to oxidative stress induced by exhaustive exercise. *Physiology & Behavior, 84*(1), 1–7.

Ahlborg, G., Felig, P., Hagenfeldt, L., Hendler, R., & Wahren, J. (1974). Substrate turnover during prolonged exercise in man: splanchnic and leg metabolism of glucose, free fatty acids, and amino acids. *Journal of Clinical Investigation, 53*(4), 1080–1090.

Akimoto, T., Pohnert, S. C., Li, P., Zhang, M., Gumbs, C., Rosenberg, P. B., . . . Yan, Z. (2005). Exercise stimulates Pgc-1α transcription in skeletal muscle through activation of the p38 MAPK pathway. *Journal of Biological Chemistry, 280*(20), 19587–19593.

Allgrove, J., Gomes, E., Hough, J., & Gleeson, M. (2008). Effects of exercise intensity on saliva antimicrobial proteins and markers of stress in active men. *Journal of Sports Sciences, 26*, 653–661. doi 10.1080/02640410701716790.

Barbieri, E., & Sestili, P. (2011). Reactive oxygen species in skeletal muscle signaling. *Journal of Signal Transduction, 2012*, 982794,.

Bishop, N., & Gleeson, M. (2009). Acute and chronic effects of exercise on markers of mucosal immunity. *Frontiers in Bioscience (Landmark edition), 14*, 4444–4456.

Blannin, A. K., Chatwin, L. J., Cave, R., & Gleeson, M. (1996). Effects of submaximal cycling and long-term endurance training on neutrophil phagocytic activity in middle aged men. *British Journal of Sports Medicine, 30*(2), 125–129.

Booth, F. W., & Lees, S. J. (2007). Fundamental questions about genes, inactivity, and chronic diseases. *Physiological Genomics, 28*(2), 146–157.

Brahmi, Z., Thomas, J. E., Park, M., Park, M., & Dowdeswell, I. R. (1985). The effect of acute exercise on natural killer-cell activity of trained and sedentary human subjects. *Journal of Clinical Immunology, 5*(5), 321–328.

Brand, M. D. (2010). The sites and topology of mitochondrial superoxide production. *Experimental Gerontology, 45*(7), 466–472.

Brandtzaeg, P. (2003). Role of secretory antibodies in the defence against infections. *International Journal of Medical Microbiology, 293*(1), 3–15.

Bratthall, D., & Widerstrom, L. (1985). Ups and downs for salivary IgA. *European Journal of Oral Sciences, 93*(2), 128–134.

Brooks, G. A., & Mercier, J. (1994). Balance of carbohydrate and lipid utilization during exercise: the "crossover" concept. *Journal of Applied Physiology, 76*(6), 2253–2261.

Bruun, J. M., Helge, J. W., Richelsen, B., & Stallknecht, B. (2006). Diet and exercise reduce low-grade inflammation and macrophage infiltration in adipose tissue but not in skeletal muscle in severely obese subjects. *American Journal of Physiology-Endocrinology And Metabolism, 290*(5), E961–E967.

Budgett, R. (1998). Fatigue and underperformance in athletes: the overtraining syndrome. *British Journal of Sports Medicine, 32*(2), 107–110.

Calabrese, E. J., & Baldwin, L. A. (2001). U-shaped dose-responses in biology, toxicology, and public health. *Annual Review of Public Health, 22*(1), 15–33.

Calabrese, E. J., & Baldwin, L. A. (2002). Defining hormesis. *Human & Experimental Toxicology, 21*(2), 91–97.

Campbell, J. P., Riddell, N. E., Burns, V. E., Turner, M., van Zanten, J. J. C. S. V., Drayson, M. T., & Bosch, J. A. (2009). Acute exercise mobilises CD8+ T lymphocytes exhibiting an effector-memory phenotype. *Brain, Behavior, and Immunity, 23*(6), 767–775.

Cardoso, A., Bagatini, M., Roth, M., Martins, C., Rezer, J., Mello, F., . . . Schetinger, M. (2012). Acute effects of resistance exercise and intermittent intense aerobic exercise on blood cell count and oxidative stress in trained middle-aged women. *Brazilian Journal of Medical and Biological Research, 45*(12), 1172–1182.

Carlson, L. A., Kenefick, R. W., & Koch, A. J. (2013). Influence of carbohydrate ingestion on salivary immunoglobulin A following resistance exercise. *Journal of the International Society of Sports Nutrition, 10*(1), 14.

Cases, N., Sureda, A., Maestre, I., Tauler, P., Aguiló, A., Córdova, A., . . . Pons, A. (2006). Response of antioxidant defences to oxidative stress induced by prolonged exercise: antioxidant enzyme gene expression in lymphocytes. *European Journal of Applied Physiology, 98*(3), 263–269.

Cherednichenko, G., Zima, A. V., Feng, W., Schaefer, S., Blatter, L. A., & Pessah, I. N. (2004). NADH oxidase activity of rat cardiac sarcoplasmic reticulum regulates calcium-induced calcium release. *Circulation Research, 94*(4), 478–486.

Chubak, J., McTiernan, A., Sorensen, B., Wener, M., Yasui, Y., Velasquez, M., . . . Potter, J. (2006). Moderate-intensity exercise reduces the incidence of colds among postmenopausal women. *The American Journal of Medicine, 119*(11), 937–942.

Coggan, A. R., & Coyle, E. F. (1989). Metabolism and performance following carbohydrate ingestion late in exercise. *Medicine and Science in Sports and Exercise, 21*(1), 59–65.

Cong, L., Ran, F. A., Cox, D., Lin, S., Barretto, R., Habib, N., . . . Marraffini, L. A. (2013). Multiplex genome engineering using CRISPR/Cas systems. *Science, 339*(6121), 819–823.

Coyle, E., Hagberg, J., Hurley, B., Martin, W., Ehsani, A., & Holloszy, J. (1983). Carbohydrate feeding during prolonged strenuous exercise can delay fatigue. *Journal of Applied Physiology, 55*(1), 230–235.

Coyle, E. F. (1995). Substrate utilization during exercise in active people. *The American Journal of Clinical Nutrition, 61*(4), 968S–979S.

Coyle, E. F., Coggan, A. R., Hemmert, M., & Ivy, J. L. (1986). Muscle glycogen utilization during prolonged strenuous exercise when fed carbohydrate. *Journal of Applied Physiology, 61*(1), 165–172.

Crottet, P., & Corthésy, B. (1998). Secretory component delays the conversion of secretory IgA into antigen-binding competent F(ab′)₂: a possible implication for mucosal defense. *The Journal of Immunology, 161*(10), 5445.

Drela, N., Kozdron, E., & Szczypiorski, P. (2004). Moderate exercise may attenuate some aspects of immunosenescence. *BMC Geriatrics, 4*(8).

Ekblom, B., Ekblom, Ö., & Malm, C. (2006). Infectious episodes before and after a marathon race. *Scandinavian Journal of Medicine & Science in Sports, 16*(4), 287–293.

Espersen, G., Elbaek, A., Ernst, E., Toft, E., Kaalund, S., Jersild, C., & Grunnet, N. (1990). Effect of physical exercise on cytokines and lymphocyte subpopulations in human peripheral blood. *APMIS: acta pathologica, microbiologica, et immunologica Scandinavica, 98*(5), 395–400.

Fehrenbach, E., & Northoff, H. (2000). Free radicals, exercise, apoptosis, and heat shock proteins. *Exercise Immunology Review, 7*, 66–89.

Flatt, J.-P. (1995). Use and storage of carbohydrate and fat. *The American Journal of Clinical Nutrition, 61*(4), 952S–959S.

Foster, C. (1998). Monitoring training in athletes with reference to overtraining syndrome. *Medicine and Science in Sports and Exercise, 30*(7), 1164–1168.

Fujii, N., Hayashi, T., Hirshman, M. F., Smith, J. T., Habinowski, S. A., Kaijser, L., . . . Witters, L. A. (2000). Exercise induces isoform-specific increase in 5′ AMP-activated protein kinase activity in human skeletal muscle. *Biochemical and Biophysical Research Communications, 273*(3), 1150–1155.

Ghosh, S., Khazaei, M., Moien-Afshari, F., Ang, L. S., Granville, D. J., Verchere, C., . . . Sharma, K. (2009). Moderate exercise attenuates caspase-3 activity, oxidative stress, and inhibits progression of diabetic renal disease in db/db mice. *American Journal of Physiology-Renal Physiology, 296*(4), F700–F708.

Gill, S., Teixeira, A., Rosado, F., Hankey, J., Wright, A., Marczak, S., . . . Costa, R. (2014). The impact of a 24-h ultra-marathon on salivary antimicrobial protein responses. *International Journal of Sports Medicine, 35*(11), 966–971.

Gillum, T. L., Keunnen, M. R., Castillo, M. N., Williams, W. N. L., Jordan-Patterson, A. T., & Gillum, T. (2015). Exercise, but not acute sleep loss, increases salivary antimicrobial protein secretion. *Journal of Strength and Conditioning Research, 29*(5), 1359–1366.

Ginsburg, G. S., O'Toole, M., Rimm, E., Douglas, P. S., & Rifai, N. (2001). Gender differences in exercise-induced changes in sex hormone levels and lipid peroxidation in athletes participating in the Hawaii Ironman triathlon: Ginsburg-gender and exercise-induced lipid peroxidation. *Clinica Chimica Acta, 305*(1), 131–139.

Giraldo, E., Garcia, J., Hinchado, M., & Ortega, E. (2009). Exercise intensity-dependent changes in the inflammatory response in sedentary women: role of neuroendocrine parameters in the neutrophil phagocytic process and the pro-/anti-inflammatory cytokine balance. *Neuroimmunomodulation, 16*(4), 237–244.

Gleeson, M., McDonald, W. A., Cripps, A. W., Pyne, D. B., Clancy, R. L., & Fricker, P. A. (1995). The effect on immunity of long-term intensive training in elite swimmers. *Clin Exp Immunol., 102*(1), 210–216.

Gleeson, M., McDonald, W. A., Pyne, D. B., Clancy, R. L., Cripps, A. W., Francis, J. L., & Fricker, P. A. (2000). Immune status and respiratory illness for elite swimmers during a 12-week training cycle. *International Journal of Sports Medicine, 21*(4), 302–307.

Gleeson, M., McDonald, W. A., Pyne, D. B., Cripps, A. W., Francis, J. L., Fricker, P. A., & Clancy, R. L. (1999). Salivary IgA levels and infection risk in elite swimmers. *Medicine and Science in Sports and Exercise, 31*(1), 67.

Gomes, R. V., Moreira, A., Lodo, L., Nosaka, K., Coutts, A. J., & Aoki, M. S. (2013). Monitoring training loads, stress, immune-endocrine responses and performance in tennis players. *Biology of Sport, 30*(3), 173.

Gomez-Cabrera, M.-C., Domenech, E., & Viña, J. (2008). Moderate exercise is an antioxidant: upregulation of antioxidant genes by training. *Free Radical Biology and Medicine, 44*(2), 126–131.

Gonenc, S., Acikgoz, O., Semin, I., & Ozgonul, H. (2000). The effect of moderate swimming exercise on antioxidant enzymes and lipid peroxidation levels in children. *Indian Journal of Physiology and Pharmacology, 44*(3), 340–344.

Gordon, P. M., Liu, D., Sartor, M. A., IglayReger, H. B., Pistilli, E.E., Gutmann, L., Nader, G. A., & Hoffman, E. P. (2012). Resistance exercise training influences skeletal muscle immune activation: a microarray analysis. *J Appl Physiol, 112*(3), 443–453.

Goto, C., Higashi, Y., Kimura, M., Noma, K., Hara, K., Nakagawa, K., . . . Nara, I. (2003). Effect of different intensities of exercise on endothelium-dependent vasodilation in humans role of endothelium-dependent nitric oxide and oxidative stress. *Circulation, 108*(5), 530–535.

Goto, C., Nishioka, K., Umemura, T., Jitsuiki, D., Sakagutchi, A., Kawamura, M., . . . Higashi, Y. (2007). Acute moderate-intensity exercise induces vasodilation through an increase in nitric oxide bioavailiability in humans. *American Journal of Hypertension, 20*(8), 825–830.

Gounder, S. S., Kannan, S., Devadoss, D., Miller, C. J., Whitehead, K. S., Odelberg, S. J., . . . Abel, E. D. (2012). Impaired transcriptional activity of Nrf2 in age-related myocardial oxidative stress is reversible by moderate exercise training. *PLoS ONE, 7*(9), e45697.

Grivennikova, V. G., & Vinogradov, A. D. (2006). Generation of superoxide by the mitochondrial Complex I. *Biochimica et Biophysica Acta (BBA)-Bioenergetics, 1757*(5), 553–561.

Handschin, C., & Spiegelman, B. M. (2006). Peroxisome proliferator-activated receptor γ coactivator 1 coactivators, energy homeostasis, and metabolism. *Endocrine Reviews, 27*(7), 728–735.

Hartmann, A., Pfuhler, S., Dennog, C., Germadnik, D., Pilger, A., & Speit, G. (1998). Exercise-induced DNA effects in human leukocytes are not accompanied by increased formation of 8-hydroxy-2′-deoxyguanosine or induction of micronuclei. *Free Radical Biology and Medicine, 24*(2), 245–251.

Hawley, J. A., Hargreaves, M., Joyner, M. J., & Zierath, J. R. (2014). Integrative biology of exercise. *Cell, 159*(4), 738–749.

Hawley, J. A., Hargreaves, M., & Zierath, J. R. (2006). Signalling mechanisms in skeletal muscle: role in substrate selection and muscle adaptation. *Essays in Biochemistry, 42*, 1–12.

He, C. S., Tsai, M. L., Ko, M. H., Chang, C. K., & Fang, S. H. (2010). Relationships among salivary immunoglobulin A, lactoferrin and cortisol in basketball players during a basketball season. *European Journal of Applied Physiology, 110*(5), 989–995.

Heath, G. W., Ford, E. S., Craven, T. E., Macera, C. A., Jackson, K. L., & Pate, R. R. (1991). Exercise and the incidence of upper respiratory tract infections. *Medicine and Science in Sports and Exercise, 23*(2), 152.

Hemmrich, K., Suschek, C. V., Lerzynski, G., & Kolb-Bachofen, V. (2003). iNOS activity is essential for endothelial stress gene expression protecting against oxidative damage. *Journal of Applied Physiology, 95*(5), 1937–1946.

Henriksen, E. J., Diamond-Stanic, M. K., & Marchionne, E. M. (2011). Oxidative stress and the etiology of insulin resistance and type 2 diabetes. *Free Radical Biology and Medicine, 51*(5), 993–999.

Henson, D., Nieman, D., Davis, J., Dumke, C., Gross, S., Murphy, A., . . . McAnulty, S. (2008). Post-160-km race illness rates and decreases in granulocyte respiratory burst and salivary IgA output are not countered by quercetin ingestion. *Int J Sports Med, 29*(10), 856–863.

Higashi, Y., & Yoshizumi, M. (2004). Exercise and endothelial function: role of endothelium-derived nitric oxide and oxidative stress in healthy subjects and hypertensive patients. *Pharmacology & Therapeutics, 102*(1), 87–96.

Hoffman, N. J., Parker, B. L., Chaudhuri, R., Fisher-Wellman, K. H., Kleinert, M., Humphrey, S. J., . . . Fazakerley, D. J. (2015). Global phosphoproteomic analysis of human skeletal muscle reveals a network of exercise-regulated kinases and AMPK substrates. *Cell Metabolism, 22*(5), 922–935.

Hoffman-Goetz, L., & Pedersen, B. K. (1994). Exercise and the immune system: a model of the stress response? *Immunology Today, 15*(8), 382–387.

Holloszy, J. O. (1967). Biochemical adaptations in muscle effects of exercise on mitochondrial oxygen uptake and respiratory enzyme activity in skeletal muscle. *Journal of Biological Chemistry, 242*(9), 2278–2282.

Hood, D. A., Tryon, L. D., Carter, H. N., Kim, Y., & Chen, C. C. (2016). Unravelling the mechanisms regulating muscle mitochondrial biogenesis. *Biochemical Journal, 473*(15), 2295–2314.

Hsu, P. D., Lander, E. S., & Zhang, F. (2014). Development and applications of CRISPR-Cas9 for genome engineering. *Cell, 157*(6), 1262–1278.

Inoue, H., Sakai, M., Kaida, Y., & Kozue, K. (2004). Blood lactoferrin release induced by running exercise in normal volunteers: antibacterial activity. *Clinica Chimica Acta, 341*(1–2), 165–172.

Jäger, S., Handschin, C., Pierre, J. St-., & Spiegelman, B. M. (2007). AMP-activated protein kinase (AMPK) action in skeletal muscle via direct phosphorylation of PGC-1α. *Proceedings of the National Academy of Sciences, 104*(29), 12017–12022.

Jamart, C., Benoit, N., Raymackers, J.-M., Kim, H. J., Kim, C. K., & Francaux, M. (2012). Autophagy-related and autophagy regulatory genes are induced in human muscle after ultraendurance exercise. *European Journal of Applied Physiology, 112*(8), 3173–3177.

Jensen, T. E., & Richter, E. A. (2012). Regulation of glucose and glycogen metabolism during and after exercise. *The Journal of Physiology, 590*(5), 1069–1076.

Jessen, N., & Goodyear, L. J. (2005). Contraction signaling to glucose transport in skeletal muscle. *Journal of Applied Physiology, 99*(1), 330–337.

Joseph, A.-M., Pilegaard, H., Litvintsev, A., Leick, L., & Hood, D. A. (2006). Control of gene expression and mitochondrial biogenesis in the muscular adaptation to endurance exercise. *Essays in Biochemistry, 42*, 13–29.

Joyner, M. J., & Casey, D. P. (2015). Regulation of increased blood flow (hyperemia) to muscles during exercise: a hierarchy of competing physiological needs. *Physiological Reviews, 95*(2), 549–601.

Kakanis, M., Peake, J., Brenu, E., Simmonds, M., Gray, B., Hooper, S., & Marshall-Gradisnik, S. (2010). The open window of susceptibility to infection after acute exercise in healthy young male elite athletes. *Exercise Immunology Review, 16*, 119–137.

Katz, A., Broberg, S., Sahlin, K., & Wahren, J. (1986). Leg glucose uptake during maximal dynamic exercise in humans. *American Journal of Physiology-Endocrinology and Metabolism, 251*(1), E65–E70.

Katz, A., Sahlin, K., & Broberg, S. (1991). Regulation of glucose utilization in human skeletal muscle during moderate dynamic exercise. *American Journal of Physiology-Endocrinology and Metabolism, 260*(3), E411–E415.

Kendig, E. L., Le, H. H., & Belcher, S. M. (2010). Defining hormesis: evaluation of a complex concentration response phenomenon. *International Journal of Toxicology, 29*(3), 235–246.

Knez, W. L., Coombes, J. S., & Jenkins, D. G. (2006). Ultra-endurance exercise and oxidative damage. *Sports Medicine, 36*(5), 429–441.

Koch, A. J., Wherry, A. D., Petersen, M. C., Johnson, J. C., Stuart, M. K., & Sexton, W. L. (2007). Salivary immunoglobulin A response to a collegiate rugby game. *The Journal of Strength & Conditioning Research, 21*(1), 86–90.

Kormanovski, A., Ibarra, F. C., Padilla, E. L., & Rodriguez, R. C. (2010). Resistance to respiratory illness and antibody response in open water swimmers during training and long distance swims. *International Journal of Medicine and Medical Sciences, 2*(3), 80–87.

Korsrud, F., & Brandtzaeg, P. (1980). Quantitative immunohistochemistry of immunoglobulin- and J-chain-producing cells in human parotid and submandibular salivary glands. *Immunology, 39*(2), 129.

Kostka, T., Berthouze, S. E., Lacour, J. R., & Bonnefoy, M. (2000). The symptomatology of upper respiratory tract infections and exercise in elderly people. *Medicine and Science in Sports and Exercise, 32*(1), 46.

Kristiansen, S., Hargreaves, M., & Richter, E. A. (1997). Progressive increase in glucose transport and GLUT-4 in human sarcolemmal vesicles during moderate exercise. *American Journal of Physiology-Endocrinology and Metabolism, 272*(3), E385–E389.

Kusaka, Y., Kondou, H., & Morimoto, K. (1992) Healthy lifestyles are associated with natural killer cell activity. *Preventive Medicine, 32*, 602–615. doi:10.1016/0091–7435(92)90068-S.

Lamm, M. E. (1998). IV. How epithelial transport of IgA antibodies relates to host defense. *American Journal of Physiology-Gastrointestinal and Liver Physiology, 274*(4), G614–G617.

LaPerriere, A., Antoni, M. H., Ironson, G., Perry, A., McCabe, P., Klimas, N., . . . Fletcher, M. A. (1994). Effects of aerobic exercise training on lymphocyte subpopulations. *International Journal of Sports Medicine, 15*(S 3), S127–S130.

Larrabee, R. C. (1902). Leucocytosis after violent exercise. *The Journal of Medical Research, 7*(1), 76.

Laufs, U., Wassmann, S., Czech, T., Münzel, T., Eisenhauer, M., Böhm, M., & Nickenig, G. (2005). Physical inactivity increases oxidative stress, endothelial dysfunction, and atherosclerosis. *Arteriosclerosis, Thrombosis, and Vascular Biology, 25*(4), 809–814.

Leeuwenburgh, C., & Heinecke, J. (2001). Oxidative stress and antioxidants in exercise. *Current Medicinal Chemistry, 8*(7), 829–838.

Levada-Pires, A., Cury-Boaventura, M., Gorjão, R., Hirabara, S., Puggina, E., Peres, C., . . . Pithon-Curi, T. (2008). Neutrophil death induced by a triathlon competition in elite athletes. *Medicine and Science in Sports and Exercise, 40*(8), 1447–1454.

Lindsay, A., Lewis, J., Scarrott, C., Gill, N., Gieseg, S., & Draper, N. (2015). Assessing the effectiveness of selected biomarkers in the acute and cumulative physiological stress response in professional rugby union through non-invasive assessment. *International Journal of Sports Medicine, 36*(6), 446–454. doi: 10.1055/s-0034-1398528

Lowder, T., Padgett, D., & Woods, J. (2005). Moderate exercise protects mice from death due to influenza virus. *Brain, Behavior, and Immunity, 19*(5), 377–380.

Lundby, C., & Jacobs, R. A. (2016). Adaptations of skeletal muscle mitochondria to exercise training. *Experimental Physiology, 101*(1), 17–22.

Mackinnon, L. T., & Hooper, S. (1994). Mucosal (secretory) immune system responses to exercise of varying intensity and during overtraining. *International Journal of Sports Medicine, 15*(3), 179.

MacKinnon, L. T., & Jenkins, D. G. (1993). Decreased salivary immunoglobulins after intense interval exercise before and after training. *Medicine and Science in Sports and Exercise, 25*(6), 678–683.

Malm, C. (2006). Susceptibility to infections in elite athletes: the S-curve. *Scandinavian Journal of Medicine & Science in Sports, 16*(1), 4–6.

Martin, S. A., Pence, B. D., & Woods, J. A. (2009). Exercise and respiratory tract viral infections. *Exercise and Sport Sciences Reviews, 37*(4), 157–164.

Mastaloudis, A., Leonard, S. W., & Traber, M. G. (2001). Oxidative stress in athletes during extreme endurance exercise. *Free Radical Biology and Medicine, 31*(7), 911–922.

Matthews, C. E., Ockene, I. S., Freedson, P. S., Rosal, M. C., Merriam, P. A., & Hebert, J. R. (2002). Moderate to vigorous physical activity and risk of upper-respiratory tract infection. *Medicine and Science in Sports and Exercise, 34*(8), 1242.

McDowell, S. L., Chaloa, K., Housh, T. J., Tharp, G. D., & Johnson, G. O. (1991). The effect of exercise intensity and duration on salivary immunoglobulin A. *European Journal of Applied Physiology and Occupational Physiology, 63*(2), 108–111.

McGee, S. L., & Hargreaves, M. (2010). AMPK-mediated regulation of transcription in skeletal muscle. *Clinical Science, 118*(8), 507–518.

Miyata, M., Kasai, H., Kawai, K., Yamada, N., Tokudome, M., Ichikawa, H., . . . Hoshino, H. (2008). Changes of urinary 8-hydroxydeoxyguanosine levels during a two-day ultramarathon race period in Japanese non-professional runners. *International Journal of Sports Medicine, 29*(1), 27–33.

Miyazaki, H., Oh-ishi, S., Ookawara, T., Kizaki, T., Toshinai, K., Ha, S., . . . Ohno, H. (2001). Strenuous endurance training in humans reduces oxidative stress following exhausting exercise. *European Journal of Applied Physiology, 84*(1–2), 1–6.

Mooren, F. C., Blöming, D., Lechtermann, A., Lerch, M. M., & Völker, K. (2002). Lymphocyte apoptosis after exhaustive and moderate exercise. *Journal of Applied Physiology, 93*(1), 147.

Mooren, F. C., Lechtermann, A., & Lker, K. V. Ö. (2004). Exercise-induced apoptosis of lymphocytes depends on training status. *Medicine and Science in Sports and Exercise, 36*(9), 1476.

Mooren, F. C., Lechtermann, A., Pospiech, S., Fromme, A., Thorwesten, L., & Völker, K. (2001). Decoupling of intracellular calcium signaling in granulocytes after exhaustive exercise. *International Journal of Sports Medicine, 22*(5), 323–328.

Moreira, A., Franchini, E., de Freitas, C. G., de Arruda, A. F. S., de Moura, N. R., Costa, E. C., & Aoki, M. S. (2012). Salivary cortisol and immunoglobulin A responses to simulated and official Jiu-Jitsu matches. *The Journal of Strength & Conditioning Research, 26*(8), 2185–2191.

Moyna, N., Acker, G., Fulton, J., Weber, K., Goss, F., Robertson, R., . . . Rabin, B. (1996). Lymphocyte function and cytokine production during incremental exercise in active and sedentary males and females. *International Journal of Sports Medicine, 17*(8), 585–591.

Navarro, A., Gomez, C., López-Cepero, J. M., & Boveris, A. (2004). Beneficial effects of moderate exercise on mice aging: survival, behavior, oxidative stress, and mitochondrial electron transfer. *American Journal of Physiology-Regulatory, Integrative and Comparative Physiology, 286*(3), R505–R511.

Nehlsen-Cannarella, S. L., Nieman, D. C., Balk-Lamberton, A. J., Markoff, P. A., Chritton, D. B., Gusewitch, G., & Lee, J. W. (1991). The effects of moderate exercise training on immune response. *Medicine and Science in Sports and Exercise, 23*(1), 64–70.

Nielsen, H. B. (2003). Lymphocyte responses to maximal exercise. *Sports Medicine, 33*(11), 853–867.

Nieman, D., Johanssen, L., Lee, J., & Arabatzis, K. (1990). Infectious episodes in runners before and after the Los Angeles Marathon. *The Journal of Sports Medicine and Physical Fitness, 30*(3), 316.

Nieman, D., Nehlsen-Cannarella, S., Markoff, P., Balk-Lamberton, A., Yang, H., Chritton, D., . . . Arabatzis, K. (1990). The effects of moderate exercise training on natural killer cells and acute upper respiratory tract infections. *International Journal of Sports Medicine, 11*(6), 467–473.

Nieman, D. C. (1994). Exercise, upper respiratory tract infection, and the immune system. *Medicine and Science in Sports and Exercise, 26*(2), 128.

Nieman, D. C., Henson, D. A., Austin, M. D., & Sha, W. (2011). Upper respiratory tract infection is reduced in physically fit and active adults. *British Journal of Sports Medicine, 45*(12), 987–992.

Nieman, D. C., Miller, A. R., Henson, D. A., Warren, B. J., Gusewitch, G., Johnson, R. L., Davis, J. M., Butterworth, D. E., & Nehlsen-Cannarella, S. L. (1993). Effects of high- vs moderate-intensity exercise on natural killer cell activity. *Medicine and Science in Sports and Exercise, 25*(10), 1126–1134.

Niess, A., Baumann, M., Roecker, K., Horstmann, T., Mayer, F., & Dickhuth, H. (1998). Effects of intensive endurance exercise on DNA damage in leucocytes. *The Journal of Sports Medicine and Physical Fitness, 38*(2), 111–115.

Okita, K., Nishijima, H., Murakami, T., Nagai, T., Morita, N., Yonezawa, K., . . . Kitabatake, A. (2004). Can exercise training with weight loss lower serum C-reactive protein levels? *Arteriosclerosis, Thrombosis, and Vascular Biology, 24*(10), 1868–1873.

Ortega, E., Barriga, C., & De la Fuente, M. (1993). Study of the phagocytic process in neutrophils from elite sportswomen. *European Journal of Applied Physiology and Occupational Physiology, 66*(1), 37–42.

Ortega, E., Collazos, M., Maynar, M., Barriga, C., & De la Fuente, M. (1993). Stimulation of the phagocytic function of neutrophils in sedentary men after acute moderate exercise. *European Journal of Applied Physiology and Occupational Physiology, 66*(1), 60–64.

Papacosta, E., & Nassis, G. P. (2011). Saliva as a tool for monitoring steroid, peptide and immune markers in sport and exercise science. *Journal of Science and Medicine in Sport, 14*(5), 424–434.

Pedersen, B. K., & Nieman, D. C. (1998). Exercise immunology: integration and regulation. *Immunology Today, 19*(5), 204–206.

Pedersen, B. K., & Ullum, H. (1994). NK cell response to physical activity: possible mechanisms of action. *Medicine and Science in Sports and Exercise, 26*(2), 140–146.

Pereira, G., Prestes, J., Tibana, R., Shiguemoto, G., Navalta, J., & Perez, S. (2012). Acute resistance training affects cell surface markers for apoptosis and migration in CD4+ and CD8+ lymphocytes. *Cellular Immunology, 279*(2), 134–139.

Peters, E., Goetzsche, J., Joseph, L., & Noakes, T. (1996). Vitamin C as effective as combinations of antioxidant nutrients in reducing symptoms of upper respiratory tract infection in ultramarathon runners. *South African Journal of Sports Medicine, 11*(3), 23–27.

Peters, E. M., Goetzsche, J. M., Grobbelaar, B., & Noakes, T. D. (1993). Vitamin C supplementation reduces the incidence of postrace symptoms of upper-respiratory-tract infection in ultramarathon runners. *The American Journal of Clinical Nutrition, 57*(2), 170–174.

Peters, E. M., Shaik, J., & Kleinveldt, N. (2010). Upper respiratory tract infection symptoms in ultramarathon runners not related to immunoglobulin status. *Clinical Journal of Sport Medicine, 20*(1), 39–46.

Powers, S. K., Duarte, J., Kavazis, A. N., & Talbert, E. E. (2010). Reactive oxygen species are signalling molecules for skeletal muscle adaptation. *Experimental Physiology, 95*(1), 1–9.

Powers, S. K., & Jackson, M. J. (2008). Exercise-induced oxidative stress: cellular mechanisms and impact on muscle force production. *Physiological Reviews, 88*(4), 1243–1276.

Powers, S. K., Ji, L. L., Kavazis, A. N., & Jackson, M. J. (2011). Reactive oxygen species: impact on skeletal muscle. *Comprehensive Physiology, 1*(2), 941–969.

Puigserver, P., Rhee, J., Lin, J., Wu, Z., Yoon, J. C., Zhang, C.-Y., . . . Spiegelman, B. M. (2001). Cytokine stimulation of energy expenditure through p38 MAP kinase activation of PPARγ coactivator-1. *Molecular Cell, 8*(5), 971–982.

Pyne, D., & Gleeson, M. (1998). Effects of intensive exercise training on immunity in athletes. *International Journal of Sports Medicine, 19*(Suppl 3), S183–191; discussion S191–194.

Pyne, D. B., Baker, M. S., Fricker, P. A., McDonald, W. A., Telford, R. D., & Weidemann, M. J. (1995). Effects of an intensive 12-wk training program by elite swimmers on neutrophil oxidative activity. *Medicine and Science in Sports and Exercise, 27*(4), 536.

Pyne, D. B., Smith, J. A., Baker, M. S., Telford, R. D., & Weidemann, M. J. (2000). Neutrophil oxidative activity is differentially affected by exercise intensity and type. *Journal of Science and Medicine in Sport, 3*(1), 44–54.

Quindry, J. C., Stone, W. L., King, J., & Broeder, C. E. (2003). The effects of acute exercise on neutrophils and plasma oxidative stress. *Medicine and Science in Sports and Exercise, 35*(7), 1139–1145.

Radak, Z., Chung, H. Y., & Goto, S. (2005). Exercise and hormesis: oxidative stress-related adaptation for successful aging. *Biogerontology, 6*(1), 71–75.

Radak, Z., Chung, H. Y., & Goto, S. (2008). Systemic adaptation to oxidative challenge induced by regular exercise. *Free Radical Biology and Medicine, 44*(2), 153–159.

Radak, Z., Chung, H. Y., Koltai, E., Taylor, A. W., & Goto, S. (2008). Exercise, oxidative stress and hormesis. *Ageing Research Reviews, 7*(1), 34–42.

Radom-Aizik, S., Zaldivar, F., Oliver, S., Galassetti, P., & Cooper, D. M. (2010). Evidence for microRNA involvement in exercise-associated neutrophil gene expression changes. *Journal of Applied Physiology, 109*(1), 252–261.

Reid, M. B., Khawli, F., & Moody, M. R. (1993). Reactive oxygen in skeletal muscle. III. Contractility of unfatigued muscle. *Journal of Applied Physiology, 75*(3), 1081–1087.

Rhind, S. G., Shek, P. N., Shinkai, S., & Shephard, R. J. (1996). Effects of moderate endurance exercise and training on *in vitro* lymphocyte proliferation, interleukin-2 (IL-2) production, and IL-2 receptor expression. *European Journal of Applied Physiology and Occupational Physiology, 74*(4), 348–360.

Rigoulet, M., Yoboue, E. D., & Devin, A. (2011). Mitochondrial ROS generation and its regulation: mechanisms involved in H_2O_2 signaling. *Antioxidants & Redox Signaling, 14*(3), 459–468.

Roach, P. J., Depaoli-Roach, A. A., Hurley, T. D., & Tagliabracci, V. S. (2012). Glycogen and its metabolism: some new developments and old themes. *Biochemical Journal, 441*(3), 763–787.

Robson-Ansley, P., Howatson, G., Tallent, J., Mitcheson, K., Walshe, I., Toms, C., . . . Ansley, L. (2012). Prevalence of allergy and upper respiratory tract symptoms in runners of the London marathon. *Medicine and Science in Sports and Exercise, 44*(6), 999–1004.

Rodriguez, A., Barriga, C., & De la Fuente, M. (1991). Phagocytic function of blood neutrophils in sedentary young people after physical exercise. *International Journal of Sports Medicine, 12*(03), 276–280.

Romijn, J., Coyle, E., Sidossis, L., Gastaldelli, A., Horowitz, J., Endert, E., & Wolfe, R. (1993). Regulation of endogenous fat and carbohydrate metabolism in relation to exercise intensity and duration. *American Journal of Physiology-Endocrinology and Metabolism, 265*(3), E380–E391.

Roschel, H., Barroso, R., Batista, M., Ugrinowitsch, C., Tricoli, V., Arsati, F., . . . Moreira, A. (2011). Do whole-body vibration exercise and resistance exercise modify concentrations of salivary cortisol and immunoglobulin A? *Brazilian Journal of Medical and Biological Research, 44*(6), 592–597.

Rose, A. J., & Hargreaves, M. (2003). Exercise increases Ca2+–calmodulin-dependent protein kinase II activity in human skeletal muscle. *The Journal of Physiology, 553*(1), 303–309.

Rose, A. J., & Richter, E. A. (2005). Skeletal muscle glucose uptake during exercise: how is it regulated? *Physiology, 20*(4), 260–270.

Santos-Silva, A., Rebelo, M. I., Castro, E. M. B., Belo, L., Guerra, A., Rego, C., & Quintanilha, A. (2001). Leukocyte activation, erythrocyte damage, lipid profile and oxidative stress imposed by high competition physical exercise in adolescents. *Clinica chimica acta, 306*(1–2), 119–126.

Saygin, O., Karacabey, K., Ozmerdivenli, R., Zorba, E., Ilhan, F., & Bulut, V. (2006). Effect of chronic exercise on immunoglobin, complement and leukocyte types in volleyball players and athletes. *Neuroendocrinology Letters, 27*(1–2), 271–276.

Scharhag, J., Meyer, T., Gabriel, H., Schlick, B., Faude, O., & Kindermann, W. (2005). Does prolonged cycling of moderate intensity affect immune cell function? *British Journal of Sports Medicine, 39*(3), 171–177.

Shephard, R., & Shek, P. (1998). Acute and chronic over-exertion: do depressed immune responses provide useful markers? *International Journal of Sports Medicine, 19*(3), 159–171.

Shimizu, K., Kimura, F., Akimoto, T., Akama, T., Otsuki, T., Nishijima, T., . . . Kono, I. (2007). Effects of exercise, age and gender on salivary secretory immunoglobulin A in elderly individuals. *Exercise Immunology Review, 13*, 55–66.

Shinkai, S., Kohno, H., Kimura, K., Komura, T., Asai, H., Inai, R., . . . Shephard, R. (1995). Physical activity and immune senescence in men. *Medicine and Science in Sports and Exercise, 27*(11), 1516–1526.

Spence, L., Brown, W. J., Pyne, D. B., Nissen, M. D., Sloots, T. P., Mccormack, J. G., . . . Fricker, P. A. (2007). Incidence, etiology, and symptomatology of upper respiratory illness in elite athletes. *Medicine and Science in Sports and Exercise, 39*(4), 577.

Steerenberg, P. A., Asperen, I. A., Amerongen, A. N., Biewenga, J., Mol, D., & Medema, G. (1997). Salivary levels of immunoglobulin A in triathletes. *European Journal of Oral Sciences, 105*(4), 305–309.

Steinbacher, P., & Eckl, P. (2015). Impact of oxidative stress on exercising skeletal muscle. *Biomolecules, 5*(2), 356–377.

Sylow, L., Kleinert, M., Richter, E. A., & Jensen, T. E. (2016). Exercise-stimulated glucose uptake – regulation and implications for glycaemic control. *Nature Reviews Endocrinology*. doi: 10.1038/nrendo. 2016.162

Tauler, P., Gimeno, I., Aguilo, A., Guix, M., & Pons, A. (1999). Regulation of erythrocyte antioxidant enzyme activities in athletes during competition and short-term recovery. *Pflügers Archiv, 438*(6), 782–787.

Tauler, P., Martinez, S., Moreno, C., Martínez, P., & Aguilo, A. (2013). Changes in salivary hormones, immunoglobulin A, and C-reactive protein in response to ultra-endurance exercises. *Applied Physiology, Nutrition, and Metabolism, 39*(5), 560–565.

Teixeira de Lemos, E., Oliveira, J., Páscoa Pinheiro, J., & Reis, F. (2012). Regular physical exercise as a strategy to improve antioxidant and anti-inflammatory status: benefits in type 2 diabetes mellitus. *Oxidative Medicine and Cellular Longevity, 2012*, 741545.

Tharp, G. D. (1991). Basketball exercise and secretory immunoglobulin A. *European Journal of Applied Physiology and Occupational Physiology, 63*(3), 312–314.

Thorpe, R., & Sunderland, C. (2012). Muscle damage, endocrine, and immune marker response to a soccer match. *The Journal of Strength & Conditioning Research, 26*(10), 2783–2790.

Tiidus, P. M., Pushkarenko, J., & Houston, M. E. (1996). Lack of antioxidant adaptation to short-term aerobic training in human muscle. *American Journal of Physiology-Regulatory, Integrative and Comparative Physiology, 271*(4), R832–R836.

Tomasi, T. B., Trudeau, F. B., Czerwinski, D., & Erredge, S. (1982). Immune parameters in athletes before and after strenuous exercise. *Journal of Clinical Immunology, 2*(3), 173–178.

Tozzi-Ciancarelli, M., Penco, M., & Di Massimo, C. (2002). Influence of acute exercise on human platelet responsiveness: possible involvement of exercise-induced oxidative stress. *European Journal of Applied Physiology, 86*(3), 266–272.

Traeger Mackinnon, L., Ginn, E., & Seymour, G. J. (1993). Decreased salivary immunoglobulin A secretion rate after intense interval exercise in elite kayakers. *European Journal of Applied Physiology and Occupational Physiology, 67*(2), 180–184.

Tsai, M. L., Chou, K. M., Chang, C. K., & Fang, S. H. (2011). Changes of mucosal immunity and antioxidation activity in elite male Taiwanese taekwondo athletes associated with intensive training and rapid weight loss. *British Journal of Sports Medicine, 45*(9), 729–734.

Tuan, T.-C., Hsu, T.-G., Fong, M.-C., Hsu, C.-F., Tsai, K. K., Lee, C.-Y., & Kong, C.-W. (2008). Deleterious effects of short-term, high-intensity exercise on immune function: evidence from leucocyte mitochondrial alterations and apoptosis. *British Journal of Sports Medicine, 42*(1), 11–15.

Turner, J., Hodges, N., Bosch, J., & Aldred, S. (2011). Prolonged depletion of antioxidant capacity after ultraendurance exercise. *Medicine and Science in Sports and Exercise, 43*(9), 1770–1776.

Turner, J. E., Bennett, S. J., Campbell, J. P., Bosch, J. A., Aldred, S., & Griffiths, H. R. (2013). The antioxidant enzyme peroxiredoxin-2 is depleted in lymphocytes seven days after ultra-endurance exercise. *Free Radical Research, 47*(10), 821–828.

Umanskaya, A., Santulli, G., Xie, W., Andersson, D. C., Reiken, S. R., & Marks, A. R. (2014). Genetically enhancing mitochondrial antioxidant activity improves muscle function in aging. *Proceedings of the National Academy of Sciences, 111*(42), 15250–15255.

Usui, T., Yoshikawa, T., Orita, K., Ueda, S.-y., Katsura, Y., & Fujimoto, S. (2012). Comparison of salivary antimicrobial peptides and upper respiratory tract infections in elite marathon runners and sedentary subjects. *The Journal of Physical Fitness and Sports Medicine, 1*(1), 175–181.

Usui, T., Yoshikawa, T., Orita, K., Ueda, S., Katsura, Y., Fujimoto, S., & Yoshimura, M. (2011). Changes in salivary antimicrobial peptides, immunoglobulin A and cortisol after prolonged strenuous exercise. *European Journal of Applied Physiology*, 1–10.

Wagner, K. H., Reichhold, S., & Neubauer, O. (2011). Impact of endurance and ultraendurance exercise on DNA damage. *Annals of the New York Academy of Sciences, 1229*(1), 115–123.

Wahren, J., Felig, P., Ahlborg, G., & Jorfeldt, L. (1971). Glucose metabolism during leg exercise in man. *Journal of Clinical Investigation, 50*(12), 2715–2725.

Walsh, N. (1999). The effects of high-intensity intermittent exercise on saliva IgA, total protein and alpha-amylase. *Journal of Sports Sciences, 17*(2), 129–134.

Walsh, N. P., Bishop, N. C., Blackwell, J., Wierzbicki, S. G., & Montague, J. C. (2002). Salivary IgA response to prolonged exercise in a cold environment in trained cyclists. *Medicine and Science in Sports and Exercise, 34*(10), 1632–1637.

Wang, J., & Huang, Y. (2005). Effects of exercise intensity on lymphocyte apoptosis induced by oxidative stress in men. *European Journal of Applied Physiology, 95*(4), 290–297.

Werner, C., Fürster, T., Widmann, T., Pöss, J., Roggia, C., Hanhoun, M., . . . Kindermann, W. (2009). Physical exercise prevents cellular senescence in circulating leukocytes and in the vessel wall. *Circulation, 120*(24), 2438–2447.

West, N., Pyne, D., Kyd, J., Renshaw, G., Fricker, P., & Cripps, A. (2010). The effect of exercise on innate mucosal immunity. *British Journal of Sports Medicine, 44*(4), 227–231.

West, N. P., Pyne, D. B., Renshaw, G., & Cripps, A. W. (2006). Antimicrobial peptides and proteins, exercise and innate mucosal immunity. *FEMS Immunology & Medical Microbiology, 48*(3), 293–304.

Widegren, U., Jiang, X. J., Krook, A., Chibalin, A. V., Björnholm, M., Tally, M., . . . Zierath, J. R. (1998). Divergent effects of exercise on metabolic and mitogenic signaling pathways in human skeletal muscle. *The FASEB Journal, 12*(13), 1379–1389.

Winder, W., & Hardie, D. (1996). Inactivation of acetyl-CoA carboxylase and activation of AMP-activated protein kinase in muscle during exercise. *American Journal of Physiology-Endocrinology and Metabolism, 270*(2), E299–E304.

Wong, C. M., Lai, H. K., Ou, C. Q., Ho, S. Y., Chan, K. P., Thach, T. Q., . . . Hedley, A. J. (2008). Is exercise protective against influenza-associated mortality? *PLoS ONE, 3*(5), e2108.

Zhao, G., Zhou, S., Davie, A., & Su, Q. (2012). Effects of moderate and high intensity exercise on T1/T2 balance. *Exercise Immunology Review, 18*(18), 98–114.

14   Psychology and physical activity

Brad H. Miles

Keywords: Psychology, exercise, physical activity, behaviour, mental health

It is exercise alone that supports the spirits, and keeps the mind in vigor.

(Cicero, 65 BCE)

How do psychological processes relate to physical activity and vice versa? Despite more than two thousand years of philosophical speculation on this question it is only since the latter part of the 20th century that a systematic and coherent body of research has emerged on the topic. Conventionally described as exercise psychology, this rapidly growing field of inquiry brings together investigators from a broad range of disciplines and perspectives, including social psychology, exercise science, physiology, clinical psychology, neuroscience, epidemiology, and public health – each with their own concomitant theories, methods, and goals. This interdisciplinary richness of exercise psychology contributes to the vitality of the field but also means that disparate goals and methods can be difficult to contextualise. This chapter identifies some of the main themes, findings, and applications of contemporary exercise psychology, discusses the strengths and limitations of current approaches, and briefly looks toward the future of the field.

Dual approaches in exercise psychology

Broadly, research into the relationship between psychology and physical activity can be characterised by two related but distinct approaches. The first approach looks to understand the consequences that physical activity can have for mental health, cognitive functioning, general well-being, and a range of lower-level psychological constructs such as self-esteem, body image, and mood. Although much, but certainly not all, of the work in this approach is correlational in nature, there is often a tacit assumption that exercise and physical activity can have a causal effect on psychological functioning. In this sense, physical activity is treated as an independent variable that has a putative causal effect on the dependent variable of psychological functioning. As an example, Broocks et al. (1998) investigated the use of exercise in the treatment of panic disorder and found regular aerobic exercise to be associated with significant reductions in symptomatology. Applications emerging from this approach use physical activity as an intervention or prevention measure to bolster or maintain psychological functioning and well-being.

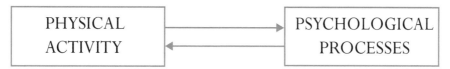

Figure 14.1 Dual approach conceptualisation of research in exercise psychology depicting a bidirectional relationship between physical activity and psychological processes

The second approach looks to understand the psychological variables that are antecedent to participation and engagement in physical activity. This approach explores the notion that certain psychological factors may function to increase or decrease the likelihood of being physically active. In this sense, physical activity is treated as a dependent variable that is causally affected by antecedent psychological factors that function as independent variables. For example, the psychological construct of self-efficacy has been found to be predictive of exercise participation in middle-aged adults (McAuley, 1992). In this approach, the application is often in terms of attempts at behaviour change with the aim of increasing the likelihood of individuals engaging in and sustaining physical activity behaviour.

This simple characterisation of research in exercise psychology, depicted in Figure 14.1, does not do justice to the breadth of the goals and methods in the field, but does provide a useful conceptual starting point for a broad examination of recent research.

Psychology as consequent: the effects of physical activity on psychology

As noted above, one of the central issues in exercise psychology concerns the impact that physical activity can have on mental health and psychological functioning. While the positive physical health benefits of regular physical activity (and conversely the negative effects of inactivity) have been well established (Bouchard, Blair, & Haskell, 2012; USDHHS, 1996), it is only relatively recently that systematic efforts to understand the mental health effects of physical activity have gained traction (Faulkner & Taylor, 2005). Motivating many of these efforts is recognition of the prevalence of mental illness and the associated individual, social, and economic costs. Indeed, one recent estimate suggests mental illness is the current largest contributor to the global burden of disease (Vigo, Thornicroft, & Atun, 2016). Depression, for example, is a commonly occurring mental health issue and a major cause of worldwide morbidity and reduction in quality of life (Richards & O'Hara, 2014). While there is much variation across countries, large-scale epidemiological studies regularly estimate life-time prevalence rates for major depressive episodes to be between 11 and 15%, with life-time rates for depression-related symptoms around 50% (Kessler & Bromet, 2013).

Not surprisingly, depression-related disorders have been one of the primary targets for investigating the preventive and mitigating effects of physical activity. Cross-sectional and longitudinal studies have typically identified a negative relationship between physical activity and depression with greater levels of physical activity being associated with the experience of fewer depressive symptoms (e.g., Abu-Omar, Rutten, & Lehtinen, 2004; Motl, Birnbaum, Kubik, & Dishman, 2004; Steptoe et al., 1997; Strohle et al., 2007). However, given that for many people depression is likely to act as a considerable barrier to physical activity, the causal implications of such findings are difficult to establish. More compelling evidence comes from a large number of randomised controlled trials (RCTs) that have investigated the efficacy of physical activity in combatting depression (Faulkner & Taylor, 2005). Detailed assessment of these studies is beyond the scope of this chapter, but importantly, many of these RCTs have been subjected to systematic and meta-analytic review (e.g., Cooney et al., 2013; Josefsson, Lindwall, & Archer, 2014; Kvam, Kleppe, Nordhus, & Hovland, 2016; Rethorst, Wipfli, & Landers, 2009; Schuch et al., 2016). Meta-analyses can be a useful tool for systematically integrating findings and deriving conclusions from multiple studies. Despite considerable variation, both in the methods and in the magnitudes of outcome effects in these studies, the recurrent theme to emerge is that physical activity produces significant antidepressant effects in both clinical and non-clinical populations. As such, physical activity appears to offer considerable value as an option for the treatment and prevention of depression that is simple, cost-effective, readily available, non-stigmatising, and associated with few negative side-effects.

Similar to depression, anxiety disorders appear to be among the most commonly experienced mental health issues with some large-scale epidemiological studies estimating 12-month prevalence rates of between 10 and 20% and life-time prevalence rates often nearing 30% (Bandelow & Michaelis, 2015; Kessler, Wai, Demler, & Walters, 2005; P. Martin, 2003). While the research examining the effects of physical activity on anxiety is far more limited than that for depression, the empirical evidence is suggestive of similar effects. Cross-sectional studies typically show a negative relationship in which regular physical exercise is associated with less experience of anxiety (e.g., De Moor, Beem, Stubbe, Boomsma, & De Geus, 2006; Goodwin, 2003), and several RCTs have identified exercise to have significant anxiolytic effects, although only a limited number of studies adopting this approach have included participants experiencing clinically significant levels of anxiety (Broocks et al., 1998; Esquivel et al., 2008; Strickland & Smith, 2014). In a recent review of RCTs and meta-analyses examining the relationship between exercise and anxiety, Stonerock and colleagues (2015) cautioned against definitive conclusions on the basis of a number of limitations in the current research, but tentatively maintained that there was evidence to suggest that exercise could have beneficial effects for anxiety reduction.

A further domain that has received attention in terms of the effects of physical activity is general cognitive functioning. Since a seminal study by Spirduso (1975), in which older men who had been regularly physically active were found to have faster reaction times than their less physically active counterparts, there has been an emerging view that exercise has a positive relationship with cognitive functioning. The general mechanism thought to underpin such relationships is that physical activity produces physiological responses that affect the brain and these in turn have measurable cognitive and behavioural effects. Across the lifespan, physical activity appears to be inversely associated with age-related cognitive decline and age-related loss of brain tissue (Bherer, Erickson, & Liu-Ambrose, 2013; Gomez-Pinilla & Hillman, 2013). Cross-sectional and longitudinal investigations typically support positive links between physical activity and cognitive function, although individual RCTs have sometimes produced inconsistent results (see Young, Angevaren, Rusted, & Tabet, 2015). Nevertheless, several narrative reviews and meta-analytic studies have concluded that there is a small but consistent effect whereby participation in physical activity can result in increased performance across a variety of cognitive tasks (Chang, Labban, Gapin, & Etnier, 2012; Etnier et al., 1997; Lambourne & Tomporowski, 2010; McMorris & Graydon, 2000).

Attention has also been given to the links between physical activity and a host of other psychological constructs, and although the evidence is not as strong as for the aforementioned domains there is a growing number of results suggestive of positive effects of physical activity on mood, self-esteem, and body image. For example, while many people claim that exercise makes them feel better and there appears to be widespread belief in the efficacy of physical activity as a contributor to positive mood and affect (Gauvin & Spence, 1996), well-designed RCTs examining the effects of physical activity on general mood state and affect are not common. Nevertheless, narrative reviews of the available literature have suggested that exercise can be associated with elevations in mood across a variety of exercise types (Gauvin & Spence, 1996; Scully, Kremer, Meade, Graham, & Dudgeon, 1998) and a recent meta-analysis found acute bouts of aerobic exercise to produce increases in positive affect (Reed & Ones, 2006).

Self-esteem reflects an individual's overall evaluation of their own worth and is often taken as having prospective impact on important life outcomes such as academic achievement, relationship satisfaction, employment status, employment satisfaction, and mental health (Orth, Robins, & Widaman, 2012). A meta-analysis of 113 studies examining the relationship between exercise and self-esteem found a small effect with participation in physical activity bringing about an increase in self-esteem, and the magnitude of the effect being positively influenced by the degree of change in physical fitness (Spence, McGannon, & Poon, 2005). A similar small effect was identified in a review of research examining the relationship between exercise and self-esteem in children and adolescents (Ekeland, Heian, Hagen, & Coren, 2005).

Efforts have also been made to examine the potential effects of physical activity on body image. Body image is conceived of as a person's internal representation (including perceptual, affective, cognitive, and behavioural dimensions) of their physical appearance and has been found to be related to a range of psychological and behavioural factors including smoking (Croghan et al., 2006), sexual functioning (Wiederman, 2002), emotional well-being (Johnson & Wardle, 2005), depression (Stice & Bearman, 2001), and eating disorders (Stice, Presnell, & Spangler, 2002). Narrative reviews of the research literature have provided some support for a positive effect of exercise on body image, but also highlighted several methodological constraints and equivocal findings (e.g., Martin & Lichtenberger, 2002). More recent meta-analyses (Campbell & Hausenblas, 2009; Hausenblas & Fallon, 2006; Reel et al., 2007) have provided evidence for small, but significant, positive effects of exercise and physical activity on body image.

While the above sections highlight some of the recent evidence suggesting that physical activity can have beneficial impacts on a number of domains of psychological functioning and well-being, many questions and issues remain unresolved. At the top of this list are questions concerning the explicit mechanisms through which physical activity exerts influence on psychological functioning. For example, if exercise can have a therapeutic, anti-depressant effect, exactly how does this effect come about? Several such explanations have been offered, including changes to monoamine neurotransmitters (e.g., Dunn & Dishman, 1991), increases in cerebral blood-flow (e.g., Etnier, 2008), changes in endorphin levels (e.g., Morgan, 1985), changes in neurotrophins (e.g., Russo-Neustadt, Beard, & Cotman, 1999), changes in body temperature (e.g., Youngstedt, Dishman, Cureton, & Peacock, 1993), protection from oxidative stress (e.g., Ji, 2002), distraction effects (e.g., Yeung, 1996), enhancement of self-efficacy (e.g., North, McCullagh, & Tran, 1990), and social interaction (e.g., North et al., 1990). Nevertheless, the mechanisms responsible for the psychological functioning effects of physical activity remain unclear. It is likely that no single mechanism accounts for any particular observed effect and that different mechanisms may interact to produce different effects. Research that further elucidates the relevant causal mechanisms will greatly enhance understanding of the effects of physical activity on psychological functioning and be an important contributor to prescribing behavioural recommendations for the promotion of psychological health and well-being.

Similarly, further insight of the moderating variables that affect the relationship between physical activity and psychological functioning will greatly improve the efficacy of physical activity as an intervention option. The current chapter has made minimal reference to such issues but the research literature is replete with considerations of moderating variables, albeit often in an inconsistent and equivocal manner. Paramount among moderating variables is consideration of the type of physical activity that is being examined. Exercise is sometimes classified as either acute or chronic, with acute exercise typically involving a single session at a specified level of intensity and duration, and chronic exercise involving multiple sessions of acute exercise repeated over a sustained period of time. Further characterisations are often made between forms of exercise that are aerobic and anaerobic in nature, and then between forms such as resistance exercise and flexibility training. Still further characterisations are made in terms of the intensity of an exercise activity and in the duration of an exercise activity. These issues are sometimes framed in terms of a dose-response relationship and essentially involve working out the exercise patterns required to best produce concomitant psychological benefits. For example, acute bouts of aerobic exercise at submaximal intensity may have differential (and potentially opposite, that is, facilitative vs. debilitative) effects on some measures of cognitive performance dependent on the duration of the exercise (Tomporowski, 2003). This example not only highlights the complexity of the relationship between exercise and cognition (and psychology in general), but also the importance of explicitly identifying and examining moderating variables. Part of the research goal here is to not only gain insight into the type of physical activity that might be most efficacious, but also to gain insight into both the minimal and optimal amount of that activity that is required to bring about positive psychological effects, and further, to gain insight into potential maximal amounts of activity at which point the psychological gains from physical activity may begin to plateau or even decline. For the most part, dose-response relationships and their associated issues remain poorly understood. Specifying the type, intensity, duration, and frequency of physical activity that best results in positive psychological outcomes is a pressing goal in exercise psychology.

A second general category of moderating variables is in terms of the individual characteristics of the exerciser. Attempts have been made to understand how broad social and demographic variables such as sex, age, ethnicity, and socioeconomic status impact on the relationship between physical activity and psychological functioning, as well as more specific individual differences that consider factors such as a person's current level of physical fitness and psychological health. A good example here is a distinction between research with clinical populations and non-clinical populations. Several lines of evidence, including RCTs, suggest that various forms of exercise may have short-term anxiolytic effects but only a small subset of this research has been conducted with participants experiencing anxiety at clinical levels. As such, conclusions regarding the efficacy of physical activity as a treatment for anxiety disorder remain tentative. Similarly, how physical activity compares and/or combines with other forms of mental health intervention such as cognitive behavioural therapy and drug therapy, and indeed how a whole range of potential moderating variables interact, is only just beginning to be examined.

Psychology as antecedent: the effects of psychology on physical activity

A second prominent approach in exercise psychology is to treat psychological factors as antecedent to physical activity behaviour. A conceptual starting point to much of this research is that despite widespread acceptance that regular physical activity has numerous health benefits (both physical and mental) and extensive efforts to promote physical activity, large numbers of people are inactive to the point that physical inactivity is considered a major contributor to ill-health (Bouchard et al., 2012). This 'puzzle of exercise' – in which physical activity is seen to offer numerous health benefits but engage insufficient levels of participation to engender many of those benefits – has become a central issue in exercise psychology. In essence, this issue is often framed in terms of attempting to understand the factors that determine the adoption and maintenance of physical activity behaviour. At the core of this approach, is the idea that understanding these determinant factors may then offer an avenue for developing effective intervention strategies and increasing the prevalence of physical activity behaviour. What then are some of the psychological factors that influence participation in physical activity and how do they do so?

One attempt used to address the question of what influences participation in physical activity has involved identifying a range of variables that are correlated with physical activity. This method was once common in the exercise psychology literature and a host of psychologically relevant correlates of physical activity have been identified. For example, age, sex, health status, social support, self-efficacy for exercise, intentions to exercise, perceived health and fitness, perceived social support, attitudes toward exercise, personality, stress, and enjoyment are some of the factors that have been linked to participation in exercise and physical activity (Bauman et al., 2012).

This correlate variable research, which is often undertaken with the use of cross-sectional studies, offers an interesting starting point for understanding the psychological determinants of physical activity but does not necessarily identify any causal relationships. As such, other approaches have often attempted to integrate understanding of correlated variables with theoretical models that endeavour to explain the causal connections of those variables to physical activity. While a number of theoretical models have been employed in attempts to account for physical activity behaviour, the most dominant approach has been through the use of psychosocial models.

One of the earliest psychological models to be applied to understanding physical activity was that of social cognitive theory (Bandura, 1977, 1986, 1997). Social cognitive theory is a theoretical approach that attempts to explain how people acquire and maintain particular patterns of behaviour and posits a three-way model of reciprocal causation between behaviour, environment, and individual cognitive factors. While a full account of social cognitive theory is not warranted here, two key constructs within the theory have been viewed as particularly relevant to understanding physical activity behaviour. The first of these constructs, self-efficacy, reflects a person's belief in their ability to achieve a particular behavioural outcome, and is sometimes viewed as a form of content specific self-confidence. More precisely, self-efficacy is concerned with an individual's perception that he or she has the necessary resources to perform a specific behaviour (Bandura, 1977). For example, an experienced and healthy middle-distance runner may have high self-efficacy for running continuously for 60 minutes, while a similarly experienced middle-distance runner who has recently suffered a broken leg may have low self-efficacy for the same task. Self-efficacy is often taken as having a causal effect on the types of activity that people engage in and is viewed as having particular utility as a determinate factor in accounting for the health-related behaviours that people choose to engage in (Luszczynska & Schwarzer, 2005). The second construct, outcome expectations, reflects the consequences that a person anticipates will follow from performing a particular behaviour. For example, an outcome expectation for a sustained resistance-training programme might be increases in strength and muscle size. Both self-efficacy and outcome expectations have been considered important antecedent factors for physical activity and both have received empirical research attention (McAuley & Blissmer, 2000), but it is self-efficacy that has received the most consistent support as a predictor of exercise participation and adherence across a variety of contexts and populations (e.g., McAuley & Blissmer, 2000; Rodgers & Brawley, 1993; Rovniak, Anderson, Winett, & Stephens, 2002; Sweet et al., 2009). The general pattern to emerge is that as self-efficacy for physical activity increases, so too does the likelihood of participation in physical activity.

Social cognitive theory, particularly the construct of self-efficacy and its consistent relationship with physical activity, has had significant impact in exercise psychology and attempts to change self-efficacy have served as a basis for efforts to ultimately change physical activity behaviour (e.g., Burke, Beilin, Cutt, Mansour, & Mori, 2008; Darker, French, Eves, & Sniehotta, 2010). Indeed, Bandura's (1977) initial account of social cognitive theory describes a number of influences on self-efficacy that provide clear targets for attempts to modify self-efficacy and some research has now turned to evaluating the effectiveness of various methods for altering self-efficacy in a physical activity context (e.g., French, Olander, Chisholm, & McSharry, 2014; Williams & French, 2011). Nevertheless, despite the emphasis on self-efficacy, physical activity interventions that have employed the full theoretical model of social cognitive theory have been limited and often produced equivocal results, and it is clear that self-efficacy is only a small part of a much larger puzzle with social cognitive theory having only limited success in accounting for physical activity behaviour.

The theory of planned behaviour (Ajzen, 1985) is another theoretical model that has received much attention in physical activity research. This approach holds that a person's behavioural intentions are the most proximate predictor of that person's actual behaviour. Behavioural intentions are influenced by the constructs of attitudes, subjective norms, and perceived behavioural control. More specifically, within this model behavioural intentions are viewed as a motivational construct that represent the degree of investment that a person is willing to make in regards to performing a particular behaviour. The other three constructs of attitudes, subjective norms, and perceived behavioural control are thought to have causal influence in determining behavioural intentions. Attitudes for example, capture a person's overall evaluation of a particular behaviour and reflect a set of behavioural beliefs about the costs and benefits of the behaviour. Subjective norms refer to a person's beliefs about how significant others would want them to behave and reflect a set of normative beliefs about the perceived social influences and pressures to perform (or not perform) a behaviour. Finally, the construct of perceived behavioural control captures a person's beliefs about their ability to perform certain behaviours and reflects a set of beliefs about the presence of factors that may facilitate or inhibit the performance of the behaviour. In a sense, the construct of perceived behavioural control operates in a similar capacity to that of self-efficacy.

The theory of planned behaviour has received much attention in exercise psychology research and individual studies have had some measure of success in using the theory to explain and predict physical activity behaviour. One of the advantages of the theory of planned behaviour is that it has been able to flexibly integrate or mediate more distal constructs and factors into its explanatory framework. For example, the perceived behavioural control component accounts for a range of commonly cited inhibitors and facilitators of physical activity such as bad weather, lack of time, and fatigue, while the attitude and subjective norm constructs may mediate the effects of a more distal construct such as personality on physical activity. Several reviews and meta-analyses have been conducted (Hagger, Chatzisarantis, & Biddle, 2002b; Hausenblas, Carron, & Mack, 1997; Symons Downs & Hausenblas, 2005) with the evidence suggesting that the theory has some general utility in accounting for physical activity behaviour. Behavioural intentions have been found to be a significant predictor of actual behaviour and all primary constructs within the theory of planned behaviour have been found to exert significant effects on behavioural intentions, with attitudes and perceived behavioural control exhibiting the largest effects. In general, the results of these meta-analytic studies suggest that the theory of planned behaviour can be a useful psychological model for explaining physical activity behaviour.

Social cognitive theory and the theory of planned behaviour represent just two examples of a larger set of psychosocial models that have been employed to examine the psychological antecedents of physical activity. While the research base is perhaps the most robust for the two examples given, other approaches such as self-determination theory (Deci & Ryan, 1985), protection motivation theory (Rogers, 1983), and the transtheoretical model (Prochaska & DiClemente, 1982) have been widely used as a theoretical base for explaining physical activity behaviour. Generally speaking, all of the previously mentioned models have shown degrees of utility in accounting for physical activity and each has particular strengths and limitations.

A full consideration of each psychosocial model is far beyond the scope of the current chapter, but three general points should be noted. First, there appears to be considerable overlap and redundancy across many of the models (Bandura, 2004). That is, several of the proposed constructs are essentially performing the same explanatory functions. As such, there have been recent attempts to integrate various elements of complementary psychosocial models both in order to reduce construct redundancy and to strengthen explanatory breadth and depth. For example, Hagger, Chatzisarantis, and Biddle (2002a) have found that motivational orientations from self-determination theory affect behavioural intentions for physical activity but do so via the constructs of attitudes and perceived behavioural control that are integral components of the theory of planned behaviour. Only a relatively small body of research has examined integrated psychosocial models for the determinants of physical activity, but the initial empirical support has been encouraging and integration offers a promising avenue for theoretical development. Second, with some exceptions, there have been relatively few examples of well-designed experimental intervention studies that have tested the full mediating capacities of the respective theories and constructs. One of the goals in the development of theoretical models in exercise psychology is to inform and guide practical efforts to promote physical activity participation (Rhodes & Pfaeffli, 2010). As such, developing and testing interventions on the basis of constructs and mechanisms that are known to mediate effects on physical activity is to be encouraged. Finally, while several psychosocial theories have shown utility in explaining the links between psychology and physical activity, they typically only account for a small proportion of the variation in observed behaviour. That is, despite their prominence in exercise psychology research, it seems reasonable to conclude that factors other than the explicit cognitive constructs identified in conventional psychosocial theories are significantly affecting physical activity participation and adherence.

An alternative approach to the social-cognitive models discussed above has been to examine exercise participation from an affective or hedonistic perspective. The central idea here is that people often do what makes them feel good and avoid what makes them feel bad, and that for many people and in many contexts, physical activity may be an aversive experience. Proponents of this approach suggest that despite widespread belief that physical activity makes people feel better, methodological limitations including failure to appropriately consider and measure negative affective states, means that negative experiences of physical activity are often neglected (e.g., Backhouse, Ekkekakis, Bidle, Foskett, & Williams, 2007). This idea could be considered an example of a broader approach to understanding the links between psychology and physical activity that begins to incorporate more implicit and automatic psychological processes alongside the more explicit and volitional processes that have typically characterised much of the research in the area. This dual-process approach has had substantial influence in many areas of psychology and holds much potential for advancing understanding of the psychological processes that affect physical activity.

Conclusion

This chapter has presented a broad overview of some of the recent research that has attempted to understand the relationships between psychology and physical activity. Synthesising this research presents inherent challenges due to the myriad goals, theories, methods, and findings that characterise the field. A further challenge is that any broad synthesis is likely to be simplifying and the scope of this chapter has limited deeper critical discussion of current issues. Nevertheless, a picture has emerged of a large and growing body of evidence demonstrating that physical activity has beneficial effects on a range of indices of psychological functioning. Understanding how these effects come about and the contexts in which physical activity is most likely to affect psychological functioning could have considerable benefits for efforts to promote health and well-being. Moreover, a host of psychological factors antecedent to physical activity have been identified and continuing progress in understanding the mechanisms of how these factors exert influence on physical activity behaviour will provide insight into how physical activity can best be promoted to achieve improvements in health and well-being.

Chapter summary

- Physical activity has a range of positive effects on mental health and psychological functioning.
- Understanding the causal mechanisms by which physical activity produces psychological effects and the factors that moderate such effects will increase the efficacy of physical activity for the promotion of psychological health and well-being.
- A number of psychological factors influence participation in physical activity.
- Interventions that target the malleable psychological determinates of physical activity offer scope for increasing participation in physical activity.

References

Abu-Omar, K., Rutten, A., & Lehtinen, V. (2004). Mental health and physical activity in the European Union. *Sozial-Und Praventivmedizin, 49*(5), 301–309.

Ajzen, I. (1985). From intentions to actions: a theory of planned behavior. In J. Kuhl & J. Beckmann (Eds.), *Action control: from cognition to behavior* (pp. 11–39). New York: Springer-Verlag.

Backhouse, S.H., Ekkekakis, P., Bidle, S.J., Foskett, A., & Williams, C. (2007). Exercise makes people feel better but people are inactive: paradox or artifact? *Journal of Sport and Exercise Psychology, 29*(4), 498–517.

Bandelow, B., & Michaelis, S. (2015). Epidemiology of anxiety disorders in the 21st century. *Dialogues in Clinical Neuroscience, 17*(3), 327–335.

Bandura, A. (1977). *Social learning theory*. Englewood Cliffs, NJ: Prentice Hall.

Bandura, A. (1986). *The foundations of thought and action*. Englewood Cliffs, NJ: Prentice Hall.

Bandura, A. (1997). *Self-efficacy: the exercise of control*. New York: Freeman.

Bandura, A. (2004). Health promotion by social cognitive means. *Health Education and Behavior, 31*(2), 143–164. doi: 10.1177/1090198104263660

Bauman, A.E., Reis, R.S., Sallis, J.F., Wells, J.C., Loos, R.J.F., & Martin, B.W. (2012). Correlates of physical activity: why are some people physically active and others not? *The Lancet, 380*(9838), 258–271. doi: 10.1016/S0140-6736(12)60735-1

Bherer, L., Erickson, K.I., & Liu-Ambrose, T. (2013). A review of the effects of physical activity and exercise on cognitive and brain functions in older adults. *Journal of Aging Research, 2013*, 657508. doi: 10.1155/2013/657508

Bouchard, C., Blair, S.N., & Haskell, W. (2012). *Physical activity and health* (2nd ed.). Champaign, IL: Human Kinetics.

Broocks, A., Bandelow, B., Pekrun, G., George, A., Meyer, T., Bartmann, U., . . . Rüther, E. (1998). Comparison of aerobic exercise, clompipramine, and placebo in the treatment of panic disorder. *American Journal of Psychiatry, 155*, 603–609.

Burke, V., Beilin, L.J., Cutt, H.E., Mansour, J., & Mori, T.A. (2008). Moderators and mediators of behaviour change in a lifestyle program for treated hypertensives: a randomized controlled trial (ADAPT). *Health Education Research, 23*(4), 583–591. doi: 10.1093/her/cym047

Campbell, A., & Hausenblas, H.A. (2009). Effects of exercise interventions on body image: a meta-analysis. *Journal of Health Psychology, 14*(6), 780–793. doi: 10.1177/1359105309338977

Chang, Y.K., Labban, J.D., Gapin, J.I., & Etnier, J.L. (2012). The effects of acute exercise on cognitive performance: a meta-analysis. *Brain Research, 1453*, 87–101. doi: http://dx.doi.org/10.1016/j.brainres.2012.02.068

Cooney, G.M., Dwan, K., Greig, C.A., Lawlor, D.A., Rimer, J., Waugh, F.R., . . . Mead, G.E. (2013). Exercise for depression. *Cochrane Database of Systematic Reviews, 9*(Cd004366). doi: 10.1002/14651858.CD004366.pub6

Croghan, I.T., Bronars, C., Patten, C.A., Schroeder, D.R., Nirelli, L.M., Thomas, J.L., . . . Hurt, R.D. (2006). Is smoking related to body image satisfaction, stress, and self-esteem in young adults? *American Journal of Health Behavior, 30*(3), 322–333. doi: 10.5555/ajhb.2006.30.3.322

Darker, C.D., French, D.P., Eves, F.F., & Sniehotta, F.F. (2010). An intervention to promote walking amongst the general population based on an 'extended' theory of planned behaviour: a waiting list randomised controlled trial. *Psychology & Health, 25*(1), 71–88. doi: 10.1080/08870440902893716

De Moor, M.H., Beem, A.L., Stubbe, J.H., Boomsma, D.I., & De Geus, E.J. (2006). Regular exercise, anxiety, depression and personality: a population-based study. *Preventive Medicine, 42*(4), 273–279. doi: 10.1016/j.ypmed.2005.12.002

Deci, E.L., & Ryan, R.M. (1985). *Intrinsic motivation and self determination in human behavior*. New York: Plenum.

Dunn, A.L., & Dishman, R.K. (1991). Exercise and the neurobiology of depression. *Exercise and Sport Sciences Reviews, 19*(1), 41–98.

Ekeland, E., Heian, F., Hagen, K., & Coren, E. (2005). Can exercise improve self esteem in children and young people? A systematic review of randomised controlled trials. *British Journal of Sports Medicine, 39*(11), 792–798. doi: 10.1136/bjsm.2004.017707

Esquivel, G., Diaz-Galvis, J., Schruers, K., Berlanga, C., Lara-Munoz, C., & Griez, E. (2008). Acute exercise reduces the effects of a 35% CO_2 challenge in patients with panic disorder. *Journal of Affective Disorders, 107*(1–3), 217–220. doi: 10.1016/j.jad.2007.07.022

Etnier, J.L. (2008). Mediators of the exercise and cognition relationship. In W.W. Spirduso, L.W. Poon, & W.J. Chodzko-Zajko (Eds.), *Aging, exercise, and cognition series: exercise and its mediating effects on cognition* (pp. 13–32). Urbana-Champaign, IL: Human Kinetics.

Etnier, J.L., Salazar, W., Landers, D.M., Petruzzello, S.J., Han, M., & Nowell, P. (1997). The influence of physical fitness and exercise upon cognitive functioning: a meta-analysis. *Journal of Sport and Exercise Psychology, 19*(3), 249–277. doi:10.1123/jsep.19.3.249

Faulkner, G.E.J., & Taylor, A.H. (2005). *Exercise, health and mental health: emerging relationships.* New York: Routledge.

French, D.P., Olander, E.K., Chisholm, A., & McSharry, J. (2014). Which behaviour change techniques are most effective at increasing older adults' self-efficacy and physical activity behaviour? A systematic review. *Annals of Behavioral Medicine, 48*(2), 225–234. doi: 10.1007/s12160-014-9593-z

Gauvin, L., & Spence, J.C. (1996). Physical activity and psychological well-being: knowledge base, current issues, and caveats. *Nutrition Reviews, 54*(4), 13.

Gomez-Pinilla, F., & Hillman, C. (2013). The influence of exercise on cognitive abilities. *Comprehensive Physiology, 3*(1), 403–428. doi: 10.1002/cphy.c110063

Goodwin, R.D. (2003). Association between physical activity and mental disorders among adults in the United States. *Preventive Medicine, 36*(6), 698–703.

Hagger, M.S., Chatzisarantis, N.L.D., & Biddle, S.J.H. (2002a). The influence of autonomous and controlling motives on physical activity intentions within the Theory of Planned Behaviour. *British Journal of Health Psychology, 7*, 283–297. doi: 10.1348/135910702760213689

Hagger, M.S., Chatzisarantis, N.L.D., & Biddle, S.J.H. (2002b). A meta-analytic review of the theories of reasoned action and planned behavior in physical activity: predictive validity and the contribution of additional variables. *Journal of Sport and Exercise Psychology, 24*(1), 3–32. doi: 10.1123/jsep.24.1.3

Hausenblas, H.A., Carron, A.V., & Mack, D.E. (1997). Application of the theories of Reasoned Action and Planned Behavior to exercise behavior: a meta-analysis. *Journal of Sport and Exercise Psychology, 19*(1), 36–51. doi: 10.1123/jsep.19.1.36

Hausenblas, H.A., & Fallon, E.A. (2006). Exercise and body image: A meta-analysis. *Psychology & Health, 21*(1), 33–47. doi: 10.1080/14768320500105270

Ji, L.L. (2002). Exercise-induced modulation of antioxidant defense. *Annals of the New York Academy of Sciences, 959*, 82–92.

Johnson, F., & Wardle, J. (2005). Dietary restraint, body dissatisfaction, and psychological distress: a prospective analysis. *Journal of Abnormal Psychology, 114*(1), 119–125. doi: 10.1037/0021-843x.114.1.119

Josefsson, T., Lindwall, M., & Archer, T. (2014). Physical exercise intervention in depressive disorders: meta-analysis and systematic review. *Scandinavian Journal of Medicine & Science in Sports, 24*(2), 259–272. doi: 10.1111/sms.12050

Kessler, R.C., & Bromet, E.J. (2013). The epidemiology of depression across cultures. *Annual Review of Public Health, 34*, 119–138. doi: 10.1146/annurev-publhealth-031912-114409

Kessler, R.C., Wai, T.C., Demler, O., & Walters, E.E. (2005). Prevalence, severity, and comorbidity of 12-month DSM-IV disorders in the National Comorbidity Survey Replication. *Archives of General Psychiatry, 62*(6), 617–627. doi: 10.1001/archpsyc.62.6.617

Kvam, S., Kleppe, C.L., Nordhus, I.H., & Hovland, A. (2016). Exercise as a treatment for depression: a meta-analysis. *Journal of Affective Disorders, 202*, 67–86. doi: http://dx.doi.org/10.1016/j.jad.2016.03.063

Lambourne, K., & Tomporowski, P. (2010). The effect of exercise-induced arousal on cognitive task performance: a meta-regression analysis. *Brain Research, 1341*, 12–24. doi: 10.1016/j.brainres.2010.03.091

Luszczynska, A., & Schwarzer, R. (2005). Social cognitive theory. In M. Conner & P. Norman (Eds.), *Predicting health behaviour* (2nd ed., pp. 127–169). Buckingham, England: Open University Press.

Martin, K.A., & Lichtenberger, C.M. (2002). Fitness enhancement and changes in body image. In T.F. Cash & T. Pruzinsky (Eds.), *A handbook of theory, research, and clinical practice* (pp. 414–421). New York: Guildford Press.

Martin, P. (2003). The epidemiology of anxiety disorders: a review. *Dialogues in Clinical Neuroscience, 5*(3), 281–298.

McAuley, E. (1992). The role of efficacy cognitions in the prediction of exercise behavior in middle-aged adults. *Journal of Behavioral Medicine, 15*(1), 65–88. doi: 10.1007/bf00848378

McAuley, E., & Blissmer, B. (2000). Self-efficacy determinants and consequences of physical activity. *Exercise and Sport Science Reviews, 28*(2), 85–88.

McMorris, T., & Graydon, J. (2000). The effect of incremental exercise on cognitive performance. *International Journal of Sport Psychology, 31*(1), 66–81.

Morgan, W.P. (1985). Affective beneficence of vigorous physical activity. *Medicine and Science in Sports and Exercise, 17*(1), 94–100.

Motl, R.W., Birnbaum, A.S., Kubik, M.Y., & Dishman, R.K. (2004). Naturally occurring changes in physical activity are inversely related to depressive symptoms during early adolescence. *Psychosomatic Medicine, 66*(3), 336–342.

North, T.C., McCullagh, P., & Tran, Z.V. (1990). Effect of exercise on depression. *Exercise and Sport Sciences Reviews, 18*(1), 379–416.

Orth, U., Robins, R.W., & Widaman, K.F. (2012). Life-span development of self-esteem and its effects on important life outcomes. *Journal of Personality and Social Psychology, 102*(6), 1271–1288. doi: 10.1037/a0025558

Prochaska, J.O., & DiClemente, C.C. (1982). Transtheoretical therapy: toward a more integrative model of change. *Psychotherapy:Theory, Research & Practice, 19*(3), 276–288.

Reed, J., & Ones, D.S. (2006). The effect of acute aerobic exercise on positive activated affect: a meta-analysis. *Psychology of Sport and Exercise, 7*(5), 477–514. doi: http://dx.doi.org/10.1016/j.psychsport.2005.11.003

Reel, J.J., Greenleaf, C., Baker, W.K., Aragon, S., Bishop, D., Cachaper, C., . . . Hattie, J. (2007). Relations of body concerns and exercise behavior: a meta-analysis. *Psychological Reports, 101*(3 Pt 1), 927–942. doi: 10.2466/pr0.101.3.927-942

Rethorst, C.D., Wipfli, B.M., & Landers, D.M. (2009). The antidepressive effects of exercise: a meta-analysis of randomized trials. *Sports Medicine, 39*(6), 491–511. doi: 10.2165/00007256-200939060-00004

Rhodes, R.E., & Pfaeffli, L.A. (2010). Mediators of physical activity behaviour change among adult non-clinical populations: a review update. *International Journal of Behavioral Nutrition and Physical Activity, 7,* 37. doi: 10.1186/1479-5868-7-37

Richards, C.S., & O'Hara, M.W. (2014). *The Oxford handbook of depression and comorbidity*. New York: Oxford University Press.

Rodgers, W.M., & Brawley, L.R. (1993). Using both self-efficacy theory and the theory of planned behavior to discriminate adherers and dropouts from structured programs. *Journal of Applied Sport Psychology, 5*(2), 195–206. doi: 10.1080/10413209308411314

Rogers, R.W. (1983). Cognitive and physiological processes in fear appeals and attitude change: a revised theory of protection motivation. In J.T. Cacioppo & R.E. Petty (Eds.), *Social psychophysiology* (pp. 153–176). New York: Guildford Press.

Rovniak, L.S., Anderson, E.S., Winett, R.A., & Stephens, R.S. (2002). Social cognitive determinants of physical activity in young adults: a prospective structural equation analysis. *Annals of Behavioral Medicine, 24*(2), 149–156.

Russo-Neustadt, A., Beard, R.C., & Cotman, C.W. (1999). Exercise, antidepressant medications, and enhanced brain derived neurotrophic factor expression. *Neuropsychopharmacology, 21*(5), 679–682. doi: 10.1016/s0893-133x(99)00059-7

Schuch, F.B., Vancampfort, D., Richards, J., Rosenbaum, S., Ward, P.B., & Stubbs, B. (2016). Exercise as a treatment for depression: a meta-analysis adjusting for publication bias. *Journal of Psychiatric Research, 77,* 42–51. doi: http://dx.doi.org/10.1016/j.jpsychires.2016.02.023

Scully, D., Kremer, J., Meade, M.M., Graham, R., & Dudgeon, K. (1998). Physical exercise and psychological well being: a critical review. *British Journal of Sports Medicine, 32*(2), 111–120.

Spence, J.C., McGannon, K.R., & Poon, P. (2005). The effect of exercise on global self-esteem: a quantitative review. *Journal of Sport and Exercise Psychology, 27*(3), 311–334. doi:10.1123/jsep.27.3.311

Spirduso, W.W. (1975). Reaction and movement time as a function of age and physical activity level. *Journal of Gerontology, 30*(4), 435–440.

Steptoe, A., Wardle, J., Fuller, R., Holte, A., Justo, J., Sanderman, R., & Wichstrom, L. (1997). Leisure-time physical exercise: prevalence, attitudinal correlates, and behavioral correlates among young Europeans from 21 countries. *Preventive Medicine, 26*(6), 845–854. doi: 10.1006/pmed.1997.0224

Stice, E., & Bearman, S.K. (2001). Body-image and eating disturbances prospectively predict increases in depressive symptoms in adolescent girls: a growth curve analysis. *Developmental Psychology, 37*(5), 597–607.

Stice, E., Presnell, K., & Spangler, D. (2002). Risk factors for binge eating onset in adolescent girls: a 2-year prospective investigation. *Health Psychology, 21*(2), 131–138.

Stonerock, G.L., Hoffman, B.M., Smith, P.J., & Blumenthal, J.A. (2015). Exercise as treatment for anxiety: systematic review and analysis. *Annals of Behavioral Medicine, 49*(4), 542–556. doi: 10.1007/s12160-014-9685-9

Strickland, J.C., & Smith, M.A. (2014). The anxiolytic effects of resistance exercise. *Frontiers in Psychology, 5*, 753. doi: 10.3389/fpsyg.2014.00753

Strohle, A., Hofler, M., Pfister, H., Muller, A.G., Hoyer, J., Wittchen, H.U., & Lieb, R. (2007). Physical activity and prevalence and incidence of mental disorders in adolescents and young adults. *Psychological Medicine, 37*(11), 1657–1666. doi: 10.1017/s003329170700089x

Sweet, S.N., Fortier, M.S., Guerin, E., Tulloch, H., Sigal, R.J., Kenny, G.P., & Reid, R.D. (2009). Understanding physical activity in adults with type 2 diabetes after completing an exercise intervention trial: a mediation model of self-efficacy and autonomous motivation. *Psychology, Health & Medicine, 14*(4), 419–429. doi: 10.1080/13548500903111806

Symons Downs, D., & Hausenblas, H.A. (2005). The theories of reasoned action and planned behavior applied to exercise: a meta-analytic update. *Journal of Physical Activity and Health, 2*(1), 76–97. doi: 10.1123/jpah.2.1.76

Tomporowski, P.D. (2003). Effects of acute bouts of exercise on cognition. *Acta Psychologica* (Amsterdam), *112*(3), 297–324.

USDHHS. (1996). *Physical activity and health: a report of the surgeon general.* Atlanta: GA: U.S. Department of Health and Human Services, Centers for Disease Control and Prevention, National Center for Chronic Disease Prevention and Health Promotion.

Vigo, D., Thornicroft, G., & Atun, R. (2016). Estimating the true global burden of mental illness. *The Lancet Psychiatry, 3*(2), 171–178. doi: 10.1016/S2215-0366(15)00505-2

Wiederman, M.W. (2002). Body image and sexual functioning. In T.F. Cash & T.T. Pruzinsky (Eds.), *Body image: a handbook of theory, research, and clinical practice* (pp. 287–294). New York: Guildford Press.

Williams, S.L., & French, D.P. (2011). What are the most effective intervention techniques for changing physical activity self-efficacy and physical activity behaviour – and are they the same? *Health Education Research, 26*(2), 308–322. doi: 10.1093/her/cyr005

Yeung, R.R. (1996). The acute effects of exercise on mood state. *Journal of Psychosomatic Research, 40*(2), 123–141. doi: http://dx.doi.org/10.1016/0022-3999(95)00554-4

Young, J., Angevaren, M., Rusted, J., & Tabet, N. (2015). Aerobic exercise to improve cognitive function in older people without known cognitive impairment. *Cochrane Database of Systematic Reviews, 4*(CD005381). doi: 10.1002/14651858.CD005381.pub4

Youngstedt, S.D., Dishman, R.K., Cureton, K.J., & Peacock, L.J. (1993). Does body temperature mediate anxiolytic effects of acute exercise? *Journal of Applied Physiology, 74*(2), 825–831.

15 Neurophysiology and physical activity

Michael J. Grey, Simon Franklin and Nick Kitchen

Keywords: Ageing, development, central nervous system, neuroplasticity, neuroprotection, peripheral nervous system

Throughout one's lifetime, physical activity has a wide variety of effects in the central and peripheral nervous systems. The effects of exercise are apparent from the molecular and cellular levels to macroscopic structural changes in neural tissue, all of which are manifested in cognitive and behavioural changes. In the last few decades there has been a surge of interest in understanding the mechanisms by which physical exercise can enhance the nervous system promoting healthy brain function and protecting it against the development of neurodegeneration. As a result, there is now a plethora of evidence from both animal and human research demonstrating that physical exercise is associated with structural and functional changes in the nervous system including angiogenesis, neurogenesis, increased synaptic plasticity, enhanced neurotransmitter release.

This chapter presents an overview of the role of physical activity in normal neurological development and the benefits of physical activity in maintaining neurological functioning across the lifespan. Whilst we touch briefly on the beneficial effects of physical activity on broad neural functioning such as cognition and behavioural change (of which there is a vast literature) our main intention here is to focus on the neurophysiological changes that underpin these phenomena. Similarly, neurodegeneration is discussed in the context of the neuroprotective effects of physical exercise, but we have specifically avoided the important role of physical activity in neurorehabilitation, neurological disorders, age-related cognitive decline and the treatment of diseases related to neurodegeneration.

Until quite recently the normal/healthy human nervous system was thought to be highly malleable for the first few years of life and thereafter fixed and immutable. We now understand that all parts of the nervous system from the brain to the neuromuscular junction undergo morphological and/or functional changes as a normal process of development, and then through experience-dependent neuroplasticity during adolescence and adulthood. Importantly, even when the nervous system undergoes the normal process of age-related neurodegeneration, it continues to be plastic and, therefore, maintains the ability to adapt and to learn. Experience-dependent neuroplasticity is best effected when the experience (training) is repeated frequently, when the stimulus is specific and intense, when it is challenging and motivating.

Gray and white matter

Chronic exposure to physical activity is linked to structural and physiological changes in the nervous system with several neuroimaging studies showing that aerobic exercise enhances both brain structure and functional connectivity. For example, the reduced brain tissue loss associated with ageing appears to be substantially alleviated with physical exercise. Aerobic fitness is associated with reduced atrophy in the prefrontal cortex, hippocampus, caudate nucleus and cerebellum in older fit adults compared with older sedentary adults (Ahlskog, Geda, Graff-Radford, & Petersen, 2011; Colcombe et al., 2003; Cotman & Berchtold, 2002; Erickson, Miller, & Roecklein, 2012; Maass et al., 2015). Similarly, diffusion tensor imaging studies suggest that the normal age-related decline in white matter integrity is limited in older adults who maintain good cardiovascular fitness (Burzynska et al., 2014; Burzynska et al., 2010; Hayes, Salat, Forman, Sperling, & Verfaellie, 2015).

Perhaps most importantly, gray matter has been shown to increase in adults who participate in an exercise programme. Colcombe et al. (2006) exposed a group of sedentary older adults (aged 60–79) to a 6-month aerobic training protocol involving brisk walking at 60–75% of their maximal heart rate. Gray matter volume in the prefrontal cortex, anterior cingulate cortex, and the lateral temporal lobes increased compared with a control group exposed to a stretching and toning programme. Subsequently, in a much larger study Erickson et al. (2011), used a very similar exercise intervention in older adults and showed that aerobic exercise training increased the size of the anterior hippocampus by 2%. They suggested this reversed the age-related loss in hippocampal volume by 1–2 years. Similarly, Voss et al. (2013) have observed increased white matter integrity following a one-year walking program, although these structural benefits did not translate to functional improvements outside of the improved physical fitness. Thomas et al. (2016) have demonstrated that hippocampus volume can increase in early to middle aged adults with as little as six weeks of aerobic exercise. Importantly, they noted that the increase is not permanent, and that it returned to baseline after a further six weeks without regular aerobic exercise.

Activity-related structural change is not restricted to adults. Kramer's group have used magnetic resonance imaging to demonstrate increased gray matter volume in the hippocampus (Chaddock, Erickson, Prakash, Kim, et al., 2010), basal ganglia (Chaddock, Erickson, Prakash, VanPatter, et al., 2010), as well as increased cortical activity (Chaddock et al., 2012) and functional connectivity (Voss et al., 2011) in frontal and prefrontal lobes in aerobically fit children compared with less fit children. Similar to the older adults, they used diffusion tensor imaging to estimate white matter fibre tract volume, showing that aerobic fitness is positively related in increased microstructure in the corpus callosum, corona radiate, and superior longitudinal fasciculus compared to less fit children (Chaddock-Heyman et al., 2014). They suggested children with higher aerobic fitness would have faster neural connectivity and therefore more efficient communication between different areas of the brain.

Whilst there is robust evidence to support the idea that exercise enhances gray matter volume during development and that it reduces gray matter atrophy associated with ageing, these effects appear to be limited to the areas of the brain responsible for cognition (i.e. executive function and memory). Similar changes have not been reported in areas of the brain responsible for sensorimotor function. However, it is notable that the literature tends to focus on areas of the brain associated with cognition rather than movement and that cortical areas such as the primary, premotor and supplementary motor cortices in addition to the visual cortex do not decline to the same extent as do the cortical areas associated with cognition (Fjell & Walhovd, 2010).

Angiogenesis, neurogenesis and synaptogenesis

Neuroplasticiy is tightly linked to angiogenesis, neurogenesis and synaptogenesis. A fundamental driver for neuroplasticity is the enriched environment, of which physical activity plays an important role. In parallel with the exercise-related increase in neural tissue, vascularisation also appears to be enhanced with exercise. Increased capillary density associated with physical activity has been demonstrated in rodents (Black, Isaacs, Anderson, Alcantara, & Greenough, 1990) and in monkeys trained to run on a treadmill (Rhyu et al., 2010). In humans, magnetic resonance angiography has demonstrated increased blood vessel diameter in elderly individuals with an aerobically active lifestyle compared with sedentary individuals (Bullitt et al., 2009). Maass et al. (2015) have demonstrated that hippocampus vascularisation also improves following a 3-month exercise intervention.

The increased vascularisation associated with exercise likely results in more than simply providing a greater oxygen and glucose supply to the neural tissue. Increased vascularisation has been correlated with increased production of neurotrophic factors, enhanced synaptic plasticity and neurogenesis (Maass et al., 2015). Furthermore, in otherwise healthy ageing rodent models vascular resistance increases and endoneurial blood flow decreases (Kihara, Nickander, & Low, 1991). This disturbs normal resting membrane potentials through impairment of ATP-dependent ion pumps and subsequently reduces the efficiency of action potential propagation. As such, the role of exercise in improving vascularisation of vessels may be important for helping to diminish the effects this may have on neural signalling in the ageing nervous system.

Synaptogenesis and neurogenesis have been directly observed in animal models particularly in the hippocampus, and indirectly in humans. Both synaptogenesis and neurogenesis are preferentially activated during learning tasks. Synaptic plasticity is largely driven by the phenomenon of long-term potentiation (LTP) – a persistent strengthening of synapses based on recent patterns of activity (Bliss & Lomo, 1973). Rodents exposed to treadmill running have exhibited significantly greater LTP in the hippocampus compared with control animals (O'Callaghan, Ohlc, & Kelly, 2007; van Praag, Christie, Sejnowski, & Gage, 1999). Exercise induced LTP is observed in both young rodents and in old rodents when compared with sedentary controls (van Praag, 2009). Dendrites in the hippocampus lengthen, synaptogenesis is increased, and the dendritic tree becomes more dense and complex following exercise (Eadie, Redila, & Christie, 2005; Farmer et al., 2004). Aerobic exercise increases the expression of N-methyl-D-aspartic acid (NMDA) receptors in the hippocampus which also enhances synaptic plasticity (Farmer et al., 2004). Black et al. (1990) were one of the first groups to demonstrate that synaptic function is influenced by the type of training. They compared synaptogenesis in adult rats exposed to voluntary wheel running, forced treadmill running and a programme of acrobatic training (balance beams, see-saws, rope bridges and other obstacles). The rats exposed to the more challenging, novel and stimulating acrobatic exercise group exhibited greater synaptic activity and synaptogenesis.

Whilst synaptogenesis occurs throughout the nervous system, in the mammalian nervous system new neurons are generated in only two areas of adult brain – the olfactory bulb in the lateral ventricles and the dentate gyrus of the hippocampus. Neurogenesis is much greater in young animals, but is not abolished with age. Numerous studies have demonstrated that aerobic exercise increases the rate of neurogenesis and this appears to be one of its strongest stimuli (e.g. Cotman, Berchtold, & Christie, 2007; van Praag et al., 1999; Vivar, Potter, & van Praag, 2013). Whilst a large proportion of newly generated neurons do not survive (Kempermann et al., 2010), exercise appears to ameliorate the loss survivability of these new neurons (Kronenberg et al., 2003). Animals who are exercised from young to middle age exhibit far less age-related decline in neurogenesis than do sedentary controls (Kronenberg et al., 2006) as do rodents who begin to be exercised when they are old (van Praag, Shubert, Zhao, & Gage, 2005). The onset of exercise-induced neurogenesis is rapid but the effect is transient, suggesting that this process is strongly related to learning. Kronenberg et al. (2006), for example, observed the rate of neurogenesis to be maximal three days after the onset of a wheel running task, returning to baseline after one month. There is no direct evidence of neurogenesis in the adult human; however, post-mortem and neuroimaging studies have provided convincing indirect evidence of human adult neurogenesis albeit this has been linked to memory and learning rather than physical activity *per se* (Erickson et al., 2011; Eriksson et al., 1998).

Neurotrophic factors

Neurotrophins are critical proteins for the nervous system development, survival and repair. Three key neurotrophins are brain derived neurotrophic factor (BDNF), insulin-like growth factor I (IGF-1), and vascular endothelial growth factor (VEGF). BDNF and IGF-1, and less commonly VEGF, are frequently used as biomarkers for neuroplasticity in animal and human studies as all of these neurotropins are up-regulated with exercise in animal and human models.

VEGF is a signalling protein known to promote angiogenesis, as well as endothelial cell survival, proliferation, and migration (Fabel et al., 2003). The hormone IGF-1 is the major mediator of growth hormone stimulated somatic growth, and has also been strongly linked to angiogenesis (Black et al., 1990). VEGF and IGF-1 are both linked to neurogenesis, playing a particular role in mediating the effects of exercise-induced neurogenesis. IGF-1 is produced peripherally in skeletal muscle and the liver and because it crosses the blood–brain barrier, it facilitates the exercise-induced up-regulation of BDNF and plays an important role in neurogenesis (Carro, Nunez, Busiguina, & Torres-Aleman, 2000; Gomez-Pinilla & Hillman, 2013). In humans, both chronic exercise interventions (e.g. Cassilhas, Tufik, & de Mello, 2016) and acute aerobic exercise interventions (Roig, Skriver, Lundbye-Jensen, Kiens, & Nielsen, 2012) as well as resistance training (Rojas Vega, Knicker, Hollmann, Bloch, & Struder, 2010) have been observed to increase IGF-1 production.

BDNF is centrally produced but found in the brain and the periphery. It plays a key role in regulating the development of synaptic connections and dendritic size; and it has been suggested to be crucial for neurogenesis and synaptogenesis (Cotman et al., 2007). BDNF facilitates both pre- and post-synaptic mechanisms and the induction of LTP. Of all the neurotrophins, BDNF responds most readily to exercise and physical activity. Experiments with animal models have consistently demonstrated that exercise up-regulates BDNF in a variety of brain areas including hippocampus, cerebral cortex, cerebellum, and basal ganglia (for a review see: Cotman & Berchtold, 2002; Erickson et al., 2012). BDNF has also been observed to increase in human studies following an aerobic training programme (Erickson et al., 2011; Ruscheweyh et al., 2011; Voss et al., 2013) after a single bout of intensive aerobic exercise (Hakansson et al., 2017; Laske et al., 2010). Although BDNF is produced in the brain, contracting muscles release myokines that enhance the synthesis of BDNF (Dishman et al., 2006). Whilst peripheral BDNF increases following exercise, it typically returns to baseline when the training stops. Early studies suggested that resistance training also enhances BDNF production, but recent systematic reviews suggest this effect is limited at best (Dinoff et al., 2016; Knaepen, Goekint, Heyman, & Meeusen, 2010). Finally, Gomez-Pinilla and Hillman (2013) have argued that because the placenta may be an important source of BDNF and other neurotrophins (e.g. Flock et al., 2016), and if neurotrophins in the placenta diffuse from the placenta to the fetus, that exercise during pregnancy may be beneficial to the developing fetal brain.

In the periphery, it has been shown that elderly frail and pre-frail women are able to increase plasma BDNF levels in response to several weeks of progressive resistance training exercise (F.M. Coelho et al., 2012), yet there is little evidence to examine the direct physiological and functional effects this might have on the PNS specifically. Other research such as rodent nerve injury models have shown that enhanced recovery in younger animals was associated with higher peripheral BDNF (Park & Hoke, 2014), and therefore this could suggest that exercising in later life may have a neuroprotective effect of the PNS by increasing circulating BDNF.

Neurotransmitter regulation

As previously noted, aerobic exercise is strongly correlated with the up-regulation of genes that mediate synaptic plasticity. Glutamate (GLU; the major excitatory neurotransmitter in the nervous system) and γ-aminobutyric acid (GABA; the major inhibitory neurotransmitter) work in concert to establish the brain's excitation–inhibition balance. As GLU is a precursor to GABA, they share a common pathway. Therefore, when the production of GLU is increased in the normally functioning brain, GABA will also be increased to restore the balance. This is important because the depletion of either of these neurotransmitters will shift the excitation–inhibition balance in the brain. For example, if the balance is shifted too far towards excitation, GLU excitotoxicity produces an inflammatory response that accelerates neurodegeneration. GLU (and therefore GABA) is enhanced by exercise (e.g. Maddock, Casazza, Fernandez, & Maddock, 2016); however, vigorous physical activity is known to shift the excitation–inhibition balance in the brain towards a state of excitability (Crabbe & Dishman, 2004). This increased neural activity is associated with increased cortical functioning and increased expression of NMDA receptors, which are crucial for synaptic transmission and LTP (Farmer et al., 2004; Molteni, Ying, & Gomez-Pinilla, 2002). This provides a basis for well-recognised relationship between exercise and learning.

Physical activity also activates the monoamine system, with noradrenaline (NA) dopamine (DA) and serotonin (5-HT, 5-hydroxytryptamine) in particular increased during exercise (Chaouloff, 1989). NA is a major neuromodulator that regulates the activity of neuronal and non-neuronal cells in the brain. It plays a role in regulating cerebral blood flow, energy metabolism of a broad range of cell types in the brain, modulating cortical connectivity, and it contributes the neuroinflammation response and to the induction of LTP. Among its many functions, DA plays a critical role in reward-motivated behaviour and motor learning. 5-HT is strongly associated with depression, neuroplasticity and neurogenesis.

These brain monoamines are strongly associated with behavioural and endocrine responses to stress. For example, chronic exposure to stress leads to increased activity of NA-mediated neurons and, as a result NA is markedly depleted (Dishman et al., 2006). Similarly, 5-HT and DA are both reduced when the animal is stressed, but to a lesser extent than has been reported for NA (Dishman et al., 2006). However, acute exercise can transiently restore these monoamines, and their levels can be maintained by chronic exercise. The exercise-induced modulation of these monoamines is one of the critical mechanisms by which exercise alleviates stress, anxiety and depression (Strohle, 2009). Aerobic exercise has been shown to produce a major antidepressant effect that is as strong a serotonergic medication (Babyak et al., 2000).

Oxidative stress

One of the main mechanisms of neurodegeneration and the subsequent decline of neural functioning is oxidative stress. Oxidative stress is particularly prominent with older adults, and refers to the damaging effects of reactive oxygen species (ROS) which are released in small amounts during normal energy production at the mitochondria. In these small amounts, the human body is able to control the degenerative effects of ROS on DNA, lipids and proteins using antioxidants. However, the accumulation of damage over time (such as with ageing) can inhibit mitochondrial function and biogenesis causing ROS production to surpass levels capable of antioxidant containment (Cui, Kong, & Zhang, 2012). In particular, recent evidence suggests that this process could occur at the level of nerve fibre myelin sheath (Ravera et al., 2015; Ravera & Panfoli, 2015) and the damaging effects of oxidative stress has been linked to neurodegenerative diseases such as Alzheimer's and Parkinson's (for a review see Kim, Kim, Rhie, & Yoon, 2015).

Physical activity induces a transient elevation of ROS by increasing the energy demand from the mitochondria. It may therefore seem counterintuitive to suggest that regular exercise may prevent oxidative stress, however current research suggests this is the case due to a process known as mitohormesis (Bo, Jiang, Ji, & Zhang, 2013; Ristow & Zarse, 2010). Mitohormesis is a term which refers to the physiological response to these transient increases in ROS which help the mitochondria to cope with similar stresses in the future. Indeed, consuming exogenous antioxidants has actually been seen to inhibit the effects of exercise-induced mitohormesis (Ristow et al., 2009) suggesting that transient ROS exposures are necessary for long-term oxidative stress resistance. Similarly, regular exercise has been shown to stimulate mitochondrial remodelling and biogenesis in rodents, which may help to prevent increased ROS production by damaged or inefficient aged mitochondria (Bo et al., 2013). This may in part explain why neurodegenerative disease risk is typically reported as higher with physical inactivity. Indeed, physical inactivity is thought to contribute to around 22% of cases of Alzheimer's disease in the UK (Norton, Matthews, Barnes, Yaffe, & Brayne, 2014), with additional epidemiological evidence showing increased physical activity can prevent the development of Parkinson's disease, particularly when adopted in middle to late adulthood (Xu et al., 2010). Collectively, these findings demonstrate that regular physical activity can improve the body's defence against oxidative stress and associated neurodegenerative processes.

Enhancing the effects of exercise

An enriched diet can facilitate normal brain health, promote neuroplasticity, and enhance neural repair. Traditionally, studies have primarily focused on the antioxidant and anti-inflammatory properties of dietary factors; however, like exercise, dietary factors can modulate the molecular and cellular processes critical to action potential propagation, neural processing, and neural repair. In contrast, poor dietary habits, such as high-caloric intake, contribute to the acceleration of neurodegeneration. Two compounds that have received considerable attention in recent years are omega-3 polyunsaturated fatty acids and plant polyphenols. Docosahexaenoic (DHA) is one of the most important forms of the omega-3 fatty acids as it is the most abundant phospholipid in the brain and is a critical component of the pre- and postsynaptic membrane. However, phospholids are highly susceptible to oxidative stress and because DHA production in mammals is inefficient, dietary DHA is critical for neuronal function as it provides the structural material for regeneration of the synaptic membranes (Gomez-Pinilla, 2011). In contrast, diets with high sugar, saturated fats, or caloric content are considered to increase oxidative stress, thus impairing neural function (Gomez-Pinilla, 2011). For example, Molteni and colleagues (2002) demonstrated that rodents exposed to a diet high in sugar and saturated fat exhibited decreased hippocampal BDNF and synaptic plastic. However, when these animals were exercised these effects were reversed (Molteni et al., 2004). Polyphenols are potent antioxidants that are found in plant-derived foods such as blueberry, green tea, red wine, cocoa and coffee. Polyphenols are neuroprotective agents that inhibit neurotoxins, reduce neuroinflammation, and promote neuroplasticity (Vauzour, 2012). van Praag et al. (2007) have suggested that the ability of polyphenols to stimulate angiogenesis may be even greater than exercise alone. Most attention has been paid to flavonoids as they represent the largest group of the polyphenols. In addition to their antioxidant properties, flavonoids activate signalling pathways that increase the expression of neurotrophins that drive LTP and therefore enhance long-term memory (Spencer, 2008). In mice, the flavanol (−)epicathechin has been shown to cross the blood–brain barrier where it increases angiogenesis and neuronal spine density in the hippocampus as well as up-regulating genes associated with learning and down-regulating markers of neurodegeneration. Interestingly, this effect was enhanced when the animals were exercised suggesting that the effects of dietary supplementation and exercise are complementary.

Much of this chapter has focused on the neurophysiological effects of aerobic exercise. In part, this reflects the overwhelming proportion of literature in this field that is devoted to aerobic exercise compared with resistance training and more complex training that challenges the sensorimotor and cognitive systems. Indeed, very few studies have attempted to specifically investigate neurophysiological effects associated with different types of physical activity and most studies investigating different exercise modalities tend to focus on the cognitive domain. Nevertheless, studies that investigate the effects of resistance training and more complex sensorimotor training do enhance different aspects of the nervous system. Resistance training is associated with improved executive function (Liu Ambrose, Nagamatsu, Voss, Khan, & Handy, 2012), as well as improved short-term memory and attention (Cassilhas et al., 2016). Cassilhas and colleagues have demonstrated that both aerobic and resistance exercise improve spatial learning and short-term memory in humans and rodents (Cassilhas et al., 2012; Cassilhas et al., 2007), although the mechanisms of action appear to depend on the type of exercise. In these experiments, aerobic exercise was associated with up-regulation of BDNF whereas resistance training up-regulated IGF-1. This result strongly supports the well-known suggestion that an exercise programme should include both aerobic and resistance training. It is important to note that, with the exception of a few studies involving participants with neurological disorders (e.g. cerebral palsy), there are no studies that have specifically investigated the neurophysiological effects of resistance training in healthy children. Furthermore, the vast majority of studies investigating neurophysiological effects of resistance training have been conducted with elderly participants in order to better understand healthy ageing and neurodegeneration. As a result, there is a dearth of knowledge about the effects of resistance training in the developing nervous system.

More complex activities are better suited to challenge the sensorimotor and cognitive systems. For example, Kattenstroth and colleagues have performed an elegant series of experiments which demonstrate that dance training with elderly participants result in better cognitive, motor and perceptual performance compared with sedentary controls (Kattenstroth, Kalisch, Holt, Tegenthoff, & Dinse, 2013; Kattenstroth, Kalisch, Kolankowska, & Dinse, 2011; Kattenstroth, Kalisch, Kowalewski, Tegenthoff, & Dinse, 2013; Kattenstroth, Kalisch, Peters, Tegenthoff, & Dinse, 2012; Kattenstroth, Kolankowska, Kalisch, & Dinse, 2010). These effects were shown in participants who had been dancing regularly for years and also in participants exposed to a short intervention (6 months, 1h/week) of dance training. Similar effects have been reported for participants who engage in Tai Chi (e.g. Tao et al., 2016; Zheng et al., 2015) and martial arts (e.g. Alesi et al., 2014; Douris et al., 2015; Krampe, Smolders, & Doumas, 2014; Pons van Dijk, Huijts, & Lodder, 2013). The enriched environment associated with more engaged activities (e.g. sport, fitness classes, exergaming) compared with exercise prescription programmes is becoming a focus of recent attention. Such activities involve learning, motor coordination and cognitive stimulation to a greater extent than is possible in traditional exercise. As a result, the nervous system is exposed to training that is repetitive yet motivating and challenging – three key principles that promote neuroplasticity. The few studies that have tested this idea have yielded promising results particularly in the emerging area of exergaming, where video or virtual reality is employed to gamify exercise in such a manner that movement is tracked and relevant feedback is provided to motivate the participant and enhance the cognitive component of the exercise (Bonetti, Drury, Danoff, & Miller, 2010). For example, BDNF has been shown to increase and executive function has improved in participants who perform stationary cycling with the aid of gamification compared with stationary cycling alone (Anderson-Hanley et al., 2012; Barcelos et al., 2015). Other studies have demonstrated improvements in balance and functional mobility in older adults (Donath, Rossler, & Faude, 2016).

Despite this compelling evidence, the guidelines or recommendations regarding physical activity for older adults (who may typically stand to gain some of the greatest neurophysiological benefits of exercise) are sparse. Small bouts of moderate intensity exercise are thought to optimise peripheral BDNF production for the elderly (F.G.D. Coelho et al., 2013), with attention to avoiding high intensity exercise as this can increase ROS levels past the adaptive tolerance of cells, inhibiting exercise-induced mitohormesis (Radak, Marton, Nagy, Koltai, & Goto, 2013). Exercises should also aim to include all areas of the body, since exercise-induced benefits (at least in terms of motor unit preservation) have been observed as limited to trained muscles alone (Power et al., 2012; Power et al., 2010). Despite being grounded in the literature, these recommendations are still relatively vague in terms of advising how to implement a beneficial exercise regime to the general public. Greater efforts should therefore be made to improve specific guidelines for physical activity in older adults to avoid confusion and subsequent inactivity.

Conclusions

Physical activity has consistent and robust effects on the nervous system that are observed in both animal and human models. Physical exercise, particularly aerobic exercise, stimulates neuroplasticity and enhances neuroprotection, both of which are critical for a healthy nervous system. Morphological changes in the brain are regionally specific, in that physical activity appears to influence areas responsible for cognition, memory and executive function to a greater extent than is observed in other cortical areas. However, the majority of our understanding in this area has been derived from studies investigating neurodegeneration associated with ageing. Furthermore, there is great deal to learn about the link between the molecular, cellular and morphological responses to exercise and the cognitive/behavioural changes we are ultimately trying to enhance.

Whilst we are beginning to have a good understanding of the effects of physical activity on the nervous system, there is a need for larger randomised controlled studies that will allow us to make better recommendations for physical activity guidelines. There is a particular need to perform more intervention studies that take place outside the laboratory in order to better elucidate the real-world effects in large groups of participants in order to inform recommendations.

Issues relating to dose (i.e. duration, frequency and intensity) are not well understood nor are age-related issues – the vast majority of study in this field has been conducted with older people although there is a growing body of evidence promoting the importance of regular physical activity in children and young to middle-aged adults. Whilst we should encourage active participation in physical activity at all ages, it needs to be acknowledged that some people make lifestyle choices that do not include physical activity. Therefore, it would be important to understand if there is an age at which exercise should be more strongly encouraged from a public health point of view in order to best enhance neuroprotection to reduce the personal socioeconomic costs associated with age-related neurodegeneration. We know that effects of an acute bout of physical activity are transient, therefore more research is needed to determine if these effects can be lengthened; and for those people who normally maintain an active lifestyle, we need to better understand for how long the beneficial effects of prior exercise is retained.

It is clear that a good exercise programme should incorporate both aerobic and non-aerobic activity. The extent to which different types of exercise enhance the nervous system is only beginning to be investigated. The majority of the literature has been focused on aerobic training, as a result we need to better understand the effects of resistance training, more complex training (e.g. sport and exergaming), and how exercise might be combined synergistically with diet to optimise the benefit.

Chapter summary

- Physical activity is associated with morphological and functional changes throughout the nervous system and across the lifespan.
- Physical activity enhances neuroplasticity and acts as a neuroprotective agent against normal age-related neurodegeneration processes such as oxidative stress.
- Aerobic and non-aerobic training have different, yet complementary effects on the nervous system.
- The beneficial effects of exercise can be enhanced when combined with other modalities (e.g. diet) and in an environment that challenges other systems (e.g. cognition, executive function, balance and coordination).

References

Ahlskog, J.E., Geda, Y.E., Graff-Radford, N.R., & Petersen, R.C. (2011). Physical exercise as a preventive or disease-modifying treatment of dementia and brain aging. *Mayo Clinic Proceedings, 86*(9), 876–884. doi:10.4065/mcp.2011.0252

Alesi, M., Bianco, A., Padulo, J., Vella, F.P., Petrucci, M., Paoli, A., . . . Pepi, A. (2014). Motor and cognitive development: the role of karate. *Muscles Ligaments Tendons J, 4*(2), 114–120.

Anderson-Hanley, C., Arciero, P.J., Brickman, A.M., Nimon, J.P., Okuma, N., Westen, S.C., . . . Zimmerman, E.A. (2012). Exergaming and older adult cognition: a cluster randomized clinical trial. *Am J Prev Med, 42*(2), 109–119. doi:10.1016/j.amepre.2011.10.016

Babyak, M., Blumenthal, J.A., Herman, S., Khatri, P., Doraiswamy, M., Moore, K., . . . Krishnan, K.R. (2000). Exercise treatment for major depression: maintenance of therapeutic benefit at 10 months. *Psychosom Med, 62*(5), 633–638.

Barcelos, N., Shah, N., Cohen, K., Hogan, M.J., Mulkerrin, E., Arciero, P.J., . . . Anderson-Hanley, C. (2015). Aerobic and Cognitive Exercise (ACE) pilot study for older adults: executive function improves with cognitive challenge while exergaming. *J Int Neuropsychol Soc, 21*(10), 768–779. doi:10.1017/S1355617715001083

Black, J.E., Isaacs, K.R., Anderson, B.J., Alcantara, A.A., & Greenough, W.T. (1990). Learning causes synaptogenesis, whereas motor activity causes angiogenesis, in cerebellar cortex of adult rats. *Proc Natl Acad Sci U S A, 87*(14), 5568–5572.

Bliss, T.V., & Lomo, T. (1973). Long-lasting potentiation of synaptic transmission in the dentate area of the anaesthetized rabbit following stimulation of the perforant path. *J Physiol, 232*(2), 331–356.

Bo, H., Jiang, N., Ji, L.L., & Zhang, Y. (2013). Mitochondrial redox metabolism in aging: effect of exercise interventions. *Journal of Sport and Health Science, 2*(2), 67–74. doi:10.1016/j.jshs.2013.03.006

Bonetti, A.J., Drury, D.G., Danoff, J.V., & Miller, T.A. (2010). Comparison of acute exercise responses between conventional video gaming and isometric resistance exergaming. *J Strength Cond Res, 24*(7), 1799–1803. doi:10.1519/JSC.0b013e3181bab4a8

Bullitt, E., Rahman, F.N., Smith, J.K., Kim, E., Zeng, D., Katz, L.M., & Marks, B.L. (2009). The effect of exercise on the cerebral vasculature of healthy aged subjects as visualized by MR angiography. *AJNR Am J Neuroradiol, 30*(10), 1857–1863. doi:10.3174/ajnr.A1695

Burzynska, A.Z., Chaddock-Heyman, L., Voss, M.W., Wong, C.N., Gothe, N.P., Olson, E.A., . . . Kramer, A.F. (2014). Physical activity and cardiorespiratory fitness are beneficial for white matter in low-fit older adults. *PLoS ONE, 9*(9), e107413. doi:10.1371/journal.pone.0107413

Burzynska, A.Z., Preuschhof, C., Backman, L., Nyberg, L., Li, S.C., Lindenberger, U., & Heekeren, H.R. (2010). Age-related differences in white matter microstructure: region-specific patterns of diffusivity. *Neuroimage, 49*(3), 2104–2112. doi:10.1016/j.neuroimage.2009.09.041

Carro, E., Nunez, A., Busiguina, S., & Torres-Aleman, I. (2000). Circulating insulin-like growth factor I mediates effects of exercise on the brain. *J Neurosci, 20*(8), 2926–2933.

Cassilhas, R.C., Lee, K.S., Fernandes, J., Oliveira, M.G., Tufik, S., Meeusen, R., & de Mello, M.T. (2012). Spatial memory is improved by aerobic and resistance exercise through divergent molecular mechanisms. *Neuroscience, 202*, 309–317. doi:10.1016/j.neuroscience.2011.11.029

Cassilhas, R.C., Tufik, S., & de Mello, M.T. (2016). Physical exercise, neuroplasticity, spatial learning and memory. *Cell Mol Life Sci, 73*(5), 975–983. doi:10.1007/s00018-015-2102-0

Cassilhas, R.C., Viana, V.A., Grassmann, V., Santos, R.T., Santos, R.F., Tufik, S., & Mello, M.T. (2007). The impact of resistance exercise on the cognitive function of the elderly. *Med Sci Sports Exerc, 39*(8), 1401–1407. doi:10.1249/mss.0b013e318060111f

Chaddock, L., Erickson, K.I., Prakash, R.S., Kim, J.S., Voss, M.W., VanPatter, M., . . . Kramer, A.F. (2010). A neuroimaging investigation of the association between aerobic fitness, hippocampal volume, and memory performance in preadolescent children. *Brain Res, 1358*, 172–183. doi:10.1016/j.brainres.2010.08.049

Chaddock, L., Erickson, K.I., Prakash, R.S., VanPatter, M., Voss, M.W., Pontifex, M.B., . . . Kramer, A.F. (2010). Basal ganglia volume is associated with aerobic fitness in preadolescent children. *Dev Neurosci, 32*(3), 249–256. doi:10.1159/000316648

Chaddock, L., Erickson, K.I., Prakash, R.S., Voss, M.W., VanPatter, M., Pontifex, M.B., . . . Kramer, A.F. (2012). A functional MRI investigation of the association between childhood aerobic fitness and neurocognitive control. *Biol Psychol, 89*(1), 260–268. doi:10.1016/j.biopsycho.2011.10.017

Chaddock-Heyman, L., Erickson, K.I., Holtrop, J.L., Voss, M.W., Pontifex, M.B., Raine, L.B., . . . Kramer, A.F. (2014). Aerobic fitness is associated with greater white matter integrity in children. *Front Hum Neurosci, 8*, 584. doi:10.3389/fnhum.2014.00584

Chaouloff, F. (1989). Physical exercise and brain monoamines – a review. *Acta Physiologica Scandinavica, 137*(1), 1–13. doi:10.1111/j.1748-1716.1989.tb08715.x

Coelho, F.G.D., Gobbi, S., Andreatto, C.A.A., Corazza, D.I., Pedroso, R.V., & Santos-Galduroz, R.F. (2013). Physical exercise modulates peripheral levels of brain-derived neurotrophic factor (BDNF): a systematic review of experimental studies in the elderly. *Archives of Gerontology and Geriatrics, 56*(1), 10–15. doi:10.1016/j.archger.2012.06.003

Coelho, F.M., Pereira, D.S., Lustosa, L.P., Silva, J.P., Dias, J.M., Dias, R.C., . . . Pereira, L.S. (2012). Physical therapy intervention (PTI) increases plasma brain-derived neurotrophic factor (BDNF) levels in non-frail and pre-frail elderly women. *Arch Gerontol Geriatr, 54*(3), 415–420. doi:10.1016/j.archger.2011.05.014

Colcombe, S.J., Erickson, K.I., Raz, N., Webb, A.G., Cohen, N.J., McAuley, E., & Kramer, A.F. (2003). Aerobic fitness reduces brain tissue loss in aging humans. *J Gerontol A Biol Sci Med Sci, 58*(2), 176–180.

Colcombe, S.J., Erickson, K.I., Scalf, P.E., Kim, J.S., Prakash, R., McAuley, E., . . . Kramer, A.F. (2006). Aerobic exercise training increases brain volume in aging humans. *J Gerontol A Biol Sci Med Sci, 61*(11), 1166–1170.

Cotman, C.W., & Berchtold, N.C. (2002). Exercise: a behavioral intervention to enhance brain health and plasticity. *Trends in Neurosciences, 25*(6), 295–301. doi:10.1016/S0166-2236(02)02143-4

Cotman, C.W., Berchtold, N.C., & Christie, L.A. (2007). Exercise builds brain health: key roles of growth factor cascades and inflammation. *Trends Neurosci, 30*(9), 464–472. doi:10.1016/j.tins.2007.06.011

Crabbe, J.B., & Dishman, R.K. (2004). Brain electrocortical activity during and after exercise: a quantitative synthesis. *Psychophysiology, 41*(4), 563–574. doi:10.1111/j.1469-8986.2004.00176.x

Cui, H., Kong, Y., & Zhang, H. (2012). Oxidative stress, mitochondrial dysfunction, and aging. *J Signal Transduct, 2012*, 646354. doi:10.1155/2012/646354

Dinoff, A., Herrmann, N., Swardfager, W., Liu, C.S., Sherman, C., Chan, S., & Lanctot, K.L. (2016). The effect of exercise training on resting concentrations of peripheral Brain-Derived Neurotrophic Factor (BDNF): a meta-analysis. *PLoS ONE, 11*(9), e0163037. doi:10.1371/journal.pone.0163037

Dishman, R.K., Berthoud, H.R., Booth, F.W., Cotman, C.W., Edgerton, V.R., Fleshner, M.R., . . . Zigmond, M.J. (2006). Neurobiology of exercise. *Obesity* (Silver Spring), *14*(3), 345–356. doi:10.1038/oby.2006.46

Donath, L., Rossler, R., & Faude, O. (2016). Effects of virtual reality training (exergaming) compared to alternative exercise training and passive control on standing balance and functional mobility in healthy community-dwelling seniors: a meta analytical review. *Sports Medicine, 46*(9), 1293–1309. doi:10.1007/s40279-016-0485-1

Douris, P., Douris, C., Balder, N., LaCasse, M., Rand, A., Tarapore, F., . . . Handrakis, J. (2015). Martial art training and cognitive performance in middle-aged adults. *J Hum Kinet, 47*, 277–283. doi:10.1515/hukin-2015-0083

Eadie, B.D., Redila, V.A., & Christie, B.R. (2005). Voluntary exercise alters the cytoarchitecture of the adult dentate gyrus by increasing cellular proliferation, dendritic complexity, and spine density. *J Comp Neurol, 486*(1), 39–47. doi:10.1002/cne.20493

Erickson, K.I., Miller, D.L., & Roecklein, K.A. (2012). The aging hippocampus: interactions between exercise, depression, and BDNF. *Neuroscientist, 18*(1), 82–97. doi:10.1177/1073858410397054

Erickson, K.I., Voss, M.W., Prakash, R.S., Basak, C., Szabo, A., Chaddock, L., . . . Kramer, A.F. (2011). Exercise training increases size of hippocampus and improves memory. *Proc Natl Acad Sci U S A, 108*(7), 3017–3022. doi:10.1073/pnas.1015950108

Eriksson, P.S., Perfilieva, E., Bjork-Eriksson, T., Alborn, A.M., Nordborg, C., Peterson, D.A., & Gage, F.H. (1998). Neurogenesis in the adult human hippocampus. *Nat Med, 4*(11), 1313–1317. doi:10.1038/3305

Fabel, K., Fabel, K., Tam, B., Kaufer, D., Baiker, A., Simmons, N., . . . Palmer, T.D. (2003). VEGF is necessary for exercise-induced adult hippocampal neurogenesis. *Eur J Neurosci, 18*(10), 2803–2812.

Farmer, J., Zhao, X., van Praag, H., Wodtke, K., Gage, F.H., & Christie, B.R. (2004). Effects of voluntary exercise on synaptic plasticity and gene expression in the dentate gyrus of adult male Sprague-Dawley rats *in vivo. Neuroscience, 124*(1), 71–79. doi:10.1016/j.neuroscience.2003.09.029

Fjell, A.M., & Walhovd, K.B. (2010). Structural brain changes in aging: courses, causes and cognitive consequences. *Rev Neurosci, 21*(3), 187–221.

Flock, A., Weber, S.K., Ferrari, N., Fietz, C., Graf, C., Fimmers, R., . . . Merz, W.M. (2016). Determinants of brain-derived neurotrophic factor (BDNF) in umbilical cord and maternal serum. *Psychoneuroendocrinology, 63*, 191–197. doi:10.1016/j.psyneuen.2015.09.028

Gomez-Pinilla, F. (2011). Collaborative effects of diet and exercise on cognitive enhancement. *Nutr Health, 20*(3–4), 165–169. doi:10.1177/026010601102000401

Gomez-Pinilla, F., & Hillman, C. (2013). The influence of exercise on cognitive abilities. *Compr Physiol, 3*(1), 403–428. doi:10.1002/cphy.c110063

Hakansson, K., Ledreux, A., Daffner, K., Terjestam, Y., Bergman, P., Carlsson, R., . . . Mohammed, A.K. (2017). BDNF responses in healthy older persons to 35 minutes of physical exercise, cognitive training, and mindfulness: associations with working memory function. *J Alzheimers Dis, 55*(2), 645–657. doi:10.3233/JAD-160593

Hayes, S.M., Salat, D.H., Forman, D.E., Sperling, R.A., & Verfaellie, M. (2015). Cardiorespiratory fitness is associated with white matter integrity in aging. *Ann Clin Transl Neurol, 2*(6), 688–698. doi:10.1002/acn3.204

Kattenstroth, J.C., Kalisch, T., Holt, S., Tegenthoff, M., & Dinse, H.R. (2013). Six months of dance intervention enhances postural, sensorimotor, and cognitive performance in elderly without affecting cardio-respiratory functions. *Front Aging Neurosci, 5*, 5. doi:10.3389/fnagi.2013.00005

Kattenstroth, J.C., Kalisch, T., Kolankowska, I., & Dinse, H.R. (2011). Balance, sensorimotor, and cognitive performance in long-year expert senior ballroom dancers. *J Aging Res, 2011*, 176709. doi:10.4061/2011/176709

Kattenstroth, J.C., Kalisch, T., Kowalewski, R., Tegenthoff, M., & Dinse, H.R. (2013). Quantitative assessment of joint position sense recovery in subacute stroke patients: a pilot study. *J Rehabil Med, 45*(10), 1004–1009. doi:10.2340/16501977-1225

Kattenstroth, J.C., Kalisch, T., Peters, S., Tegenthoff, M., & Dinse, H.R. (2012). Long-term sensory stimulation therapy improves hand function and restores cortical responsiveness in patients with chronic cerebral lesions. Three single case studies. *Front Hum Neurosci, 6*, 244. doi:10.3389/fnhum.2012.00244

Kattenstroth, J.C., Kolankowska, I., Kalisch, T., & Dinse, H.R. (2010). Superior sensory, motor, and cognitive performance in elderly individuals with multi-year dancing activities. *Front Aging Neurosci, 2*. doi:10.3389/fnagi.2010.00031

Kempermann, G., Fabel, K., Ehninger, D., Babu, H., Leal-Galicia, P., Garthe, A., & Wolf, S.A. (2010). Why and how physical activity promotes experience-induced brain plasticity. *Front Neurosci, 4*, 189. doi:10.3389/fnins.2010.00189

Kihara, M., Nickander, K.K., & Low, P.A. (1991). The effect of aging on endoneurial blood flow, hyperemic response and oxygen-free radicals in rat sciatic nerve. *Brain Res, 562*(1), 1–5.

Kim, G.H., Kim, J.E., Rhie, S.J., & Yoon, S. (2015). The role of oxidative stress in neurodegenerative diseases. *Exp Neurobiol, 24*(4), 325–340. doi:10.5607/en.2015.24.4.325

Knaepen, K., Goekint, M., Heyman, E.M., & Meeusen, R. (2010). Neuroplasticity – exercise-induced response of peripheral brain-derived neurotrophic factor: a systematic review of experimental studies in human subjects. *Sports Med, 40*(9), 765–801. doi:10.2165/11534530-000000000-00000

Krampe, R.T., Smolders, C., & Doumas, M. (2014). Leisure sports and postural control: can a black belt protect your balance from aging? *Psychol Aging, 29*(1), 95–102. doi:10.1037/a0035501

Kronenberg, G., Bick-Sander, A., Bunk, E., Wolf, C., Ehninger, D., & Kempermann, G. (2006). Physical exercise prevents age-related decline in precursor cell activity in the mouse dentate gyrus. *Neurobiol Aging, 27*(10), 1505–1513. doi:10.1016/j.neurobiolaging.2005.09.016

Kronenberg, G., Reuter, K., Steiner, B., Brandt, M.D., Jessberger, S., Yamaguchi, M., & Kempermann, G. (2003). Subpopulations of proliferating cells of the adult hippocampus respond differently to physiologic neurogenic stimuli. *J Comp Neurol, 467*(4), 455–463. doi:10.1002/cne.10945

Laske, C., Banschbach, S., Stransky, E., Bosch, S., Straten, G., Machann, J., . . . Eschweiler, G.W. (2010). Exercise-induced normalization of decreased BDNF serum concentration in elderly women with remitted major depression. *Int J Neuropsychopharmacol, 13*(5), 595–602. doi:10.1017/S1461145709991234

Liu-Ambrose, T., Nagamatsu, L.S., Voss, M.W., Khan, K.M., & Handy, T.C. (2012). Resistance training and functional plasticity of the aging brain: a 12-month randomized controlled trial. *Neurobiol Aging, 33*(8), 1690–1698. doi:10.1016/j.neurobiolaging.2011.05.010

Maass, A., Duzel, S., Goerke, M., Becke, A., Sobieray, U., Neumann, K., . . . Duzel, E. (2015). Vascular hippocampal plasticity after aerobic exercise in older adults. *Molecular Psychiatry, 20*(5), 585–593. doi:10.1038/mp.2014.114

Maddock, R.J., Casazza, G.A., Fernandez, D.H., & Maddock, M.I. (2016). Acute modulation of cortical glutamate and GABA content by physical activity. *J Neurosci, 36*(8), 2449–2457. doi:10.1523/JNEUROSCI.3455-15.2016

Molteni, R., Barnard, R.J., Ying, Z., Roberts, C.K., & Gomez-Pinilla, F. (2002). A high-fat, refined sugar diet reduces hippocampal brain-derived neurotrophic factor, neuronal plasticity, and learning. *Neuroscience, 112*(4), 803–814.

Molteni, R., Wu, A., Vaynman, S., Ying, Z., Barnard, R.J., & Gomez-Pinilla, F. (2004). Exercise reverses the harmful effects of consumption of a high-fat diet on synaptic and behavioral plasticity associated to the action of brain-derived neurotrophic factor. *Neuroscience, 123*(2), 429–440.

Molteni, R., Ying, Z., & Gomez-Pinilla, F. (2002). Differential effects of acute and chronic exercise on plasticity-related genes in the rat hippocampus revealed by microarray. *Eur J Neurosci, 16*(6), 1107–1116.

Norton, S., Matthews, F.E., Barnes, D.E., Yaffe, K., & Brayne, C. (2014). Potential for primary prevention of Alzheimer's disease: an analysis of population-based data. *Lancet Neurol, 13*(8), 788–794. doi:10.1016/S1474-4422(14)70136-X

O'Callaghan, R.M., Ohle, R., & Kelly, A.M. (2007). The effects of forced exercise on hippocampal plasticity in the rat: a comparison of LTP, spatial- and non-spatial learning. *Behav Brain Res, 176*(2), 362–366. doi:10.1016/j.bbr.2006.10.018

Park, J.S., & Hoke, A. (2014). Treadmill exercise induced functional recovery after peripheral nerve repair is associated with increased levels of neurotrophic factors. *PLoS ONE, 9*(3), e90245. doi:10.1371/journal.pone.0090245

Pons van Dijk, G., Huijts, M., & Lodder, J. (2013). Cognition improvement in Taekwondo novices over 40. Results from the SEKWONDO study. *Front Aging Neurosci, 5*, 74. doi:10.3389/fnagi.2013.00074

Power, G.A., Dalton, B.H., Behm, D.G., Doherty, T.J., Vandervoort, A.A., & Rice, C.L. (2012). Motor unit survival in lifelong runners is muscle dependent. *Med Sci Sports Exerc, 44*(7), 1235–1242. doi:10.1249/MSS.0b013e318249953c

Power, G.A., Dalton, B.H., Behm, D.G., Vandervoort, A.A., Doherty, T.J., & Rice, C.L. (2010). Motor unit number estimates in masters runners: use it or lose it? *Med Sci Sports Exerc, 42*(9), 1644–1650. doi:10.1249/MSS.0b013e3181d6f9e9

Radak, Z., Marton, O., Nagy, E., Koltai, E., & Goto, S. (2013). The complex role of physical exercise and reactive oxygen species on brain. *Journal of Sport and Health Science, 2*(2), 87–93. doi:10.1016/j.jshs.2013.04.001

Ravera, S., Bartolucci, M., Cuccarolo, P., Litame, E., Illarcio, M., Calzia, D., . . . Panfoli, I. (2015). Oxidative stress in myelin sheath: the other face of the extramitochondrial oxidative phosphorylation ability. *Free Radic Res, 49*(9), 1156–1164. doi:10.3109/10715762.2015.1050962

Ravera, S., & Panfoli, I. (2015). Role of myelin sheath energy metabolism in neurodegenerative diseases. *Neural Regen Res, 10*(10), 1570–1571. doi:10.4103/1673-5374.167749

Rhyu, I.J., Bytheway, J.A., Kohler, S.J., Lange, H., Lee, K.J., Boklewski, J., . . . Cameron, J.L. (2010). Effects of aerobic exercise training on cognitive function and cortical vascularity in monkeys. *Neuroscience, 167*(4), 1239–1248. doi:10.1016/j.neuroscience.2010.03.003

Ristow, M., & Zarse, K. (2010). How increased oxidative stress promotes longevity and metabolic health: the concept of mitochondrial hormesis (mitohormesis). *Exp Gerontol, 45*(6), 410–418. doi:10.1016/j.exger.2010.03.014

Ristow, M., Zarse, K., Oberbach, A., Kloting, N., Birringer, M., Kiehntopf, M., . . . Bluher, M. (2009). Antioxidants prevent health-promoting effects of physical exercise in humans. *Proc Natl Acad Sci U S A, 106*(21), 8665–8670. doi:10.1073/pnas.0903485106

Roig, M., Skriver, K., Lundbye-Jensen, J., Kiens, B., & Nielsen, J.B. (2012). A single bout of exercise improves motor memory. *PLoS ONE, 7*(9), e44594. doi:10.1371/journal.pone.0044594

Rojas Vega, S., Knicker, A., Hollmann, W., Bloch, W., & Struder, H.K. (2010). Effect of resistance exercise on serum levels of growth factors in humans. *Horm Metab Res, 42*(13), 982–986. doi:10.1055/s-0030-1267950

Ruscheweyh, R., Willemer, C., Kruger, K., Duning, T., Warnecke, T., Sommer, J., . . . Floel, A. (2011). Physical activity and memory functions: an interventional study. *Neurobiol Aging, 32*(7), 1304–1319. doi:10.1016/j.neurobiolaging.2009.08.001

Spencer, J.P. (2008). Food for thought: the role of dietary flavonoids in enhancing human memory, learning and neuro-cognitive performance. *Proc Nutr Soc, 67*(2), 238–252. doi:10.1017/S0029665108007088

Strohle, A. (2009). Physical activity, exercise, depression and anxiety disorders. *J Neural Transm* (Vienna), *116*(6), 777–784. doi:10.1007/s00702-008-0092-x

Tao, J., Liu, J., Egorova, N., Chen, X., Sun, S., Xue, X., . . . Kong, J. (2016). Increased hippocampus-medial prefrontal cortex resting-state functional connectivity and memory function after Tai Chi Chuan practice in elder adults. *Front Aging Neurosci, 8*, 25. doi:10.3389/fnagi.2016.00025

Thomas, A.G., Dennis, A., Rawlings, N.B., Stagg, C.J., Matthews, L., Morris, M., . . . Johansen-Berg, H. (2016). Multi-modal characterization of rapid anterior hippocampal volume increase associated with aerobic exercise. *Neuroimage, 131*, 162–170. doi:10.1016/j.neuroimage.2015.10.090

van Praag, H. (2009). Exercise and the brain: something to chew on. *Trends Neurosci, 32*(5), 283–290. doi:10.1016/j.tins.2008.12.007

van Praag, H., Christie, B.R., Sejnowski, T.J., & Gage, F.H. (1999). Running enhances neurogenesis, learning, and long-term potentiation in mice. *Proc Natl Acad Sci U S A, 96*(23), 13427–13431.

van Praag, H., Lucero, M.J., Yeo, G.W., Stecker, K., Heivand, N., Zhao, C., . . . Gage, F.H. (2007). Plant-derived flavanol (-)epicatechin enhances angiogenesis and retention of spatial memory in mice. *J Neurosci, 27*(22), 5869–5878. doi:10.1523/JNEUROSCI.0914-07.2007

van Praag, H., Shubert, T., Zhao, C., & Gage, F.H. (2005). Exercise enhances learning and hippocampal neurogenesis in aged mice. *J Neurosci, 25*(38), 8680–8685. doi:10.1523/JNEUROSCI.1731-05.2005

Vauzour, D. (2012). Dietary polyphenols as modulators of brain functions: biological actions and molecular mechanisms underpinning their beneficial effects. *Oxid Med Cell Longev, 2012*, 914273. doi:10.1155/2012/914273

Vivar, C., Potter, M.C., & van Praag, H. (2013). All about running: synaptic plasticity, growth factors and adult hippocampal neurogenesis. *Curr Top Behav Neurosci, 15*, 189–210. doi:10.1007/7854_2012_220

Voss, M.W., Chaddock, L., Kim, J.S., Vanpatter, M., Pontifex, M.B., Raine, L.B., . . . Kramer, A.F. (2011). Aerobic fitness is associated with greater efficiency of the network underlying cognitive control in preadolescent children. *Neuroscience, 199*, 166–176. doi:10.1016/j.neuroscience.2011.10.009

Voss, M.W., Heo, S., Prakash, R.S., Erickson, K.I., Alves, H., Chaddock, L., . . . Kramer, A.F. (2013). The influence of aerobic fitness on cerebral white matter integrity and cognitive function in older adults: results of a one-year exercise intervention. *Human Brain Mapping, 34*(11), 2972–2985. doi:10.1002/hbm.22119

Xu, Q., Park, Y., Huang, X., Hollenbeck, A., Blair, A., Schatzkin, A., & Chen, H. (2010). Physical activities and future risk of Parkinson disease. *Neurology, 75*(4), 341–348. doi:10.1212/WNL.0b013e3181ea1597

Zheng, Z., Zhu, X., Yin, S., Wang, B., Niu, Y., Huang, X., . . . Li, J. (2015). Combined cognitive-psychological-physical intervention induces reorganization of intrinsic functional brain architecture in older adults. *Neural Plast, 2015*, 713104. doi:10.1155/2015/713104

16 Biomechanics and physical activity

Neil D. Reeves and Steven J. Brown

Keywords: Biomechanics, forces, movement, walking, lower limb

Introduction

Biomechanics is the study of the movement of living organisms per the mechanical laws of motion. This involves understanding how forces act on the organism from the environment (external forces) and how forces act within the organism's body (internal forces) to bring about movement of the organism. When applied to humans, biomechanics allows us to quantify the motions of the body during a range of movements and activities. Biomechanics can help us to quantify and define specific patterns of movement and help us identify alterations to 'normal' movement as a result of clinical conditions or interventions. The application of forces on and within the body have multiple effects: body parts are accelerated, soft tissues within the body undergo deformation and damage to tissues can also result when forces exceed the body's capacity for dissipation and/or when these tissues fail to adapt over time in response to chronic application of such forces.

Biomechanics allows us to understand the impact of forces acting on and within the body and how they bring about movement. Understanding these issues through biomechanics enables identification of impairments to movement resulting from a number of possible causes such as chronic disease, musculoskeletal injury, or the natural ageing processes. Biomechanics can therefore be used as a 'diagnostic tool' for identifying where specific limitations exist and in understanding how known limitations impact upon movement. Another application of biomechanics is in understanding how specific movements and activities might lead to injury by for example, causing excessively high loads on particular parts of the body. Furthermore, biomechanics is used extensively for understanding the 'natural' or 'normal' loads and demands placed on the body by various different activities. This is with a view to understanding 'normal' behaviour and recognising pathology, but also with the aim of optimising safety and performance during such activities.

Biomechanical analysis is utilised across numerous different populations, including clinical and sports populations. The purpose of biomechanical testing could be diagnostic, to inform decision making, optimise performance and to track progress or rehabilitation. Typically, when biomechanics is applied to tasks involving variants of locomotion it is termed gait analysis.

Example: biomechanical analysis of a patient with foot problems may reveal why certain areas of the foot are predisposed to injury or a cyclist may understand their optimal bicycle dimensions to maximise the efficiency of their pedalling.

Biomechanical fundamentals and measurement

Fundamentals

Biomechanics is concerned with the behaviour of the 'segments' of the body, in terms of how forces and movements occur and interact with these body segments. This can be broken into two separate fields, which are tightly related: **kinematics** describes the motion of the body segments without reference to the forces which cause this motion; **kinetics** describes the forces acting on the body segments and the resulting effects of these forces. As a basic example, a kinematic analysis will tell us that a person running is moving their joints faster than a person walking; whereas a kinetic analysis will further inform us that there are higher forces acting around the joints in the legs of the person running compared to the person walking.

To analyse the biomechanical performance of a system requires equipment capable of quantifying the movements and the forces applied upon and created within the human body. This will include interactions with the surrounding environment, forces generated by the muscles with the body, mass and positions of different body segments, etc. The list of contributing factors to motion within the human body is in fact enormous. A single skeletal joint for instance experiences forces upon it from muscles connected via tendons, ligaments, and contact forces with surrounding soft tissue/cartilage/bone. With more than 300 skeletal joints in the human body, as well as countless mechanical interactions between and within the soft tissue of the body, a completely precise and comprehensive biomechanical analysis to current technologies is difficult to achieve. Therefore, biomechanical analysis techniques rely upon a few basic assumptions to achieve accurate representations of the overall behaviour of targeted interactions within the body.

The most traditional technique of biomechanical analysis is through rigid body mechanics. As the most rigid component of the body, the skeleton is responsible for the majority of force transfer to alter body position, apply forces externally and have external forces work upon the body. The science of rigid body mechanics assumes an ideal of a solid skeleton where deformation is neglected, therefore in human analysis we can treat the human body as a set of rigid segments, e.g. the leg may be treated as three rigid segments: a foot, shank and thigh. Deformations such as twisting, bending and displacement of these body segments are typically considered minimal in comparison to the overall movements of the human body during an activity such as walking, therefore when studying these larger movements, it is considered acceptable to ignore these very small movements within these body segments and consider the segment rigid.

Investigation of the human body as a set of rigid segments has been common over the period of the last century in biomechanics. During walking for instance, familiar kinematic and kinetic patterns can be described for the lower limb joints (Figure 16.1). Kinematic investigation allows the positions of the lower limbs to be tracked and described throughout the movement. Joint angular changes and joint angular velocities for instance are very commonly investigated biomechanical parameters, and during a cyclic repetitive motion such as walking in a straight line, common patterns can be observed within the same person and also between different people. Similarly, kinetic parameters may also be considered such as those

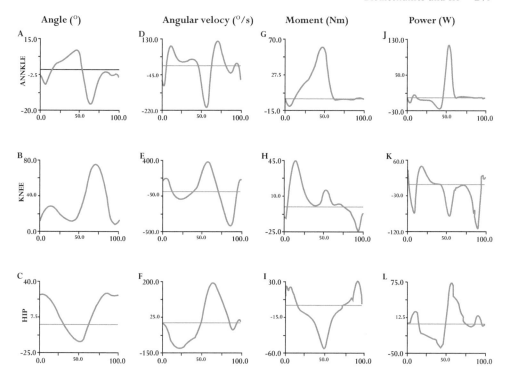

Figure 16.1 Exemplar kinematic and kinetic traces during walking. Joint angles, angular velocities, internal moments and powers for ankle, knee and hip during a single gait cycle. Traces are presented as 0–100% of a gait cycle. Panels A–C: joint angles, positive-joint flexion (dorsi-flexion for ankle), negative-joint extension (plantar-flexion at ankle). Panels D–F: joint angular velocity, positive-joint flexion (dorsi-flexion for ankle), negative-joint extension (plantar-flexion at ankle). Panels: G–I: joint moments, positive-extension moment (plantar-flexion at ankle), negative-flexion moment (dorsi-flexion for ankle). Panels: J–L: joint powers, positive-concentric contraction, negative-eccentric contraction.

causing joint moments (i.e., the rotational force acting around a joint) and power (rate of energy generation/use), which allow description of the forces acting upon the lower limb joints. By understanding the movement and causes of movement these biomechanical parameters can allow us to draw insight regarding differences between populations or individuals.

> *Example: an inactive elderly individual may have lower muscular strength and stiffer joints, during activities such as walking therefore a biomechanist may observe a smaller range of joint motion due to the increased joint stiffness. Additionally decreased muscular strength will limit the ability to generate the forces required for walking, thereby limiting the magnitude of joint moments experienced around a joint.*

The techniques and equipment for measuring biomechanical parameters have evolved dramatically over the past century. Early biomechanical analysis revolved around basic measures of the outcomes of mechanical changes, for instance temporal-spatial parameters.

During walking this might include step lengths, step times, walking speeds, etc. Kinematic techniques were then developed in the early 20th century by filming movement using video cameras and measuring joint positions from the images taken, before the development of computer modelling allowing for multi-camera analysis of 3-dimensional kinematics.

> *Example: muscle weakness limits the forces an individual can generate, therefore an individual with muscle weakness may walk slower than a healthy, strong individual, which is easily measurable with biomechanical techniques.*

Equipment

To collect kinematic (movement) and kinetic (force) data, techniques that allow measurement of body positions and measurement of forces acting on the body are required. Many of these techniques may be applied to the whole body during a range of activities. Within this section we will discuss the application of these techniques mostly focused upon the lower body during common activities such as standing or walking. One common technique to assess kinematics utilises a camera system and reflective or illuminated markers placed on specific anatomical locations of the body. Placement of markers at specific anatomical positions, commonly bony landmarks, allows the definition of body segments and joint centres of rotation. Multi-camera systems allow for 3-dimensional measurement of these marker positions. Knowledge of the location of the skeletal anatomy relative to marker placements thereby allows the position of body segments to be calculated from the positions of the markers (Figure 16.2). Therefore, the positions of body segments in space can be measured, and changes in the positions of these segments are determined so that calculation of movements relative to other body segments can be used to calculate relative angles (i.e. joint angles such as the knee angle are calculated from the relative positions of shank and thigh body segments). Figure 16.1a–f show examples of ankle, knee and hip joint angular changes and angular velocities over the gait cycle (defined as foot contact until the same foot contacts the ground again, i.e., left foot contact through to left foot contact again) during walking, that have been calculated using the technique described.

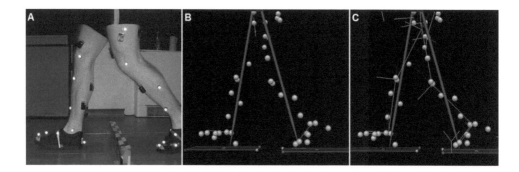

Figure 16.2   Stages of biomechanical modelling. A – the lower limbs with reflective markers placed to define body segments (black boxes are sensors to detect electromyographic activity from the muscles). B – the marker positions with ground reaction force vectors indicated. C – lower limb segments modelled to marker positions, with 3-dimensional axes indicated.

Whilst kinematic measurements are often useful measures by themselves, kinetic measures may be acquired by measurement of the force interactions between the body and the surrounding environment. During walking this involves measurement of the forces applied to the ground underneath the feet, which can be measured using force platforms. According to Newton's third law of motion, which states that 'for every action there is an equal and opposite reaction', a force applied to the ground will have a force *equal in magnitude* and *opposite in direction* that comes back up from the ground and acts on the body through the foot of the individual. This *reaction* force is known as the *ground reaction force* and can be measured using force platforms that are set into the laboratory floor. Ground reaction forces represent the force exerted upon the body from the environment and the magnitude and direction of these forces are dependent upon both how the body moves and the forces being generated by the muscles within the body. The ground reaction force data itself is an informative biomechanical variable.

Calculation of body segment kinetics such as joint moments and powers require knowledge of the forces experienced by each segment and integration of the kinetic and kinematic data. Methods such as inverse dynamics allow the calculation of joint moments based upon the assumption that the major influences upon each segment are the external force interactions and the mass of the segment. Where body segments interact with the surroundings, external force interactions may be measured by force transducers. The ground reaction forces are an example of this. The mass of individual body segments is difficult to measure directly. Modern imaging techniques may allow individual body segment masses to be approximated based upon tissue volume and densities, however, this is a long process requiring imaging and processing time for every individual. More commonly, body segment masses have been approximated using regression equations based upon cadaver data, scaled to an individual's specific anthropometric characteristics to estimate the individual mass of each body segment and the position of the segment's centre-of-mass. Therefore, when investigating a body segment interacting with the surroundings, measurement of interaction forces and knowledge of the position and properties of the segment allow for calculation of force interactions throughout the segment. Commonly this would include kinetic quantities at the joint (e.g. for a foot in contact with the floor, inverse dynamics allows calculation of force interactions at the ankle joint).

When considering additional segments, without direct interactions with the surroundings, inverse dynamics treats the body as a series of linked segments. When considering the walking example, calculation of the forces acting around the ankle provide the external forces acting upon the distal end of the shank, thereby allowing calculation of the forces acting around the proximal end of the segment. By this method joint kinetics may be calculated for each stage in the linked segment chain (Figure 16.3), so long as no additional external interactions take place (e.g. during stair walking an individual may utilise a handrail, thereby providing an additional external interaction which may provide force interactions that transfer throughout the body, in this example inverse dynamics would no longer provide an accurate calculation of joint kinetics, unless the forces interacting with the handrail were measured as well as the foot-ground reaction forces).

Figure 16.1g–l demonstrates some of the joint kinetic variables that may be calculated during walking including joint moments and joint powers using motion analysis and force platforms. Joint moments represent the overall forces acting around a joint, thereby indicating the muscular force requirements from major groups during a given activity. Joint powers provide indications of energy usage and absorption, which can provide indications of the type of muscle contractions occurring. When a joint is moving there are two main types of muscle

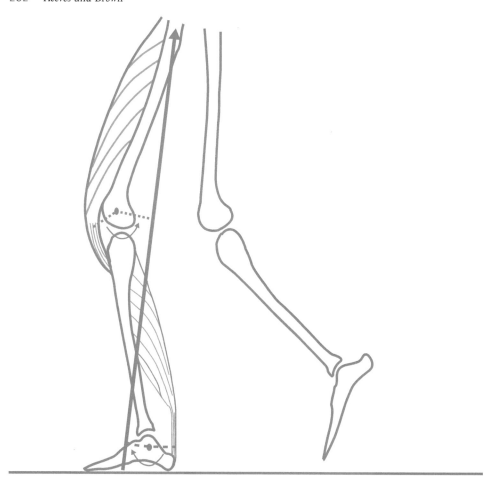

Figure 16.3   Diagram illustrating the development of joint moments around the knee and ankle joints. The thick arrow arising from the ground indicates the magnitude (height) and direction of the ground reaction force. The ground reaction force passes in front of the ankle joint centre of rotation (shown by the small circle) and behind the knee joint centre of rotation, causing an 'external' joint moment that if unopposed would dorsiflex the ankle and flex the knee. The direction of this external joint moment of the ground reaction force is shown by the clockwise arrow at the ankle and the anti-clockwise arrow at the knee. This external joint moment at the knee and ankle is opposed by an 'internal' joint moment developed by the quadriceps and plantar flexor muscle groups, respectively. Both external and internal joint moments act around a lever arm, which is defined as the perpendicular distance between the action line of the force and the joint centre of rotation (external and internal lever arms shown by the dotted lines at the knee and the ankle).

contraction: *concentric*, where the muscle is shortening while developing tension and *eccentric*, where a muscle is lengthening while developing tension. For example, eccentric contractions occur at the ankle throughout most of the stance phase of walking (i.e., when the foot is on the ground), where the ankle plantar flexor muscles (calf muscles) lengthen to control movement of the foot and the rest of the body above it. In contrast, there is a propulsive phase towards the end of the stance phase of walking where a concentric contraction of the ankle plantar flexors occurs as the foot pushes off the floor to provide propulsion to move the body and the leg forwards.

Additional biomechanical techniques

Three-dimensional motion capture and measurement of ground reaction forces are commonly utilised techniques within biomechanics and gait analysis. This approach provides detailed information on how the whole body moves and how forces act on the body to bring about specific movements. However, the study of biomechanics encompasses the understanding of how forces and motion are produced throughout the body during various activities. Whilst the techniques described above provide an indication of how forces act within the body, by for example, understanding the joint moments produced by major muscle groups acting around joints, these measurements alone do not allow for direct calculation of such forces (i.e. how forces are transferred within the soft tissues of the foot). Calculation of how forces or movements occur within a body, whether a rigid body (i.e. a bone) or soft tissue (e.g. calcaneal fat pad) require knowledge of both forces applied and tissue properties, including how tissue properties and shape alter throughout the body. If this information can be gathered using imaging techniques and mechanical testing, processes such as finite element modelling can be used to measure force behaviours within a body/segment.

Whilst we can infer which muscle groups are active to bring about a certain movement from joint kinetics, this technique alone is not capable of directly quantifying muscle activity, or the presence of co-contractions. Electromyography is a technique that uses small sensors to measure the electrical activity produced within muscles when they are actively contracting. Typically, this technique is known as surface electromyography since the sensors are secured onto the skin directly above the muscle of interest (Figure 16.2a). Electromyography may be used in isolation or in combination with the kinetic and kinematic techniques described above. The main purpose of electromyography is to assess which muscles are active and when these muscles are active during the gait cycle. This technique essentially functions as a 'window' into the muscle to enable understanding of which muscles are responsible for causing or controlling certain movements at specific joints during various activities. The data from electromyography typically correlates very closely with inferences of muscle activity from inverse dynamics. Electromyography might also provide complimentary and more detailed information when used in conjunction with inverse dynamics techniques, for example, it might highlight dysfunction within a particular muscle, or muscle group, during walking, that might otherwise have gone undetected from inverse dynamics alone.

Dynamometry is a technique used to measure joint moments around specific joints during movement in a single plane. Using this method, we may infer the forces generated by the major muscle groups and transferred by connective tissues such as tendons.

> *Example: measurement of joint moment at the ankle during plantar flexion allows us to calculate the force produced by the ankle plantar flexor muscles and transmitted through the Achilles tendon. Force transmitted by the tendon is calculated by division of the joint moment by tendon lever arm length, which may be measured by imaging techniques (i.e. magnetic resonance imaging) as the distance between ankle joint centre and tendon action line (i.e. internal lever arm, as shown in Figure 16.3).*

Given the variety of methods available to biomechanists, it is important to understand the capabilities and limitations of individual techniques.

Example: joint kinetics is a useful method for measuring lower limb joint activity during walking where external interactions can be limited to contact with the floor and the forces measured. When swimming external force interactions occur wherever the body is in contact with the water, thereby removing the utility of inverse dynamics for calculating joint forces. However, electromyography can allow for measurement of muscular activity during swimming and information about the joint forces may be inferred from muscular activity.

Biomechanics during different activities

Activities of daily living

Different daily activities pose vastly different biomechanical demands upon the body. During quiet standing, the body moves very little and kinematic analysis shows motion restricted to a small magnitude postural sway, with only very minimal movement occurring at the lower limb joints. Muscles do however need to remain active during quiet standing, particularly those of the lower limbs, to maintain upright posture and resist the effects of gravity 'pulling' the body towards the ground, as well as to control the level of sway within certain limits and maintain balance. In contrast, during walking postural control of balance remains a factor. Cyclic movements of the limbs are required to move the body in the direction of progression, therefore producing larger kinematic alterations at the joints, and larger kinetic requirements from the muscles.

Due to the small movements of balance control that occur during quiet standing, joint motions are rarely investigated. Instead, an emphasis is placed upon understanding the position of the body segments and whole body centre-of-mass. Motions are typically assessed only of natural sway of the whole-body; either by movement of the body centre-of-mass or of the application of force to the ground, typically measured by the centre-of-pressure, the range of which is typically in the region of 2cm (Gatev et al., 1999). Therefore, whilst changes in joint movement and forces are often too small for alterations due to physiological changes to be reliably identified, observation of the movement of the body as a whole allows us to infer how postural or mechanical changes impact upon the postural control of the body.

During locomotion such as walking: the biomechanics of the body differ greatly compared to those of standing. The lower limbs follow a series of cyclic motions, adapting according to alterations in terrain and or/changes of direction. Figure 16.1 shows the typical patterns of lower-limb motion associated with 'normal' walking on a smooth flat surface. Initial contact with the ground is typically termed 'heel-strike' and is considered to be the 'normal' initial contact between the foot and the ground during gait. Initial ground contact may not be a heel-strike in certain pathological gaits and also during running. Immediately after initial contact of the foot with the floor, it can be seen that the foot plantar flexes, allowing the foot to flatten to the ground, resulting in the first negative peak shown in Figure 16.1a. At this same point, the knee is beginning to flex to 'absorb' the impact of ground contact and the hip is at its most extended as the leg is out-stretched to lengthen the step and advance the body forwards. With progression through the gait cycle, the ankle joint dorsiflexes in response to the forward movement of the body over the foot and as the shank progresses forward, whilst the foot is maintained in a flat supportive position to optimise the base of support.

The forces acting around the lower limb joints during physical activity contribute to the joint moments, as shown for walking in Figure 16.1g–i. The association between joint moments and joint movements can be observed by comparing the effects of the two. For example after heel-strike there is a short period where the foot plantar flexes to become flat on the floor (Figure 16.1a), during this time there is a dorsiflexor moment observed at the ankle, Figure 16.1g. This is caused by the ground reaction force being directed behind the ankle joint, which means that the muscles on the opposite side of the joint, i.e., the dorsiflexors, need to act to control or overcome this 'external moment'. This dorsiflexion moment is in opposition to the direction of movement of the foot, which is confirmed by observing a negative eccentric joint power magnitude at the ankle at this point. Therefore, we can understand that whilst the ankle joint is plantar flexing, the action of the dorsiflexor muscles is in opposition to overall muscle action around the joint. This means they are acting *eccentrically* to slow and control the motion. In comparison, if we consider ankle movement during 40–60% gait cycle, both joint moment (Figure 16.1g) and joint motion (Figure 16.1d) are in the plantar flexion direction. When the joint moment is acting in the direction of motion at a specific joint we can determine that this joint moment is being generated by a *concentric* muscle action to produce the movement and overcome the external moment, and hence a positive, concentric joint power can be observed (Figure 16.1j). From 60% onwards in Figure 16.1 the limb of interest is no longer in contact with the ground (termed the stance phase), but is now in the air in the phase of the gait cycle known as the swing phase. This is when the limb is moved through the air to produce the step length that will advance the body forwards in the direction of progression. It can be observed that during this phase the knee and hip joints flex and the ankle dorsiflexes to ensure the foot and/or toes clear the ground as they 'swing' through the air. The foot/toes are actually closest to the ground during what is known as the mid-swing phase when the swinging foot passes next to the standing leg. After this and towards the end of the swing phase, the knee is then extended out to optimise the length of the stride and the heel is presented for contact with the ground.

When intensity of activity increases

As an activity performed with very little conscious thought, and during the course of any typical day, walking is a highly analysed activity. However, when we increase the intensity of our activity further to include running, cycling or many other activities, the biomechanical demands upon our body alter. Running shares similarities to walking, depending upon the speed of running, the lower-limb joint patterns shown in Figure 16.1 remain similar. As the speed of running increases, the muscular demands increase to generate the forces necessary to 'absorb' the ground impacts and to propel the body forwards. As running speed increases, the period of time available for ground contact decreases, which means a greater force needs to be applied to the ground in a shorter time-period. Large increases in the ground reaction forces can immediately be seen. Vertical ground reaction forces during walking normally reach approximately 1–1.5 times body weight (Nilsson & Thorstensson, 1989), whereas during running these ground reaction forces increase to three times body weight (Nilsson & Thorstensson, 1989) or higher. Similarly, horizontal ground reaction forces, which are indicative of the forces contributing to forward motion increase four-fold when comparing running to walking, increasing from about 0.1 times body weight during walking, to over 0.4 times body weight during running (Nilsson & Thorstensson, 1989).

As we run faster the pattern of movement changes at the lower limbs: step length increases causing foot placement changes, with feet landing further forward. The foot lands in a more plantar flexed position, creating a mid-foot landing, or at faster speeds a forefoot landing. Placing the feet closer to the centre-of-mass and in a plantar flexed position removes the

Table 16.1   Peak sagittal ankle and knee joint moments during walking/ running at different speeds. Values are representative values of healthy, young individuals (Speed: m/s; Ankle and knee joint moment: Nm/kg)

Speed	Ankle	Knee
1.1	1.70	0.50
2.2	2.25	2.15
3.3	2.80	2.60
4.4	3.00	2.65

initial period of plantar flexion, which can act as a braking force, which is seen during walking (Figure 16.1a). Therefore, running gait minimises the braking effects of foot contact allowing for more efficient forward motion. When running slowly there are changes to gait cycle time and magnitudes of different variables, but similar kinematic and kinetic patterns of motion are present when compared to walking. As running speed increases, however, and limb placement alters to improve running efficiency, these kinematic patterns alter (e.g. when forefoot running the ankle may remain in plantar flexion throughout the stance period) with knock-on alterations to the kinetic control.

The key factor that remains throughout during increasing intensity of activity such as running faster is that the muscular requirement increases with increasing intensity of activity to generate adequate joint moments to produce and control movements. Examples of the increase in peak joint moment requirements for different running speeds can be seen in Table 16.1. The faster the running speed, the greater the requirement from muscles such as the quadriceps and calf muscles to provide the forward motion and maintain upright support despite the decreased time in which each limb is in contact with the ground. Therefore, the joint moments at each lower limb joint increase with increasing ground reaction forces and a corresponding increase in the contribution from the muscles is required to produce and control movements.

Biomechanics when people are less active

When people become less active, whether due to lifestyle, age and/or illness it has a consequent effect on the biomechanics of movement. The key physiological effects resulting from inactivity are commonly sarcopenia (a loss of muscle mass) and weight gain, however, if illness is a factor there may be physiological changes to the size and function of skeletal muscle, the nervous system, skeletal structures, and many other factors that can alter biomechanical behaviour during movement.

Age

As we get older there is an inevitable decrease in muscle size and function, which is compounded when decreased capabilities result in individuals decreasing their daily physical activities, leading to a downward spiral of decreasing muscle function and reducing physical activity levels. Additionally, as we age some joint structures become stiffer, reducing the range-of-motion at joints, thereby impacting upon kinematic behaviour. Therefore, older people are commonly seen to walk with shorter steps, which allows for reduced lower-limb joint range of motion. Step times also increase, with longer times spent in double-support (where two feet are in contact with the ground) to maximise balance control. Increased step-widths allow for a larger base-of-support during double stance, compensating for compromised balance control, due to impaired vision and hearing, as well as the reduced body centre-of-mass stability associated with slower walking and less forward momentum (Bhatt, Wening, & Pai, 2005).

As adequate muscular contributions are key to completing daily activities, reduced muscular size and strength results in difficulties and/or inabilities meeting the 'normal' biomechanical demands. Therefore, to allow activities to be undertaken and optimise efficiency, people may alter their biomechanical strategy during certain activities (Reeves et al., 2008; Brown et al., 2014). People tend to walk slower, older runners tend to run slower: this is because faster motions are associated with higher demands for joint moments and muscle forces as mentioned previously. Therefore, as muscular capabilities reduce with ageing we become unable to attain such high intensity of activity with their associated high muscular demands and need to alter the nature of the biomechanical demands associated with the activity by employing altered biomechanical strategies.

Chronic disease, illness and injury

Chronic disease, illness and musculoskeletal injuries may all impact upon factors that affect how an individual moves, altering their biomechanical strategy. Many chronic diseases, illnesses and injuries will impact upon aspects of the sensory or motor systems that bring about alterations to the biomechanics of walking and other activities. For example, some may cause impairments to the motor system and muscle directly, resulting in lower muscular capabilities than 'healthy' individuals, with similar impacts upon biomechanics as ageing, limiting the ability to produce adequately high joint moments, and requiring slower, less 'demanding' movements to be employed.

Almost any conditions that impact upon the mechanisms used for movement will have a resultant change to the biomechanical behaviour of the individual. Whilst muscle weakness is a common factor, any changes to various bodily systems will have an impact. This can include the sensory control systems (e.g. peripheral sensation, inner ear balance control, visual input, etc.), soft tissues, or alterations to skeletal structure (e.g. deformation of joint surfaces in arthritis) which may all impact upon how a movement is performed.

> *Example: an individual with diabetes may experience multiple complications. Decreased muscle strength is common, reducing physical capabilities, causing the individual to walk slower, generating lower joint moments. Presence of Diabetic Peripheral Neuropathy (damage to the peripheral nerves) will reduce sensory feedback from the plantar surface of the foot, as well as reducing proprioception (the ability to detect joint position) thereby reducing balance control and encouraging shorter steps with longer time spent in stance and double stance to maximise the support during walking. Further, diabetes is associated with stiffening of soft tissues, resulting in stiffer tendons and thinner less absorptive fat pads on the sole of the foot, which may further limit the range-of-motion of the joints contributing to shorter step lengths as well as reducing the shock absorption properties of the sole.*

Practical applications

Applications of biomechanics feature in a range of situations including healthcare and sports. Either of these applications may be directed towards population specific or individual specific goals. When considering a population, the key objective is typically identification of factors influencing or impairing a given movement task, for example, understanding how muscular weakness impacts upon walking, or how a particular training regimen impacts muscle strength. Biomechanical knowledge gleaned from population-based approaches is enabling screening techniques for specific health conditions and is optimising physical performance in various sporting disciplines. Practical applications of biomechanics will likely expand further into the future with advances in equipment, software and individual expertise.

Chapter summary

- Human biomechanics is the study of forces acting on and within the human body and the motion resulting from such forces.
- Human motion is dependent upon the resultant of both external forces acting upon the body and internal forces acting within the body.
- As the intensity of the activity increases, higher forces are placed upon the body to generate faster/stronger movements.
- Prolonged physical inactivity, chronic disease and musculoskeletal injury may all impact upon physical capabilities and/or the mechanical properties of body tissues, resulting in alterations from the typical 'normal' movement strategy.

References

Bhatt T., Wening J.D., & Pai, Y.-C. (2005). Influence of gait speed on stability: recovery from anterior slips and compensatory stepping. *Gait Posture, 21*(2), 146–156. Available from: www.sciencedirect. com/science/article/pii/S0966636204000232

Brown, S.J., Handsaker, J.C., Bowling, F.L., Maganaris, C.N., Boulton, A.J.M., & Reeves, N.D. (2014). Do patients with diabetic neuropathy use a higher proportion of their maximum strength when walking? *J Biomech, 47*(15), 3639–3644. Available from: www.sciencedirect.com/science/article/pii/S0021929014005247

Gatev, P., Thomas, S., Kepple, T., & Hallett, M. (1999). Feedforward ankle strategy of balance during quiet stance in adults. *J Physiol,* 1999 (pt 3): 915–928. Available from: www.ncbi.nlm.nih.gov/pubmed/9882761

Nilsson, J., & Thorstensson, A. (1989). Ground reaction forces at different speeds of human walking and running. *Acta Physiol Scand, 136*(2): 217–227. Available from: www.ncbi.nlm.nih.gov/pubmed/2782094

Reeves, N.D., Spanjaard, M., Mohagheghi, A.A., Baltzopoulos, V., & Maganaris, C.N. (2008). The demands of stair descent relative to maximum capacities in elderly and young adults. *J Electromyogr Kinesiol, 18*(2), 218–227. Available from: www.sciencedirect.com/science/article/pii/S1050641107001034

17 Sociology and physical activity

Ross Neville

Keywords: exercising, gym-going, health and fitness, body lessons, consumer culture, digital media technologies

The sociological perspective

Introduction and working definition

The context for a sociological understanding of physical activity has been in the pipeline for some time now – a long time, perhaps (Boudreau, 1978; cf. Freund & Martin, 2004). Some will argue that sociologists have always had important things to say about physical activity. This is true, particularly in relation to the division of labour in modern societies and how movement is subsequently (and differentially) organised and experienced in relation to both work and non-work (or leisure) time (see Harvey, 2000, pp. 97–116).

The majority of readers and contributors to this volume will be aware of the recent shift away from behavioural science approaches to understanding physical activity towards the use of broader social-ecological (or systems-based) models (Kennedy & Blair, 2014; Kohl et al., 2012; cf. McLeroy et al., 1988; Sallis, Bauman, & Pratt, 1998). This shift provides an appropriate context for situating physical activity in relation to the *sociological perspective*, which is defined for the purposes of this chapter simply, and broadly, as encompassing research on social *units*, social *processes*, and social *products* (Hirschman, 1986, p. 238).[1] The interrelationship between social process and social product components (of the sociological perspective) will be the main focus of this chapter.

Why sociology? Why now?

As for the presence of a chapter on the *sociology* of physical activity in the present volume: is there any indication that the relevance of the discipline has become more widely accepted in recent years? An important position statement from Das and Horton (2012) seems to indicate that there is.

In what is now regarded as a landmark publication for advocating physical activity as a concern in its own right and a unique speciality in public health (published in *The Lancet* [2012, cf. Hallal et al., 2012a, 2012b; Kohl et al., 2012; Lee et al., 2012] entitled 'Rethinking our approach to physical activity'), Das and Horton (2012) open by stating:

> Physical activity is not a medical or pathological predicament but more a cultural challenge: to create a lifestyle inclusive of physical activity . . . But the first step in what must

be a social revolution towards an active, and away from a passive, physical and mental life should be to assemble the best experts in the field and the best evidence to understand what we know about human health and physical activity.

(p. 189)

As far as creating lifestyles inclusive of physical activity, we will proceed in this chapter on the basis that sociology, and the work of the sociologist in particular, is a relevant resource, both to this cultural challenge, and to the need for a monumental shift in the social organisation of movement.

Sociology of physical activity as exercise

While the chapter is framed broadly in relation to social process- and product-related components of the sociological perspective, in the sections that follow, the proposal is to draw readers' direct attention to the most established body of research evidence that exists within sociology on physical activity. Namely, research on exercising, health and fitness culture, or 'gym-going' more colloquially, as these represent what sociologists would regard, without qualification, as advanced modern society's primary *institutionalisation* of physical activity.

While it does not exhaust the current state of research on the sociology of physical activity to focus on health and fitness- (or gym-) culture, this chapter will no doubt provide readers with a useful and, hopefully, interesting introduction to: (i) research perspectives in sociology, and (ii) critical considerations about how the place and role of physical activity in modern society is uniquely interpreted from the sociological view.

The sociological perspective –*product* and *process* aspects

Social products

Research on actual products which span the health and fitness sector is too vast an issue to do justice to in this section (see Andreasson & Johansson, 2014; Millington, 2016; Bordo, 1993; Pronger, 2002; Smith Maguire, 2007). What's more, the introduction of digital media-based products into the market in recent years is such that the sociology of self-tracking in health has required book-length treatment to do it justice[2] (Lupton, 2014). The focus in this section is on the role of the media more broadly – on the role of *mediation* in physical activity and exercise contexts, broadly conceived. The process by which knowledge regarding physical activity is 'translated' (Latour, 1987, pp. 108–121) into information that is actionable for individuals in the form of exercise will be considered here.

Fitness media – or: What mediates knowledge about fitness?

The work of consumption and media studies scholar, Jennifer Smith Maguire (2001, 2002, 2006, 2007, 2008a, 2008b) is the authority in this area. As such, this section draws out key points and practical implications from her work, which specifies the ways in which individuals *typically* engage with the output, or with the *products*, of scientific knowledge as 'body lessons' (Smith Maguire 2002, p. 450).

Clearly, some body lessons which are *accessible to* and being *accessed by* individuals today, particularly in consumer culture (Baudrillard, 1998; Sassatelli, 2010), are not at all the product of (or even related to) empirical scientific research! (Glassner, 1989, 1990, 1992) Even where body lessons have a scientific basis or warrant, research indicates that there is often reluctance to follow-up on more recent developments beyond headline-grabbing initial findings (particularly where falsification is concerned) (see Bourdaa et al., 2015).

Being fit, or being fit for consumption?

Smith Maguire's (2002) research establishes a basic premise which has far-reaching consequences in this context. That is, despite the origin, or genus, of body lessons – despite benefits which accrue to society in terms of objective health (Trost, Blair, & Khan, 2014) or to individuals in the form objective health *plus* personal subjective wellbeing (Garcia et al., 2012) – physical activity and exercising are, for the most part in modern society, presented to individuals: (i) as motivational problems to be overcome; (ii) promoted as a means to extrinsic ends and/or source of calculable rewards; and (iii) therefore just another object of and for consumption activity (Baudrillard, 1998; Bauman, 2007).

Drawing on a systematic document analysis of lifestyle media through which body lessons are commonly transmitted (Duncan, 1994; Dworkin & Wachs, 2009; Lloyd, 1996; Mansfield, 2011; Markula, 2003), Smith Maguire (2002) observes that physical activity and exercising, while good for one's 'health', in reality, are promoted, bought and sold for the purposes of enhancing 'fitness'. And she simply asks, 'Fit for what?' and 'Fit for whom?' (Smith Maguire, 2007). The answer to this question, it turns out, exits in some tension with the view that would typically be ascribed to physical activity and exercise in ordinary language and therefore in the context of everyday life (Blaxter, 2003).

Far from being a simple matter of objective health and of personal subjective wellbeing, according to Smith Maguire (2007), physical activity taken as exercise has become associated with a form of social fitness that she neatly refers to as the project of 'being fit for consumption' – of 'being fit to consume, and fit to be consumed by others' (p. 196; cf. Scott, 2006).

Knowledge as body lessons, information as rules to go by

In order to elaborate on this, Smith Maguire indicates that, for the most part, public exposure to scientific knowledge in the area of physical activity and exercising comes in the form of (and is subsequently internalised as) 'ensembles of rules' as opposed to 'ensembles of facts' (Foucault, 1980, p. 132; cf. Glassner, 1990, pp. 215–216). That is to say: in relation to taking physical activity *as* exercise, public understanding of science is based on *information* as opposed to *knowledge*; this information comes in the form of *rules to go by*, or simple *instructions*; and, because of this, body lessons are presented to individuals as practical guides which combine a multitude of affiliated consumption behaviours. This rationalisation of physical activity as exercise in the form of consumer behaviour, as opposed to simply healthy behaviours, has some interesting implications, as we will see.

Cumulatively, when solutions to motivational problems are sought on the basis of *information* and *instruction*, as opposed to *knowledge*, and when these instructions are translated for individuals in the form of practical guides for consumption behaviour or 'consumption scripts' (LaRose, 2010, p. 198; Wansink, 2004, p. 464), a 'culture of expertise' (Giddens, 1991, p. 31) emerges. In the present context, so-called 'expertise' ranges from those practising basic science in the public interests at one end of the spectrum, to fitness crusaders, zealots and moral entrepreneurs (Andreasson & Johansson, 2014; Monaghan, Hollands, & Pritchard, 2010) practising in the name of commercial interests at the other.

Experts of the first kind practise basic science in relative obscurity in the belief that facts speak for themselves. This has the resulting effect of naturalising physical activity and exercise in forms that are often not yet made accessible by the public (Hunter et al., 2014; Kay et al., 2014; Knox, Musson, & Adams, 2015). The latter practises marketing campaigns on behalf of the public interest much more aggressively. This has quite a different effect, as it translates the meaning of 'exercise' in many and varied senses of the term: as exercising control and practising self-restraint; as making personal investments and being more productive; as a form of emotional labour and therefore evidence of emotional intelligence; and as an opportunity or obligation to conduct *self-work* in one's own leisure time (Smith Maguire, 2008b; Hochschild, 1983; Rojek, 2010). In short, from the sociological perspective, there is much more at stake in physical activity than simple bodily movement produced by skeletal muscle resulting in energy expenditure! (Caspersen, Powell, & Christenson, 1985)

Physical activity as exercise; exercise as compensatory consumption behaviour

Crucial to the sociological perspective is recognition that body lessons are more than a matter of activity and energy expenditure. What's more, these body lessons serve to instruct the consuming public that physical activity and exercise need not be pleasurable, or even worth doing for their own sake. To clarify the message: they can be pleasurable . . . they are worth doing for their own sake . . . but they simply don't have to be. This, by and large, is how the physical activity is presented to individuals in modern society (as Smith Maguire sees it). Because of this lack of *necessity* for pleasure or enjoyment, social products owing to physical activity and exercise have a tendency to be largely extrinsic, and based on the notion that investing time and energy will result in subsequent, 'calculable', rewards (Smith Maguire, 2002, p. 451).

Physical activity and exercising are thus reconciled on terms that are relevant to participating in consumer culture. One must balance the requirement for self-discipline with a desire for instant-gratification – i.e. what Featherstone (1982) referred to in the initial sociological studies of the body in consumer culture as 'calculating hedonism' (p. 18). Since physical activity and exercise do not lend themselves immediately or easily to intrinsic rewards, 'material self-reward' becomes the standard technique through which to promote and habituate these healthy behaviours (Smith Maguire, 2002, p. 461). Individuals are instructed that the consumption of subsequent pleasures outside of the gym is made permissible through the discipline of exercising within it (Smith Maguire, 2007, p. 196). This involves the prospects of *shopping in* and *shopping for* a newly fit body, Smith Maguire observes. To reiterate: there is so much more to physical activity than simple bodily movement produced by skeletal muscle resulting in energy expenditure. Forget health, energy expenditure creates more room for consumption! Expend more here now, and you can spend more somewhere else later. Or, phrased as a body lesson that everyone can understand: 'Exercise now; go shopping and eat cake later'.

Social processes

The elements of the sociological perspective do not exist in isolation. Any sharp distinction between the components is arbitrary, but it is necessary to frame the analysis. The focus in this section is on the boundary, or transition, from *social products* to *social processes*, of which physical activity taken as exercise is an excellent example.[3]

Reflexive embodiment

As far as empirical research is concerned, there is little doubt (in my mind at least) that the formative work in this area comes from Nick Crossley. Crossley's (2004a, 2004b, 2005, 2006a, 2006b, 2006c, 2008; cf. Sassatelli, 1999, 2010) ethnographies of exercising, or 'gym-going', as he phrases it (2006b, p. 23), provide lucid, 'rich', descriptions of exercising as an emergent and pervasive social practice, and as a reflection of the broader process of 'reflexive embodiment' (2006c, pp. 1–3) which operate in contemporary society. According to Crossley, reflexive embodiment is the capacity of individuals and their tendency as social agents to perceive, emote about, and reflect back upon their own body in order to modify or maintain it in some way. Reflexive embodiment therefore encompasses both body-image (Featherstone, 1982, 2010) and body-work (Gimlin, 2002, 2007) aspects, both of which are necessary if individual social agents are to engage with body lessons and subsequently put them into action.

Reflexive body techniques (RBTs)

Within the context of this broad process of reflexive embodiment, Crossley (2006b) situates gym-going along a continuum of habitual and/or routine bodily practices and modification strategies, which he subsequently defines as 'reflexive body techniques' (p. 40; Crossley, 2004a, p. 39), or RBTs, which are specific actions or activities aimed at the fulfilment of some body lesson. Change is a fundamental component of RBTs, and individuals will tend to make use of a range of resources from the external environment in order to manage this process. The crucial 'reflexive' component here, of course, is that the changes at stake within reflexive embodiment are much less about changes to the external environment than they are about changes to the individual or social agent themselves.

The notion of 'body lessons' and 'compensatory consumption', that were introduced in the previous section, are being built on here by Crossley. What his research contributes is a further understanding of how the body lessons which are being instructed, or prescribed, to individuals in modern consumer societies are getting translated, and play out, in actual practical settings. His research informs us about how physical activity taken as exercise becomes translated further in what Baudrillard (1998) referred to as a process of 'managed consumption' (pp. 131–132, 134).

Managed consumption – the role and language of motivation

Crossley (2006b) begins his ethnography by stating the defining feature of gym-going, as he sees it: '[J]oining a gym is different from sticking at it. Many more agents manage the former than the latter . . . [A] new set of motives kicks in for regular gym-goers and . . . these motives are accessible to them, in some part, on account of the [learning experiences] that go along with a gym career.' (pp. 46–47). His research therefore takes up where Smith Maguire left off in that he too recognises in gym-going a fundamental motivational problem to be overcome: a problem to be managed, and that can, if *adequately* or *appropriately* motivated, develop over time into a 'gym career' (p. 47).

But by what authority can a sociologist discuss adequacy and appropriateness of motivational dispositions? Beyond, say, what is already, and perhaps more legitimately, covered at length in psychology? To understand the answer to this question requires a brief detour, which we will return to, to truly understand the nuance, and value, that exists in Crossley's account.

Crossley's treatment of motivation shares similarities with psychological perspectives in that motives are not conceived here as either singular or static: 'There are many motives for gym-going. It cannot be reduced down to a single factor' (Crossley, 2006b, p. 45) 'which remains static, and which is identical for all people' (p. 25). In order to develop on this notion that motivates can be multiple, and that motivation is a fluid process, Crossley invokes Mills' (1940) notion, 'vocabularies of motive' (p. 904).

Mills' vocabularies of motive specifies that the language of motivational ascription does not inhabit the inner life of individuals who act autonomously. The language of motivation is not, according to Mills, based on descriptions of inner feelings, needs, wants or desires (not exclusively, at least). Rather, motives inhabit the social world around us. Motivational structures, to borrow from Brandom (1995) operate according to a 'deontic' (as opposed to a 'consequentialist') logic. In other words: we do not have motives as a consequence of this or that inner feeling, urge, or desire. Motives, in themselves, do not, strictly speaking, *have* reasons. Rather, motives are *themselves* reasons. Crossley elaborates motives are the reasons we have, and give, for entering and inhabiting a shared social space with others. Motives operate with the 'space of reasons', according to Brandom (1995, p. 899), and according to what he subsequently (1995) refers to as the simple logic of 'giving and asking for reasons' (p. 902). Such a view of motivation, i.e. as part of a social process of giving and asking for reasons, is, according to Crossley, a fundamental aspect of gym-going.

'Motive talk'

Newcomers are particularly implicated in this process, and Crossley observes that talking about motives is a fundamental aspect of the initial gym-going experience. But, talk of motives is not necessarily a reflection of social agents opening up, or sharing the innermost depths of their psyche to strangers. Rather, talk of motives is simply the first in a series of ongoing steps where the gym-goer will have to account for their presence (Crossley, 2006b, p. 27). Relatedness is not, strictly speaking, or exclusively, a motive which drives individuals towards the act of gym-going (cf. Gill, 2000). Rather, in the social milieu of the gym, and in social milieus in general, talk of motives serve a relatedness function. Talk of motives is for convincing others as to why you are inhabiting this or that social space; or at least reaffirming to them what they already suspect (based on prior experience with other people like you) or expect (based on their initial observations of you).

Supplementing psychological perspectives then, this might, usefully, be referred to as ritualising, as opposed to the rationalising, function of motivation. We *share* motives as opposed to simply *having* them. This recognises, and utilises, the dual meaning of the word *share* to come to terms with the way motivation operates in this context – i.e. as an interplay between giving reasons and having reasons in common.

Crossley's rich descriptions of gym-going as a lived experience herein, though grounded in empirical observations (Crossley, 2004a, 2006b, 2008), are very much a function of looking at gym culture through these two theoretical lenses. This enables him to show how RBTs, such as exercising, require, for their initial establishment and maintenance over time, a broad repertoire of motives. From here, participants will have to draw one, many, *or all* of them on occasions, perhaps, in order to account for their presence in the gym, at any given point in time: account for their presence both to themselves, and to others whom they now aspire to be like (cf. Crossley, 2006b, pp. 27–29).

From here, the crux of Crossley's observations, and his contribution to the sociology of physical activity and exercise, can be summarised as follows: (i) taking physical activity as exercise is an expression of the reflexive embodiment which extends to and affects individuals in modern society; (ii) reflexive body techniques such as gym-going, though prevalent in modern societies, remain a motivational problem that social agents attempt to overcome; (iii) starting at the gym and sticking at it require fundamentally different motivational structures, vocabularies or repertoires; (iv) those who manage to stick to it over time are (very much the exception as opposed to the rule) do this constantly establishing new meanings and/or new incentives; (v) this makes space for, or situates, gym-going as a natural feature within their everyday lives; (vi) one must, therefore, acquire a taste, or a thirst, for gym-going (like one would establish or refine their palate in relation to gastronomic or culinary settings, for example; Bourdieu, 1984); (vi_a) one must learn when and how to interpret the initial antagonistic-agonistic nature of the task in question (i.e. expending energy, exerting physical effort, *working*) (vi_b) as either positive and/or even pleasant, or at least as a signal to them of the necessity for exercising (Crossley, 2006b, p. 40; cf. Neville et al., 2015, pp. 293–295; Sassatelli, 1999, pp. 233–237). Finally, and for persevering with all of this, individuals are (vii) rewarded with a psycho-bio-social state (Hanin & Ekkekakis, 2014) known to those of a psychoanalytic persuasion as an experience of tension-release (Crossley, 2006b, pp. 41–42; cf. Elias & Dunning, 1986; Maguire, 1992; Malcolm & Mansfield, 2013).

I have built on the work of Smith Maguire and Crossley in my own modest research endeavours, published elsewhere (De Lyon, Neville, & Armour, 2016; Neville, 2013a, 2013b; Neville, Gorman, Flanagan, & Dimanche, 2015; Neville & Gorman, 2016). The overall point from these studies that is relevant to our purposes here now, and which summarise a latent observation in Crossley's research, can be stated briefly as follows: motives for joining a gym, i.e. motives for initiating and initiation into this social process, are very much related to the nature of the *activities,* and to the *outcomes* which are on offer. Motives for actually going to gym, sticking with it, and managing to do this over time relate more broadly to lifestyle considerations and to the nature of the *process* or *experience* itself.

The following, penultimate, section of this chapter makes a slight change in direction in order to address current issues within the sociology of physical activity – issues, however, that, while under-researched, are likely to be having a substantial bearing transition from *activity* to *experience*, too.

Current issues in the sociology of physical activity

Digital mediation

Without exception, the most topical current issue in the sociology of physical activity and exercise is the introduction of digital media technologies (DMTs) into the market. The issue falls under the remit of what sociologists are referring to as '*digital mediation*', which represents the increased filtering of everyday social life through remote, interactive, and otherwise 'new' media (Lupton, 2014; Orton-Johnson & Prior, 2013). Digital mediation acknowledged the dual role that DMTs play in both supporting greater interconnectivity in social life and in feeding back into the organisation of social life itself (Burrows & Savage, 2014).

Preliminary evidence base

Despite research in the area being nascent, there is already a growing multi-disciplinary agreement that the formative role played by DMTs in social life has the potential to enhance the promotion, monitoring, and support of meaningful engagement, in physical activity and exercise. Recent reviews, for example, indicate that interventions incorporating DMTs are effective in supporting people to achieve recommended levels of physical activity, and stick to this over time (Foster et al., 2013; Middelweerd et al., 2014). Recent evidence suggests that DMTs offer increased social support for exercising when compared with other intervention strategies (Kinnafick, Thøgersen-Ntoumani, & Duda, 2016). From the perspective of the sociology of physical activity, there is also a growing consensus that the formative role played by DMTs is enhancing the production and (in particular) the display of cultural-, social-, even economic-capital. This is particularly evident in the use of social media and, to paraphrase the famous idiom from Goffman (1971) in the presentation of the self, or 'selfie!', in everyday life (Lupton, 2014; Millington, 2016).

In sum: there is clearly a wealth of information now available online to support health-enhancing behaviours. Consider too the cost-effectiveness of public health messaging in this medium; the pervasiveness, frequency and intensity of daily internet usage; and even the potential for public health messages to have penetration at a global level. The potential for DMTs to support increased physical activity is therefore substantial. This is why recent developments in social media, despite their commercial basis, are being welcomed, by and large (Williams et al., 2014; Laranjo et al., 2014; Vaterlaus et al., 2015).

Mounting concerns

There are, however, mounting concerns here too. DMT-use alerts attention even more so to the discrepancy that exists between *information* and *knowledge* (Woolgar, 2002). Building on traditional concerns about the intentions of fitness crusaders, zealots and moral entrepreneurs (Andreasson & Johansson, 2014; Monaghan, Hollands, & Pritchard, 2010), in the digital age, we have potentially entered into 'outlaw territory', Serres (*in* Obrist, 2014) observes. Increasingly, Serres warns, market transactions take place with little or no presumption or regard for source, or for the professional qualifications and competence of source providers. The discrepancy between information and knowledge addressed in previous sections is therefore potentially doubled: by an unbounded outlaw territory, on the one hand, and a lack of regulation as to the types of body lessons which are produced and consumed online, on the other. When it comes to the role of DMTs in public health promotion, so-called advances – namely, the potential for promoting increased physical activity – also pose substantial challenges from the perspective of social and pedagogical relations (Casey, Goodyear, & Armour, 2016a; Gard, 2015; Lupton, 2015).

The concern for adolescent health and wellbeing has particular urgency in this context (Casey, Goodyear, & Armour, 2016b). The need for taking exercise, perceptions about the need for weight loss, and broader body-reflexive considerations that stigmatise and lead to interpersonal judgments by size have affected western, body-conscious, societies for some time – particularly for females (Bartky, 1993; Bordo, 1993; Gimlin, 2002, 2007). These issues now appear to be affecting those of an increasingly younger age, regardless of gender (van den Berg et al., 2010), with the passing of every academic review and damning governmental department inquiry and subsequent report (Livingstone et al., 2017). The dangers to adolescents are apparent, but the full extent of the consequences of unsolicited health-related information (which is being shared and accessed through social media) remains largely unknown.

Opportunities arising

It is encouraging that, in the digital age, individuals are seeking health-related information more autonomously than in previous generations. However, a major concern in this context is that the reflexive body techniques (RBTs) being engaged in, and the body lessons being sought, are aimed less at health than at social status gains and the display of conspicuous consumption. Increasing research seems to indicate that individuals – again, adolescents in particular – are exercising in a way that is very much in spite of their health, and not contributing towards it (for an example, see Boardley, Grix, & Dewar, 2014; Boardley, Grix, & Harkin, 2015; Boardley et al., 2016).

Granted, some of these are not new issues by sociological standards (Bartky, 1993; Beck, 1992; Bordo, 1993; Bourdieu, 1984; Featherstone, 1982). They are not an outcome of, or caused by, DMTs, or digital mediation – but they are important current issues, nonetheless – exacerbated by digital mediation at a magnitude which makes seminal remarks about lifestyle media and consumer culture quaint, and frankly, trivial by comparison.

To conclude this section on a positive note, let's affirm DMTs can potentially be a resource for promoting physical activity, as opposed to disavowing them outright. Three positive notes to be more precise:

1. In research conducted in other areas of social life, where digital mediation is prevalent, evidence indicates that new forms of personal agency and social (re-) engagement are developing and being enacted online (Marres, 2016);
2. Engagement with new media technologies has been shown to facilitate civic learning:

    *   by mobilising public interest and popular opinion into broader collective sentiment or collective representations;
    *   and by offering a shared platform from which to participate in public issues, which affect society as a whole (Marres, 2016);

3. There is even evidence to suggest that the networked structure and networking capabilities of digital media culture at large, can be harnessed to offer previously socially-isolated individuals increased opportunities for engaging in meaningful social action (Brauer, 2011).

Prospects

The prospects for digital media technologies to enhance the efforts of social-ecological (or systems-based) approaches to increasing physical activity is, therefore, easy to establish, when we consider these recent developments with the sociology of science and technology studies. For now, however, the ways in which they can be leveraged or 'repurposed' (Rogers, 2013) so as to serve the public as opposed to solely serving commercial interests is not yet very well understood.

Conclusions and practical implications

Rethinking our approach to physical activity

Das and Horton's (2012) remarks in our opening sections come with a health warning which relates to the contents and directs the conclusions of this chapter: '[P]hysical activity is not about sport and it is more than just exercise. It is not about running on a treadmill, whilst staring at a mirror listening to your iPod' (p. 189).

What needs to be recognised here, however, and what the sociological perspective alerts our attention to, is a subtle distinction. What Das and Horton are really saying is that:

> Physical activity doesn't have to be, and perhaps shouldn't be, just about these things.

This is true, at least in part: for a significant proportion of people, institutionalised forms of physical activity such as sport and exercise will never be an appropriate means of achieving the weekly recommended guidelines. However, for a significant proportion of people, they are enough.[4] This is what they think physical activity is about: going to the gym and working out, getting fit, losing a bit of weight, or toning up. In other words, for them, physical activity *is about* sport and exercise. Perhaps this is what they *want* physical activity to be about. For whatever reason: they want to be with or make friends; they want to learn how to like exercise, and how to use it for pleasure and relaxation; because it is most convenient *for them*. And, perhaps they want to be able to do these things better.

Why sociology? What next?

So, with Das and Horton, let's offer alternatives to physical activity as sport and exercise. However, let's also not lose sight of, and cease offering support to, people who want to be able to achieve their recommended weekly dose of physical activity in these forms. For whatever reason, these might simply represent *meaningful forms of physical activity for them*. So, let's consider meeting people *where they are at*, and not simply presenting them *with what we know*. A person's inability to achieve recommended weekly levels of physical activity does not need to be coupled with accusations of ignorance about what physical activity is actually about. Our personal, and even our academic, preferences for a particular form of physical activity should not be the only basis for a reduction in policies, provision or promotions regarding it. *Physical activity is about sport and exercise too* . . . So let's also consider this when 'rethinking our approach to physical activity' (Das & Horton, 2012, p. 189).

Balancing these goals will no doubt benefit from insights based on the sociological perspective – what C. Wright Mills (1959) referred to as 'the sociological imagination' (p. 5). Let's use it critically, but also constructively. This will enable us to better translate our research into forms which are actionable for individuals: i.e. into body lessons to go by as opposed to facts by which they must abide. As Smith Maguire's research has taught us, if nothing else, given the inclination for information and instruction over knowledge, we cannot be confident that individuals are going to be willing, able, or are even going to want to access it on any other terms anyway!

> Knowing is not enough; we must apply . . .
> Willing is not enough; we must do.
>
> Goethe

Chapter summary

1. **Why sociology?**
   Shift away from behavioural science approaches to understanding physical activity is drawing attention to the importance of sociology

   • The science of social systems

2. **Physical activity and exercising**
   Sociological research to date has focused on physical activity taken as exercise

   • Exercising represents an institutionalised form of physical activity for advanced modern societies

3. **Social products – physical activity *as* exercise**
   Lack of exercise is a motivational problem to be overcome

   • This involves rules for conduct known as 'body lessons', including

       ○ *Exercising* control
       ○ *Practising* self-restraint
       ○ *Working* on yourself, or, working on *your self*

   • When exercise is framed as self-work

       ○ Material rewards become standard for habituating exercise, which
       ○ Results in understanding health as 'being fit for consumption'

4. **Social processes – gym-going and working out**
   Physical activity taken as exercise in commercial health clubs, or 'gyms'

   • Distinction between motives for joining and for sticking to it

       ○ Latter requires establishing new meanings and incentives
       ○ Developing 'a taste for it'
           ▪ Learning to reinterpret antagonistic nature of activities
           ▪ Framing as positive, pleasant, or at least necessary
           ▪ Rewarded by experiencing tension-release

5. **Current issues – digital mediation**
   Digital media technologies support interconnectivity and feed back into the organisation of social life

   • This affects physical activity

       ○ positively, through relatedness pathways
       ○ negatively, due to a lack of regulation

6. **Summary and practical applications**
   Sport and exercise may never be an appropriate means for some people to achieve recommended physical activity levels

   • Need to better translate scientific knowledge about physical activity into body lessons which are actionable (by them), and accommodating of their preferences

Notes

1 A useful preliminary reading on the sociological perspective is Delaney and Madigan (2015), Chapter 1, and/or Delaney (2015). Chapters 1–6 of Giulianotti (2015) will also provide the reader with additional background information beyond what is feasible in this chapter.

2 Remarks on how increased '*digital mediation in social life*' affects physical activity, fitness and health are made in the next section (in the context of *Current issues*).

3 The fact that so many prominent sociologists have dedicated time within their broader analyses of social relations to explaining health and fitness culture is a testament to this point (for a review, see Crossley, 2006a).

4 *Potentially* 150 million people if industry report figures of annual gym and sports-club memberships from 2015 are anything to go by (IHRSA, 2016). The International Health, Racquet and Sportsclub Association (IHRSA) report that, globally, in 2015, 187,000 clubs had 150 million members, many of whom were new members, and that the total number of visits across the sector was in excess of 5 billion!

References

Andreasson, J., & Johansson, T. (2014). The fitness revolution: Historical transformations in the global gym and fitness culture. *Sport Science Review, 23*, 91–111.

Bartky, S. (1993). *Gender and domination*. London: Routledge.

Baudrillard, J. (1998). *The consumer society: Myths and structures*. London: Sage.

Bauman, Z. (2007) *Consuming life*. Cambridge: Polity.

Beck, U. (1992). *Risk society: Towards a new modernity*. London: Sage.

Blaxter, M. (2003). *Health and lifestyles*. London: Routledge.

Boardley, I.D., Allen, N., Simmons, A., & Laws, H. (2016). Nutritional, medicinal, and performance enhancing supplementation in dance. *Performance Enhancement & Health, 4*, 3–11.

Boardley, I.D., Grix, J., & Dewar, A.J. (2014). Moral disengagement and associated processes in performance-enhancing drug use: A national qualitative investigation. *Journal of Sports Sciences, 32*, 836–844.

Boardley, I.D., Grix, J., & Harkin, J. (2015). Doping in team and individual sports: A qualitative investigation of moral disengagement and associated processes. *Qualitative Research in Sport, Exercise and Health, 7*, 698–717.

Bordo, S. (1993). *Unbearable weight*. Berkeley, CA: University of California Press.

Boudreau, T. (1978). Physical activity, health and social policies. In F. Landry & W. Orban (Eds.), *Physical activity and human well-being* (pp. 239–250). Miami: Symposium Books.

Bourdaa, M., Konsman, J.P., Sécail, C., Venturini, T., Veyrat-Masson, I., & Gonon, F. (2015). Does television reflect the evolution of scientific knowledge? The case of attention deficit hyperactivity disorder coverage on French television. *Public Understanding of Science, 24*, 200–209.

Bourdieu, P. (1984). *Distinction: A social critique of the judgement of taste*. Cambridge, MA: Harvard University Press.

Brandom, R. (1995). Knowledge and the social articulation of the space of reasons. *Philosophy and Phenomenological Research, 55*, 895–908.

Brauer, C. (2011). *Netmodern: Interventions in digital sociology* (Unpublished doctoral dissertation), Goldsmiths, University of London, London UK.

Burrows, R., & Savage, M. (2014). After the crisis? Big Data and the methodological challenges of empirical sociology. *Big Data & Society, 1*, 1–6.

Casey, A., Goodyear, V.A., & Armour, K.M. (2016a). Rethinking the relationship between pedagogy, technology and learning in health and physical education. *Sport, Education and Society, 22*, 288–304.

Casey, A., Goodyear, V.A., & Armour, K.M. (Eds.). (2016b). *Digital technologies and learning in physical education: Pedagogical cases*. London: Routledge.

Caspersen, C.J., Powell, K.E., & Christenson, G.M. (1985). Physical activity, exercise, and physical fitness: Definitions and distinctions for health-related research. *Public Health Reports, 100*, 126–131.

Crossley, N. (2004a). The circuit trainer's habitus: Reflexive body techniques and the sociality of the workout. *Body & Society, 10*, 37–69.

Crossley, N. (2004b) Fat is a sociological issue: Obesity rates in late modern, 'body conscious' societies. *Social Theory & Health, 2*, 222–253.

Crossley, N. (2005) Mapping reflexive body techniques: On body modification and maintenance. *Body & Society, 11*, 1–35.

Crossley, N. (2006a) The networked body and the question of reflexivity. In D.D. Waskul & P. Vannini (Eds.), *Body / embodiment: Symbolic interaction and the sociology of the body* (pp. 21–34). Hampshire: Ashgate.

Crossley, N. (2006b). In the gym: Motives, meaning and moral careers. *Body & Society, 12*, 23–50.

Crossley, N. (2006c). *Reflexive embodiment in contemporary society*. Maidenhead: Open University Press.

Crossley, N. (2008) (Net)working out: Social capital in a private health club. *British Journal of Sociology, 59*, 475–500.

Das, P., & Horton, R. (2012). Rethinking our approach to physical activity. *The Lancet, 380*, 189–190.

De Lyon, A.T., Neville, R.D., & Armour, K.M. (2016). The role of fitness professionals in public health: A review of the literature. *Quest*, 1–18. doi: http://dx.doi.org/10.1080/00336297.2016.1224193

Delaney, T. (2015). The functionalist perspective on sport. In R. Giulianotti (Ed.), *The Routledge handbook of the sociology of sport* (pp. 18–28). New York: Routledge.

Delaney, T., & Madigan, T. (2015) *The sociology of sports: An introduction*. Jefferson, NC: McFarland & Company, Inc., Publishers.

Duncan, M.C. (1994). The politics of women's body images and practices: Foucault, the panopticon, and Shape magazine. *Journal of Sport and Social Issues, 18*, 48–65.

Dworkin, S.L., & Wachs, F.L. (2009). *Body panic: Gender, health, and the selling of fitness*. New York: NYU Press.

Elias, N., & Dunning, E. (1986). *Quest for excitement: Sport and leisure in the civilizing process*. Oxford: Blackwell.

Featherstone, M. (1982). The body in consumer culture. *Theory, Culture & Society, 1*, 18–33.

Featherstone, M. (2010). Body, image and affect in consumer culture. *Body & Society, 16*, 193–221.

Foster, C., Richards, J., Thorogood, M., & Hillsdon, M. (2013). Remote and web 2.0 interventions for promoting physical activity. *Cochrane Database of Systematic Reviews, 2013*(9), 1–83. doi: 10.1002/14651858.CD010395.pub2.

Foucault, M. (1980). *Power/knowledge: Selected interviews and other writings, 1972–1977*. New York: Pantheon.

Francombe, J., & Silk, M. (2012). Pedagogies of fat: The social currency of slenderness. In M.L. Silk & D.L. Andrews (Eds.), *Sport and neoliberalism* (pp 225–241). Philadelphia, PA: Temple University Press.

Freund, P., & Martin, G. (2004). Walking and motoring: Fitness and the social organisation of movement. *Sociology of Health & Illness, 26*, 273–286.

Garcia, D., Archer, T., Moradi, S., & Andersson-Arntén, A.C. (2012). Exercise frequency, high activation positive affect, and psychological well-being: Beyond age, gender, and occupation. *Psychology, 3*, 328–336.

Gard, M. (2015). They know they're getting the best knowledge possible: Locating the academic in changing knowledge economies. *Sport, Education and Society, 20*, 107–121.

Giddens, A. (1991). *Modernity and self-identity: Self and society in the late modern age*. Stanford, CA: Stanford University Press.

Gill, D.L. (2000). *Psychological dynamics of sport and exercise*. Champaign, IL: Human Kinetics.

Gimlin, D. (2002). *Body work: Beauty and self-image in American culture*. Berkeley, CA: University of California Press.

Gimlin, D. (2007). What is 'body work'? A review of the literature. *Sociology Compass, 1*, 353–370.

Giulianotti, R. (Ed.). (2015) *The Routledge handbook of the sociology of sport.* New York: Routledge.

Glassner, B. (1989). Fitness and the postmodern self. *Journal of Health and Social Behavior, 30*, 180–191.

Glassner, B. (1990). Fit for postmodern selfhood. In H.S. Becker & M.M. McCall (Eds.), *Symbolic Interaction and Cultural Studies* (pp. 215–243). Chicago, IL: University of Chicago Press.

Glassner, B. (1992). *Bodies: Overcoming the tyranny of perfection.* Los Angeles, CA: Lowell House.

Goffman, I. (1971) *The presentation of the self in everyday life.* Harmondsworth, London UK: Penguin.

Hallal, P.C., Andersen, L.B., Bull, F.C., Guthold, R., Haskell, W., Ekelund, U., & Lancet Physical Activity Series Working Group. (2012a). Global physical activity levels: Surveillance progress, pitfalls, and prospects. *The Lancet, 380*, 247–257.

Hallal, P.C., Bauman, A.E., Heath, G.W., Kohl 3rd, H.W., Lee, I.M., & Pratt, M. (2012b). Physical activity: More of the same is not enough. *The Lancet, 380*, 190.

Hanin, J., & Ekkekakis, P. (2014). Emotions in sport and exercise settings. In A.G. Papaioannou & D. Hackfort (Eds.), *Routledge companion to sport and exercise psychology: Global perspectives and fundamental concepts* (pp. 83–104). New York: Routledge.

Harvey, D. (2000). *Spaces of hope.* Berkeley, CA: University of California Press.

Hirschman, E.C. (1986). Humanistic inquiry in marketing research: Philosophy, method, and criteria. *Journal of Marketing Research, 23*, 237–249.

Hochschild, A.R. (1983). *The managed heart.* Berkeley, CA: University of California Press.

Hunter, R.F., Tully, M.A., Donnelly, P., Stevenson, M., & Kee, F. (2014). Knowledge of UK physical activity guidelines: Implications for better targeted health promotion. *Preventive Medicine, 65*, 33–39.

International Health, Racquet and Sportsclub Association (IHRSA) (2016). *The IHRSA global report 2016: The state of the health club industry.* Boston, MA: IHRSA.

Kay, M.C., Carroll, D.D., Carlson, S.A., & Fulton, J.E. (2014). Awareness and knowledge of the 2008 Physical Activity Guidelines for Americans. *Journal of Physical Activity and Health, 11*, 693–698.

Kennedy, A.B., & Blair, S.N. (2014). Motivating people to exercise. *American Journal of Lifestyle Medicine, 8*, 324–329.

Kinnafick, F.E., Thøgersen-Ntoumani, C., & Duda, J. (2016). The effect of need supportive text messages on motivation and physical activity behaviour. *Journal of Behavioral Medicine, 39*, 574–586.

Knox, E.C., Musson, H., & Adams, E.J. (2015). Knowledge of physical activity recommendations in adults employed in England: Associations with individual and workplace-related predictors. *International Journal of Behavioral Nutrition and Physical Activity, 12*, 69–76.

Kohl, H.W., Craig, C.L., Lambert, E.V., Inoue, S., Alkandari, J.R., Leetongin, G., . . . & Lancet Physical Activity Series Working Group. (2012). The pandemic of physical inactivity: Global action for public health. *The Lancet, 380*, 294–305.

Laranjo, L., Arguel, A., Neves, A.L., Gallagher, A.M., Kaplan, R., Mortimer, N., . . . & Lau, A.Y. (2014). The influence of social networking sites on health behavior change: A systematic review and meta-analysis. *Journal of the American Medical Informatics Association, 22*, 243–256.

LaRose, R. (2010). The problem of media habits. *Communication Theory, 20*, 194–222.

Latour, B. (1987). *Science in action: How to follow scientists and engineers through society.* Cambridge, MA: Harvard University Press.

Lee, I.M., Shiroma, E.J., Lobelo, F., Puska, P., Blair, S.N., Katzmarzyk, P.T., & Lancet Physical Activity Series Working Group. (2012). Effect of physical inactivity on major non-communicable diseases worldwide: An analysis of burden of disease and life expectancy. *The Lancet, 380*, 219–229.

Livingstone, S., Ólafsson, K., Helsper, E.J., Lupiáñez-Villanueva, F., Veltri, G.A., & Folkvord, F. (2017). Maximizing opportunities and minimizing risks for children online: The role of digital skills in emerging strategies of parental mediation. *Journal of Communication, 67*, 82–105.

Lloyd, M. (1996). Feminism, aerobics and the politics of the body. *Body & Society, 2*, 79–98.

Lupton, D. (2014). *Digital sociology.* London: Routledge.

Lupton, D. (2015). Data assemblages, sentient schools and digitised health and physical education (response to Gard). *Sport, Education and Society, 20*, 122–132.

Maguire, J. (1992). Towards a sociological theory of sport and the emotions: A process-sociological perspective. In E. Dunning & C. Rojek (Eds.), *Sport and leisure in the civilizing process* (pp. 96–120). Hampshire, UK: Palgrave Macmillan.

Malcolm, D., & Mansfield, L. (2013). The quest for exciting knowledge: Developments in figurational sociological research on sport and leisure. *Política y Sociedad, 50*, 397–419.

Mansfield, L. (2011). 'Sexercise': Working out heterosexuality in Jane Fonda's fitness books. *Leisure Studies, 30*, 237–255.

Markula, P. (2003). Postmodern aerobics: Contradiction and resistance. In A. Bolin & J. Granskog (Eds.), *Athletic intruders: Ethnographic research on women, culture, and exercise* (pp. 53–78). New York: State University of New York Press.

Marres, N. (2016). *Material participation: Technology, the environment and everyday publics.* Basingstoke, Hampshire UK: Palgrave Macmillan.

McLeroy K.R., Bibeau, D., Steckler, A., & Glanz, K. (1988). An ecological perspective on health promotion programs. *Health Education & Behavior, 15*, 351–377.

Middelweerd, A., Mollee, J.S., van der Wal, C.N., Brug, J., & te Velde, S.J. (2014). Apps to promote physical activity among adults: A review and content analysis. *International Journal of Behavioral Nutrition and Physical Activity, 11*, 97–105.

Millington, B. (2016). Fit for prosumption: Interactivity and the second fitness boom. *Media, Culture & Society, 38*, 1184–1200.

Mills, C.W. (1940). Situated actions and vocabularies of motive. *American Sociological Review, 5*, 904–913.

Mills, C.W. (1959). *The sociological imagination.* New York: Oxford University Press.

Monaghan, L.F., Hollands, R., & Pritchard, G. (2010). Obesity epidemic entrepreneurs: Types, practices and interests. *Body & Society, 16*, 37–71.

Neville, R.D. (2013a). Exercise is medicine: Some cautionary remarks in principle as well as in practice. *Medicine, Health Care and Philosophy, 16*, 615–622.

Neville, R.D. (2013b). Considering a complemental model of health and fitness. *Sociology of Health & Illness, 35*, 479–492.

Neville, R.D., & Gorman, C. (2016). Getting 'in' and 'out of alignment': Some insights into the cultural imagery of fitness from the perspective of experienced gym adherents. *Qualitative Research in Sport, Exercise and Health, 8*, 147–164.

Neville, R.D., Gorman, C., Flanagan, S., & Dimanche, F. (2015). Negotiating fitness, from consumption to virtuous production. *Sociology of Sport Journal, 32*, 284–311.

Obrist, H.U. (2014). Michel Serres. *032c, 25*(Winter), 119–123. Retrieved from: https://032c.com/2014/michel-serres/

Orton-Johnson, K., & Prior, N. (Eds.). (2013). *Digital sociology: Critical perspectives.* Basingstoke, Hampshire UK: Palgrave Macmillan.

Pronger, B. (2002). *Body fascism: Salvation in the technology of physical fitness.* Toronto, ON: University of Toronto Press.

Rogers, R. (2013). *Digital methods.* Cambridge, MA: MIT Press.

Rojek, C. (2010). *The labour of leisure: The culture of free time.* London: Sage.

Sallis, J.F., Bauman, A., & Pratt, M. (1998). Environmental and policy interventions to promote physical activity. *American Journal of Preventative Medicine, 15*, 379–397.

Sassatelli, R. (1999). Interaction order and beyond: A field analysis of body culture within fitness gyms. *Body & Society, 5*, 227–248.

Sassatelli, R. (2010). *Fitness culture: Gyms and the commercialisation of discipline and fun.* Basingstoke, Hampshire UK: Palgrave Macmillan.

Scott, S. (2006). The medicalisation of shyness: From social misfits to social fitness. *Sociology of Health & Illness, 28*, 133–153.

Smith Maguire, J. (2001). Fit and flexible: The fitness industry, personal trainers and emotional service labor. *Sociology of Sport Journal, 18*, 379–402.

Smith Maguire, J. (2002). Body lessons: Fitness publishing and the cultural production of the fitness consumer. *International Review for the Sociology of Sport, 37*, 449–464.

Smith Maguire, J. (2006). Exercising control: Empowerment and the fitness discourse. In L. Fuller (Ed.), *Sport, rhetoric, and gender: Historical perspectives and media representations* (pp. 119–129). New York: Palgrave Macmillan.

Smith Maguire, J. (2007). *Fit for consumption: Sociology and the business of fitness*. London and New York: Routledge.

Smith Maguire, J. (2008a). Leisure and the obligation of self-work: An examination of the fitness field. *Leisure Studies, 27*, 59–75.

Smith Maguire, J. (2008b). The personal is professional: Personal trainers as a case study of cultural intermediaries. *International Journal of Cultural Studies, 11*, 211–229.

Trost, S.G., Blair, S.N., Khan, N.M. (2014). Physical inactivity remains the greatest public health problem of the 21st century: Evidence, improved methods and solutions using the '7 investments that work' as a framework. *British Journal of Sports Medicine, 48*, 169–170.

van den Berg, P.A., Mond, J., Eisenberg, M., Ackard, D., & Neumark-Sztainer, D. (2010). The link between body dissatisfaction and self-esteem in adolescents: Similarities across gender, age, weight status, race/ethnicity, and socioeconomic status. *Journal of Adolescent Health, 47*, 290–296.

Vaterlaus, J.M., Patten, E.V., Roche, C., & Young, J.A. (2015). #Gettinghealthy: The perceived influence of social media on young adult health behaviors. *Computers in Human Behavior, 45*, 151–157.

Wansink, B. (2004). Environmental factors that increase the food intake and consumption volume of unknowing consumers. *Annual Review of Nutrition, 24*, 455–479.

Williams, G., Hamm, M.P., Shulhan, J., Vandermeer, B., & Hartling, L. (2014). Social media interventions for diet and exercise behaviours: A systematic review and meta-analysis of randomised controlled trials. *BMJ Open, 4*, 1–16.

Woolgar, S. (2002). *Virtual society? Technology, cyberbole, reality*. Oxford: Oxford University Press.

Part III

Applied physical activity

18 Physical activity in natural environments

Carly Wood, Miles Richardson and Jo Barton

Keywords: Nature, physical activity, green exercise, health, well-being

Introduction

Physical inactivity is the fourth leading cause of death worldwide (Kohl et al., 2012) and costs the economy at least $67.5 billion per annum (Ding et al., 2016). Despite government recommendations and campaigns to raise public awareness, the physical inactivity pandemic is gathering momentum. Although UK gym membership continues to rise (9 million members; Leisure database, 2016), 63% of new members usually stop attending within 3 months and less than 4% remain active one year later (Sperandei, Vieira & Reis, 2016). Recent evidence also suggests that 24 million English adults visit green spaces at least once a week (White et al., 2016). Of these, 8.23 million adults make at least one weekly 'active' visit to green spaces, equating to an annual health value of £2.2 billion (White et al., 2016). This suggests that parks and countryside can play a key role in increasing PA. Evidence indicates that individuals are more active when accessing green spaces compared to alternative settings; thus providing nature and green spaces to facilitate physical activity (PA) may offer one solution to address this international crisis.

Natural environments for physical activity

Access to nature and physical activity

Regular PA is essential to health and well-being (Janssen and Leblanc, 2010; World Health Organization, 2010; Janz et al., 2010; Larson, Whiting, Green & Bowker, 2015); yet a large proportion of UK adults do not meet the recommendation of 150 minutes of moderate-intensity PA (MPA) per week (Townsend, Wickramasinghe, Williams, Bhatnagar & Rayner, 2015). Similarly, only 21% of boys and 16% of girls (aged 5–15 years) engage in the recommended 60 minutes of daily moderate to vigorous PA (MVPA) (Townsend et al., 2015). Declines in child fitness are also evident (Sandercock, Voss, McConnell & Rayner, 2010) in parallel with increasing levels of sedentariness (Colley et al., 2011). The negative impact of this physical inactivity is vast and is estimated to cost worldwide health care systems $53.8 billion per year (Ding et al., 2016).

There is evidence to suggest that the environment can play a key role in influencing PA levels. Evidence regarding the impact of nature/green space on PA has generally been presented in two forms: i) a direct environmental comparison; and ii) examination of the impact of nature close to the home.

Direct environmental comparison

A relatively small number of studies have been conducted comparing PA in different environments; and of these, the majority are on young people. One such study compared PA levels during playtime on the playground and field, with playtime on the field resulting in 40% more MVPA (Wood, Gladwell & Barton, 2014a). Similar findings were demonstrated in a study comparing PA during urban and rural orienteering. Participants were significantly more active during rural orienteering, spending half of their time in the natural environment in MVPA compared to only a quarter in the built environment (Wood, Sandercock & Barton, 2014b). These studies also indicated that the use of natural environments for PA might be effective in reducing the gap in male and female PA levels and encouraging girls to be more active (Wood et al., 2014a, b); engaging the less fit children in PA (Barton, Sandercock, Pretty & Wood, 2014); and making PA seem easier and more enjoyable to children who are less physically active (Reed et al., 2013). Wheeler, Cooper, Page and Jago (2010) also reported differences in children's PA when in green and non-green areas, with the odds of being active in green space being 1.37 and 1.08 times greater than the odds of being active in non-green space, for boys and girls, respectively. In a recent systematic review, children were found to be more physically active outdoors compared to indoors (Gray et al., 2015) with studies in the review reporting outdoor PA levels to be between 2.2 and 3.3 times higher than indoor patterns (Cooper et al., 2010; Dunton, Liao, Intille, Wolch & Pentz, 2011; Raustorp et al., 2012; Vanderloo, Tucker, Johnson & Holmes, 2013).

Nature close to the home

By comparison, a wealth of research has been conducted to determine the influence of neighbourhood greenness/proximity to green space on levels of PA. However, work in this area is far from conclusive with some weak and contradictory evidence (Mytton, Townsend, Rutter & Foster, 2012). Early research conducted in the UK by Hillsdon and colleagues (2006) reported no clear relationship between PA and access to greenspace. However, other research reported a significant reduction in the odds of achieving PA recommendations and an increase in the odds of being overweight or obese with increasing distance from a formal greenspace (Coombes, Jones & Hillsdon, 2010). Mytton et al. (2012) supported this finding reporting that the odds of achieving PA recommendations were 1.24 times greater for individuals living in the greenest compared to the least green neighbourhoods. This relationship was even stronger when restricted to urban areas; indicating that the relationship cannot be explained by people living in rural areas being more active and that there may be an essential role of urban green space in increasing PA.

However, a similar pattern of contradictory evidence occurs across the globe. In Australia, proximity to green spaces are associated with higher levels of walking; with adults in the greenest areas being 44% more likely to meet PA recommendations than adults in the least green areas (Coombes et al., 2010; Richardson, Mitchell & Kingham, 2013). In children, the percentage of total park area in a community is a significant predictor of PA, with a

1.4% increase in PA for every 1% increase in park area (Roemmich et al., 2006; Timperio et al., 2008). These findings are supported by Lachowycz, Jones, Page, Wheeler and Cooper (2012) who found that time spent in green space contributes over one third of all children's outdoor MVPA on weekday evenings, over 40% on Saturdays and 60% on Sundays; indicating that green space may be an important contributor to overall PA. Each additional hour spent outdoors is associated with an extra 26.5 and 21 minutes of MVPA per week in girls and boys, respectively (Cleland et al., 2008). During weekends each additional hour spent outdoors at baseline is associated with an additional five minutes of MVPA per week in girls and boys three years later. So, green space availability facilitates PA particularly in girls, whose PA is more susceptible to decline during adolescence.

Toftager et al. (2011) also reported that the odds of engaging in MVPA in the Nether-lands are significantly reduced in individuals who are greater than 300 m from a greenspace. It is however important to note that, whilst people with good access to green space may be more likely to use it for PA (Lee & Maheswaran, 2010); it may also be that a greater desire for PA drives individuals to self-select areas with high levels of green space (Cohen-Cline, Turkheimer & Duncan, 2015). In addition, other Danish studies have indicated no relation-ship between green space proximity and engagement in PA (Maas, Verheij, Spreeuwenberg & Groenewegen, 2008; Schipperijn, Bentsen, Troelsen, Toftager & Stigsdotter, 2013). The latter study focused specifically on urban green spaces and reported no association between outdoor PA and the size of, distance to and number of features in the nearest urban green space; or amount/number of urban green spaces within 1 km of the home (Schipperijn et al., 2013). However, the study did reveal positive associations between the amount of PA performed in the nearest urban green spaces and the size of the space, the number of walking and cycling routes, wooded areas, water features, lights, pleasant views, bike racks and parking, indicating that there may be key features of urban green spaces that promote PA.

It has also been suggested that PA mediates the relationship between green space and health; that is, individuals who have easy access to green space have better health as a result of the impact of the environment on PA levels (Richardson et al., 2013). In Adelaide, increased walking explained the relationship between perceived greenness of the surroundings and physical health and also partly explained the relationship between perceived greenness and mental health. However, this relationship may only hold true for set activity types (Richardson et al., 2013).

Overall, the evidence regarding the impact of nature on PA is mixed, likely due to a num-ber of factors. Firstly, there are inconsistencies in the use of natural environments with age. In particular teenagers and the elderly may be less frequent users of green space due to concerns over factors such as safety; whilst it is expected that young adults are the most frequent users of green space (Lee & Maheswaran, 2011). Thus, the sample group might heavily influence study findings. Research methodologies can also impact findings. Some studies have used objective methods to assess both green space proximity/use and engagement in PA, whilst others have used questionnaires. Whilst questionnaires are susceptible to socially desirable responding and are therefore thought to be less reliable than objective measures such as GPS and accelerome-ters, wearing monitors might also influence an individual's behavioural choices.

The country in which the study is performed may also influence findings due to differ-ences in environmental characteristics, definitions of and types of green spaces, culture and also weather. For example, Maas et al. (2008) suggested that individuals in the Netherlands with lots of surrounding green space may be less active due to the need to use a car to reach facilities which are further away. Whilst this may hold true for rural areas, Maas et al. (2008)

also suggested that this is true for urban areas in the Netherlands with lots of green space as facilities are typically less dense. Thus, it is feasible that living in a rural location is somewhat restrictive of PA.

Nature and exercise characteristics

The exercise environment might also influence an individual's selection, and experience of PA. Research indicates that the outdoor environment provides distraction from fatigue, and disassociation from exercise-related thoughts, therefore helping exercise to feel easier and more enjoyable and enabling participants to engage in more intense activities (LaCaille, Masters & Heath, 2004; Plante et al., 2007; Dasilva et al., 2011; Reed et al., 2013).

Early research in this area by Ceci and Hassmen (1991) examined heart rate, RPE and blood lactate concentrations at three different exercise intensities on a treadmill and outdoor track. They reported significantly lower values outdoors, at all exercise intensities. Later research by LaCaille et al. (2004) supported these findings, reporting that participants performed a 5 km run significantly slower on the treadmill compared to an indoor track and outdoor route, with the fastest time in the outdoor route. RPE was also significantly lower during the outdoor route. However, in all of studies mentioned above, the authors did not specify how much green space was in the outdoor environment and it is therefore difficult to determine the exact role that nature might have played in influencing EE, RPE or enjoyment.

More recent studies assessing RPE and EE during PA in different environments have produced contrasting findings. Focht (2009) examined exercise intensity and RPE in 35 college age women during a 10-minute self-paced outdoor walk and indoor treadmill walk and found no differences in either RPE or selected intensity. Rogerson and Barton (2015), who conducted a laboratory study which allowed exercise intensity to be rigorously controlled, found that there were no significant differences between EE, respiratory exchange ratio or RPE during two bouts of exercise conducted under three different experimental conditions: a natural video, a built video and no video (control). However, time to exhaustion was 12.7% and 6.9% longer in the green condition compared to the built and control conditions, respectively. In the case of this study in particular, the inconsistent findings could be a result of the different modes of exercise utilised and the fact that viewing scenes of nature may not effectively simulate the experience of being outdoors.

Despite the contrasting evidence regarding the effect of the environment on RPE and EE, a number of the studies discussed revealed that the environment can influence enjoyment and adherence to the PA. Focht (2009) found that participants reported greater enjoyment and intention for future participation following the outdoor walk; whilst LaCaille et al. (2004) reported significantly greater satisfaction following the outdoor run compared to either the indoor track or treadmill run. These findings were supported by a recent randomised trial comparing a 12-week indoor and outdoor training programme which revealed that outdoor exercise was associated with enhanced affective responses and greater likelihood of adherence (Lacharite-Lemieux, Brunelle & Dionne, 2015). It could also be that the psychological benefits derived from exercise in nature (see below) drive individuals to repeatedly be active in a natural environment. However, these observations are speculative and further research is required to confirm these hypotheses.

Overall the evidence regarding the impact of the environment on exercise characteristics such as RPE, exercise intensity, enjoyment and adherence are limited, with some mixed findings. It is important for further research to be conducted in this area, as the ability to alter these characteristics may have a significant impact on the number of people meeting PA guidelines and thus important implications for health and well-being.

Green exercise and psychological well-being

Does exercising in different environments effect psychological well-being?

Pretty and colleagues (2005) have hypothesised that there could be an additive psychological benefit of engaging in PA whilst exposed to nature (Green Exercise: GE). In order to examine the idea, Pretty et al. (2005) performed a laboratory study whereby participants exercised on a treadmill whilst viewing rural pleasant, urban pleasant, rural unpleasant or urban unpleasant scenes (unpleasant scenes were those spoiled by pollutants or visual impediments). In order to infer changes in psychological well-being (PWB), measures of self-esteem (SE) and mood were examined before and after each condition. The results revealed that whilst exercise alone resulted in improvements in SE and mood, via reductions in confusion and tension and increases in vigour, viewing urban and rural pleasant scenes whilst exercising had greater effects than exercise alone. When viewing the urban pleasant scenes participants saw the greatest improvements in confusion, tension and vigour. Thus, the findings of this study indicated that there is a synergistic benefit of taking part in GE.

Following this study, numerous field studies were conducted to examine the impact of 'real' GE activities on PWB as it was unclear whether laboratory-based findings are fully applicable to real-world scenarios. This has involved the comparison of outdoor built and green environments and indoor and outdoor environments. These two approaches provide a wide evaluation of the psychological benefits of GE and provide an ecologically valid comparison of different environments in which individuals may often exercise (Barton, Wood, Pretty & Rogerson, 2016). However, in field settings such as these it can be difficult to rigorously control the exercise intensity (Ekkekakis, Parfitt & Petruzzello, 2011; Ekkekakis & Petruzzello, 1999). Given that the characteristics of the exercise may influence health outcomes, the ability to control exercise intensity is likely to be important.

Despite these limitations, the results are indicative of an additive benefit of GE for PWB. A review by Bowler et al. (2010) comparing exercise in natural and built environments found that exercise in a natural setting resulted in lower negative emotions such as anger and sadness and improved attention. This was supported by numerous studies reporting less stress and negative affect, improved mood and SE, reduced frustration and arousal, and better well-being following exercise in a natural setting (Roe and Aspinall, 2011; Marselle, Irvine & Warber, 2013; Aspinall, Mavros, Coyne & Roe, 2015; Tyrvainen et al., 2014). Furthermore, Mitchell (2013) found that people who regularly use the natural environment for PA have half the risk of poor mental health compared to those who do not.

A review by Thompson and colleagues (2011) also compared the benefits of indoor and outdoor PA. The authors reported that outdoor walking was associated with more positive mood outcomes, improved SE, vitality and energy and reduced fatigue, frustration, worry and depression. Similarly, running outdoors was also associated with greater reductions in anxiety, depression, anger and hostility than running indoors. In addition, a single bout of exercise outdoors was associated with greater levels of affect, excitement and activation compared to an indoor exercise session and a sedentary control condition (Fruhauf et al., 2016), whilst an outdoor 12-week exercise programme led to increased levels of PA and reduced feelings of depression compared to a 12-week indoor exercise group (Lacharite-Lemieux et al., 2015). These findings are suggestive of a role of the exercise setting in manipulating self-motivated exercise behaviours. National survey data from Finland also showed that being active in outdoor green spaces was more positively associated with emotional well-being compared to indoor and built settings (Pasanen, Tyrvainen & Korpela, 2014).

In addition to the increasing body of evidence regarding the psychological benefits of GE, Barton and Pretty (2010) conducted a multi-study analysis in order to determine the optimal 'dose' of GE. The analysis revealed that all types of GE improved SE and mood but that the greatest improvements were experienced in the first five minutes of GE, decreasing for activities between 10 and 60 minutes and half a day, but increasing for whole day activity. A similar response was found for mood and exercise intensity, with the greatest benefits coming from light and vigorous activity; however, for SE higher-intensity exercise resulted in diminishing benefits. Improvements in PWB were also greatest in environments containing water. Conversely, Rogerson, Brown, Sandercock, Wooler and Barton (2015) reported that there were no significant differences in the psychological benefits of running in four different park locations: beachside, riverside, grassland and heritage. However, the exercise performed in the latter study was more intense and structured than most previous GE activities, perhaps causing participants to take less notice of their surrounding environment.

The evidence discussed is primarily concerned with the psychological benefits of GE for adult populations. There is also good evidence to suggest that GE is effective at improving PWB in vulnerable groups. Barton and Pretty (2010) found that health benefits were greatest for those with declared mental ill-health, whilst Roe and Aspinall (2011) found that people with mental health problems experienced greater reductions in stress following a rural walk than people with a good level of mental health. However, evidence regarding the psychological impact of GE on children's PWB has produced contrasting findings. Wood, Angus, Pretty, Sandercock and Barton (2012) found no differences between the change in SE and mood when cycling whilst viewing either rural or urban scenes. These findings are supported by Duncan et al. (2014) who found that cycling whilst viewing a forest video provided no additive benefits for the mood of primary school children compared to cycling alone. Several studies have also examined the effect of being directly exposed to different environment types. Reed et al. (2013) compared the effects of running in a natural and urban environment and found that whilst the PA improved SE, there were no differences in the improvements in SE between the two environments. These findings are supported by Wood et al. (2014a), Barton et al. (2014) and Wood, Sandercock and Barton (2014b) who also found no differences in SE when performing PA in natural and built settings. This lack of additional benefit could be attributed to the types of activities included in these studies. Adult studies have primarily included walking activities which are of light intensity and enable participants to interact with the environment. The exercise included in the studies with children primarily include running and cycling and might have been too intense to enable them to take notice of their surrounding environment (Wood et al., 2014a).

Despite the potential lack of GE effect in children, large proportions of the psychological benefits of GE appear to be universally obtainable and independent of demographic, performance level, climatic and other environmental characteristics (Rogerson et al., 2015; Barton et al., 2016); indicating that GE is a valuable tool for improving the health and well-being of a variety of different cohorts.

Why does green exercise result in additive benefits of psychological well-being?

There are numerous theories as to why GE might result in additive benefits for PWB. In terms of the health benefits of having contact with nature there are three key theories that might explain the benefits: i) The Biophilia Hypothesis (Wilson, 1984); ii) The Psycho-Evolutionary Stress Reduction Theory (Ulrich, 1981); and iii) The Attention Restoration Theory (Kaplan and Kaplan, 1989).

The Biophilia Hypothesis suggests that '*humans have an inherent inclination to affiliate with nature*' (Grinde & Patil, 2009, p. 2332) which is genetically based (Kahn, 1997), and that contact with nature stems from an evolutionary competitive advantage in having superior knowledge about the natural world (Kellert & Wilson, 1993). It is this knowledge that contributes to improved well-being and mental development. Whilst research seems to support the theory, it is unclear exactly how it might work and which genetic mechanisms are involved (Kellert & Wilson, 1993; Kahn, 1997; White & Heerwagen, 1998; Fawcett & Gullone, 2001; Joye, 2007; Grinde & Patil, 2009; Windhager, Atzwanger, Bookstein & Schaefer, 2011).

The Psycho-Evolutionary Stress Reduction theory hypothesises that exposure to nature reduces stress by promoting stress recovery (Ulrich, 1981; Herzog & Strevey, 2008; Ewert Overholt, Voight & Wang, 2011). Natural environments provide positive distractions from daily stresses, thereby reducing stress symptoms and promoting positive affect (Ulrich, 1981; Herzog & Strevey, 2008; Ewert et al., 2011). This reduction in stress can restore physical and mental well-being through affective or emotional changes. The theory has been supported by numerous studies documenting reductions in stress measures following exposure to nature (Ulrich 1991, 1993; Hartig, Evans, Jamner, David & Garling, 2003; Laumann, Garling & Stormark, 2003; Herzog & Strevey, 2008; Ward Thompson et al., 2012). However, it fails to take into account the effect of stress on cognitive functioning and the role of the natural environment in replenishing mental fatigue.

The Attention Restoration Theory (ART) is more commonly used to explain the relationship between nature and health (Kaplan & Kaplan, 1989; Taylor & Kuo, 2009). The theory proposes that there are two types of attention: directed attention (DA) and involuntary attention. DA requires mental effort and if overused leads to DA fatigue (Kaplan, 1995; Taylor, Kuo & Sullivan, 2001; Berman, Jonids & Kaplan, 2008; Herzog & Strevey, 2008; Taylor & Kuo, 2009; Ewert et al., 2011; Rogerson & Barton, 2015). This fatigue is more common in times of stress, illness and grief and can lead to a reduction in well-being. Natural environments promote the use of involuntary attention, which requires no mental effort, and therefore provides an opportunity for recovery from mental fatigue (Berman et al., 2008; Taylor & Kuo, 2009; Rogerson & Barton, 2015). A number of studies have emerged in support of this theory. Ottosson and Grahn (2005) reported that resting for one hour in an outdoor garden resulted in greater improvements in DA than equivalent rest indoors, whilst nature views or the presence of plants within the workplace have been demonstrated to reduce mental fatigue (Kaplan, 1993; Berto, 2005; Raanaas, Evensen, Rich, Sjöström & Patil, 2011).

PA has also been linked with attention restoration via the transient hypofrontality hypothesis (Dietrich & Sparling, 2004; Dietrich, 2006; Rogerson & Barton, 2015). The hypothesis suggests that DA is associated with prefrontal cortex activation and that PA results in prefrontal cortex restoration; to allow the brain structures concerned with motor cortex activity to be activated (Daffner et al., 2000; Miller & Cohen, 2001; Dietrich & Sparling, 2004; Dietrich, 2006; Rogerson & Barton, 2015). Whilst this decreased prefrontal cortex activity may be detrimental to cognition during PA (Dietrich & Sparling 2004; Labelle, Bosquet, Mekary & Bherer, 2013), the opportunity for restoration can result in improved executive function following PA (Yanagisawa et al., 2010; Byun et al., 2014). Measures of brain activity have also supported the role of environmental settings for psychological restoration. Electroencephalogram data showed that in line with ART, movement from an urban shopping street to a green space was associated with changes in brain activity patterns indicative of reductions in arousal, frustration and engagement, and increased meditation (Aspinall, Mavros, Coyne & Roe, 2015).

However, Beute and Kort (2014) challenged the proposition that nature primarily provides restorative benefits and thus the focus on ART as a means of explaining GE health benefits. This challenge was based on results revealing that nature provides beneficial health effects even when mental resources have not been depleted (Beute & Kort, 2014). Furthermore, the theories discussed fail to consider the link between PWB, positive affect and physiology. A recent theory takes these links into account, considering the well-being benefits of GE within an evolutionary model of affect regulation (Richardson, McEwan, Maratos & Sheffield, 2016). The model proposes that there are 'three circles' of affect regulation: drive, contentment and threat (Gilbert, 2014). Drive is stimulating, about fun and excitement, but also includes competitive drives. Drive seeking is linked to the sympathetic nervous system, an over-reliance on which can increase vulnerability to depression (Gilbert, 2014). Contentment is linked to the parasympathetic nervous system, and is associated with affiliation, calming and connection. It can bring balance, toning down the drive system, and the third element of the three circles model, threat. GE can bring joy and competition, and contentment and affiliation; both of which are needed to bring a balanced emotional state, which ultimately impacts on our physiology and health.

The importance of connection to nature

An additional hypothesis is that in order for GE to provide additive benefits for PWB a connection with nature is required. In adults, it is suggested the magnitude of psychological benefits might be mediated by specific individual-environmental and exercise related variables such as enjoyment and nature connection. In fact, Rogerson et al. (2015) reported that participants who were more connected to nature and who reported greater enjoyment of their GE experienced the greatest number of health benefits. Richardson, Cormack, McRobert and Underhill (2016) found that an increase in connection with nature mediated the relationship between improved happiness and health from undertaking nature-based activities. However, there is a paucity of research into the links between nature connectedness, PA and exercise (Wolsko & Lindberg, 2013). Initial findings suggest that nature connectedness is associated with greater participation in outdoor activities and improved well-being (Wolsko & Lindberg, 2013), but there is clearly a need for further investigation into how an individual's subjective sense of being of, and within nature, impacts on GE. For example, those who are more connected with nature are more likely to be active in seeking out green space, and therefore, exercise in green spaces (Cooper et al., 2010). However, natural environments might also provide meaning and interest during the exercise, for example noticing the good things in nature (Richardson and Sheffield, 2017). Such appreciative recreation can cultivate greater nature connection bringing about associated benefits for PWB (Lumber, Richardson & Sheffield, 2017; Wolsko & Lindberg, 2013).

Summary and practical applications

Overall, the evidence implies that natural environments are more effective at promoting PA, reducing psychological stress and improving well-being in comparison to synthetic settings. Despite this, increasing amounts of time are spent indoors engaging in sedentary activities (Larson, Green & Cordell, 2011; Gray et al., 2015). Therefore, an effective strategy for restricting sedentary behaviour and promoting PA could be to simply increase the amount of time spent outdoors (Barber et al., 2013; Ngo et al., 2014) and to provide accessible green spaces nearby the home. This has implications for planners and local authorities to ensure communities have accessible, safe green spaces (including urban parks, allotments, urban farms) within walking distance. These research findings are also of note for policy makers in the public health sphere, because they are suggestive of a role for GE in increasing PA participation and influencing affective responses to exercise, intentions, and future exercise behaviours (Williams et al., 2008; Kwan & Bryan, 2010a; Kwan & Bryan, 2010b; Ekkekakis, Parfitt & Petruzzello, 2011). Adherence to PA programmes could not only increase if they were delivered in the outdoors, but by adopting a self-selected pace programme could also foster adherence, compared to prescribed high-intensity exercise (Perri et al., 2002). This approach leads to more positive affective responses via a greater sense of autonomy (Wardwell, Focht, Courtney Devries, O'Connell & Buckworth, 2013).

Chapter summary

- There is a growing body of evidence to indicate that natural settings can promote participation in PA in both adults and youth.
- Natural environments might also influence exercise-related characteristics such as intensity, perceived exertion, adherence and enjoyment; which can have important implications for future exercise intention.
- There is also evidence to indicate that GE can provide additive benefits for PWB above exercise in other settings; a large proportion of which appear be universally obtainable.
- Planners, local authorities and policy makers should seek to provide accessible green spaces close to the home in order address and overcome the global physical inactivity pandemic.

References

Aspinall, P., Mavros, P., Coyne, R., & Roe, J. (2015). The urban brain: analysing outdoor physical activity with mobile EEG. *British Journal of Sports Medicine, 49*, 272–276. doi: 10.1136/bjsports-2012-091877

Barber, S.E., Jackson, C., Akhtar, S., Bingham, D.D., Ainsworth, H., Hewitt, C., Richardson, G., Summerbell, C.D., Pickett, K.E., Moore, H.J., Routen, A.C., O'Malley, C.L., Brierley, S., & Wright, J. (2013). "Pre-schoolers in the playground" an outdoor physical actvity intervention for children aged 18 months to 4 years old: study protocol for a pilot cluster randmised controlled trial. *Trials, 14*. doi: 10.1186/1745-6215-14-326

Barton, J., & Pretty, J. (2010). What is the best dose of nature and green exercise for improving mental health. A multi-study analysis. *Environmental Science and Technology, 44*, 3947–3955. doi: 10.1021/es903183r

Barton, J., Sandercock, G., Pretty, J., & Wood, C. (2014). The effect of playground- and nature-based playtime interventions on physical activity in self-esteem in UK school children. *International Journal of Environmental Health Research, 12*, 1–11. doi: 10.1080/09603123.2014.915020

Barton, J., Wood, C., Pretty, J., & Rogerson, M. (2016). Green exercise for health. In J. Barton, R. Bragg, C. Wood, & J. Pretty (Eds). *Green Exercise: Linking nature, health and well-being* (pp. 26–36). Abingdon: Routledge.

Berman, M.G., Jonids, J., & Kaplan, S. (2008). The cognitive benefits of interacting with nature. *Psychological Science, 19*, 1207–1212. doi: 10.1111/j.1467–9280.2008.02225.x

Berto, R. (2005). Exposure to restorative environments helps restore attentional capacity. *Journal of Environmental Psychology, 25*, 249–259. doi: 10.1016/j.jenvp.2005.07.001

Beute, F., & Kort, Y. A. (2014). Salutogenic effects of the environment: review of health protective effects of nature and daylight. *Applied Psychology: Health and Well-Being, 6*(1), 67–95.

Bowler, D.E. Buyung-Ali, L.M., Knight, T.M. & Pullin, A.S. (2010). A systematic review of the added benefits to health of exposure to natural environments. *BMC Public Health, 10*, 456–466. doi: 10.1186/1471-2458-10-456

Byun, J., Hyodo, K., Suwabe, K., Ochi, G., Sakairi, Y., Kato, M., Dan, I., & Soya, H. (2014). Positive effect of acute mild exercise on executive function via arousal-related prefrontal activations: an fNIRS study. *Neuroimage, 98*, 336–345. doi: 10.1016/j.neuroimage.2014.04.067

Ceci, R., & Hassmen, P. (1991). Self-monitored exercise at three different RPE intensities in treadmill vs field running. *Medicine and Science in Sports and Exercise, 23*(6), 732–738.

Cleland, V., Crawford, D., Baur, L.A., Hume, C., Timperio, A., & Salmon, J. (2008). A prospective examination of children's time spent outdoors, objectively measured physical activity and overweight. *International Journal of Obesity, 32*, 1685–1693. doi: 10.1038/ijo.2008.171

Cohen-Cline, H., Turkheimer, E., & Duncan, G.E. (2015). Access to green space, physical activity and mental health: a twin study. *Journal of Epidemiology and Community Health, 69*, 523–529. doi: 10.1136/jech-2014-204667

Colley, R., Garriguet, D., Janssen, I., Craig, C.L., Clarke, J., & Tremblay, M.S. (2011). Physical activity of Canadian children and youth: accelerometer results from the 2007 to 2009 Canadian Health Measures Survey. *Health Reports, 22*(1), 15–23.

Coombes, E., Jones, A.P., & Hillsdon, M. (2010) The relationship of physical activity and overweight to objectively measured green space accessibility and use. *Social Science and Medicine, 70*, 816–822. doi: 10.1016/j.socscime.2009.11.020

Cooper, A.R., Page, A.S., Wheeler, B.W., Hillsdon, M., Griew, P., & Jago, R. (2010). Patterns of GPS measured time outdoors after school and objective physical activity in English children: the PEACH project. *International Journal of Behavioral Nutrition and Physical Activity, 7*, 31. doi: 10.1186/1479-5868-7-31

Daffner, K.R., Mesulam, M., Scinto, L., Acar, D., Calvo, V., Faust, R., Chabrerie, A., Kennedy, B., & Holcomb, P. (2000). The central role of the prefrontal cortex in directing attention to novel events. *Brain, 123*(5), 927–939.

Dasilva, S.G., Guidetti, L., Buzzachera, C.F., Elsangedy, H.M., Krinski, K., De Campos, W., Goss, F.L., & Baldari, C. (2011). Psychophysiological responses to self-paced treadmill and overground exercise. *Medicine and Science in Sports and Exercise, 43*, 1114–1124. doi: 10.1249/MSS.0b013e318205874c

Dietrich, A. (2006). Transient hypofrontality as a mechanism for the psychological effects of exercise. *Psychiatric Research, 145*, 79–83. doi: 10.1016/j.psychres.2005.07.033

Dietrich, A., & Sparling, P.B. (2004). Endurance exercise selectively impairs prefrontal-dependent cognition. *Brain Cognition, 55*, 516–524. doi: 10.1016/j.bandc.2004.03.002

Ding, D., Lawson, K.D., Kolbe-Alexander, T.L., Finkelstein, E.A., Katzmarzyk, P.T., van Mechelen, W., & Pratt, M. (2016). The economic burden of physical inactivity: a global analysis of major noncommunicable diseases. *Lancet, 388*, 1311–1324. doi: 10.1016/20140-6736(16)30383-x

Duncan, M.J., Clarke, N.D., Birch, S.L., Tallis, J., Hankey, J., Byrant, E., & Eyre, E.L. (2014). The effect of green exercise on blood pressure, heart rate and mood state in primary school children. *International Journal of Environmental Research and Public Health, 2*, 3678–3688. doi: 10.3390/ijerph110403678

Dunton, G.F., Liao, Y., Intille, S., Wolch, J., & Pentz, M.A. (2011) Physical and social contextual influences on children's leisure-time physical activity: an ecological momentary assessment study. *Journal of Physical Activity and Health, 8*(1), 103–108.

Ekkekakis, P., Parfitt, G., & Petruzzello, S.J. (2011). The pleasure and displeasure people feel when they exercise at different intensities. *Sports Medicine, 41*, 641–671. doi: 10.2165/11590680-000000000-00000

Ekkekakis, P., & Petruzzello, S.J. (1999). Acute aerobic exercise and affect. *Sports Medicine, 28*, 337–347. doi:10.2165/00007256-199928050-00005

Ewert, A., Overholt, J., Voight, A., & Wang, C.C. (2011). Understanding the transformative aspects of the wilderness and protected lands experience upon human health. *USDA Forest Service Proceedings, 1*, 140–146.

Fawcett, N.R., & Gullone, E. (2001). Cute, cuddly and a whole lot more? A call for empirical investigation into the therapeutic benefits of human-animal interaction for children. *Behaviour Change, 18*, 124–133. doi: 10.1375/bech.18.2.124

Focht, B.C. (2009). Brief walks in outdoor and laboratory environments. *Research Quarterly for Exercise and Sport, 80*, 611–620. doi: 10.1080/02701367.2009.10599600

Fruhauf, A., Niedermeier, M., Elliot, L.R., Ledochowski, L., Marksteiner, J., & Kopp, M. (2016). Acute effects of outdoor physical activity on affect and psychological well-being in depressed patients – a preliminary study. *Mental Health and Physical Activity, 10*, 4–9.

Gilbert, P. (2014). The origins and nature of compassion focused therapy. *British Journal of Clinical Psychology, 53*, 6–41. doi: 10.1111/bjc.12043

Gray, C., Gibbons, R., Larouche, R., Sandseter, E.B.H., Bienenstock, A., Brussoni, M., Chabot, G., Herrington, S., Janssen, I., Pickett, W., Power, M., Stanger, N., Sampson, M., & Tremblay, M.S. (2015). What is the relationship between outdoor time and physical activity, sedentary behaviour, and physical fitness in children? A systematic review. *International Journal of Environmental Research and Public Health, 12*, 6455–6474. doi: 10.3390/ijerph120606455

Grinde, B.R., & Patil, G. (2009). Biophilia: does visual contact with nature impact on health and well-being? *International Journal of Environmental Research and Public Health, 6*, 2332–2343. doi: 10.3390/ijerph6092332

Hartig, T., Evans, G.W., Jamner, L.D., David, D.S., & Garling, T. (2003). Tracking restoration in natural and urban settings. *Journal of Environmental Psychology, 23*, 109–123. doi: 10.1016/S0272-4944(02)00109-3

Herzog, T.R., & Strevey, S.J. (2008). Contact with nature, sense of humor, and psychological well-being. *Environment and Behaviour, 40*, 747–776. doi: 10.1177/0013916507308524

Hillsdon, M., Panter, J., Foster, C., & Jones, A. (2006). The relationship between access and quality of urban green space with population physical activity. *Public Health, 120*, 1127–1132. doi: 10.1016/j.puhe.2006.10.007

Janssen, I., & Leblanc, A.G. (2010). Systematic review of the health benefits of physical activity and fitness in school-aged children and youth. *International Journal of Behavioural Nutrition and Physical Activity, 11*, 7. doi: 10.1186/1479-5868-7-40

Janz, K.F., Letuchy, E.M., Gilmore, J.M., Burns, T.L., Torner, J.C., Willing, M.C., & Levy, S. (2010). Early physical activity provides sustained bone health benefits later in childhood. *Medicine and Science in Sports and Exercise, 42*, 1072–1078. doi: 10.1249/MSS.0b0133181c619b2

Joye, Y. (2007). Architectural lessons from environmental psychology: the case of biophilic architecture. *Review of General Psychology, 11*, 305–328. doi: 10.1037/1089-2680.11.4.305

Kahn, P. (1997). Developmental psychology and the Biophilia Hypothesis: children's affiliation with nature. *Developmental Review, 17*, 1–61. doi: 10.1006/drev.1996.0430

Kaplan, R. (1993). The role of nature in the context of the workplace. *Landscape and Urban Planning, 26*, 193–201. doi:10.1016/0169-2046(93)90016-7

Kaplan, R., & Kaplan, S. (1989). *The experience of nature: A psychological perspective*. Cambridge: Cambridge University Press.

Kaplan, S. (1995). The restorative benefits of nature: toward an integrative framework. *Journal of Environmental Psychology, 15*, 169–182. doi: 10.1016/0272-4944(95)90001-2

Kellert, S.R., & Wilson, E.O. (1993). *The Biophilia Hypothesis*. Washington, DC: Island Press.

Kohl, H.W., Craig, C.L., Lambert, E.V., Inoue, S., Alkandari, J.R., Leetongin, G., Kahlmeier, S., & LPASW Group. (2012). The pandemic of physical inactivity: global action for public health. *The Lancet, 380*, 294–305. doi: 10.1016/S0140-6736(12)60898-8

Kwan, B.M., & Bryan, A. (2010a). In-task and post-task affective response to exercise: translating exercise intentions into behaviour. *British Journal of Health Psychology, 15*, 115–131. doi: 10.1348/135910709X433267

Kwan, B.M., & Bryan, A.D. (2010b). Affective response to exercise as a component of exercise motivation: attitudes, norms, self-efficacy, and temporal stability of intentions. *Psychology of Sport and Exercise, 11*(1), 71–79.

Labelle, V., Bosquet, L., Mekary, S., & Bherer, L. (2013). Decline in executive control during acute bouts of exercise as a function of exercise intensity and fitness level. *Brain Cognition, 81*, 10–17. doi: 10.1016/j.bandc.2012.10.001

LaCaille, R.A., Masters, K., & Heath, E.M. (2004). Effects of cognitive strategy and exercise setting on running performance, perceived exertion, affect and satisfaction. *Psychology of Sport and Exercise, 5*, 461–476. doi: 10.1016/S1469-0292(03)00039

Lacharite-Lemieux, M., Brunelle, J.P., & Dionne, I.J. (2015). Adherence to exercise and affective responses: comparison between outdoor and indoor training. *Menopause, 22*, 731–740. doi: 10.1097/GME.0000000000000366

Lachowycz, K., Jones, A.P., Page, A.S., Wheeler, B.W., & Cooper, A.R. (2012). What can global positioning systems tell us about the contribution of different types of urban greenspace to children's physical activity? *Health and Place, 18*, 586–594. doi: 10.1016/j.healthplace.2012.01.006

Larson, L.R., Green, G.T., & Cordell, H.K. (2011). Children's time outdoors: results and implications of the national kids survey. *Journal of Park and Recreation Administration, 29*(2), 1–20.

Larson, L.R., Whiting, J.W., Green, G.T., & Bowker, J.M. (2015). Contributions of non-urban state parks to youth physical activity: a case study in Northern Georgia. *Journal of Park and Recreation Administration, 33*(2), 20–36.

Laumann, K., Garling, T., & Stormark, K.M. (2003). Selective attention and heart rate responses to natural and urban environments. *Journal of Environmental Psychology, 23*, 125–134. doi: 10.1016/S0272-4944(02)00110-X

Lee, A.C.K., & Maheswaran, R. (2011). The health benefits of urban green spaces: a review of the evidence. *Journal of Public Health, 33*, 212–222. doi: 10.1093/pubmed/fdq068

Leisure Database (2016). 2016 state of the UK fitness industry report. Available at: www.leisuredb.com/blog/2016/5/11/press-release-2016-state-of-the-uk-fitness-industry-report

Lumber, R., Richardson, M., & Sheffield, D. (2017). Beyond knowing nature: Contact, emotion, compassion, meaning, and beauty are pathways to nature connection. *PLoS ONE, 12*(5), e0177186.

Maas, J., Verheij, R.A., Spreeuwenberg, P., & Groenewegen, P. (2008). Physical activity as a possible mechanism behind the relationship between green space and health: a multilevel analysis. *BMC Public Health, 8*, 206. doi: 10.1186/1471-2458-8-206

Marselle, M.R., Irvine, K.N., & Warber, S.L. (2013). Walking for well-being: are group walks in certain types of natural environments better for well-being than group walks in urban environments? *International Journal of Environmental Research and Public Health, 10*, 5603–5628. doi: 10.3390/ijerph10115603

Miller, E.K., & Cohen, J.D. (2001). An integrative theory of prefrontal cortex function. *Annual Review of Neuroscience, 24*, 167–202. doi: 10.1146/annurev.neuro.24.1.167

Mitchell, R. (2013). Is physical activity in natural environments better for mental health than physical activity in other environments? *Sports Science and Medicine, 91*, 130–134. doi: 10.1016/j.socscimed.2012.04.012

Mytton, O.T., Townsend, N., Rutter, H., & Foster, C. (2012). Greenspace and physical activity: an observational study using Health Survey for England data. *Health and Place, 18*, 1034–1041. doi: 10.1016/j.healthplace.2012.06.003

Ngo, C.S., Pan, C., Finkelstein, E., Lee, C., Wong, I., Ong, J., Ang, M., Wong, T., & Saw, S. (2014). A cluster randomised controlled trial evaluating an incentive based outdoor physical activity programme to increase outdoor time and prevent myopia in children. *Opthalmic & Physiological Optics, 34*, 362–368. doi: 10.1111/opo.12112

Ottosson, J., & Grahn, P. (2005). A comparison of leisure time spent in a garden with leisure time spent indoors: on measures of restoration in residents in geriatric care. *Landscape Research, 30*, 23–55. doi: 10.1080/0142639042000324758

Pasanen, T.P., Tyrvainen, L., & Korpela, K.M. (2014). The relationship between perceived health and physical activity indoors, outdoors in built environments, and outdoors in nature. *Applied Psychology: Health and Well-Being, 6*, 324–346. doi: 10.1111/aphw.12031

Perri, M.G., Anton, S.D., Durning, P.E., Ketterson, T.U., Sydeman, S.J., Berlant, N.E., & Martin, A.D. (2002). Adherence to exercise prescriptions: effects of prescribing moderate versus higher levels of intensity and frequency. *Health Psychology, 21*, 452–458. doi: 10.1037/0278-6133.21.5.452

Plante, T.G., Gores, C., Brecht, C., Carrow, J., Imbs, A., & Willemsen, E. (2007). Does exercise environment enhance the psychological benefits of exercise for women? *International Journal of Stress Management, 14*, 88–98. http://dx.doi.org/10.1037/1072-5245.14.1.88

Pretty, J., Peacock, J., Sellens, M., Griffin, M. (2005). The mental and physical health outcomes of green exercise. *International Journal of Environmental Health Research, 15*, 319–337. doi: 10.1080/09603120500155963

Raanaas, R.K., Evensen, K.H., Rich, D., Sjöström, G., & Patil, G. (2011). Benefits of indoor plants on attention capacity in an office setting. *Journal of Environmental Psychology, 31*, 99–105. doi: 10.1016/j.jenvp.2010.11.005

Raustorp, A., Pagels, P., Boldemann, C., Cosco, N., Söderström, M., & Mårtensson, F. (2012). Accelerometer measured level of physical activity indoors and outdoors during preschool time in Sweden and the United States. *Journal of Physical Activity and Health, 9*, 801–808. doi: http://dx.doi.org/10.1123/jpah.9.6.801

Reed, K., Wood, C., Barton, J., Pretty, J., Cohen, D., & Sandercock, G.R.H. (2013). A repeated measures experiment of green exercise to improve self-esteem in UK school children. *PLoS ONE, 8*, e69176. doi: 10.1371/journal.pone.0069176

Richardson, M., Cormack, A., McRobert, L., & Underhill, R. (2016). 30 Days Wild: development and evaluation of a large-scale nature engagement campaign to improve well-being. *PLoS ONE, 11*(2), e0149777

Richardson, M., McEwan, K., Maratos, F., & Sheffield, D. (2016). Joy and calm: how an evolutionary functional model of affect regulation informs positive emotions in nature. *Evolutionary Psychological Science, 2*(4), 308–320.

Richardson, E.A., Mitchell, J.P., & Kingham, M.S. (2013). Role of physical activity in the relationship between urban green space and health. *Public Health, 127*, 318–324. doi: 10.1016/j.puhe.2013.01.004

Richardson, M., & Sheffield, D. (2017). Three good things in nature: noticing nearby nature brings sustained increases in connection with nature. *Psyecology, 8*(1), 1–32. doi: 10.1080/21711976.2016.1267136

Roe, J., & Aspinall, P. (2011). The restorative benefits of walking in urban and rural settings in adults with good and poor mental health. *Health and Place, 17*, 103–113. doi: 10.1016/j.healthplace.2010.09.003

Roemmich, J.N., Epstein, L.H., Raja, S., Yin, L., Robinson, J., & Winiewicz, D. (2006). Association of access to parks and recreational facilities with physical activity of young children. *Preventive Medicine, 43*, 437–441. doi: 10.1016/j.ypmed.2006.07.007

Rogerson, J., Brown, D., Sandercock, G., Wooler, J., & Barton, J. (2015). A comparison of four typical green exercise environments and prediction of psychological health outcomes. *Perspectives in Public Health, 136*, 171–180. doi: 10.1177/1757913915589845

Rogerson, M., & Barton, J. (2015). Effects of the visual exercise environments on cognitive directed attention, energy expenditure and perceived exertion. *International Journal of Environmental Research and Public Health, 12*, 7321–7336. doi: 10.3390/ijerph120707321

Sandercock, G., Voss, C., McConnell, D., & Rayner, P. (2010). Ten year secular declines in the cardiorespiratory fitness of affluent English children are largely independent of changes in body mass index. *Archives of Disease in Childhood, 95*, 46–47. doi: 10.1136/adc.2009.162107

Schipperijn, J., Bentsen, P., Troelsen, J., Toftager, M., & Stigsdotter, U.K. (2013). Associations between physical activity and characteristics of urban green space. *Urban Forestry and Urban Greening, 12*, 109–116. doi: 10.1016/j.ufug.2012.12.002

Sperandei, S., Vieira, M.C., & Reis, A.C. (2016). Adherence to physical activity in an unsupervised setting: explanatory variables for high attrition rates among fitness center members. *Journal of Science and Medicine in Sport, 19*, 916–920. doi: 10.1016/j.jsams.2015.12.522

Taylor, A.F., & Kuo, F.E. (2009). Children with attention deficits concentrate better after walk in the park. *Journal of Attention Disorders, 12*, 402–409. doi: 10.1177/1087054708323000

Taylor, A.F., Kuo, F.E., & Sullivan, W.C. (2001). Coping with ADD: the surprising connection to green play settings. *Environment and Behaviour, 33*, 54–77. doi: 10.1177/00139160121972864

Thompson Coon, J., Boddy, K., Whear, R., Barton, J., & Depledge, M.H. (2011). Does participating in physical activity in outdoor natural environments have a greater effect on mental well-being than physical activity indoors? A systematic review. *Environmental Science and Technology, 45*, 1761–1772. doi: 10.1021/es102947t

Timperio, A., Giles-Corti, B., Crawford, D., Andrianopoulos, N., Ball, K., Salmon, J., & Hume, C. (2008). Features of public open spaces and physical activity among children: findings from the CLAN study. *Preventive Medicine, 47*, 514–518. doi: 10.1016/j.ypmed.2008.07.015

Toftager, M., Ekholm, O., Schipperijn, J., Stigsdotter, U., Bentsen, P., Groobaek, M., Randrup. T.B., & Kamper-Jorgensen, F. (2011). Distance to green space and physical activity: a Danish national representative survey. *Journal of Physical Activity and Health, 8*(6), 741–749.

Townsend, N., Wickramasinghe, K., Williams, J., Bhatnagar, P., & Rayner, M. (2015). *Physical Activity Statistics 2015*. London: British Heart Foundation.

Tyrvainen, L., Ojala, A., Korpela, K., Lanki, T., Tsunetsugu, Y., Kagawa, T. (2014). The influence of urban green environments on stress relief measures: a field experiment. *Journal of Environmental Psychology, 38*, 1–9. doi: 10.1016/j.jenvp.2013.12.005

Ulrich, R.S. (1981). Natural versus urban scenes: some psychophysiological effects. *Journal of Environment and Behaviour, 13*, 523–556. doi: 10.1177/0013916581135001

Vanderloo, L.M., Tucker, P., Johnson, A.M., Holmes, J.D. (2013). Physical activity among preschoolers during indoor and outdoor childcare play periods. *Applied Physiology, Nutrition and Metabolism, 38*, 1173–1175. doi: 10.1139/apnm-2013-0137

Ward Thompson, C., Roe, J., Aspinall, P., Mitchell, R., Clow, A., & Miller, D. (2012). More green space is linked to less stress in deprived communities: evidence from salivary cortisol patterns. *Landscape and Urban Planning, 105*, 221–229. doi: 10.1016/j.landurbplan.2011.12.015

Wardwell, K.K., Focht, B.C., Courtney Devries, A., O'Connell, A.A., & Buckworth, J. (2013). Affective responses to self-selected and imposed walking in inactive women with high stress: a pilot study. *The Journal of Sports Medicine and Physical Fitness, 53*(6), 701–712.

Wheeler, B.W., Cooper, A.R., Page, A.S., & Jago, R. (2010). Greenspace and children's physical activity: a GPS/GIS analysis of the PEACH project. *Preventive Medicine, 51*, 148–152. doi: 10.1016/j.ypmed.2010.06.001

White, M.P., Elliott, L.R., Taylor, T., Wheeler, B.W., Spencer, A., Bone, A., Depledge, M.H., & Fleming, L.E. (2016). Recreational physical activity in natural environments and implications for health: a population based cross-sectional study in England. *Preventive Medicine, 91*, 383–388. doi: 10.1016/j.ypmed.2016.08.023

White, R., & Heerwagen, J. (1998). Nature and mental health: biophilia and biophobia. In A. Lundberg, (Ed.). *The environment and mental health: A guide for clinicians*. New Jersey: Lawrence Erlbaum Associates.

Williams, D.M., Dunsider, S., Ciccolo, J.T., Lewis, B.A., Albrecht, A.E., & Marcus, B.H. (2008). Acute affective response to a moderate-intensity exercise stimulus predicts physical activity participation 6 and 12 months later. *Psychology of Sport and Exercise, 9*, 231–245. doi: 10.1016/j.psychsport.2007.04.002

Wilson, E.O. (1984.). *Biophilia*. London: Harvard University Press.

Windhager, S., Atzwanger, K., Bookstein, F., & Schaefer, K. (2011). Fish in a mall aquarium – an ethological investigation of biohpilia. *Landscape and Urban Planning, 99*, 23–30. doi: 10.1016/j.landurbplan.2010.08.008

Wolsko, C., & Lindberg, K. (2013). Experiencing connection with nature: the matrix of psychological well-being, mindfulness, and outdoor recreation. *Ecopsychology, 5*(2), 80–91.

Wood, C., Angus, C., Pretty, J., Sandercock, G., & Barton, J. (2012). A randomized control trial of physical activity in a perceived environment on self-esteem and mood in adolescents. *International Journal of Environmental Health Research, 23*, 311–320. doi: 10.1080/09603123.2012.733935

Wood. C., Gladwell, V., & Barton, J.L. (2014a). A repeated measures experiment of school playing environment to increase physical activity and enhance self-esteem in UK school children. *PLoS ONE, 9*, e108701. doi: 10.1371/journal.pone.0108701

Wood, C., Sandercock, G., Barton, J.L. (2014b). Interactions between physical activity and the environment to improve adolescent psychological wellbeing: a randomized controlled trial. *International Journal of Environment and Health, 7*, doi: 10.1504/IJENVH.2014.067359

World Health Organization (2010). *Global recommendations on physical activity for health*. Geneva: World Health Organization.

Yanagisawa, H., Dan, I., Tsuzuki, D., Kato, M., Okamoto, M., Kyotoku, Y., & Soya, H. (2010). Acute moderate exercise elicits increased dorsolateral prefrontal activation and improves cognitive performance with stroop test. *Neuroimage, 50*, 1702–1710. doi: 10.1016/j.neuroimage.2009.12.023

19 Urban physical activity

Brad Harasymchuk and Chris North

Keywords: Physical activity, neighbourhood, place-based approaches, health, well being

Introduction

In this chapter we explore the benefits of neighbourhood and place-based physical activity (PA); it is important to look at some basic definitions and frame the problem briefly. 'Physical inactivity has been identified as the fourth leading risk factor for global mortality causing

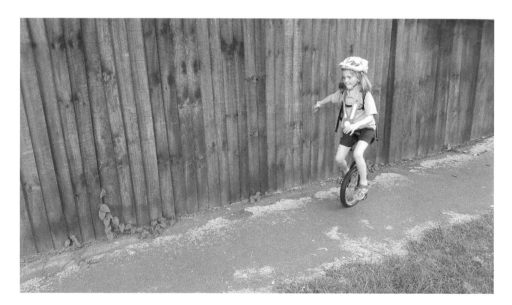

Figure 19.1 My youngest daughter is eight years old and she took up unicycling last year. Now every trip to school, to the local park or shops is a challenge to see how far she can get without falling off, what obstacles she can negotiate and what opportunities for adventure lurk in the neighbourhood. Instead of me trying to convince her to get outside, she now calls me to come and see her latest trick on the footpath, jumping the gutter or some other new skill she has learnt. In addition, I had no idea when she started unicycling that it was a ticket to get into conversations with everyone we meet. She is very active and I know the people in our neighbourhood so much better thanks to my unicycling eight year old.

an estimated 3.2 million deaths globally' (World Health Organization, n.d.). These effects are not only felt by adults; over 41 million children under the age of 5 are considered obese (WHO, 2016). Clearly the situation is critical with significant implications for healthcare, their associated costs, and more importantly, for health related quality of life.

We argue that rather than seeing physical activity as an end in itself, we see physical activity as a means to enhance well-being of individuals and communities. We do not doubt that there are significant dangers resulting from widespread physical inactivity, but we will argue here that physical activity in our neighbourhoods – in other words a place-based approach to physical activity – has the potential to enhance individual *and* communal well-being *and* bring benefits to local neighbourhoods by enhancing social capital. We begin by identifying the importance of a place-based understanding of neighbourhood that can facilitate physical activity. We then use place-based approaches to examine examples from our experiences.

Urban physical activity

Neighbourhood defined

Both individual factors and social factors affect physical activity levels (Bauman et al., 2012). One of the more important determinants of physical activity is a person's immediate environment – one's neighbourhood (King et al., 2000). A neighbourhood is a community within a larger city, town or other geographic area. Moreover neighbourhoods have a geographic dimension that is integrated with socio-cultural constructs. Within this construct, neighbourhoods are social communities where people often come together and interact for the mutual benefit of all those who are part of the community settings. Further, neighbourhoods facilitate situations where people interact socially for the mutual benefit of all that are part of that community (Bernard et al., 2007; World Health Organization, 1998). According to the WHO (2006), neighbourhoods are natural settings for active living that differ from other organisational settings such as schools, healthcare facilities and workplaces. Neighbourhoods are shaped by the built environment and the social context and are the arena for everyday life for all citizens: young and old, men and women, workers and students, artists and migrants. This definition of neighbourhood means that it is more than a physical space, it is a place.

Place and neighbourhoods

The definition of 'place' varies and has been used synonymously with 'community' (Gruenewald & Smith, 2008) and 'the commons' (Bowers, 2005). When discussing place, Casey (1997) stated:

> We are immersed in it and could not do without it. To be at all – to exist in any way – is to be somewhere, and to be somewhere is to be in some kind of place. Place is as requisite as the air we breathe, the ground on which we stand, the bodies we have. We are surrounded by places. We walk over and through them. We live in places, relate to others in them, die in them. Nothing we do is unplaced.
>
> (p. ix)

The ways in which we live in our neighbourhoods and connect to them transform them from simply spaces, into places 'by giving them meaning through experiences, understanding, and relationship' (Harasymchuk, 2015). Perhaps the neighbourhoods in which we live and work are some of the most meaningful and influential places in our lives. Kallus and Law-Yone

(2000) extend our understanding of neighbourhood as having three components that are part of a process of transformation. Viewing the neighbourhood as a place rather than simply as space 'emphasizes the neighbourhood as a unique urban phenomenon. Its significance is seen to stem from its conventional everyday function (residential) which involves continuity and permanence and which fixes the neighbourhood sense of place in the urban collective memory' (p. 815). Based on this view, neighbourhoods are more than geographically bounded spaces but are shared places for neighbours to commune.

For the purpose of this chapter neighbourhoods are defined as shared living places with unique histories and which can be traversed/navigated using modes of physical activity and human powered transport. Due to the emphasis on shared places, we consider physical activity conducted indoors or on one's own property to fall outside of the scope of neighbourhoods. Neighbourhoods come in many different sizes with different architectural settings. But one thing that most neighbourhoods have in common is that they are part of an urban environment.

Influence of our urban neighbourhood environment on physical activity

Increasingly, the most accessible physical environments are the urban areas – the neighbourhoods – in which we live. The United Nations estimates that by 2030, more than two-thirds of the total world population will live in urban areas (United Nations, 2014). Most of this increase will take place in the megacities and newly emerging urban regions of the developing world (Hutchison, 2010). This urbanisation requires considerable planning, engineering and architectural expertise to allow so many people to live in close proximity and still deal with waste, transport and provide various facilities. What is high on the agenda are opportunities for recreation and physical activity. In response, authors such as Franzini et al. (2009) argue that neighbourhood social factors and physical environment should be considered in the development of health policy and interventions to reduce obesity. Urban planning can create wastelands or wonderlands that can either discourage or encourage physical activities (Kneeshaw-Price et al., 2013). However, most neighbourhoods lie on the continuum somewhere between a wasteland and a wonderland, therefore individual and group agency is required to reclaim space and turn it into accessible lived places which attract people pursuing well-being enhancing activities. In their research into the experiences of children in Auckland city, New Zealand, Carroll, Witten, Kearns, and Donovan (2015) found that neighbourhoods profoundly influence the physical activity of children:

> Many children spoke of enjoying walking, cycling or scootering to school and other destinations. The street was more than just a thoroughfare, providing many opportunities for play: children jumped on walls, balanced on kerbs and avoided stepping on cracks; they ran, skipped and spun in circles; and they played various games incorporating manhole covers, shadows and other street features.
>
> (p. 428)

Note in this quote that the features children played with were not designed to enhance PA, but were used by the children for play. This is not simply relevant for the play of children, human creativity has co-opted engineering and architectural works to develop creative and adventurous opportunities for physical activity in the urban environment. Borden (2010) discusses how urban skateboarders enact 'a radical subversion of the intended use of architecture – that is, using architecture in a way that is different from that originally intended by architects, planners, building owners, and urban managers.' He explains how 'these new urban skate-boarders skated over fire hydrants and curbs, onto bus benches and planters, and down steps and handrails.' This is only one of several examples of physical activities that have actually emerged from the architecture and environment of urban areas. Another example is Parkour a new activity, where participants aim to move around an area such as a city or park without stopping (Edwardes, 2009). Parkour can involve running, jumping, and climbing over build-ings and obstacles. It is a truly urban activity, and it is high intensity. Low intensity activities, such as walking or rollerblading also take well to the paved surfaces of the urban environment. Table 19.1 lists over 50 physical activities that can take place in an urban neighbourhood.

It is evident that our neighbourhoods are important for encouraging physical activity and hold multiple benefits: neighbourhoods are accessible to people of all ages and most abilities; equipment is unnecessary (even shoes are optional). This is in contrast to much of the organ-ised opportunities for PA or the remote extremes of the green and blue spaces which often require thousands of dollars of specialised equipment to participate. These features make neighbourhoods the most democratic of all PA sites.

The benefits of PA in our neighbourhoods are important for our health. The following sec-tion examines how physical activity in one's own neighbourhood can affect our mental state.

The relationship between psychological well-being and physical activity in one's neighbourhood

Psychological well-being is a multi-faceted and complex concept that is sometimes used inter-changeably with the concept of mental health. Good mental health is a sense of well-being, confidence and self-esteem (Western Australia Mental Health Commission, n.d.). It enables us to fully enjoy and appreciate other people, day-to-day life and our environment. It also enables us to form positive relationships, use our abilities to reach our potential, and deal with life's challenges. Several studies have demonstrated that physical activity can have a positive impact on mental health (International Society of Sport Psychology, 1992; Mutrie & Biddle,

Table 19.1   List of activities in a neighbourhood

Parkour	Backyard cricket	Circuit training
Skateboarding	Basketball	Pilates
Scootering	Volleyball	Climb stairs
Bicycling	Badminton	Tennis
Unicycling	Hockey	Make a snowman
Walking	Ice hockey	Snow fight
Jogging	Street hockey	Community service projects
Dog-walking	Touch rugby	Plant flowers
Geocaching	Baseball	Plant a tree
Frisbee	Football	Water the flowers
Frisbee golf	Wiffle ball	Rollerblading
Hide and seek	Bocce ball	Run through sprinkler
Capture the flag	Horseshoes	Urban camping
Tag	Croquet	Roll down a hill
Tai chi	Trampoline	Boot camp
Yoga	Fly a kite	Four square
Jump rope	Hand ball	

1995; Scully, Kremer, Meade, Graham, & Dudgeon, 1998; Weir, 2011). It can also improve energy expenditure rates compared to exercising indoors, which will be discussed further below. If physical activity in the outdoors has benefits to both mental health and exercising outcomes, then how does physical activity in one's own neighbourhood affect one's psychological well-being?

Familiar places and our mental state

Environmental psychologists Low and Altman (1992) suggested that it is the ways in which people create relationships with places that form attachments. Yi-Fu Tuan (1977) argued that the emotions people attach to locations move the experience of a particular place to a layer of meaning beyond the practical functions associated with other locations (such as workplaces or schools). Tuan postulated that familiar places provoke a stronger fondness 'in the same sense that an old raincoat can be said to have character' (Tuan, 1974, p. 234). Places are infused with the character that is given to them by those who experience specific places over long periods of time. Hutson (2011) stated that 'places, like the old raincoat, may represent objective use and meaning that over time transforms into something comforting, dependable and nurturing with a personality that can be only understood with a history of experience.' This dependability and comfort that familiar places can elicit is part of the positive psychological effect that our local environment can have on us. Mah (2016) alluded to the importance of familiar places for their ability to instil calmness, rhythm and flow into our activities. Indeed the American College of Sports Medicine (2010) recommends getting out to pursue physical activity into one's own neighbourhood, (a place that is familiar and well known), to improve one's mental state, and as treatment for those experiencing anxiety and depression.

Neighbourhood physical activity has been associated with enhanced social capital as measured by greater participation in community activities, greater trust in others and decreased reliance on TV for entertainment (Rogers, Halstead, Gardner, & Carlson, 2011). The literature also includes personal accounts which shed light on the power of neighbourhood PA. For example Robert (2002), discusses how his memories of running in his neighbourhood are moments that he will cherish forever – including playing tag with his children and going running for exercise. Dinkens (2002) tells the story of how she began running in her own neighbourhood after spending many mornings 'sitting on [her] porch and watching others participate in life'. She went on to describe the self-motivation that ensued from her 'dreadfully gratifying trek' down her neighbourhood street. During the process of writing this chapter we were spurred to investigate the experiences of others in our neighbourhoods:

> *Glenys is an elderly woman who I saw walking down my street. I noticed her walking several days in a row and eventually we stopped to talk while I was outside playing with my children. Glenys told me that she wants to walk regularly because she is aware of 'use it or lose it' when it comes to aging and physical activity. What's more, she walks for 60 minutes each day which involves 6 full laps of our street. During this time she has gotten to know all the residents.*
>
> *Now as she walks along, she tells me, as she passes each house, she says a small prayer for the people inside and asks God to look after them. Through talking with Glenys, I realised that neighbourhood walking means much more than simply being physically active.*
>
> *(Reflection Chris North)*

These stories illustrate experiences of enjoying physical activity in one's own neighbourhood resulting in positive psychological benefits. Part of psychological well-being involves our relationships with others. Social engagement is often an intricate part of being physically active in our neighbourhood, which brings about the subject of social capital.

Social capital and psychological well-being

Social capital, according to Grootaert and van Bastelaer (2001), refers to the 'internal social and cultural coherence of society, the norms and values that govern interactions among people and the institutions in which they are embedded'. Social capital is rooted into our neighbourhoods through social networks and community involvement. Physical activity within a neighbourhood, such as group walking, can generate social capital (Lee, 2014), and this social capital is linked to well-being. Research has shown that the more integrated we are with our community, the less likely we are to experience colds, heart attacks, strokes, cancer, depression and premature deaths of all sorts (Putnam, 2000). Yamaguchi (2013) empirically validated the relationship between social capital and psychological well-being of adolescents.

Physical activity within neighbourhoods has a positive effect on psychological well-being through our unique ties to place and the potential to build social capital. But how does physical activity in a neighbourhood differ physiologically from exercise that takes place elsewhere?

Neighbourhoods, physical activity and energy expenditure (physiological)

For the majority of the population, sending a child to a sports club is considered a valuable way to increase her/his physical activity and lies in contrast to the bookishness of schools and the commonly criticised digital immersion of home life (sometimes called 'Minecraft™ baby-sitting'). Interestingly, Mackett and Paskins (2008) used accelerometers to measure physical activity of children aged 10–13 and found that they used more calories per minute in neighbourhood play, than at home, school or club sports. In organised sports, children spend a great deal of time listening to instructions and waiting for their turn. By contrast, the informal play occurring in neighbourhoods has much to offer children seeking physical activity. Children are significantly different to adults. While we were unable to locate research similar to Mackett and Paskin's work contrasting physical activity in different activities for adults, research in adult populations (18–65 y) has shown consistent positive relationships between neighbourhood walkability and several types of PA, in particular transport-related walking (Frank et al., 2006) has resulted in less obesity (Frank, Andresen, & Schmid, 2004), and this held true regardless of socio-economic-status. Neighbourhood PA is clearly important also for adults. The research strongly supports the benefits of neighbourhood PA, which requires us to ask 'why are there not more people out being physically active in neighbourhoods?'

Barriers to neighbourhood physical activity

There are numerous studies which highlight the challenges and barriers to PA in local urban environments. This section examines fear and poor urban design as potential barriers.

Fear

Statistics show us that most abductions of children are carried out by someone the child knows or a relative, yet there is a persistent fear of letting children go unsupervised in the neighbourhood because of a fear of strangers. Perhaps reflecting this state of anxiety, Kearns and Collins (2006) found that middle-income children from the suburbs were often confined to the 'semi-fortified space of home' and shuttled from one activity to the next by parents (Kearns and Collins 2006, p. 108). In addition, the research by Carroll et al. (2015) revealed that children were also fearful, in particular those that had little unsupervised time away from home. A child of a new immigrant who had lived for 10 years in the area stated that 'I don't know a lot of places in my neighbourhood. I think I want to go back 'cause there's not much to look around. [. . .] I don't want to get lost.' (p. 430). Such research identifies the looming threat that this could be the age of the 'last child left in the neighbourhood'.

Such fears are not only the concern of parents and children. Separating adults from their neighbourhoods has a combined effect of reducing PA and increasing fear. Research suggests that people rated the trustworthiness of their neighbours lower if they were out less often in their neighbourhoods (Rogers, Halstead, Gardner, & Carlson, 2011). While one could argue that there are good reasons for not being out in some neighbourhoods, Rogers and colleagues' (2011) study controlled for socio-economic-status indicating that neighbourhood PA is effective in reducing fear and enhancing social connectedness. PA can turn spaces into places.

This is not to suggest that if people in ALL neighbourhoods spent more time on the streets that they would feel safer, indeed there are some neighbourhoods that are less safe by objective measures: red-light districts, areas with many bars. A certain level of diligence is necessary in our opinion before releasing unsupervised children into neighbourhood streets; however, the more people who are on the streets, the safer they are and the safer people tend to feel (Rogers et al., 2011).

Poor urban design

To this point, we have largely focused on individual factors that provide barriers to PA in neighbourhoods. There are also urban design factors that are influential. In particular, busy roads with high speed vehicles are likely to limit possibilities for neighbourhood PA. Car culture in today's society appears to promote the ability to drive everywhere and park, which places constraints on other forms of PA that do not involve vehicles. The responsibility for ensuring that the neighbourhoods become walkable is a democratic project. It requires the advocacy of individuals in society as well as leadership by politicians and the vision of urban planners to see beyond a myopic car-culture focus.

But we could wait forever for the perfect neighbourhood to be designed to entice us outdoors. The future realisation of neighbourhoods as sites for rich experiences of socially connected PA rests jointly with individuals, society and designers of neighbourhoods.

Summary and practical applications

> 'In fact, parkour can be picked up at any time, in any place, by anybody. And it is precisely this level of access to a progressive and holistic method of practice that provides a whole new arena for human development on a mass scale'
>
> (Edwardes, 2010 p. 375)

While often neglected in the PA research, we have argued that neighbourhoods offer the most egalitarian and accessible forms of physical activity. We see a future where in addition to adventures in parks and the wilderness, participating in sports, exercising in gyms and other amenities, neighbourhoods are filled with people taking physical activity opportunities and participating in society. PA envisioned through neighbourhoods offers a means to minimise the 'exporting' of responsibility for PA onto external factors such as sub-optimal urban planning, unaffordability of expensive gym memberships, inaccessibility to locate remote green or blue space or time-poverty. The time has come for us to step outside our property and start taking regular non-motorised outings. The adventure starts at the kerb. It is up to us to turn the largely unknown neighbourhood space into a life-enhancing place. We need to make this a societal project, one that uses PA as a ticket to more than physical health, but as a ticket to well-being in its widest sense, constrained only by the limits of human creativity. We wish for you the same level of enjoyment that we have found in our place-based explorations and connections.

Chapter summary

- Neighbourhoods are highly accessible for physical activity (PA).
- Research indicates that children are more active in the neighbourhood than at sports clubs, school or home.
- Drawing on the work of place-based experiences, neighbourhood PA has the potential to convert unknown spaces into familiar and comforting places.
- Neighbourhood PA has the potential to build connections with others and enhance well-being more generally.
- Barriers to neighbourhood PA include fear and inadequate urban design.
- Such barriers can largely be overcome through more frequent neighbourhood PA and creative approaches to PA.

References

American College of Sports Medicine. (2010). Exercising with anxiety and depression. Excersizeismedicine. org. http://exerciseismedicine.org/assets/page_documents/EIM%20Rx%20series_Exercising% 20with%20Anxiety%20and%20Depression_2.pdf

Bauman, A., Seis, R., Sallis, J., Well, J., Loos, R., & Martin, B. (2012). Correlates of physical activity: Why are some people physically active and others not? *The Lancet, 380*(9838), 258–271.

Bernard, P., Charafeddine, R., Frohlich, K., Daniel, M., Kestens, Y., & Potvin, L. (2007). Health inequalities and place: A theoretical conception of neighbourhood. *Social Science & Medicine, 65*, 1839–1852.

Borden, I. (2010). Skateboarding. In R. Hutchison (Ed.), *Encyclopedia of urban studies* (pp. 729–773). Thousand Oaks, California: SAGE Publications, Inc.

Bowers, C. (2005). *Revitalizing the commons: Cultural and educational sites of resistance and affirmation.* Lanham, MD: Lexington Books.

Carroll, P., Witten, K., Kearns, R., & Donovan, P. (2015). Kids in the city: Children's use and experiences of urban neighbourhoods in Auckland, New Zealand. *Journal of Urban Design, 20*(4), 417–436.

Casey, E. (1997). *The fate of place: A philosophical history.* Berkeley, CA: University of California Press.

Dinkens, L. (2002). One block at a time. In G. Battista (Ed.), *How running changed my life: True stories of the power of running.* Halcottsville, NY: Breakaway Books.

Edwardes, D. (2009). *Parkour.* New York, NY: Crabtree Publishing Company.

Edwardes, D. (2010). Encouraging physical activity through parkour. *British Journal of School Nursing, 5*(8), 375–376.

Frank, L., Andresen, M., & Schmid, T. (2004). Obesity relationships with community design, physical activity, and time spent in cars. *American Journal of Preventative Medicine, 27*(2), 87–96.

Frank, L., Sallis, J., Conway, T., Chapman, J., Saelens, B., & Bachman, W. (2006). Many pathways from land use to health: Associations between neighborhood walkability and active transportation, body mass index, and air quality. *Journal of the American Planning Association, 72*(1), 75–87. doi: 10.1080/01944360608976725

Franzini, L., Elliott, M.N., Cuccaro, P., Schuster, M., Gilliland, M.J., Grunbaum, J., Franklin, F., & Tortolero, S.R. (2009). Influences of physical and social neighborhood environments on children's physical activity and obesity. *American Journal of Public Health, 99*(2): 271–278.

Grootaert, C., & van Bastelaer, T. (2001). Understandings and measuring social capital: A synthesis of findings and recommendations from the social capital initiative. Social Capital Working Paper Number 24. The World Bank Social Development Family Environmentally and Socially Sustainable Development Network.

Gruenewald, D., & Smith, G. (Eds.). (2008). *Place-based education in the global age: Local diversity*. New York, NY: Taylor & Francis Group.

Harasymchuk, B. (2015). Place-based education & critical pedagogies of place: Teachers challenging the neocolonizing processes or the New Zealand and Canadian schooling system. (Doctoral dissertation). Retrieved from University of Canterbury Research Repository. http://hdl.handle.net/10092/10662

Hutchison, R. (2010). *Encyclopedia of urban studies*. Thousand Oaks, CA: Sage Publications Inc.

Hutson, G. (2011). Remembering the roots of place meanings for place-based outdoor education. *Pathways: The Ontario Journal of Outdoor Education, 23*(3), 19–25.

International Society of Sport Psychology. (1992). Physical activity and psychological benefits: A position statement. *The Sport Psychologist, 6*, 199–204.

Kallus, R., & Law-Yone, H. (2000). What is a neighbourhood? The structure and function of an idea. *Environment and Planning B: Planning and Design, 27*, 815–826.

Kearns, R., & Collins, D. (2006). Children in the intensifying city: Lessons from Auckland's walking school buses. In B. Gleeson & N. Sipe (Eds.), *Creating child friendly cities: Reinstating kids in the city* (pp. 105–120). London: Routledge.

King, A., Castro, C., Wilcox, S., Eyler, A., Sallis, J., & Brownson, R. (2000). Personal and environmental factors associated with physical inactivity among different racial-ethnic groups of U.S. middle-aged and older-aged women. *Health Psych, 19*(4), 354–364.

Kneeshaw-Price, S., Saelens, B., Sallis, J., Glanz, K., Frank, L., Kerr, J., & Cain, K. (2013). Children's objective physical activity by location: Why the neighborhood matters. *Pediatric Exercise Science, 25*(3), 468–486.

Lee, H. (2014). Physical activity and thriving community: Can social group-walking generate social capital? A literature review. Master of Applied Positive Psychology (MAPP) Capstone Projects, Paper 61. University of Pennsylvania Scholarly Commons.

Low, S., & Altman, I. (1992). Place attachment: A conceptual inquiry. In I. Altman & S.M. Low (Eds.), *Place attachment* (pp. 1–12). New York, NY: Plenum Press.

Mackett, R.L., & Paskins, J. (2008). Children's physical activity: The contribution of playing and walking. *Children & Society, 22*(5), 345–357.

Mah, M. (2016). *Take up your mat and walk: Applying the metaphor of walking to the spiritual life*. Eugene, OR: Wipf and Stock.

Mutrie, N., & Biddle, S. (1995). The effects of exercise on mental health in nonclinical populations. In S.J.H. Biddle (Ed.), *European perspectives on exercise and sport psychology*. Champaign, IL: Human Kinetics.

Putnam, R. (2000). *Bowling alone: The collapse and revival of American community*. New York, NY: Simon & Schuster.

Robert, C. (2002). The run. In G. Battista (Ed.), *How running changed my life: True stories of the power of running*. Halcottsville, NY: Breakaway Books.

Rogers, S., Halstead, J., Gardner, K., & Carlson, C. (2011). Examining walkability and social capital as indicators of quality of life at the municipal and neighborhood scales. *Applied Research in Quality of Life, 6*(2), 201–213.

Scully, D., Kremer, J., Meade, M., Graham, R., & Dudgeon, K. (1998). Physical exercise and psychological well-being: A critical review. *British Journal of Sports Medicine, 32*(2), 111–120.

Tuan, Y. (1974). Space and place: Humanistic perspective. *Philosophy in Geography*, 6.

Tuan, Y. (1977). *Space and place: The perspective of experience.* Minneapolis, MN: University of Minnesota Press.

United Nations (2014). *World urbanization prospects.* Department of Economic and Social Affairs, New York, NY: United Nations.

Van Dyck, D., Cardon, G., Deforche, B., Sallis, J., Owen, N., & Bourdeaudhuij, I. (2010). Neighborhood SES and walkability are related to physical activity behavior in Belgian adults. *Preventive Medicine, 50*, S74–S79.

Weir, K. (2011). The exercise effect. *American Psychology Association*, *27*(11).

Western Australia Mental Health Commission (n.d.). What is mental health? Retrieved from www.mentalhealth.wa.gov.au/mental_illness_and_health/mh_whatis.aspx

World Health Organization (n.d.). Physical activity fact sheet. Retrieved from www.who.int/mediacentre/factsheets/fs385/en/

World Health Organization (1998). Social capital. In D. Nutbeam (Ed.), *Health promotion glossary.* Geneva: WHO, Division of Health Promotion, Education and Communication.

World Health Organization, Regional Office for Europe (2006). Promoting physical activity and active living in urban environments: The role of local governments. In P. Edwards & A. Tsouros, (Eds), *The solid facts series.* Copenhagen, Denmark.

World Health Organization (2016). Obesity and overweight fact sheet. Mediacentre. Retrieved from www.who.int/mediacentre/factsheets/fs311/en/

Yamaguchi, A. (2013). Impact of social capital on the psychological well-being of adolescents. *International Journal of Psychological Studies, 5*(3), 100–109.

20 School Gym and physical activity

A case study in whole school approach to physical activity

Dylan Blain and Mark Bellamy

Keywords: Physical education, gamified health and fitness intervention, motivation, physical literacy, movement competence

Introduction/background of School Gym

The School Gym concept was originally developed by staff within the physical education department who viewed the traditional practices within physical education as not meeting the needs of the broad range of pupils they were teaching. Observations of skill and fitness levels of pupils commencing secondary school, highlighted the need for them to 'do something different'. It was with this backdrop that the department identified the Health, Fitness and Well-being activity area of the National Curriculum for physical education in Wales (WAG, 2008a), as a basis for the development of an innovative approach to physical education. This centred on supporting all pupils, irrespective of their ability level and interest in different sports, with an opportunity to develop their motivation towards, and participation in, regular and purposeful physical activity. Additionally, and in line with wider educational aims, supporting the development of well-rounded young people, through a holistic approach that addressed learning within cognitive, social and affective domains, alongside physical development (Bailey, 2006; Bailey et al., 2009) was also targeted. This inclusive approach, providing for the unique learning needs of all pupils, formed the basis of the School Gym concept.

The School Gym concept is a result of extensive action-research by teachers and collaborative work between students and staff. Together with support from the school's senior management and governing body teams, extensive fundraising and sponsorship was sought in order to enable the project to continually evolve. Partnership with industry experts in the fitness (Indigo Fitness Ltd) and software development (Writemedia Ltd) fields, enabled the School Gym project to be developed into the whole school case study presented in this chapter. Prior to a detailed description of School Gym, a brief outline of key literature used to underpin and inform decisions made in the creation of School Gym is provided.

School Gym – an overview of the underpinning theory

The promotion of lifelong participation in physical activity is often described as the predominant aim for physical education (Fairclough & Stratton, 2005; Kirk, 2011). Relatedly, and more recently, physical literacy has been proposed as an outcome that physical education should aim to support in all pupils (UNESCO, 2015). Broadly considered as the building blocks to a physically active life (Longmuir & Tremblay, 2016), physical literacy encompasses a range of psychological, social and physical traits and behaviours that target healthy living and development (Robinson et al., 2015). Described as the 'motivation, confidence, physical competence, knowledge and understanding to value and take responsibility for engagement in physical activities for life' (Whitehead, 2016), physical literacy is considered a lifelong disposition that requires continual work in order to maintain (Whitehead, 2010; 2012). The schooling years can be considered an important time period in the development and future maintenance of physical literacy. Indeed, evidence of physical activity habits tracking from adolescence into later life has emerged (Telema et al., 2014). Developing programmes of study, or interventions, that effectively support pupils in developing physical literacy (Longmuir & Tremblay, 2016) and to engage with regular and purposeful physical activity have been identified as an important area of research (Gillis et al., 2013). Such complex interventions should be based on the best available evidence and appropriate theory (Craig et al., 2008). In accordance with this, the School Gym programme applied concepts related to the development of physical literacy, particularly in relation to the development of motivation from a self-determination theory (SDT; Deci & Ryan, 1985; 2000; Ryan & Deci, 2000) perspective. Figure 20.1 provides a conceptual overview outlining the theoretical constructs utilised to provide a theoretical base for both the content and delivery approach used within the programme.

Central to excelling on one's physical literacy journey is having the motivation to 'value and take responsibility for engagement in physical activities for life' (Whitehead, 2016). Motivation is often considered as an energiser and driver of one's behaviour (Hagger & Chatzisarantis, 2007, p. xi). It thus impacts behavioural choices, persistence and intensity and continuation of involvement (Biddle, Mutrie, & Gorely, 2015). One prominent motivational theory that has been extensively used to explore physical activity behaviours is SDT (Deci & Ryan, 1985; 2000; Ryan & Deci, 2000).

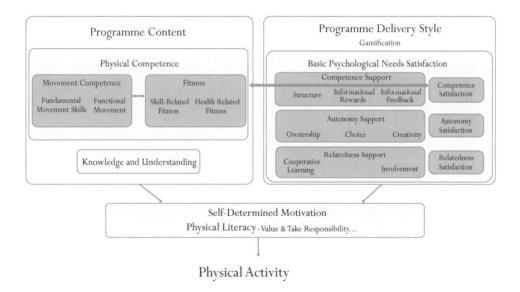

Figure 20.1 Conceptual model outlining the theoretical background underpinning School Gym

Originally developed by Deci and Ryan (1985; 2000), SDT is considered a macro-theory of human motivation, personality and development. Central to SDT is the extent to which individual behaviour is autonomous or self-determined (Deci & Ryan, 2000). As such, in addition to accounting for the quantity of one's motivation, SDT also distinguishes between different types of motivation. Autonomous forms of motivation, characterised by an individual fully endorsing one's actions, consistently lead to more positive outcomes, better functioning and positive development within a range of different fields (for a review see Standage & Ryan, 2012). In contrast, controlled motivational regulations involve individuals acting in order to satisfy external factors. Such controlled motivational regulations have been associated with a range of negative outcomes. Empirical evidence within a range of physical activity related fields support the tenets forwarded within SDT (for a review see Standage & Ryan, 2012 or Ntoumanis & Standage, 2009 for a review of SDT within physical education specifically). As such, developing more autonomous or self-determined forms of motivation towards physical activity is seen as a productive strategy to promote positive physical activity behaviours and physical literacy. Within its sub-theory, basic psychological needs theory, SDT proposes that when an individual's social environment is supportive of the basic psychological needs for autonomy (i.e., experiencing a sense of volition or self-endorsing one's actions), competence (i.e., feeling effective in one's environment) and relatedness (i.e., feeling a sense of being cared for and belonging), they will develop more autonomous forms of motivation (Deci & Ryan, 2000). In contrast when the social environment is not supportive, or is thwarting of the psychological needs, more controlled forms of motivation develop (Deci & Ryan, 2000). Consequently, basic psychological need support within physical activity related contexts can be considered an essential component of programmes aiming to promote physical activity motivation and physical literacy. As such, and as depicted on the right-hand side of Figure 20.1, the social environment created within School Gym targets the satisfaction of the basic psychological needs for all pupils, through utilising need supportive delivery approaches and interactions with pupils. These are described in the detailed description of School Gym.

At the heart of both physical literacy and SDT is the core role of one's physical competence. Psychological theories such as SDT provide a framework outlining the role of the social environment in supporting one's satisfaction of the need for competence or their perceived competence. The role of one's actual competence however is posited to influence, and be influenced by, one's perceived competence (Stodden et al., 2008; Robinson et al., 2015). Thus consideration of the components of young people's actual competence is vital in order to ensure the content of physical education based programmes are suitable and meaningful for this age group. This is outlined on the left-hand side of Figure 20.1.

An individual's level of actual physical competence encompasses a range of components related to skills and fitness. Movement competence (or similar derivatives of the term, such as motor competence or movement proficiency) has been used to describe the quality of one's goal-directed human movement (Robinson et al., 2015). Research has proposed that a base level of motor competence is required prior to learning the performance of more advanced movements (Clark & Metcalfe, 2002; Seefeldt, 1980). Generally, this work postulates that the development of fundamental movement skills (FMS) is necessary in order to become competent in more advanced physical activity contexts such as sports. Competence within FMS, classified as locomotor (e.g., running, hopping and skipping), object control (e.g., throwing, catching, striking and kicking) and stability (e.g., balancing and twisting) (Gallahue, Ozmun, & Goodway, 2011) are positively associated with physical activity in both children and adolescents (Lubans et al., 2010). Extending the work on FMS, Tompsett and colleagues (2014) argue for the consideration of foundational movements as a prerequisite to FMS. They propose that the foundational movements of the squat, lunge, push (up), pull (up), hinge, rotation and brace underpin the performance of FMS (Tompsett, Burkett & McKean, 2014). That is, the development of effective foundational movement is required in order to successfully complete FMS such as jumping, hopping, landing and running. The development of movement competence may therefore require a consideration of foundational movements alongside, and in support of FMS development. Health-based physical education programmes are well positioned to address such movement competency.

Literature on the foundational movements is largely based within the field of strength and conditioning, specifically resistance training. When undertaking resistance training with young people, appropriately designed programmes are essential (Lloyd et al., 2014). Lloyd and Faigenbaum (2016) suggest utilising a range of activities that target the full range of fitness components and a variety of movement patterns. Thus alongside the development of movement competency and strength development, a young person's exercise programme should also target different components of fitness such as cardiovascular endurance, flexibility, speed, agility, coordination and balance. These components of fitness can also be considered an important aspect of an individual's overall physical competency and are likely to impact, and be impacted by, physical activity behaviours (Stodden et al., 2008).

In addition to 'learning to move', 'moving to learn' is also highlighted as a key aspect of physical education (AfPE, 2015). In his seminal work, Arnold (1979) proposed that education could be achieved in, about and through movement. Thus in addition to learning within the psychomotor domain, learning within cognitive, social and affective domains are highlighted as educational benefits that can be achieved through movement within physical education (Bailey et al., 2009). Learning within the cognitive domain could involve developing knowledge and understanding of various health and fitness based topics. Learning within the social domain, requires the provision of opportunities for social interaction and personal responsibility (Bailey, 2006). The importance of supporting this wider and holistic learning is specifically highlighted within curriculum documentation in Wales, for example the National Curriculum for PE (WAG, 2008a) and the National Skills Framework (WAG, 2008b). Given physical education's unique position in providing a structured physical experience to all young people, it is seen as an ideal vehicle to engage young people in holistic learning experiences that first and foremost hold physical development at their core, but also incorporate broader educational aims. The provision of holistic learning experiences within physical, social, cognitive and affective domains outlined in the above sections form the theoretical backdrop for School Gym.

School Gym – the environment

School Gym was initially developed as an environmental intervention, whereby a traditional, 1950s school gym environment was transformed into a modern and unique, open plan, health and fitness environment. Final design of the environment along with the incorporated equipment base was achieved through observation and analysis of pupils working within early versions of School Gym, regular discussions with pupils, and literature from fields of study previously discussed.

The space was *zonally designed* in order to provide distinctive spaces within the overall, open-plan environment. The zonal spaces provide more private and safe workspaces for pupils, aiming to limit any feelings of anxiety pupils may experience from being directly observed by their peers. This may be particularly important for pupils lacking in confidence. Each zone was provided a specific title based on a specific area of fitness. For example, cardio zone, power zone, speed and agility zone, lifting and lowering zone and core zone. These zones provide pupils with a constant reminder that fitness is multi-faceted and provides a practical approach to enhance pupils' knowledge and understanding of health related fitness based topics.

The *cardiovascular zone* contains a range of cardiovascular equipment including stationary bikes and rowing machines. In addition to providing a unique space for pupils to work on aerobic based activities individually or in small groups, the cardiovascular zone also provides a useful start point for lessons as pupils can begin their warm up immediately upon arriving into the venue. This ensures that time spent undertaking moderate intensity physical activity is maximised within limited lesson time. Additionally, by pupils warming up together, initial pulse-raising activity can be undertaken while teacher instruction is provided. The track at the centre of School Gym forms the *speed and agility zone*. This purpose made surface, overlaid on the traditional sprung floor, provides an ideal surface for young people to safely learn more high intensity/impact activities that involve moving at speed, jumping, hopping, sidestepping and turning. Additional training equipment such as hurdles and jump mats can be incorporated onto this surface. The track is marked at 1-metre and 5-metre intervals allowing recording and target setting to be easily, and accurately, undertaken by teachers and pupils as part of lessons. The track also forms part of School Gym's incorporation of numeracy skills, as it provides a useful reference point for mental arithmetic work. One example is when pupils have to run the distance of a particular sum or multiplication table. For example, a pupil may call out a sum to their peer and they have to run the answer in meters on the track. As such, the track has also been labelled 'table track' to represent a physical form of learning times tables.

The range of *equipment* incorporated into the different zones of School Gym comprises traditional fitness based equipment such as resistance bands, suspension trainers, skipping ropes, power bags, medicine balls, slam balls, light barbell sets, and boxercise equipment. In contrast to machine-based gym equipment, this type of equipment aims to create an environment that supports the development of good fundamental and foundational movement and overall fitness. Additionally, the range of equipment is available in each zone in order to provide pupils with extensive choice.

In addition to the traditional fitness equipment, School Gym also incorporates a range of bespoke products. The bespoke products were designed in order to complement traditional gym-based products. This aimed to create a more age-appropriate environment and positive and holistic learning experience for young people by enabling them to undertake a range of fundamental and foundational movement exercises in a playful and fun way. Table 20.1 provides an overview of the products used within School Gym together with the learning targeted through their design.

The open plan zonal environment and unique equipment base that forms School Gym is drawn together by the innovative use of *graphics and colour*. Each zone is distinctly identified through its own unique graphic board which clearly distinguishes specific zones (i.e., power zone, speed and agility zone, lifting lowering zone). These graphics boards also provide subtle cues to the different movements and areas of the body that can be worked within each zone. Specific graphic boards also display the activity matrix (Figure 20.3) and points ladder (Figure 20.2) so that they can be referred to by teachers and pupils when undertaking the programmes of study created for School Gym.

Table 20.1 Overview of bespoke products targeting wider learning within School Gym

Equipment Name	Description	Uses	Purpose/Aim of Product
Resistance Rack	A wall-mounted frame which provides an attachment point for resistance bands in order to provide assistance and/or resistance for a range of activities.	A variety of assisted and resisted based activities (e.g., pull ups, alternate leg drives).	Provide differentiated options catering for all pupil needs and abilities. Trigger/cue pupils to undertake a range of activities within the activity matrix.
Push up frames (variety of shapes and sizes)	A variety of different shaped and sized frames for undertaking push up based activities.	Provides a specific focused equipment piece for a range of push up based activities.	Provide differentiated options for push up based activities. Trigger/cue pupils to undertake push up based activities within zones.
Pull up frames	A variety of different shaped and sized frames for undertaking pull up based activities.	Provides a specific focused equipment piece for a range of pull up based activities.	Provide specific frames for pull up based activities as in activity matrix (Figure 20.3). Provide frames for the attachment of assistance bands to create easier/differentiated options for pull up based activities as in activity matrix (Figure 20.3) Trigger/cue pupils to undertake pull up based activities within zones.
Maze Maker	Rectangular blocks with a range of markings including domino dots and scrabble numbers and letters.	Pupils create physical games/challenges for each other by combining physical activities they have learnt with the equipment.	Key skill development & wider learning: • Creativity • Problem solving • Communication • Teamwork • Leadership • Numeracy
Alpha Mat/ Core keyboard	Training mat with lettered markings.	Pupils can physically tap the letters using their hands (e.g., from the front support position) or feet (e.g., by hopping or jumping). This allows different spelling or question and answer games to be played.	Key skill development & wider learning: • Literacy • Problem solving • Communication • Creativity

(Continued)

Table 20.1 (Continued)

Equipment Name	Description	Uses	Purpose/Aim of Product
Digi Mat	Training mat with numbered markings.	Pupils can physically tap the numbers using their hands (e.g., from the front support position) or feet (e.g., by hopping or jumping). This allows different mental arithmetic/mathematical question and answer games to be played.	Key skill development & wider learning: • Numeracy • Problem solving • Communication • Creativity
Power Board	Wall mounted board with lettered and/or numbered markings.	Pupils can use as targets in combination with a variety of balls (including medicine balls). A variety of games can be undertaken/created similar to those with Alpha and Digi mat. A variety of throwing techniques can be used from the activity matrix (e.g., chest pass, overhead throw, lateral twisting throw).	Key skill development & wider learning: • Numeracy • Literacy • Problem solving • Communication • Creativity

School Gym – the programmes (School Fitness 3T)

Alongside the environmental developments, programmes of study were devised, aiming to develop pupils holistically and support them on their physical literacy journeys (Whitehead, 2010). At the heart of these programmes of study is the creation of a need supportive environment (Deci & Ryan, 2000) for all pupils (Figure 20.1). The main programme of study, School Fitness 3T, utilises principles of Gamification to create an engaging and need supportive environment for all pupils. Gamification is described as 'the use of game design elements in non-game contexts' (Deterding, Dixon, Khaled, & Nacke, 2011). Much of this game thinking and mechanics emerges from video games that are considered engaging and motivating for a high proportion of the population. Indeed, 98% of young people reported to regularly play video games (IAB, 2011). The motivational nature of video games has been attributed to their ability to extensively nurture the basic psychological needs for autonomy, competence and relatedness reported within SDT (Przybylski, Rigby, & Ryan, 2010; Ryan, Rigby, & Przybylski, 2006). As such transferring the need supportive strategies utilised within video games into the pedagogical approach used within a health and fitness-based physical education programme appeared a productive strategy for motivating and engaging pupils in physical education.

School Fitness 3T – game elements

School Fitness 3T utilises the core game elements of *points and levelling up* in order to provide consistent feedback to support feelings of progression and competence. Within the School Fitness 3T programme, points are awarded for time spent, or repetitions completed on activities within the matrix (Figure 20.3). The activity matrix provides a series of activities based on fundamental and foundational movements and broader exercise activities. Each category within the matrix contains a series of ten progressive activities starting with the simplest form (level 1) and progressing to the most difficult (level 10). To enable pupils to work independently at a developmentally appropriate and optimally challenging level within the activity matrix, an electronic resource card is provided on an online platform for each activity (i.e., 170 electronic activity cards in total). The resource card provides still images and video footage with annotated teaching points for each activity. The choice of activities included in the activity matrix and supporting online resources, accessed through mobile devices, aim to provide support for the development of good technique and competent movers and exercisers, in a structured yet autonomy supportive way (Jang, Reeve, & Deci, 2010; Reeve, 2006).

Through completing the range of activities, pupils acquire points and progress through a series of levels towards Olympic Gold mode on the points ladder (Figure 20.2). The constant levelling up provides a clear pathway for success for all. To ensure all pupils are able to experience success in the programme, equal points are awarded for all activities on the matrix, irrespective of their difficulty. Points accumulate as pupils log their activity using the online software. This aims to create a personalised and structured pathway for competence development (Jang, Reeve, & Deci, 2010). Alongside the points ladder, pupils can unlock a range of *unlockable achievements* (Figure 20.4) for displaying certain positive behaviours. These are awarded by the teacher using their teacher login on the online software and appear for pupils to see when they log in. To promote specific behaviours and subsequent achievement of the unlockables, the teacher can utilise structured activities (outlined in a set of lesson plans) that allow pupils opportunities to demonstrate the specific behaviours. For example, to support pupils

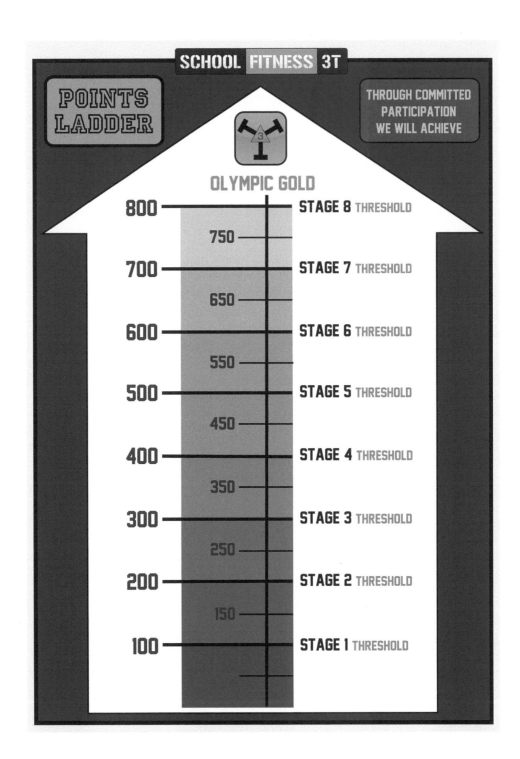

Figure 20.2 The points and levelling up ladder

SCHOOL FITNESS 3T

ACTIVITY LADDER

	LOWER BODY			UPPER BODY			JUMPS AND LANDING			CARRIES	THROWS	CORE		AEROBIC DEVELOPMENT	SPEED		COORDINATION
	SQUAT	HIP	SINGLE LEG	PUSH	PULL		HORIZONTAL	VERTICAL	MULTI DIRECTIONAL			FRONT PLANK	SIDE PLANK		LINEAR	MULTI DIRECTIONAL	
					HORIZONTAL	VERTICAL											
10	OVERHEAD PARALLEL SQUAT	SNATCH GRIP DEADLIFT FROM FLOOR	SINGLE LEG BOX SQUAT PARALLEL RESISTED	BARBELL BENCH PRESS	INVERTED ROW RESISTED FEET ON BOX	ROPE PULL NO LEGS	3 HOPS FOR DISTANCE	MULTIPLE HURDLE HOPS	SINGLE LEG MULTIDIRECTIONAL HOP MATRIX	WAITERS CARRY SINGLE ARM	EXPLOSIVE MED BALL SQUAT DIVE	FRONT PLANK 1 ARM 1 FOOT OFF FLOOR PARTNER RESISTED FOR REPS	SIDE PLANK WITH LEG AND ARM RAISE	RUNNING AEROBIC INTERVALS	MAX SPEED TECHNIQUE	REACTIVE MULTIPLE CHANGE OF DIRECTION	ALTERNATE SINGLE LEG SQUAT THRUST
9	OVERHEAD HALF SQUAT	DEADLIFT FROM FLOOR	SINGLE LEG BOX SQUAT PARALLEL BODYWEIGHT	BARBELL FLOOR PRESS	INVERTED ROW RESISTED FEET ON FLOOR	CHIN / PULL UP RESISTED	BROAD JUMPS 3 JUMPS FOR DISTANCE	MULTIPLE HURDLE JUMPS INCREASE HEIGHT	MULTIDIRECTIONAL HOP MATRIX	WAITERS CARRY DOUBLE ARM	EXPLOSIVE MED BALL OVERHEAD BACKWARD	FRONT PLANK PARTNER RESISTED HOLD	SIDE PLANK WITH LEG RAISE	RUNNING 30 MINS	ACCELERATION TECHNIQUE	REACTIVE SINGLE CHANGE OF DIRECTION	JUMPING JACKS ONTO BOX
8	RESISTED PARALLEL BACK SQUAT	DEADLIFT FROM BLOCKS / OFF PINS	SINGLE LEG BOX SQUAT HALF RESISTED	NEUTRAL GRIP DB FLOOR PRESS	INVERTED ROW BW FEET ON BOX REPS	PULL UP	REPEATED HURDLE HOP AND STICK	MULTIPLE HURDLE JUMPS LOW HURDLES	45 DEGREE REPEATED HOP	SINGLE ARM FARMERS WALK	EXPLOSIVE MED BALL OVERHEAD FORWARD	FRONT PLANK 1 ARM 1 FOOT OFF FLOOR FOR REPS	SIDE PLANK HOLD 60'S	RUNNING 20 MINS	A DRILL RUNNING	PROGRAMMED MULTIPLE CHANGE OF DIRECTION	BACK STEPS BOUNCING
7	RESISTED PARALLEL FRONT SQUAT	KETTLEBELL SWING	SINGLE LEG BOX SQUAT HALF BODYWEIGHT	RESISTED PRESS UP FEET ELEVATED	INVERTED ROW BW FEET ON FLOOR REPS	CHIN UP	REPEATED HURDLE JUMP AND STICK	HURDLE JUMP AND STICK INCREASE HEIGHT	45 DEGREE REPEATED STEP	DOUBLE ARM FARMERS WALK	EXPLOSIVE MED BALL OVERHEAD SLAM	FRONT PLANK 1 ARM 1 FOOT OFF FLOOR HOLD	SIDE PLANK HOLD 40'S	RUNNING 10 MINS	A DRILL SKIPPING	PROGRAMMED SINGLE CHANGE OF DIRECTION	BACK STEPS WITH ARMS
6	RESISTED HALF BACK SQUAT	GOOD MORNING	RESISTED WALKING LUNGE	RESISTED PRESS UP FEET ON FLOOR	INVERTED ROW BW FEET ON BOX ISOMETRIC HOLD	PULL UP BAND ASSISTED	SINGLE HURDLE HOP AND STICK	HURDLE JUMP AND STICK LOW HURDLE	45 DEGREE REPEATED JUMP	POWERBAG OVER SHOULDER CARRY 1 SIDE	STANDING LATERAL THROW AGAINST WALL	FRONT PLANK 1 ARM OFF FLOOR FOR REPS	SIDE PLANK HOLD 20'S	BIKE / CROSS TRAINER / ROWER 30 MINS	LOCKOUT SKIPPING	LADDER / HURDLE DRILLS FULL SPEED	BACK STEPS HANDS ON HIPS
5	RESISTED HALF FRONT SQUAT	ROMANIAN DEADLIFT	SPLIT SQUAT BACK LEG ELEVATED	STABILITY BALL PRESS UPS	INVERTED ROW BW FEET ON FLOOR ISOMETRIC HOLD	CHIN UP BAND ASSISTED	SINGLE HURDLE JUMP AND STICK	BOX JUMP INCREASE HEIGHT	LATERAL HOPS OVER HURDLES	POWERBAG OVER SHOULDER CARRY BOTH SHOULDERS	STANDING OVERHEAD THROW AGAINST WALL	FRONT PLANK 1 ARM OFF FLOOR HOLD	SIDE PLANK REPS	BIKE / CROSS TRAINER / ROWER 20 MINS	LOCKOUT WALKING PLATE RESISTED	LADDER / HURDLE DRILLS HALF SPEED	ALTERNATE HEEL TO BUM JUMPING
4	GOBLET PARALLEL SQUAT REPS	BAND GOOD MORNING	LUNGE VARIATIONS REPS	PRESS UPS REPS FEET ELEVATED	30 DEGREE ROW UP TO 20 REPS	PULL UP ISOMETRIC HOLD	60CM HOP AND STICK	BOX JUMP LOW BOX	LATERAL JUMPS OVER HURDLES	SINGLE ARM WEIGHTED HOLD INCREASE RESISTANCE	STANDING CHEST PASS AGAINST WALL	FRONT PLANK HOLD 60'S	KNEELING SIDE PLANK HOLD 60'S	BIKE / CROSS TRAINER / ROWER 10 MINS	LOCKOUT WALKING	LADDER OR HURDLE DRILLS WALKING	ALTERNATE HEEL TO BUM WALKING
3	GOBLET HALF SQUAT REPS	RESISTANCE BAND PULL THROUGH REPS	90/90 SPLIT SQUAT REPS	PRESS UPS REPS FEET ON FLOOR	ISOMETRIC HOLD 30 DEGREE ANGLE	CHIN UP ISOMETRIC HOLD	60CM BROAD JUMP AND STICK	VERTICAL JUMP AND STICK WITH ARMS	LATERAL HOP AND STICK	SINGLE ARM WEIGHTED HOLD	KNEELING LATERAL THROW AGAINST WALL	FRONT PLANK HOLD 40'S	KNEELING SIDE PLANK HOLD 40'S	WALKING 30 MINS	ACCELERATION WALL DRILL FULL SPEED	LATERAL SHUFFLE FULL SPEED	SPOTTY DOGS
2	GOBLET PARALLEL SQUAT ISOMETRIC HOLD	GOOD MORNING / WAITERS BOW REPS	90/90 SPLIT SQUAT HOLD BACK KNEE OFF FLOOR	PRESS UP ISO HOLD FEET ELEVATED	45 DEGREE ROW UP TO 20 REPS	ASSISTED PULL UP ISOMETRIC HOLD	30CM HOP AND STICK	VERTICAL JUMP AND STICK HANDS ON HIPS	LATERAL STEP AND STICK	DOUBLE ARM WEIGHTED HOLD INCREASE RESISTANCE	KNEELING OVERHEAD THROW AGAINST WALL	FRONT PLANK HOLD 20'S	KNEELING SIDE PLANK HOLD 20'S	WALKING 20 MINS	ACCELERATION WALL DRILL MARCHING	LATERAL SHUFFLE HALF SPEED	DOUBLE JUMPING JACKS
1	GOBLET HALF SQUAT ISOMETRIC HOLD	GOOD MORNING / WAITERS BOW ISOMETRIC HOLD	90/90 SPLIT SQUAT HOLD BACK KNEE ON FLOOR	PRESS UP ISO HOLD FEET ON FLOOR	ISOMETRIC HOLD 45 DEGREE ANGLE	ASSISTED CHIN UP ISOMETRIC HOLD	30CM BROAD JUMP AND STICK	LANDING MECHANICS STEP OFF BOX AND STICK	LATERAL JUMP AND STICK	DOUBLE ARM WEIGHTED HOLD	KNEELING CHEST PASS AGAINST WALL	KNEELING PLANK HOLD 20'S	KNEELING SIDE PLANK REPS	WALKING 10 MINS	ACCELERATION WALL DRILL POSTURE HOLD	LATERAL SHUFFLE WALKING	SINGLE JUMPING JACKS

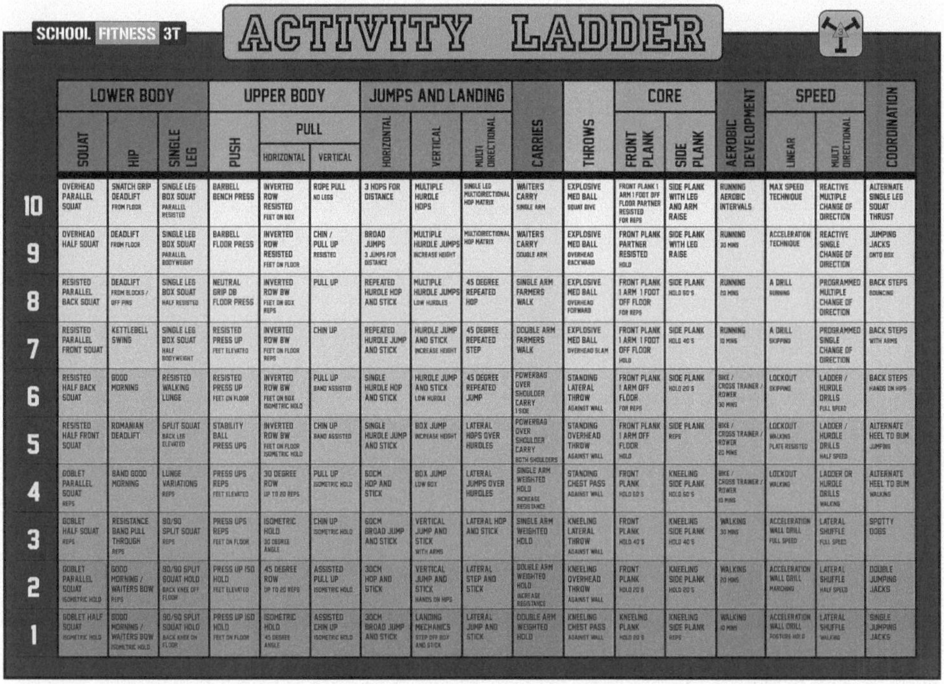

Figure 20.3 The activity matrix

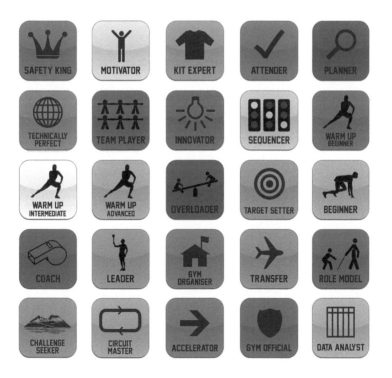

Figure 20.4 The achievement unlockables

in achieving their innovator badge, the teacher can set tasks that require pupils to use their existing knowledge (gained through following activities within the activity matrix) to create new activities of their own. This provides opportunities for pupils to have input and a sense of autonomy within lessons. Additionally, problem solving and creativity skills are fostered. Many of these activities involve pupils working cooperatively in pairs or small groups providing opportunities for pupils to experience a sense of relatedness. Thus in addition to providing further support for the basic psychological needs postulated within SDT, the achievement unlockables serve as a means of teachers providing holistic learning opportunities that enable pupils to develop broader skills within a range of domains (i.e., social, cognitive).

To support pupils in making a positive and safe start on the School Fitness 3T programme, the core game design element of a *beginner tutorial* is used. The beginner tutorial involves pupils completing the level one activity of each category of the activity matrix. This ensures pupils have an understanding of the basic movement techniques within the programme. These activities are devised at a basic level to emphasise the core techniques of each movement activity (e.g., alignment during a squat). The teaching points used at these level one activities progressively develop to more advanced activities in each column. This approach provides a constant thread of teaching cues as pupils progress through the levels. Not only does this approach aid in developing movement competency, it also enhances pupils' ability to provide effective feedback to their peers within reciprocal learning tasks (Mosston & Ashworth, 2008).

In addition to the video game elements described above, the School Fitness 3T programme also integrates more traditional, playful game components incorporated within board games. For example, through individual and team challenges. This aims to engage and enthuse pupils and enable them to develop their movement competence and fitness in a more playful and enjoyable way. Additionally, pupils are encouraged to modify these activities and create their own games by utilising their pre-existing knowledge of fundamental and foundational movements and exercise activities, into games for their peers. This aims to engage and enthuse pupils by giving them ownership over the learning tasks so that the physical competency elements are built into their activities in a fun and enjoyable way. The bespoke equipment (Table 20.1) provides game like triggers for pupils to utilise in this process. In combination, utilisation of the range of game elements described aim to create a need supportive environment (Deci & Ryan, 2000) for all pupils to develop their fundamental and foundational movement competency and overall fitness.

School Fitness 3T – core principles

The School Fitness 3T programme was named around the central elements (and 3 Ts) of Training, Testing and Technique. The first T, for *Technique*, reflects the importance placed upon good movement and physical competence development within the programme. Additionally, the development of all-round fitness through the incorporation of a well-rounded exercise programme aids in the development of technique. *Training* or exercising forms the second T, highlighting the core role that physical activity takes within the School Fitness 3T programme. The programme aims to motivate pupils of all abilities to exercise and practise purposefully and regularly. The points system that levels up to the highest level of Olympic Gold rewards pupils for their effort. The structured progression to more difficult activities on the activity matrix supports the development of movement competency and aims to develop fitness within the different components. The programme aims to provide pupils with an optimal level of challenge and as such encourage them to exercise at a level appropriate to them. The final T represents the natural integration of *Testing* contained within the programme. In contrast to formal fitness testing procedures, School Fitness 3T includes a natural process of testing through the creation of self-monitoring using the online platform. This allows pupils to observe their progress through the accumulation of points achieved by consistently applying effort within lessons. Additionally, as their competence develops they will make progress up the activity matrix to more advanced movements and exercises. This provides pupils with self-referenced targets and informational feedback that they have control over (Jang, Reeve, & Deci, 2010). Additionally, the software allows pupils to capture and upload video footage of activities so that teacher or peer assessment can be undertaken. This can be used to ensure effective feedback is provided. In addition to monitoring effort and movement competency, the programme also allows pupils and teachers to monitor more holistic development through the achievement unlockables. Using the online platform, teachers and pupils are able to monitor progress and specify areas for improvement. For example, some pupils may have unlocked several achievements related to leadership or teamwork demonstrating their competence in this area. Others, who may be progressing well with their physical development on the other aspects of the programme may not be working so well with others and therefore will not have unlocked the relevant achievement. Armed with this ability to monitor pupils holistically, the teacher can modify their practice accordingly through the provision of informational feedback (Jang, Reeve, & Deci, 2010) or setting of specific tasks, based on pupil needs.

Present day impact

From the outset, the School Gym environment has engaged pupils of all abilities through its appealing look and feel, the extensive choice provided by the equipment base and integrated use of technology within the programme of study. Physical education teachers also note the significant impact School Gym has had on pupils with lower ability. Teachers particularly noted how pupils of all abilities were motivated to return in their leisure time (lunch times or after school) to use the environment during the designated extra-curricular clubs. For many of these pupils, the traditional extra-curricular sport-based programme had not been enticing enough to draw them in their free time. This was seen as a particular success of the project given the negative spiral of physical activity engagement posited for pupils with low perceptions of competence (Stodden et al., 2008). Additionally, adolescent girls, a group identified as at risk of disengagement from physical education and physical activity more broadly (Biddle, Brehm, Verheijden, & Hopman-Rock, 2012) have appeared motivated and engaged within the environment, with one session per week being set aside for girls due to the popularity of School Gym with this group. Physical education staff have also noted how the environment provided higher ability pupils, who were engaged in competitive sport programmes ranging from regional to international level, with a high quality environment for them to work on their movement quality and more specific conditioning programmes to support their progress in their chosen sports. For example, an under 16 international level athlete was often observed undertaking a core conditioning programme in preparation for major events and other high level sports players have commented on the benefit of the gym to their sporting aspirations.

In addition to the school staff's observations, a variety of external visitors have commented positively on the innovative approach taken within School Gym. Firstly, as part of a recent school inspection, the inclusive nature and holistic approach was noted as a particular strength.

> The recently refurbished gym area (installed three years previously but still looking brand new) is an attractive, high quality learning environment and is used in an innovative way to develop pupils learning skills. The health, fitness and well-being programme motivates pupils to a very high level and, irrespective of their ability, encourages them to get involved in physical education.
>
> (Estyn Inspection Report, 2013)

This strength of School Gym in supporting wider educational aims was also noted by experts within the field.

> Not only is the facility absolutely fantastic but also the educational thinking that underpins almost every item of equipment or area in the gym suggests deep educational thinking and the application of significant craft knowledge. The ability to differentiate learning and then apply key principles of literacy and numeracy and integrate technology into physical education warrants further support.
>
> (Professor Gareth Stratton)

Currently, School Gym continues to enthuse and engage a range of classes as part of their broader physical education programme.

Conclusion

Lifestyle changes have engineered considerable physical activity out of daily lives, leaving individual motivation to participate in regular and purposeful physical activity an important area of concern. Effective approaches to enhance the physical activity levels of young people have been called for (Gillis et al., 2013). This chapter has provided an outline of one school's attempt to positively impact young people's physical activity behaviours through the School Gym programme for physical education. Firstly, the chapter sought to provide an overview of the key theories underpinning the design and development of School Gym. Specifically, motivational theory from a SDT perspective was reviewed as a basis for the strategies and approaches used within School Gym to support physical literacy and engagement in purposeful physical activity. Secondly, the broad areas of movement and fitness competence were addressed to provide a rationale for the content of the programmes. This centred on developing differentiated programmes of study focusing on fundamental and foundational movement and well-rounded exercise activities. With this theoretical basis in mind, the chapter then described the School Gym concept in detail, with the aim of mapping the theoretical concepts onto the practical implementation strategies used. Here, the use of gamification was specifically outlined. The impact of School Gym to date was then addressed. Through its integration of the old (traditional school gym infrastructure) with the new (innovative environment, and technological based, gamified programme of study) School Gym aims to provide an innovate alternative to traditional health and fitness activities within physical education. At the heart of this development was a whole school acknowledgement of the importance of physical education within young people's school experience, and the motivation to provide a meaningful experience that supports all pupils on their physical literacy journeys. The continued development of School Gym aspires to provide a more prosperous future for health and fitness activities within physical education, in order to provide positive physical education experiences that encourage all pupils to engage in regular health-enhancing physical activity.

Chapter summary

- This chapter provides an overview of one school's innovative approach to supporting young people's development of physical literacy and engagement with regular and purposeful physical activity.
- The School Gym programme utilises an evidence-based and theoretically driven approach, and involves the redevelopment of a traditional school-based gym environment and the creation of motivational, health-related exercise programmes of study for physical education.
- Motivational theory from a SDT perspective supported the implementation strategies used within the School Gym programme.
- Based on literature from the broad area of physical competence, fundamental and foundational movement and well-rounded exercise activities formed the basis for the content of the School Gym programme.
- Through integrating the old (traditional school gym infrastructure) with the new (innovative, and technology-based gamified programme of study), School Gym provides an innovative alternative to traditional health and fitness activities within physical education.
- Future work on School Gym aims to further develop the provision of positive health and fitness-based physical education experiences for young people.

References

AfPE/Association for Physical Education (2015). *Health Position Paper*. AfPE.

Arnold, P.J. (1979). Education, movement and the curriculum. In P.J. Arnold (Ed.), *Meaning in movement, sport, and physical education,* London: Heinemann.

Bailey, R. (2006). Physical education and sport in schools: A review of benefits and outcomes. *Journal of School Health, 76*(8), 397–401. doi:10.1111/j.1746-1561.2006.00132.x

Bailey, R., Armour, K., Kirk, D., Jess, M., Pickup, I., & Sandford, R. (2009). The educational benefits claimed for physical education and school sport: An academic review. *Research Papers in Education, 24*(1), 1–27. doi:10.1080/02671520701809817

Biddle, S.J.H., Mutrie, N., & Gorely, T. (2015). *The psychology of physical activity: Determinants, well-being and interventions* (3rd ed.). London, United Kingdom: Routledge.

Biddle, S.J.H., Brehm, W., Verheijden, M., & Hopman-Rock, M. (2012). Population physical activity behaviour change: A review for the European college of sport science. *European Journal of Sport Science, 12*(4), 367–383. doi:10.1080/17461391.2011.635700

Clark, J.E., & Metcalfe, J.S. (2002). The mountain of motor development: A metaphor. In J.E. Clark & J.H. Humphrey (Eds.), *Motor development: Research and reviews* (Vol. 2) (pp. 163–190). Reston, VA: National Association of Sport and Physical Education.

Craig, P., Dieppe, P., Macintyre, S., Michie, S., Nazareth, I., & Petticrew, M. (2008). Developing and evaluating complex interventions: The new medical research council guidance. *BMJ, 337*(Sep 29 1), a1655–a1655. doi:10.1136/bmj.a1655

Deci, E.L., & Ryan, R.M. (1985). *Intrinsic motivation and self-determination in human behavior* (3rd ed.). New York: Plenum Publishing Co.

Deci, E.L., & Ryan, R.M. (2000). The 'what' and 'why' of goal pursuits: Human needs and the self-determination of behavior. *Psychological Inquiry, 11*(4), 227–268. doi:10.1207/s15327965pli1104_01

Deterding, S., Dixon, D., Khaled, R., & Nacke, L. (2011). From game design elements to gamefulness: Defining 'Gamification'. Proceedings of the 15th International Academic MindTrek Conference: Envisioning Future Media Environments, September 28–30, 2011, Tampere, Finland.

Estyn Inspection Report (2013). A Report on Dyffryn Taf School. Retrieved November 20, 2016 from www.estyn.gov.wales/sites/default/files/documents/Inspection%20report%20Dyffryn%20Taf%20School%202013_0.pdf

Fairclough, S., & Stratton, G. (2005). 'Physical education makes you fit and healthy'. Physical education's contribution to young people's physical activity levels. *Health Education Research, 20*(1), 14–23. doi:10.1093/her/cyg101

Gallahue, D.L., Ozmun, J.C., & Goodway, J.D. (2011). *Understanding motor development: Infants, children, adolescents, adults* (7th ed.). New York: McGraw Hill Higher Education.

Gillis, L., Tomkinson, G., Olds, T., Moreira, C., Christie, C., Nigg, C., . . . Van Mechelen, W. (2013). Research priorities for child and adolescent physical activity and sedentary behaviours: An international perspective using a twin-panel Delphi procedure. *International Journal of Behavioral Nutrition and Physical Activity, 10*(1), 112. doi:10.1186/1479-5868-10-112

Hagger, M., & Chatzisarantis, N.L.D. (2007) (Eds.). *Intrinsic motivation and self-determination in exercise and sport*. Champaign, IL: Human Kinetics.

IAB/Internet Advertising Bureau UK (2011). *Gaming Britain: A nation united by digital play*. IAB: UK.

Jang, H., Reeve, J., & Deci, E.L. (2010). Engaging students in learning activities: It is not autonomy support or structure but autonomy support and structure. *Journal of Educational Psychology, 102*(3), 588–600. doi:10.1037/a0019682

Kirk, D. (2011). *Physical education futures*. London: Taylor & Francis.

Lloyd R.S., & Faigenbaum, A.D. (2016). Age and sex-related differences and their implications for resistance exercise. In G.G. Haff & T.N. Triplett (Eds.), *Essentials of strength training and conditioning*. United States: Human Kinetics.

Lloyd, R.S., Faigenbaum, A.D., Stone, M.H., Oliver, J.L., Jeffreys, I., Moody, J.A., . . . Myer, G.D. (2014). Position statement on youth resistance training: The 2014 international consensus. *British Journal of Sports Medicine, 48*(7), 498–505. doi:10.1136/bjsports-2013-092952

Longmuir, P.E., & Tremblay, M.S. (2016). Top 10 research questions related to physical literacy. *Research Quarterly for Exercise and Sport, 87*(1), 28–35. doi:10.1080/02701367.2016.1124671

Lubans, D.R., Morgan, P.J., Cliff, D.P., Barnett, L.M., & Okely, A.D. (2010). Fundamental movement skills in children and adolescents. *Sports Medicine, 40*(12), 1019–1035. doi:10.2165/11536850-000000000-00000

Mosston, M., & Ashworth, S. (2008). *Teaching physical education* (First Online Edition). Retrieved November 27, 2016, from www.spectrumofteachingstyles.org/

Ntoumanis, N., & Standage, M. (2009). Motivation in physical education classes: A self-determination theory perspective. *Theory and Research in Education, 7*(2), 194–202. doi:10.1177/1477878509104324

Przybylski, A.K., Rigby, C.S., & Ryan, R.M. (2010). A motivational model of video game engagement. *Review of General Psychology, 14*(2), 154–166. doi:10.1037/a0019440

Reeve, J. (2006). Teachers as facilitators: What autonomy-supportive teachers do and why their students benefit. *The Elementary School Journal, 106*(3), 225–236. doi:10.1086/501484

Robinson, L.E., Stodden, D.F., Barnett, L.M., Lopes, V.P., Logan, S.W., Rodrigues, L.P., & D'Hondt, E. (2015). Motor competence and its effect on positive developmental trajectories of health. *Sports Medicine, 45*(9), 1273–1284. doi:10.1007/s40279-015-0351-6

Ryan, R.M., & Deci, E.L. (2000). Self-determination theory and the facilitation of intrinsic motivation, social development, and well-being. *American Psychologist, 55*(1), 68–78. doi:10.1037/0003-066x.55.1.68

Ryan, R.M., Rigby, C.S., & Przybylski, A. (2006). The motivational pull of video games: A self-determination theory approach. *Motivation and Emotion, 30*(4), 344–360. doi:10.1007/s11031-006-9051-8

Seefeldt, V. (1980). Developmental motor patterns: Implications for elementary school physical education. In C. Nadeau, W. Holliwell, K. Newell, & G. Roberts (Eds.), *Psychology of motor behavior and sport* (pp. 314–323). Champaign, IL: Human Kinetics.

Standage, M., & Ryan, R.M. (2012). Self-determination theory and exercise motivation: Facilitating self-regulatory processes to support and maintain health and well-being. In G.C. Roberts & D.C. Treasure (Eds.), *Advances in motivation in sport and exercise* (3rd ed.) (pp. 233–270). Champaign, IL: Human Kinetics.

Stodden, D.F., Goodway, J.D., Langendorfer, S.J., Roberton, M.A., Rudisill, M.E., Garcia, C., & Garcia, L.E. (2008). A developmental perspective on the role of motor skill competence in physical activity: An emergent relationship. *Quest, 60*(2), 290–306. doi:10.1080/00336297.2008.10483582

Telema, R., Yang, X., Leskinen, E., Kankaanpaa, A., Hirvensalo, M., Tammelin, T., . . . Raitakari, O.T. (2014). Tracking of physical activity from early childhood through youth into adulthood. *Medicine and Science in Sports and Exercise, 46*(5), 955–962. doi:10.1249/mss.0000000000000181

Tompsett, C., Burkett, B., & McKean, M.R. (2014). Development of physical literacy and movement competency: A literature review. *Journal of Fitness Research, 3*(2), 53–74.

UNESCO/United Nations Educational, Scientific and Cultural Organization (2015). *Quality physical education: Guidelines to policy-makers*. Paris: UNESCO Publishing.

WAG/Welsh Assembly Government (2008a). *Physical education in the national curriculum for Wales*. WAG: Cardiff.

WAG/Welsh Assembly Government (2008b). *Skills framework for 3 to 19-year-olds in Wales*. WAG: Cardiff.

Whitehead, M. (Ed.) (2010). *Physical literacy: Throughout the lifecourse*. New York: Routledge.

Whitehead, M. (2012). What is physical literacy and how does it impact on physical education? In S. Capel & M. Whitehead (Eds.), *Debates in physical education teaching* (pp. 37–52). New York: Routledge.

Whitehead, M. (2016). Definition of physical literacy. International physical literacy association. Retrieved November 27, 2016, from www.physical-literacy.org.uk/

21 Physical activity promotion strategies

Clover Maitland and Michael Rosenberg

Keywords: Ottawa Charter for Health Promotion, ecological model, physical activity promotion, community-wide campaigns, public education campaigns

Introduction

Have you ever wondered why some people don't do enough physical activity for good health? Regular physical activity provides physical, mental and social health benefits to individuals, reduces the burden of chronic disease, and has other co-benefits for the whole community (Giles-Corti, Foster, Shilton, & Falconer, 2010; Janssen & LeBlanc, 2010; World Health Organization, 2009a). However, physical activity has been engineered out of daily lives, such that work, travel and leisure activities are more sedentary than ever and we have lost many easy opportunities to be active every day. Many people know that physical activity is good for them. Yet knowledge alone is not enough as changing physical activity behaviour requires sustained motivation, skills and support over a long time.

Many interventions have tried to get people to be more physically active with varying success. Key challenges facing those who wish to promote physical activity include: What strategies work best to drive physical activity behaviour change? Can strategies that work for individuals be scaled up to effect change in groups or a whole population? Will strategies that work for people in one context, successfully work in another? There exist a number of frameworks, theories and strategies that new population level physical activity interventions can build upon to increase the chances of success. Principles that are common to many successful physical activity promotion interventions, and will be discussed throughout this chapter, include:

- Strategies are designed with, and tailored to, the target individuals, groups and/or populations;
- A comprehensive mix of strategies is included to target multiple levels of influence on physical activity behaviour;
- Strategies are developed using relevant health promotion frameworks and behaviour change theories; and
- Strategies are informed by research evidence about what is already known.

Overview of global health promotion and physical activity

Successful physical activity promotion has built upon a long history of health promotion frameworks that help construct and combine physical activity promoting strategies. *Health promotion* is, 'the process of enabling people to increase control over, and to improve their health' (World Health Organization, 1986). It, 'not only embraces actions directed at strengthening the skills and capabilities of individuals, but also action directed towards changing social, environmental and economic conditions so as to alleviate their impact on public and individual health' (World Health Organization, 1998). Thus, a health promotion approach to physical activity goes beyond just targeting individuals with educational and behavioural strategies, to considering a wider range of strategies that aim to change the social, organizational, physical and policy environments in which people live, work and recreate.

The 1986 *Ottawa Charter for Health Promotion* redefined how health pomotion was approached and provides an overarching framework for action that is still relevant for physical activity promotion today (World Health Organization, 1986). The Charter comprises five core action areas for health promotion: 1) building public policy; 2) creating supportive environments; 3) strengthening community action; 4) developing personal skills; and 5) reorientating health services for health promotion (Table 21.1). Advocating for health, empowering people, and mediating between health and other sectors, are key ways of working outlined by the Charter that are highly relevant for physical activity promotion practitioners. This multi-strategy approach is evident in physical activity interventions across the world.

There have been several updates to enhance the original Ottawa Charter to be more relevant in contemporary global settings. Key themes are evident throughout this evolution of health promotion that are particularly relevant for how physical activity promotion strategies should be designed and delivered.

A comprehensive approach – Health promotion programmes that include strategies to address all five core action areas are more successful than those implementing a single strategy. Settings, such as cities, local communities, workplaces and schools provide a realistic opportunity to implement this comprehensive approach.

Community empowerment – The people within a setting need to be empowered through involvement in decision making and implementation of strategies. Improving health literacy will also help sustain health promotion effects. Digital technology is a promising mechanism for increasing people's health literacy and control over their health.

Partnerships – Working in partnership is vital to changing the organisational, built and policy environments that are controlled by agencies outside of health. For example, walking path installation is controlled by government planners, and education department policies mandate requirements for physical education in schools.

Social determinants of health – Unequal distribution of power, income and access to services, employment and housing, reduces the chances of poorer people leading a healthy life (WHO Commission on Social Determinants of Health & World Health Organization, 2008). These social determinants of health and the inequity they create should be considered and addressed through health promotion strategies. For physical activity, examples include ensuring supportive environments for physical activity and opportunities for participation in sport are accessible to people on lower incomes (Ball, Carver, Downing, Jackson, & O'Rourke, 2015).

Applying a health promotion framework to physical activity

While many of these health promotion concepts may seem very big picture, they can and have been tangibly applied to physical activity promotion all over the world. The Ottawa Charter provides a framework for a comprehensive mix of physical activity promotion strategies that may be applied in a school, a community or an entire country. When designing physical activity promotion strategies across the five action areas you will need to work in partnership with

Table 21.1   The Ottawa Charter for Health Promotion applied to contemporary physical activity promotion

Action areas of the Ottawa Charter*	Application to physical activity promotion
1. Build Healthy Public Policy	Transport polices that prioritise walking, cycling and public transport Planning policies that ensure equitable access to quality community, recreational and active transport infrastructure Urban design policies that ensure local streets and communities are designed to support walking and cycling Education policies that mandate quality physical education in schools
2. Create Supportive Environments	Built environments that include quality parks, walking and cycling infrastructure, sporting facilities, and walkable communities
3. Strengthen Community Action	Community-wide programmes to facilitate community action for physical activity Community engagement in developing physical activity promotion strategies Community capacity building to deliver physical activity promotion strategies
4. Develop Personal Skills	Mass media led campaigns to deliver physical activity messages Behaviour change programmes in schools, workplaces and community settings Physical activity and health literacy development
5. Reorientate Health Services	Health services prescribe physical activity for prevention of chronic disease Schools, workplaces and other organisations include policies and practices that support and promote physical activity

* Action areas taken from Ottawa Charter for Health Promotion (World Health Organization, 1986).

other sectors, and with your target group to develop and implement the strategies. Also, consider how your strategies address the social determinants of health – are they likely to reduce or increase inequity? Table 21.1 presents the action areas of the Ottawa Charter for Health Promotion and examples of how they can be applied to developing a comprehensive mix of strategies for physical activity promotion at a population level.

Designing interventions for physical activity promotion

Physical activity behaviour is a complex interaction between people and their environment. No single physical activity promotion strategy is likely to result in behaviour change across the entire population. The Ottawa Charter provides an overall framework of what a comprehensive physical activity promotion intervention might look like and is useful for constructing and ordering different strategies. Nonetheless, many practical questions remain. How do you determine whom you should be targeting? What strategies should be selected? And how should you design and implement the strategies? This will depend on who is the focus of your programme, the theoretical approach of your programme, and the specific and measurable changes you hope to see as a result. Some commonly used approaches, theories and physical activity promotion strategies are discussed in the following section.

Focusing on individual, groups and populations

Physical activity promotion strategies can focus on individuals, groups and populations. The emphasis of this chapter is on physical activity promotion at a population level. However, many strategies delivered 'on the ground' focus on individuals or groups, and are often included as part of broad population level programmes.

Individual approaches – Providing information and skills at the individual (one-on-one) level has been used to raise awareness and change attitudes and intentions for a range of health behaviours (Golden & Earp, 2012). For physical activity promotion, strategies delivered through health care providers and targeting those with higher risk of chronic disease are a common and effective individual approach (Sims, Huang, Pietsch, & Naccarella, 2004). One-on-one approaches are not usually the sole focus of health promotion-based physical activity initiatives, as they are not generally cost-effective for the broader community and do not address the environmental barriers to physical activity that people face (Egger, Spark, & Lawson, 1990; Sallis & Glanz, 2006). However, mobile computers, phones and sensors may provide opportunities to personalise educational and behavioural strategies without requiring one-on-one human interaction, reducing costs and enabling uptake by larger numbers of individuals (Direito, Carraça, Rawstorn, Whittaker, & Maddison, 2017; Free et al., 2013). See Box 21.1 for more information on the use of mobile technology for physical activity promotion.

Box 21.1 Mobile technology for physical activity promotion

The application of technology in health is not new. Overwhelmingly, technological advances have led to better health (Free et al., 2013; Montague & Perchonok, 2012). However, electronic media, motorised transport and labour-saving devices have all contributed to reductions in physical activity. How can we better utilise new technologies to help people to change their physical activity behaviours?

Contemporary mobile technologies provide opportunities to convey physical activity messages to large numbers of people and encourage them to interact with our strategies. Text-messaging, smart phone apps and social networking-based interventions have potential for physical activity promotion but have shown only small effects on physical activity, walking and sedentary behaviour (Bort-Roig, Gilson, Puig-Ribera, Contreras, & Trost, 2014; Direito et al., 2017). Recommendations to improve mobile technology interventions include using theory-based behavioural strategies and tailoring messaging for individuals (Direito et al., 2017; Sullivan & Lachman, 2017). Advances in computing, sensors and data analysis will provide better opportunities to personally tailor interventions through real time feedback in future (Lupton, 2013).

The evidence around how best to use mobile technologies for physical activity promotion is growing and technology is likely to feature more prominently in future physical activity promotion strategies.

Group approaches – Group interventions have been used to increase knowledge, build skills, create social networks and support, and change behaviour amongst those who participate, across a range of health behaviours including physical activity (Goldfield, Epstein, Kilanowski, Paluch, & Kogut-Bossler, 2001; Heath et al., 2012). Group-based approaches for physical activity promotion may necessitate forming new groups or be implemented through already established groups (World Health Organization, 2009). Group-based interventions are generally easier to implement and more cost-effective when compared with one-on-one programmes (Heath et al., 2012). They are also conducted in workplaces and community settings as part of broader population physical activity programme (S.M. Matsudo et al., 2003).

Population approaches – Population approaches implement strategies to reach and effect change in large numbers of people thereby producing the best health outcomes for a population. Such interventions are most successful when multiple strategies are used to educate, teach skills, and address the social, physical and policy environmental influences on physical activity and other health behaviours (Centers for Disease Control and Prevention, 2011; Golden & Earp, 2012). Mass media communication to raise awareness and change attitudes in large numbers of people is a cornerstone of population health and physical activity promotion (Bauman & Chau, 2009; Wakefield, Loken, & Hornik, 2010). Environmental and policy strategies to create more supportive evironments, outside of the health sector, are also an important component of population approaches and are required to improve population physical activity levels (Gielen & Green, 2015; Global Advocacy for Physical Activity (GAPA) the Advocacy Council of the International Society for Physical Activity and Health (ISPAH), 2012).

Applying theory to physical activity promotion

Theories underpin best practice health promotion and lead to a greater chance of achieving success (Glanz, Rimer, & Viswanath, 2015). Physical activity promoters apply theories to design physical activity promotion strategies to effect change for individuals, groups and populations. By knowing what is theorised to influence and lead to physical activity behaviour (or not), we can better target and tailor physical activity promotion strategies to address those factors that have most influence. Below is a brief introduction to behavioural theories and models most relevant to physical activity and used in Case Study 1: Community-wide programmes (p. 356), and Case Study 2: Public education including mass media campaigns (p. 358). For further reading see *Health Behaviour: Theory, Research and Practice* (Glanz et al., 2015).

Health promotion has historically relied upon behavioural theories developed in psychology focusing on processes *within the individual*, such as how knowledge, attitudes and intentions lead to changing behaviour (Glanz et al., 2015). Theories that have been used to explain the individual processes that precede physical activity behaviour, and thereby identify opportunities for intervention (King et al., 1992), include the *Health Belief Model* (Rosenstock, 1974), *Theory of Reasoned Action/Theory of Planned Behaviour* (Ajzen & Fishbein, 1980), and *Transtheoretical Model* (TTM) (Prochaska & Velicer, 1997).

Social Cognitive Theory (SCT) (Bandura, 1977) emphasises interactions *between individuals, their environment and health behaviours*, assuming that human behaviour is a result of dynamic relationships between these three elements. The explicit inclusion of the environment (social and physical) as an influence on behaviour makes it particularly relevant for physical activity promotion. SCT includes the concepts: *reciprocal determinism* – the environment influences people who in return influence their environment; *self-efficacy* – the belief an individual has that they can perform a behaviour despite barriers; and *outcome expectancy* – the belief that performing a behaviour will lead to a specific outcome. Interventions developed around SCT include strategies such as encouraging physical activity with friends to increase social support (reciprocal determinism); the use of goal setting and establishment of rewards (outcome expectations); and building confidence and behavioural skills, such as planning ahead, to perform physical activity despite potential barriers (self-efficacy).

Ecological Models have been embraced by contemporary physical activity promotion (Sallis, Floyd, Rodriguez, & Saelens, 2012; Stokols, 1996). Comprehensive ecological approaches to physical activity promotion consider both the individual and the environments in which physical activity is performed (Sallis et al., 2006). A simple ecological model showing the levels of influence on physical activity behaviour is displayed in Figure 21.1. Ecological models shape the selection of strategies by identifying the multiple levels that impact on a physical activity behaviour. Interventions that include strategies to address these multiple levels of the ecological model - individual, and social, organisational, physical and policy environments – and target a specific physical activity behaviour (e.g., walking for recreation, cycling for transport), are the more likely to be effective in the short- and long-term than those that do not (Golden & Earp, 2012; Sallis, Owen, & Fisher, 2008).

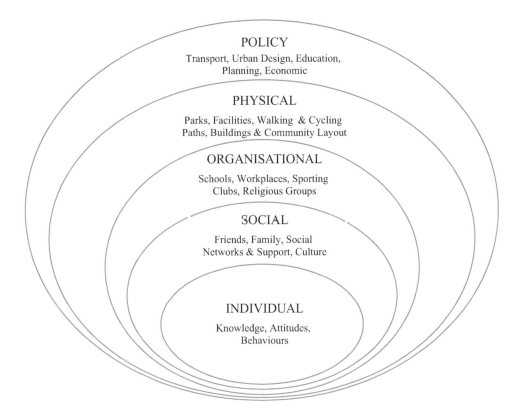

Figure 21.1 A simple ecological model for conceptualising individual and environmental influences on physical activity behaviour

Adapted from Sallis et al., 2012

Selecting strategies for physical activity promotion

In practice, physical activity practitioners employ a range of theoretically-based educational, behavioural and environmental strategies to target populations, groups and individuals within an overall framework such as the Ottawa Charter (Table 21.1) or ecological model (Figure 21.1).

Strategies to change individual knowledge and attitudes

Educational strategies aim to change knowledge, beliefs and attitudes – the personal factors that are theorised to precede changes in physical activity. Educational strategies were the foundation of early health promotion efforts and they remain a core component of physical activity promotion today (Egger et al., 1990; Golden & Earp, 2012). Mass media on television and other media channels is the most prominent educational strategy employed to reach whole populations with physical activity messages. However, mass media and other educational strategies, such as informational lectures, brochures, posters and websites implemented on their own do not usually change physical activity behaviour over the longer term as they require complementary environmental strategies and community-based programmes to be effective (Brown et al., 2012; World Health Organization, 2009b). A detailed summary of the strategies, effectiveness and recommendations for interventions that utilise mass media as part of broader physical activity promotion is contained in Case Study 1: Community-wide programmes (p. 356), and Case Study 2: Public education including mass media campaigns (p. 358).

Strategies to change individual behavioural skills

Behavioural strategies aim to develop the personal behavioural skills necessary for adopting and maintaining physical activity. Strategies are usually delivered using an individual or group approach, such as delivering counselling or group-based instruction, but also can be promoted through mass media communications. Behavioural interventions are often based on SCT, so they typically include behavioural skills such as setting physical activity goals, building social support for physical activity and reinforcing behaviour with rewards (Kahn et al., 2002). Behavioural strategies have been successful in changing physical activity behaviour as part of workplace interventions, and within community group-based physical activity programmes, in the short and medium term (Murray et al., 2017; World Health Organization, 2009b). Also, behavioural strategies targeting people with chronic disease risk and incorporated into primary health care have successfully increased physical activity, although the longer term effects are less certain (Sims et al., 2004; World Health Organization, 2009). More recently, using mobile health technologies, such as phones, health trackers and computer tablets, to deliver behavioural strategies has resulted in small increases in physical activity and walking in randomised control trials (Direito et al., 2017). The most effective behavioural strategies are theory-based, delivered with educational strategies, and tailored to an individual's readiness, interests and lifestyle (Centers for Disease Control and Prevention, 2011; World Health Organization, 2009b).

Strategies to change the social environment

Social environmental strategies aim to create and utilise social networks to facilitate physical activity behaviour and environmental change. Group-based social support interventions, such as walking groups, that involve building and maintaining social networks to support people's participation in physical activity have typically been effective in increasing physical activity for participants (Kahn et al., 2002). Furthermore, this approach has specifically shown moderate effectiveness in increasing physical activity for older adults within a social structure already in place (e.g., a religious group) (World Health Organization, 2009). Community-wide and mass media led campaigns can also effect changes in the social environment at a population level by shifting social attitudes towards physical activity, and mobilising communities to bring about environmental change needed to facilitate physical activity (Centers for Disease Control and Prevention, 2011; S.M. Matsudo et al., 2003).

Strategies to change the organisational, physical and public policy environments

Environmental strategies aim to change the structure of organisational, physical and public policy environments to provide places and systems that support participation in physical activity. Implementing these strategies requires not only physical activity and health professionals, but multiple government and community organisations in sectors such as transport, planning and education. Strategies to improve environments also have the capacity to reduce disparities in physical activity and health when implemented equitably so that those with the greatest need receive the benefits (Lieberman, Golden, & Earp, 2013).

Organisational strategies are directed at organisations to implement health-promoting policies, practices and programmes in the settings they control (Kok, Gurabardhi, Gottlieb, & Zijlstra, 2015). They allow physical activity promoters to reach and influence people through existing organisational structures where they spend their time, and are therefore likely to produce more sustainable effects (Swerissen & Crisp, 2004). Multi-level physical activity interventions targeting school settings have been effective in increasing children's physical activity (Kriemler et al., 2011; World Health Organization, 2009b). Effective interventions in schools include a combination of physical education delivered by skilled teachers, targeting families to support physical activity, providing opportunities for children to participate in physical activity programmes, and changing the local school physical and policy environment to support walking, cycling and outdoor play. Effective organisational strategies targeting workplaces involve workers in the strategy design, deliver behaviour change programmes, and provide and promote opportunities to be active (World Health Organization, 2009b). However, results of physical activity promotion in workplace settings are inconsistent to date, as many interventions are weighted towards educational and behavioural strategies and do not address organisational policies and practices (Malik, Blake, & Suggs, 2014).

Physical environmental strategies aim to change the structure of physical environments to be more supportive of physical activity participation. The built environment includes elements designed by humans such as buildings, transport infrastructure, parks and community layouts that can either act as a barrier to or be conducive for a range of physical activities. Multiple factors within the built environment have been associated with increased physical activity, including access and proximity to recreational facilities, green spaces and walking paths (Sallis et al., 2012). Additionally, having a variety of destinations nearby to walk to and safe footpaths are associated with increased walking for transport. A review of studies that either created new or improved access to places, such as recreation facilities and walking paths, found a median 25% increase in the proportion of people physically active at least three times a week (Centers for Disease Control and Prevention, 2011). Built environment and public policy strategies are often considered together as healthier public policy in transport and planning can result in improvements in the built environment. To improve the effectiveness of physical environmental strategies it is recommended they are complemented by educational strategies to promote the use of environments (Centers for Disease Control and Prevention, 2011; Sallis et al., 2012).

Policy environmental strategies typically target government organisations to change public policy, including economic, legislative, organisational and planning policy, so that physical activity becomes the easier choice. Public policy change is often the pinnacle of population health promotion, as evidence shows these strategies can result in sustained built and organisational environmental change, as well as changes in attitudes and behaviour (Gielen & Green, 2015). Recommended policy interventions to increase population level physical activity include urban planning and design policy (community and street level), to improve availability and access to parks and other recreational spaces, and to provide connected street networks to facilitate walking. Transport planning policies that prioritise walking, cycling and public transport, including the provision of walking and cycling paths, are also recommended (Centers for Disease Control and Prevention, 2011; Global Advocacy for Physical Activity (GAPA) the Advocacy Council of the International Society for Physical Activity and Health (ISPAH), 2012).

Case Study 1: Community-wide programmes

Strategies: Community-wide programmes integrate multiple strategies across a region, city or local community. This approach is also applied to settings that could be considered a community such as a school, workplace, or university (Centers for Disease Control and Prevention, 2011). Community-wide programmes are typically branded with a primary promotional health message that links all strategies together. The most common strategies of communitywide programmes are: 1) *Public education* delivered through mass media, and individual and group programmes, to change knowledge and attitudes; 2) *Programmes and initiatives* that include individual, group or population engagement to educate, motivate and provide opportunities for physical activity participation; facilitate social networks; and generate community support and action for physical activity and environmental change; 3) *Policy and environmental strategies* focusing on organisations to prioritise physical activity in their planning and government legislation, and create environmental change that provides places for physical activity (Global Advocacy for Physical Activity (GAPA) the Advocacy Council of the International Society for Physical Activity and Health (ISPAH), 2012).

Effectiveness: Community-wide programmes that involve multiple sectors and settings will generally be more effective in increasing population physical activity than any single focus or strategy (Global Advocacy for Physical Activity (GAPA) the Advocacy Council of the International Society for Physical Activity and Health (ISPAH), 2012). Community-wide approaches are based on the ecological model to target multiple levels of influence (individual and environmental) on physical activity to reduce barriers and promote participation (Centers for Disease Control and Prevention, 2011; Mummery & Brown, 2009). A review of community-wide programmes found a median 4% increase in the proportion of people participating in physical activity in the target communities, across a diverse range of settings and populations of varying income (Kahn et al., 2002). Further evaluation of the strategies implemented through community-wide programmes has been recommended to improve effectiveness (Mummery & Brown, 2009).

Recommendations to enhance success

- Formative evaluation with the community is vital to develop effective messages;
- The overarching brand needs to be recognisable to link programme strategies together;
- Target communities need to be a part of the planning, delivery and evaluation to strengthen their capacity for action to support physical activity;
- Partnerships across multiple sectors (e.g., health, transport, planning, sport and recreation, education) are required to implement the range of strategies; and
- A sustained high level of resources is required to ensure the whole community receives an adequate dose of strategies over a long enough period to effect change.

(Centers for Disease Control and Prevention, 2011; Global Advocacy for Physical Activity (GAPA) the Advocacy Council of the International Society for Physical Activity and Health (ISPAH), 2012; Mummery & Brown, 2009).

An example: *Agita São Paulo*

Introduction: Agita São Paulo is one of the most documented and effective community-wide programmes for physical activity promotion in the world. Commencing 1996 in Brazil, it has formed the basis of similar programmes in developing countries (S.M. Matsudo et al., 2003).

Objectives and target group: The programme aimed to increase knowledge of the benefits and participation in moderate physical activity in residents of São Paulo, Brazil. The programme primarily targeted students, workers and seniors (V. Matsudo et al., 2002).

Theory: Agita São Paulo is a multi-level community-wide intervention based on an ecological model (V. Matsudo et al., 2002). Multiple behavioural theories, including the Trans-theoretical Model (TTM) and Social Cognitive Theory (SCT), were used to underpin the development of programme strategies. The TTM model was used to segment the target audiences into sub-groups to apply relevant strategies to support each group according to their readiness to change.

Strategies: The term 'Agita' means to move or agitate, and is a clear and simple message for promoting physical activity. Agita is also a 'call to action', meaning the message itself communicates the desired behavioural action. The programme included mega-events such as 'Active Community Day', media and publicity, and educational materials to increase knowledge of the benefits of physical activity. Through partnerships with local organisations, *Agita São Paulo* incorporated individual and group educational and behavioural strategies delivered through primary health care providers and trained exercise professionals, into its overall population approach. Events provided opportunities for participation and to enhance community action and support for physical activity. The campaign focused on partnership development across diverse sectors to amplify programme reach and delivery, and implement environmental strategies. For example, partnerships with transport authorities delivered educational strategies to sedentary transport drivers, while partnerships with government agencies facilitated changes in the built environment, such as additional walking paths (V. Matsudo, 2012).

Evaluation and results: Evaluation included population level surveys and measurement of changes in physical activity in individuals attending programmes. A face-to-face campaign evaluation survey with 645 São Paulo residents in 2002 showed 57.7% of people were aware of *Agita*. For those who were aware, meeting physical activity guidelines was higher, although not significantly (V. Matsudo et al., 2002). Evaluation of individual and group programmes found positive changes in self-reported physical activity by people with a chronic disease, and for people participating in community, school and workplace-based group interventions (S.M. Matsudo et al., 2003). Cross-sectional surveys of over 2,000 adults found the proportion of people in São Paulo not meeting physical activity guidelines significantly decreased from 44% in 2002 to 12% in 2008 due to increases in walking and other moderate-intensity physical activity (V. Matsudo et al., 2010). However, it is difficult to know how much of this change was attributable to the *Agita São Paulo* programme.

Lessons learned: Success has been attributed to several factors including: 1) An ecological multi-sectoral approach; 2) A broad range of partnerships to deliver educational messages, behavioural programmes, and social and environmental change; 3) Clear and achievable messaging for everyone, but culturally adapted to the local level; and 4) The use of evidence and theory to inform the programme. There is now a global *Agita Mundo* network that focuses on social mobilisation to promote physical activity and motivate people to call for change to support physical activity (V.K.R. Matsudo & Lambert, 2017).

Case Study 2: Public education including mass media campaigns

Strategies: Mass media led public education campaigns are an effective way to reach large segments of the population with physical activity messages (Bauman & Chau, 2009). Campaigns commonly use paid mass media channels such as television, radio, print and online and social media. Other channels for promotion include outdoor billboards, signage on public transport and promotion at large community events. Free media coverage is usually generated by public relations activities including media releases, high-profile spokespeople and events, and through partnerships with media and other agencies. Educational strategies such as informational websites, brochures and posters deliver campaign messages at an individual, group and community level.

Effectiveness: Mass media campaigns have been used successfully to raise awareness, increase knowledge, motivate people to take action and change social and community attitudes in relation to a range of health risk behaviours including physical activity (Wakefield et al., 2010). However, physical activity mass media campaigns have shown inconsistent results overall, with awareness of campaign messages ranging from 17% to 95% and less than half of campaigns increasing physical activity behaviours (Leavy, Bull, Rosenberg, & Bauman, 2011). Inconsistencies are likely due to differences in campaign target groups, the design and implementation of the campaigns, and the physical activity outcomes measured (Bauman & Chau, 2009; Leavy et al., 2011; Yun, Ori, Younghan, Sivak, & Berry, 2017). To change physical activity behaviour, mass media strategies are best employed alongside environmental and community-based strategies that educate, build skills and reduce barriers to physical activity, rather than as a stand-alone strategy (Brown et al., 2012). Most physical activity mass media campaigns have been conducted in higher income countries (Abioye, Hajifathalian, & Danaei, 2013; Leavy et al., 2011).

Recommendations to enhance success

- Use theory and formative research with the target group to inform the campaign content;
- Deliver mass media educational strategies as part of a comprehensive health promotion approach including community programmes and policy and environmental strategies, if the goal is physical activity behaviour change;

- Campaigns need to be adequately resourced and sustained over a long period of time to ensure results are not short term; and
- More rigorous evaluation is required to better understand how physical activity mass media campaigns work best.

(Abioye et al., 2013; Bauman & Chau, 2009; Brown et al., 2012; Leavy et al., 2011; Wakefield et al., 2010).

An example: The Find Thirty® every day campaign

Introduction: The *Find Thirty® every day* campaign is an example of a mass media led physical activity campaign.

Objectives and target group: Campaign objectives were to increase the awareness, knowledge and physical activity of adults in Western Australia (WA), particularly those in priority populations who participated in less physical activity than recommended, including women, people from regional and rural locations, and people living in lower socioeconomic areas (Leavy et al., 2013).

Theory: The first WA physical activity campaign, *Find Thirty®*, promoted the duration component of the Australian physical guidelines for adults – *30 minutes* of physical activity on five or more days a week (Department of Health and Aged Care, 1999). The tagline, *It's Not a Big Exercise*, aimed to improve self-efficacy, a key concept in SCT, by communicating there are many easy ways to be physically active. In 2007, the campaign was recommissioned with new media advertising and a new tagline – *Find Thirty® every day*. The *every day* tagline was based on research that showed people were not doing enough *sessions* of physical activity each week. This new advertising was also built around SCT by promoting physical activity participation with others (social support) and the benefits of physical activity (outcome expectancies). People from priority populations informed and reviewed the mass media advertising prior to campaign launch.

Strategies: Television, radio, print and outdoor advertising, along with a website, informational materials, and community and workplace activities were implemented as part of the campaign. Figure 21.2 shows the strategy mix weighted towards mass media.

Evaluation and results: A random sample of over 900 WA adults completed a telephone survey on three occasions. Awareness of the *Find Thirty® every day* campaign increased from 30% before the launch of the new media to 49% two years later, and was higher in women and adults of lower socioeconomic status (Leavy et al., 2013). Intention to do something related to the *Find Thirty® every day* message doubled from baseline to 21%. There were positive significant increases in self-reported physical activity one year later ($p < 0.05$) for walking (30 minutes), vigorous activity (20 minutes) and total physical activity (50 minutes). However, two years later only the significant increase in walking remained. Results are limited as there was no comparison group in the research design.

Lessons learned: Despite promising results, the campaign's strategies were not enough to sustain improvements in WA population physical activity. While there were many physical activity initiatives including environmental strategies and behavioural programmes happening in WA at the time, the *Find Thirty® every day* brand was not linked to these. Changes in campaign messaging and uncertainty of future funding were challenges for developing productive long-term partnerships with health agencies and other sectors. The mass media educational strategies could have been better integrated with behavioural and environmental strategies to support long-term increases in population physical activity.

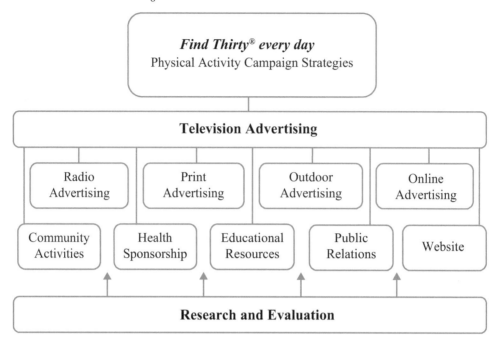

Figure 21.2   Find Thirty® every day physical activity campaign strategy mix

A global consensus on what works in physical activity promotion

Taking a global lens to the future of physical activity promotion, there is good evidence to support the use of a range of strategies to promote physical activity on a worldwide scale. The World Health Organization and Global Advocacy for Physical Activity (GAPA) (the Advocacy Council of the International Society for Physical Activity and Health), have played key roles in gathering and assessing the evidence on strategies for physical activity promotion and advocating for their implementation at a global level. WHO's *Interventions on Diet and Physical Activity: What Works Summary Report* (World Health Organization, 2009b) summarises interventions for promoting physical activity in a range of settings that have been rigorously evaluated and demonstrated effectiveness as determined by: a strong research design; achieving changes in physical activity knowledge, attitudes and/or behaviour; and applicability to other settings, especially in middle and low-income countries. Many of these intervention strategies have been outlined in this chapter.

The Toronto Charter for Physical Activity: A Global Call to Action was developed to help mobilise physical activity practitioners across the world to advocate for health enhancing physical activity in their own countries and settings (Global Advocacy Council for Physical Activity International Society for Physical Activity and Health, 2010). Developed in consultation with participants from 55 countries and drawing upon a health promotion approach, The Toronto Charter establishes guiding principles and country level action areas for physical activity promotion at a population level (Bull, 2011). It also outlines the health benefits and contribution to sustainable development and the economy of investing in policy and programmes that promote physical activity.

NCD (Non-Communicable Disease) Prevention: Investments that Work for Physical Activity is a companion document to the Toronto Charter (Global Advocacy for Physical Activity (GAPA) the Advocacy Council of the International Society for Physical Activity and Health (ISPAH), 2012) that provides seven specific strategies considered the best investments that have global applicability to increase population physical activity. Table 21.2 outlines the best investments and aligns them with their

Table 21.2 Investments for increasing population physical activity aligned to focus and strategies

Investment area*	Focus	Strategies
1 'Whole-of-school' programmes	Population focus with group focused programmes in a school setting	Comprehensive strategy mix including education, behavioural and participation programmes, and organisational, built and policy environmental strategies
2 Transport policies and systems that prioritise walking, cycling and public transport	Population focus in a broad community setting	Policy strategies with education to encourage active transport
3 Urban design regulations and infrastructure that provide for equitable and safe access for recreational physical activity, and recreational and transport-related walking and cycling across the life course	Population focus in a broad community setting	Built environmental and policy strategies
4 Physical activity and NCD prevention integrated into primary health care systems	Individual and group focus in primary health care setting	Behavioural strategies, with education
5 Public education, including mass media campaigns to raise awareness and change social norms on physical activity	Population focus in a broad community setting	Educational strategies, with social environmental strategies
6 Community-wide programmes involving multiple settings and sectors and that mobilise and integrate community engagement and resources	Population focus in a broad or local community setting	Comprehensive strategy mix including education via mass media, behavioural and participation programmes, and organisational, built and policy environmental strategies
7 Sports systems and programmes that promote 'sport for all' and encourage participation across the life span	Population focus with group focused programmes in a sports setting	Policy strategies, with education, participation and skill-building programmes, and organisational strategies

* Investments taken from *NCD Prevention: Investments that Work for Physical Activity* (Global Advocacy for Physical Activity (GAPA) the Advocacy Council of the International Society for Physical Activity and Health (ISPAH), 2012).

focus and the types of strategies that are utilised by each. Some concentrate more strongly on one category of strategy, such as educational (e.g., mass media campaigns) or environmental (e.g., changing the built environment to support walking), but several include multiple strategies. Together the investments and their strategies provide a comprehensive ecological approach to global physical activity promotion by targeting multiple levels to effect change. Still, to increase the chances of success at the country, city or community level it is important to adapt the strategies to the local context, use existing social groupings, and involve the community or other participants, as well as policy makers, in developing and implementing the strategies for physical activity promotion (World Health Organization, 2009b).

Chapter summary

The study of physical activity behaviour and the fields of health and physical activity promotion are still evolving. Despite much evidence on what strategies are more or less likely to be effective, challenges to changing physical activity behaviour in populations remain. Contemporary physical activity promotion still draws heavily on the Ottawa Charter framework, ecological models and behavioural theories. They help to design and implement multi-strategy interventions that address both the individual and the broader environment in which people live, and are more likely to succeed. This chapter has highlighted the frameworks and theories that can be applied when designing a physical activity intervention and selecting strategies, as well as providing examples of the types of physical activity promotion strategies for which there is evidence of effectiveness, with a focus on physical activity campaigns including mass media. It has also provided a global view of the strategies that can increase population levels of physical activity, reduce the burden of chronic disease and improve well-being through healthier environments, if implemented sufficiently. As such the chapter is a useful overview for those who are designing and implementing physical activity promotional strategies to increase population physical activity.

- Population level physical activity promotion strategies are based upon the Ottawa Charter framework, ecological models and behavioural theories.
- Effective physical activity promotion generally includes a comprehensive mix of strategies to target multiple levels of influence on physical activity behaviour.
- Physical activity promotion strategies can be broadly categorised as influencing the individual (educational and behavioural) or the environment (social, organisational, physical and policy) although there is interaction between all the levels of influence.
- Community-wide programmes that integrate multiple strategies including mass media under an overarching physical activity message, are recommended to increase physical activity in a range of communities.
- Stand-alone mass media campaigns can increase knowledge and influence social attitudes around physical activity but are less likely to result in sustained physical activity behaviour change without associated environmental strategies.
- There is good evidence of effectiveness to support investment in the seven broad approaches to physical activity promotion outlined in '*NCD Prevention: Investments that Work for Physical Activity*, to increase physical activity globally (Global Advocacy for Physical Activity (GAPA) the Advocacy Council of the International Society for Physical Activity and Health (ISPAH), 2012).

References

Abioye, A.I., Hajifathalian, K., & Danaei, G. (2013). Do mass media campaigns improve physical activity? A systematic review and meta-analysis. *Archives of Public Health, 71*(1), 20. doi:https://doi.org/10.1186/0778-7367-71-20

Ajzen, I., & Fishbein, M. (1980). *Understanding attitudes and predicting social behaviour.* New Jersey: Prentice-Hall.

Ball, K., Carver, A., Downing, K., Jackson, M., & O'Rourke, K. (2015). Addressing the social determinants of inequities in physical activity and sedentary behaviours. *Health Promotion International, 30*(s2), ii8-ii19. doi:https://doi.org/10.1093/heapro/dav022

Bandura, A. (1977). Self-efficacy: Toward a unifying theory of behavioral change. *Psychological Review, 84*(2), 191. doi:http://dx.doi.org/10.1037/0033-295X.84.2.191

Bauman, A., & Chau, J. (2009). The role of media in promoting physical activity. *Journal of Physical Activity and Health, 6*(s2), S196–210. doi:https://doi.org/10.1123/jpah.6.s2.s196

Bort-Roig, J., Gilson, N.D., Puig-Ribera, A., Contreras, R.S. & Trost, S.G. (2014). Measuring and influencing physical activity with smartphone technology: A systematic review. *Sports Medicine., 44*(5), 671–686. doi: 10.1007/s40279-014-0142-5

Brown, D.R., Soares, J., Epping, J.M., Lankford, T.J., Wallace, J.S., Hopkins, D., . . . Orleans, C.T. (2012). Stand-alone mass media campaigns to increase physical activity: A community guide updated review. *American Journal of Preventive Medicine, 43*(5), 551–561. doi:https://doi.org/10.1016/j.amepre.2012.07.035

Bull, F.C. (2011). Global advocacy for physical activity-development and progress of the Toronto Charter for Physical Activity: A Global Call for Action. *Research in Exercise Epidemiology, 13*(1), 1–10.

Centers for Disease Control and Prevention. (2011). *Strategies to prevent obesity and other chronic diseases: The CDC guide to strategies to increase physical activity in the community.* Atlanta: U.S. Department of Health and Human Services.

Department of Health and Aged Care. (1999). *National physical activity guidelines for adults.* Canberra: Australian Government.

Direito, A., Carraça, E., Rawstorn, J., Whittaker, R., & Maddison, R. (2017). Mhealth technologies to influence physical activity and sedentary behaviors: Behavior change techniques, systematic review and meta-analysis of randomized controlled trials. *Annals of Behavioral Medicine, 51*(2), 226–239. doi:https://doi.org/10.1007/s12160-016-9846-0

Egger, G., Spark, R., & Lawson, L. (1990). *Health promotion strategies & methods.* Sydney: McGraw-Hill.

Free, C., Phillips, G., Galli, L., Watson, L., Felix, L., Edwards, P., . . . Haines, A. (2013). The effectiveness of mobile-health technology-based health behaviour change or disease management interventions for health care consumers: A systematic review. *PLoS Medicine, 10*(1), e1001362. doi:https://doi.org/10.1371/journal.pmed.1001362

Gielen, A.C., & Green, L.W. (2015). The impact of policy, environmental, and educational interventions: A synthesis of the evidence from two public health success stories. *Health Education and Behavior, 42*(s1), 20S–34S. doi:https://doi.org/10.1177/1090198115570049

Giles-Corti, B., Foster, S., Shilton, T., & Falconer, R. (2010). The co-benefits for health of investing in active transportation. *New South Wales Public Health Bulletin, 21*(6), 122–127. doi:http://dx.doi.org/10.1071/NB10027

Glanz, K., Rimer, B.K., & Viswanath, K. (Eds.). (2015). *Health behaviour: Theory, research and practice* (5th ed.). San Fransisco: Jossey-Bass.

Global Advocacy Council for Physical Activity International Society for Physical Activity and Health. (2010). *The Toronto Charter for Physical Activity: A Global Call to Action.* Retrieved from www.globalpa.org.uk/pdf/torontocharter-eng-20may2010.pdf.

Global Advocacy for Physical Activity (GAPA) the Advocacy Council of the International Society for Physical Activity and Health (ISPAH). (2012). NCD prevention: Investments that work for physical activity. *British Journal of Sports Medicine, 46*(10), 709–712. doi:http://dx.doi.org/10.1136/bjsm.2012.091485

Golden, S.D., & Earp, J.A.L. (2012). Social ecological approaches to individuals and their contexts: Twenty years of health education & behavior health promotion interventions. *Health Education and Behavior, 39*(3), 364–372. doi:https://doi.org/10.1177/1090198111418634

Goldfield, G., Epstein, L., Kilanowski, C., Paluch, R., & Kogut-Bossler, B. (2001). Cost-effectiveness of group and mixed family-based treatment for childhood obesity. *International Journal of Obesity, 25*(12), 1843. doi:https://doi.org/10.1038/sj.ijo.0801838

Heath, G.W., Parra, D.C., Sarmiento, O.L., Andersen, L.B., Owen, N., Goenka, S., . . . Brownson, R.C. (2012). Evidence-based intervention in physical activity: Lessons from around the world. *Lancet, 380*, 272–281. doi:http://dx.doi.org/10.1016/S0140-6736(12)60816-2

Janssen, I., & LeBlanc, A. (2010). Systematic review of the health benefits of physical activity and fitness in school-aged children and youth. *International Journal of Behavioral Nutrition and Physical Activity, 7*(1), 40. doi:https://doi.org/10.1186/1479-5868-7-40

Kahn, E.B., Ramsey, L.T., Brownson, R.C., Heath, G.W., Howze, E.H., Powell, K.E., . . . Briss, P.A. (2002). The effectiveness of interventions to increase physical activity: A systematic review. *American Journal of Preventive Medicine, 22*(4), 73–108. doi:http://dx.doi.org/10.1016/S0749-3797(02)00434-8

King, A.C., Blair, S.N., Bild, D.E., Dishman, R.K., Dubbert, P.M., Marcus, B.H., . . . Yeager, K.K. (1992). Determinants of physical activity and interventions in adults. *Medicine and Science in Sports and Exercise, 24*(s6), S221–S236. doi:http://dx.doi.org/10.1249/00005768-199206001-00005

Kok, G., Gurabardhi, Z., Gottlieb, N.H., & Zijlstra, F.R.H. (2015). Influencing organizations to promote health. *Health Education and Behavior, 42*(s1), 123S–132S. doi:https://doi.org/10.1177/1090198115571363

Kriemler, S., Meyer, U., Martin, E., van Sluijs, E.M., Andersen, L.B., & Martin, B.W. (2011). Effect of school-based interventions on physical activity and fitness in children and adolescents: A review of reviews and systematic update. *British Journal of Sports Medicine, 45*(11), 923–930. doi:https://doi.org/10.1177/1090198115571363

Leavy, J.E., Bull, F.C., Rosenberg, M., & Bauman, A. (2011). Physical activity mass media campaigns and their evaluation: A systematic review of the literature 2003–2010. *Health Education Research, 26*(6), 1060–1085. doi:https://doi.org/10.1093/her/cyr069

Leavy, J.E., Rosenberg, M., Bauman, A.E., Bull, F.C., Giles-Corti, B., Shilton, T., . . . Barnes, R. (2013). Effects of Find Thirty every day®: Cross-sectional findings from a Western Australian population-wide mass media campaign, 2008–2010. *Health Education and Behavior, 40*(4), 480–492. doi:https://doi.org/10.1177/1090198112459515

Lieberman, L., Golden, S.D., & Earp, J.A.L. (2013). Structural approaches to health promotion: What do we need to know about policy and environmental change? *Health Education and Behavior, 40*(5), 520–525. doi:https://doi.org/10.1177/1090198113503342

Lupton, D. (2013). Quantifying the body: Monitoring and measuring health in the age of mHealth technologies. *Critical Public Health, 23*(4), 393–403. doi:https://doi.org/10.1080/09581596.2013.794931

Malik, S.H., Blake, H., & Suggs, L.S. (2014). A systematic review of workplace health promotion interventions for increasing physical activity. *British Journal of Health Psychology, 19*(1), 149–180. doi:https://doi.org/10.1111/bjhp.12052

Matsudo, S.M., Matsudo, V.R., Araujo, T.L., Andrade, D.R., Andrade, E.L., de Oliveira, L.C., & Braggion, G.F. (2003). The Agita São Paulo Program as a model for using physical activity to promote health. *Revista Panamericana de Salud Publica, 14*(4), 265–272.

Matsudo, V. (2012). The role of partnerships in promoting physical activity: The experience of Agita São Paulo. *Health and Place, 18*(1), 121–122. doi:http://dx.doi.org/10.1016/j.healthplace.2011.09.011

Matsudo, V., Matsudo, S., Andrade, D., Araujo, T., Andrade, E., de Oliveira, L.C., & Braggion, G. (2002). Promotion of physical activity in a developing country: The Agita São Paulo experience. *Public Health Nutrition, 5*(1a), 253–261. doi:https://doi.org/10.1079/PHN2001301

Matsudo, V., Matsudo, S.M., Araújo, T.L., Andrade, D.R., de Oliveira, L.C., & Hallal, P.C. (2010). Time trends in physical activity in the state of São Paulo, Brazil: 2002–2008. *Medicine and Science in Sports and Exercise, 42*(12), 2231–2236. doi:https://doi.org/10.1249/MSS.0b013e3181e1fe8e

Matsudo, V.K.R., & Lambert, E.V. (2017). Bright spots, physical activity investments that work: Agita Mundo global network. *British Journal of Sports Medicine.* doi:10.1136/bjsports-2016–097291

Montague, E., & Perchonok, J. (2012). Health and wellness technology use by historically underserved health consumers: Systematic review. *Journal of Medical Internet Research. 31*, 14(3):e78. doi: 10.2196/jmir.2095

Mummery, W.K., & Brown, W.J. (2009). Whole of community physical activity interventions: Easier said than done. *British Journal of Sports Medicine, 43*(1), 39–43. doi:http://dx.doi.org/10.1136/bjsm.2008.053629

Murray, J.M., Brennan, S.F., French, D.P., Patterson, C.C., Kee, F., & Hunter, R.F. (2017). Effectiveness of physical activity interventions in achieving behaviour change maintenance in young and middle aged adults: A systematic review and meta-analysis. *Social Science and Medicine, 192*, 125–133. doi:https://doi.org/10.1016/j.socscimed.2017.09.021

Prochaska, J.O., & Velicer, W.F. (1997). The transtheoretical model of health behavior change. *American Journal of Health Promotion, 12*(1), 38–48. doi:https://doi.org/10.4278/0890-1171-12.1.38

Rosenstock, I.M. (1974). Historical origins of the Health Belief Model. *Health Education Monographs, 2*(4), 328–335. doi:https://doi.org/10.1177/109019817400200403

Sallis, J.F., Cervero, R.B., Ascher, W., Henderson, K.A., Kraft, M.K., & Kerr, J. (2006). An ecological approach to creating active living communities. *Annual Review of Public Health, 27*, 297–322. doi:https://doi.org/10.1146/annurev.publhealth.27.021405.102100

Sallis, J.F., Floyd, M.F., Rodriguez, D.A., & Saelens, B.E. (2012). Role of built environments in physical activity, obesity, and cardiovascular disease. *Circulation, 125*(5), 729–737. doi:https://doi.org/10.1161/CIRCULATIONAHA.110.969022

Sallis, J.F., & Glanz, K. (2006). The role of built environments in physical activity, eating, and obesity in childhood. *The Future of Children*, 89–108.

Sallis, J.F., Owen, N., & Fisher, E.B. (2008). Ecological models of health behaviour. In K. Glanz, B.K. Rimer, & K. Viswanath (Eds.), *Health behaviour and health education: Theory, research and practice* (4th ed.) (pp. 465–485). San Francisco: Jossey-Bass.

Sims, J., Huang, N., Pietsch, J., & Naccarella, L. (2004). The Victorian Active Script Programme: Promising signs for general practitioners, population health, and the promotion of physical activity. *British Journal of Sports Medicine, 38*(1), 19–25. doi:https://dx.doi.org/10.1136%2Fbjsm.2003.001297corr1

Stokols, D. (1996). Translating social ecological theory into guidelines for community health promotion. *American Journal of Health Promotion, 10*(4), 282–298. doi:https://doi.org/10.4278/0890-1171-10.4.282

Sullivan, A.N., & Lachman, M.E. (2017). Behavior change with fitness technology in sedentary adults: A review of the evidence for increasing physical activity. *Frontiers in Public Health, 4*, 289. doi: 10.3389/fpubh.2016.00289

Swerissen, H., & Crisp, B.R. (2004). The sustainability of health promotion interventions for different levels of social organization. *Health Promotion International, 19*(1), 123–130. doi:https://doi.org/10.3389/fpubh.2016.00289

Wakefield, M.A., Loken, B., & Hornik, R.C. (2010). Use of mass media campaigns to change health behaviour. *Lancet, 376*(9748), 1261–1271. doi:http://dx.doi.org/10.1016/S0140-6736(10)60809-4

CSDH. (2008). *Closing the gap in a generation: Health equity through action on the social determinants of health. Final Report of the Commission on Social Determinants of Health. Geneva.* World Health Organization.

World Health Organization. (1986). *The Ottawa Charter for Health Promotion.* Retrieved from www.who.int/healthpromotion/conferences/previous/ottawa/en/index.html.

World Health Organization. (1998). *Health promotion glossary*. Retrieved from www.who.int/entity/healthpromotion/about/HPR%20Glossary%201998.pdf?ua=1

World Health Organization. (2009a). *Global health risks: Mortality and burden of disease attributable to selected major risks*. Retrieved from www.who.int/healthinfo/global_burden_disease/GlobalHealth Risks_report_full.pdf

World Health Organization. (2009b). *Interventions on diet and physical activity:What works summary report*. Geneva:World Health Organization.

Yun, L., Ori, E.M.,Younghan, L., Sivak, A., & Berry,T.R. (2017). A systematic review of community-wide media physical activity campaigns: An update from 2010. *Journal of Physical Activity and Health, 14*(7), 552–570. doi:https://doi.org/10.1123/jpah.2016-0616

22 School physical education and physical activity

Gareth Stratton and Nick Draper

Keywords: Physical education, health related exercise, physical literacy, physical competency, academic achievement, teaching approaches, physical fitness, technology

Introduction

For thousands of years the rational and intuitive relationship between education, *physical activity* and health has pervaded the scripts of philosophers. Moreover, *health related physical activity* is not a new concept, Nelson Mandela, stated that '*exercise was the key to physical health and peace of mind,*' Hippocrates said that individuals who '*receive the right balance of nourishment and exercise follow the safest route to good health*' and John F. Kennedy was quoted as saying that '*physical fitness is not only the most important key to a healthy body, it is the basis of dynamic and creative intellectual activity*'. Plato perhaps made the best link between physical activity and education when he proffered that '*God provided man with two means, education and physical activity. Not separately, one for the soul and the other for the body, but for the two together. With these two means man can attain perfection.*'

Epistemologically health has always had an association with physical activity, exercise, fitness and by extension physical education. In a historiography of health and fitness the aim of physical education at the turn of the 20th century was to promote *physical fitness* through military drill, in a 'make our soldiers fit for war' paradigm (Williams, 1988). Teaching the population how to keep fit was core to a 'military drill' styled physical education curriculum until the 1920s. In the mid 1920s thought was given to a curriculum that prepared a more affluent population to make use of an increase in leisure time. This change in the curriculum never materialised as the predicted increase in leisure time was undermined by the 'great depression' of the 1930s, a period that had a similar effect on the economy as the global recession in 2007. Physical education's close relationship with fitness pervaded the curriculum through to the 1960s particularly in the USA where President Kennedy founded the President's Fitness Council in response to the finding that American children had poorer levels of fitness than their European counterparts. Physical activity as we define it today was barely a flickering light in the minds of physical educators through the 1960s and 70s. Curiously, Jerry Morris's (Morris, Heady, Raffle, Roberts, & Parks, 1953) seminal findings on the relationship between physical activity and health went largely unnoticed by the physical education profession where an emphasis on the Victorian notion of sport, and the Swedish influence of gymnastics pervaded the curriculum. During the 1990s health-related exercise (HRE) finally

gained precedence over health-related fitness (HRF) ending a near 100 years of fitness dominated curricula. Twenty years later, health related physical activity emerged as a key objective
of the physical education curriculum (Cale & Harris, 2006a).

Pedagogical changes in physical education and health related exercise

During the 1980s leading physical educators such as Martin Underwood (Exeter, UK) and
Wally Mellor (Kingston, Canada) were influenced by Mosston and Ashworth's 'spectrum of
teaching styles' approach that promoted a deeper understanding of the delivery of an 'inclusive pedagogical approach' in physical education as opposed to an elite, sport dominated competitive model (Mosston & Ashworth, 2008). These leading physical educators were joined by
physical activity and health proponents Len Almond (Loughborough) and Bob Laventure who
were at one in promoting cutting edge pedagogical approaches to teaching physical education
and its constituent curriculum including health related exercise. These approaches placed high
value on more individual 'lifetime activities' that had better 'carryover value' and a delivery
style that differentiated curriculum content based on individual need.

These pedagogical changes resonated with goals of health promoting physical education
and its curriculum content. The goals of a health related exercise curriculum are clearly
outlined in the following definition proposed by Cale and Harris (Cale & Harris, 2006a)
'Health related exercise is the teaching of knowledge, understanding, physical competence
and behavioural skills, and the creation of positive attitudes and confidence associated with
current and lifelong participation in physical activity.' The definition was well matched to the
inclusive, individualised and differentiated pedagogical approaches promoted by leading academics in physical education at the time.

Whilst these changes in pedagogical approaches were clearly defined, agreement on the
most effective way to deliver a health related exercise remains elusive. Currently curriculum
content in the UK is delivered through dance, competitive games, gymnastics, aquatics, outdoor and adventurous activities and athletics and leaving little space for a direct focus on health
related physical activity. This approach is inherently problematic as students only experience
physical activity 'through' these activities. This sport related pedagogical approach has been
criticised given the wider competences and behavioural skills related to physical activity, such
as active transport, planning activity opportunities into daily living and more fitness related
competences such as developing strength, flexibility and aerobic fitness required from health
related exercise (Stratton, 1995). Moreover the public health impact of physical education
continues to be severely limited by a traditional curriculum that favours competitive team
sports over lifetime activities, motor over behavioural skills, and physical fitness over physical
activity (Trost, 2004). There is evidence of some change in the activities delivered in the curriculum. In one investigation heads of physical education departments reported that pedagogical approaches to the delivery of health related exercise were not consistent across boys and
girls curricula (Fairclough & Stratton, 2005). The dominance of 'team games' over 'lifetime
activities' was apparent in boys' physical education but the opposite was true in girls. So whilst
change in health related exercise and its influence on the physical education curriculum was evident in policy, a parallel change in practice was less clear, certainly in boys' physical education.
More worryingly the ambiguous nature of the national curriculum for physical education,
has also led to educationally undesirable pedagogical practices in health related exercise and
confusion on how best to deliver health related content (Cale & Harris, 2006b). Most recently

Lubans has suggested using 'SAAFE' principles (Supportive, Active, Autonomous, Fair, Enjoyable) for teaching physical education and after school sport and physical activity programmes that used an evidence-based framework designed to guide the planning, delivery and evaluation of organised physical activity sessions in school and community (Lubans et al., 2017). The premise of the SAAFE approach is that if physical education and after school sessions are to make a difference to young people's physical activity levels and physical literacy, they need to be of high quality, active and engaging.

Policy, the curriculum and health related exercise

It is in fact disappointing that over twenty years ago, when the national curriculum for physical education was in its infancy in England and Wales, I outlined the tensions in developing a curriculum that included a rhetoric for health but maintained a sport dominated approach, policed by a government directed national inspectorate for physical education that simply maintained the status quo (Stratton, 1995). Twenty years on health related exercise has gained momentum and now there is much greater advocacy that combines both a health related approach and a creative and individualised curriculum that engages students and motivates participation in physical activity, exercise and fitness activities (see Table 22.1).

A key driver behind this momentum is the fact that the promotion of health and physical activity is a main objective of the physical education curriculum (Whitehead, 2010) and supported by the World Health Organization (WHO, 2010). WHO have outlined seven investments for promoting physical activity and advocate that all countries include policies that promote 'high quality physical education' that supports children to develop behaviour patterns that will keep them physically active throughout their lives. More recently surveillance data summarised in a Global Matrix has helped to establish an evidence base on the quality of school physical education worldwide. The second Global matrix of Active Healthy Kids (Tremblay et al., 2016) included school physical education as a quality indicator at country level. Of the 38 participating countries only one country received an A grade, eight countries were allocated a B grade or higher, 10 a C and 9 a D grade. Lower grades tended to be in middle and lower income countries with a few exceptions. These data suggest that schools (including physical education) are arguably the strongest infrastructure

Table 22.1   The purpose of the national curriculum for physical education in England and Wales

The national curriculum for physical education (England and Wales)
Purpose of the curriculum is to deliver a high-quality physical education curriculum that inspires all pupils to succeed and excel in *competitive sport* and other physically demanding activities. It should provide opportunities for pupils to become physically confident in a way that supports their *health and fitness*. Opportunities to compete in sport and other activities build character and help to embed values such as fairness and respect.   **Aims**   The national curriculum for physical education aims to ensure that all pupils: • develop competence to excel in a broad range of physical activities   • are physically active for sustained periods of time   • engage in competitive sports and activities   • lead healthy, active lives

for promoting physical activity in young people worldwide and much research evidence supports this (van Sluijs & Kriemler, 2016). The problem lies of course in the gap between policy, implementation of a physical education curriculum and physical activity levels at the country level. For example in the USA physical education is included in the 'Health of the Nation' targets (CDC, 2016) yet a self assessed score of D+ was in the lower tertile of quality scores in the global matrix (Tremblay et al., 2016). There were many other examples of countries where school scores were relatively high but physical activity, sport participation, active transport and play were low.

Physical literacy, health related exercise and behaviour change

Recently 'physical literacy' has emerged as a central pillar in the physical education curriculum particularly in an educational era that purports to exert a lifelong influence on independent learning and achieving. Whitehead (2013) has defined physical literacy as 'the motivation, confidence, physical competence, knowledge and understanding to value and take responsibility for engagement in physical activities for life'. The concept of physical literacy has attracted significant attention and proponents suggest that it should be given the same level of educational importance as literacy and numeracy. Physical literacy captures the essence of the physical education curriculum regardless of delivery model and has become enmeshed with physical activity and is constituent in the vision for a curriculum including health related exercise. Moreover developing physical literacy satisfies the aims of lifelong learning, and the achievement of physical competence in activities that have value across the life course. The debate on the ontology of physical literacy continues to develop and clarification on its antecedents and applicability in physical education has recently been first articulated and second reduced into a number of properties (Edwards, Bryant, Keegan, Morgan, & Jones, 2017). These properties were summarised under seven sub-themes: affective, cognitive, physical capabilities, progression/developmental pathway, target audience, holistic concept and related constructs. While Edwards and colleagues (2017) included seven properties of physical literacy we will focus on Bloom's (1957) psychomotor, cognitive, affective learning and development domains. The *psychomotor* domain captures dimensions of skills and fitness, the *cognitive* domain knowledge and understanding and the *affective* domain relationships and working together. A *behavioural* domain is not included in Bloom's taxonomy but aligns with the concept of physical literacy whereby development in the psychomotor, cognitive and affective domains manifest themselves in day to day behaviours and their maintenance across a lifetime of engagement in physical activity. Edwards et al. (2017) recognised the need to include the behavioural domain in a broad definition of physical literacy because physically active behaviours are key in a process of lifelong learning. Moreover, models of behaviour change are the panacea of health promotion and arguably the physical education national curriculum is the largest most well organised behaviour change programme for physical activity that has ever existed! One of the more popular models of behaviour change that has relevance for physical education and health related exercise is the COM-B model (Michie & West, 2013) The COM-B model is central to a 'wheel of behaviour change' and suggests that a **b**ehaviour can only be demonstrated if the 3 elements of **c**ompetence and **c**apability, **o**pportunity and **m**otivation are in place. The physical education curriculum and its focus on physical literacy has significant overlap with the COM-B model.

Edwards and colleagues (2017) proposed that physical literacy is associated with behavioural, psychological, social and physical variables, and the contexts in which they occur, yet they fell short of proposing a behaviour 'change' approach that has been espoused by others (Jurbala, 2015). This is important as academics working in the area of physical literacy are polyvocal (Sparkes, 1991) and are aligned to specific philosophical approaches. A behaviour change approach, sustainable across the life course is but one perspective in a myriad of potential approaches available to physical educators when promoting physical activity and physical literacy through the physical education curriculum (Corbin, 2016).

Research into the effects of physical education on physical activity behaviour in children

In 2010 the United Nations suggested that it was timely to review the evidence-base for effective PE and updated these in their Millennium goals (United Nations, 2015). There have been significant developments in physical education over the past 20 years yet few of these have a sound evidence base. Moreover defining a set of outcome measures for physical education overall is problematic given its multiple educational goals (see Table 22.2).

Table 22.2 Broad aims for each key stage of the national curriculum for physical education in England and Wales

Key Stage	Age (y)	School level	Aims: Pupils should
1	4–7	Infant	develop fundamental movement skills, become increasingly competent and confident and access a broad range of opportunities to extend their agility, balance and coordination, individually and with others. They should be able to engage in competitive (both against self and against others) and co-operative physical activities, in a range of increasingly challenging situations
2	8–11	Junior	continue to apply and develop a broader range of skills, learning how to use them in different ways and to link them to make actions and sequences of movement. They should enjoy communicating, collaborating and competing with each other. They should develop an understanding of how to improve in different physical activities and sports and learn how to evaluate and recognise their own success.
3	12–14	Lower secondary	build on and embed the physical development and skills learned in key stages 1 and 2, become more competent, confident and expert in their techniques, and apply them across different sports and physical activities. They should understand what makes a performance effective and how to apply these principles to their own and others' work. They should develop the confidence and interest to get involved in exercise, sports and activities out of school and in later life, and understand and apply the long-term health benefits of physical activity.
4	15–16	Higher secondary	tackle complex and demanding physical activities. They should get involved in a range of activities that develops personal fitness and promotes an active, healthy lifestyle.

In particular the evidence base for the direct effect of a focused health related exercise curriculum on physical activity behaviour is at best limited. Subsequently, we are unable to report directly on the effectiveness of the health related exercise curriculum but we are able to discuss the effect of generic physical education on the psychomotor, cognitive and affective domain outcomes in addition to changes in behaviour. In one of the first reviews and meta-analyses of research in this area Dudley and colleagues (Dudley, Okely, Pearson, & Cotton, 2011) suggested three areas through which physical education effectiveness could be established:

1. Promoting high levels of physical activity participation.
2. Movement skill instruction and practice.
3. Active learning strategies with an emphasis on enjoyment.

These three areas also have indirect relevance to health related exercise in that participation in physical activity, development of fundamental movement skills and learning in an environment that promotes enjoyment closely align to lifelong participation, competence and motivation captured in physical literacy and behaviour change theories. In their review Dudley and colleagues screened 27,000 article titles, a total of 23 studies met inclusion criteria and the effect of physical education and school sport interventions on physical activity participation, movement skills, and enjoyment of physical activity are reported below:

Physical activity: An increase in physical activity was reported in 80% of studies and 70% found that these increases were significant. Two studies included follow-up measures post-intervention and found differences between the intervention group and the control group at both time points but only one of these studies showed statistically significant differences at both time points.

Fundamental movement skills: All four studies reported significant increases in movement skill proficiency, although the one study that included follow-up measures post-intervention, reported no differences between the intervention group and the control group at 6-month or 12-month post intervention. Three-quarters of the studies reported results separately for boys and girls but only girls experienced significant changes at both time points.

Enjoyment: Four intervention studies reported no significant increase in enjoyment. Conversely, of the three studies that reported improvements, only one reported statistically significant findings. Further there were significant differences in enjoyment between the intervention and the control group at 6- and 12-month post intervention, but only in boys at both time points.

Teaching approaches and curriculum delivery

In the interventions that targeted physical activity and movement proficiency, physical educators who adopted direct or explicit teaching strategies were most effective whilst the provision of professional development programmes for teachers using a well-designed prescribed curriculum also had a positive effect. Other key ingredients were the availability of quality resources such as equipment, curriculum materials, internet-resources and, for non physical education specialists, mentors or in-school consultants. The limited effect of physical education on enjoyment is consistent with the literature as it is intertwined with terms such as, fun, liking and intrinsic motivation. Enjoyment is also a nebulous term in education in that it is linked to engagement but is not an educational outcome. Rather enjoyment is a key part of the physical educators process to engage students in learning and academic achievement and lifelong engagement in 'enjoyable' health promoting physical activity.

In addition Dudley and colleagues review more detailed reviews on the effectiveness of physical education on movement proficiency, cognition and academic achievement, and physical activity during physical education lessons and physical fitness. These reviews are also contextualised in relation to teaching styles and approaches.

Physical education and movement proficiency

Morgan and colleagues (2013) systematically reviewed and meta-analysed the effect of fundamental movement skill interventions in elementary and primary schools. These interventions had a significant effect on gross motor proficiency (Effect size = 1.42) and locomotor skill competency (Effect size = 1.42) and a smaller but still significant effect on object control skill competency (Effect size = 0.63).

The mode of intervention varied significantly. A number of study designs delivered (i) an 'enhanced' physical education curriculum with a focus on fundamental movement skills and compared this approach to traditional physical education, (ii) measured the effect of increased curriculum time allotted to physical education or (iii) a combination of them both. While insufficient details on theoretical or pedagogical approaches were reported common approaches included a mastery motivational climate, competence motivation theory, self-learning, movement exploration, self-testing and self paced activity and/or direct instruction and covered the whole spectrum of Mosston and Ashworth teaching styles (Mosston & Ashworth, 2008). There are three main sections under fundamental movement, including locomotor, object control and stability skills. Morgan and co-workers (Morgan et al., 2013) reported larger effect sizes for locomotor skills than object control skills. There may be a number of reasons for this, first object control skills are more difficult to improve than locomotor skills, or that there was greater time spent teaching locomotor than object control skills. While these results are encouraging many studies were limited and follow up times in particular were very short.

Prioritising movement skill development

The scientific evidence confirms that physical education improves fundamental movement skills and physical competences. Competence is a key pillar in both the COM-B model and self determination theory (Ryan & Deci, 2000). In support of a competence focused physical education curriculum Dudley et al. (Dudley, Okely, Pearson, & Cotton, 2011) confirmed that movement skill development should be a key focus of physical education as movement proficiency has high 'carryover value' for long-term engagement in an active lifestyle. However, while movement proficiency and physical activity participation and engagement should underpin an effective pedagogical strategy, these should be encapsulated in the broader notion of 'physical literacy'. Therefore, more research into physical literacy using a range of paradigms would help clarify the effect of physical education programmes on physical literacy. This research should be informed by the debate articulated on physical literacy, physical education and health (Edwards et al., 2017; Lundvall, 2015; Jurbala, 2015).

Physical activity cognition and academic achievement

Plato and Kennedy recognised the effect of physical activity on thinking and cognition. Unfortunately over the past 20 years there has been significant pressure on the 'satellite subjects' in the curriculum to give up time to support the 'alleged' more important goals of numeracy, literacy, science and engineering curricula (Stratton, 1995). Fortunately there is a growing body of science that has quantified the effect of physical activity on learning, academic achievement, concentration and cognitive function. Donnelly and colleagues (Donnelly et al., 2016) systematically reviewed the literature and found 64 studies that met inclusion criteria for the relationship between physical activity and cognition or learning, and 73 studies that met inclusion criteria for physical activity and academic achievement or concentration. The majority of studies support the positive effects of physical fitness, single bouts of physical activity, and physical activity interventions on children's cognitive function with insufficient evidence to gain insight into the effect of physical activity on learning. On the other hand correlational and determinant studies on physical activity and academic achievement have reported impressive results, but cause and effect results are mixed. There is also a lack of well-designed studies that have sufficient length and detailed measures and research designs to give deeper insight into the issue. Moreover, the dose-response relationship between physical activity and cognition needs further exploration, and particularly on how to implement strategies in real life contexts in schools. For example do schools that include three recess breaks per day have children with better concentration levels than schools that have two? Are active classrooms that use standing desks and minimise sitting behaviour as effective as physical education programmes? What pedagogical approaches, declarative and procedural knowledge do teachers need to manage these changes? There are many professional approaches that do not have enough scientific evidence to be conclusive. On a positive note, and importantly for politicians, physical activity in school '*does not have a negative effect*' on academic achievement, concentration or cognition.

Physical activity levels during physical education lessons

Physical education is unique in the school curriculum as it offers the greatest opportunity for physical activity and development in the psychomotor domain. In one of the first publications in the area, I reported that children engaged in MVPA for 33% of physical education lesson time but that this depended on the ability level of a child, the activity being taught and the teaching style adopted by the physical educator (Stratton, 1997), a finding supported by others (Lonsdale et al., 2013). Following this research targets for the recommended amount of MVPA in physical education lessons were proposed by the United States' Centre for Disease Control and Prevention and the United Kingdom's (UK) Associations for Physical Education. Both organisations recommended that physical education lessons should engage children in MVPA for 50% of lesson time to gain appropriate health and academic benefits (Lonsdale et al., 2013). The evidence base has also developed in this area over the past 20 years. Hollis and colleagues (Hollis et al., 2016) undertook a systematic review and meta-analysis on physical activity in physical education lessons. After screening over 5,000 articles a total of 28 publications from 25 projects published between 2005 and 2014 met the inclusion criteria for further review. Five of these studies were conducted in middle and 10 in high schools. Half of the studies included were from the USA, a quarter from Australia, whilst Portugal, Brazil, the UK and Poland contributed to a dataset derived from 609 middle school PE lessons and 837 high school PE lessons. Middle and high school students spent 48.6% and 35.9% of physical education lesson time in MVPA. The amount of MVPA recorded varied by methodology. In studies that used accelerometers, students spent 34.7% (25.1–44.4%) of lesson time in MVPA compared to 44.4% (38.3–50.5%), 43.1% (24.3–61.9%) and 35.9% (31.0–40.8%)

when measured using observational methods, heart rate monitors and pedometers, respectively. Levels of MVPA by lesson type or delivery mode were not reported. An analysis to examine whether MVPA in lesson time differed by lesson type was not conducted due to a lack of data. Further, nine of the 15 studies included in the meta-analysis provided details on activity types but the majority of studies reported data from multiple categories (fitness orientated activities, team invasion games, dance and gymnastics or net game activities) without splitting data by lesson type or mode of delivery. In summary the proportion of time spent in MVPA varied considerably between 12.9 and 68.2% of lessons. The meta-analysis of 15 studies found that the proportion of lesson time spent in MVPA fell below 50% of physical education lesson time. In secondary schools 40.5% of lesson time was spent in MVPA compared to 48.6% in middle schools. The scientific evidence clearly suggests that a recommended quantity of that MVPA delivered during physical education lessons is an ambitious target that gets harder to reach as children move from junior, middle to secondary school (Lonsdale et al., 2013). More recently a set of 'SHARP' teaching principles effective at increasing MVPA during physical educations have been proposed (Powell, Woodfield, & Nevill, 2016) and are worthy of serious practical consideration.

Physical fitness

Over the past 20 years physical fitness has decreased significantly in children and adolescents (Tomkinson & Olds, 2007; Stratton et al., 2007) and with it an increase in cardiovascular risk (Boddy, Fairclough, Atkinson, & Stratton, 2012). A lack of physical activity and in particular vigorous physical activity has been implicated in these decreases (Parikh & Stratton, 2011). School physical activity programmes, in particular physical education, are arguably the best place to effect increases in children's fitness. To investigate the effect of school physical activity and physical education programmes on cardiorespiratory fitness Minatto and colleagues (Minatto, Barbosa Filho, Berria, & Petroski, 2016) completed a meta-analysis of 25 studies. Interventions significantly increased cardiorespiratory fitness (effect size of 0.68) although the magnitude of the effect (0.4–0.9) varied by age group, gender, sample size, environment, strategies to prioritise cardiorespiratory fitness, measurement method, session length, and frequency and duration of sessions. Minatto and colleagues concluded that interventions in school physical education increased cardiorespiratory fitness although study characteristics such as exercise sessions in addition to physical education classes, lesson focus on fitness, the inclusion of a combination of aerobic and resistance exercises and a duration of ≥60 min, and frequency of three lessons per week were key factors (Minatto et al., 2016).

A technology driven curriculum

Over the past 10 years there has been an exponential increase in children's participation in exergaming and in particular e-sports. This 21st-century phenomenon has also pervaded all aspects of life including teaching. Such has been the investment in computer games that many of these are now highly relevant resources that can be used to augment teaching particularly in physical education. Almost 20 years ago I commented on the influence of information technology in physical education and outlined the potential that digital 'movies, pictures and sounds' had to influence teaching and learning within a competence-based physical education curriculum and this has been supported by an exponential growth in the resources available (Lavay, Sakai, Ortiz, & Roth, 2015). Moreover, Thomas and Stratton (Thomas & Stratton, 2006) coined the term 'edutainment' which captured the combination of education and entertainment that computer games add to the learning environment and concur with Papastergiou (2009) who positively supports the positive effect of active video games on children's academic achievement.

In a systematic review on active video games in schools and effects on physical activity and health, Norris and colleagues (Norris, Hamer, & Stamatakis, 2016) identified 22 studies 11 of which assessed physical activity, 5 assessed motor skill, and 6 assessed both physical activity and health. Nine out of 14 studies found greater physical activity during school time when comparing data from children who took part in active video game sessions with controls. Motor skills also improved in children who took part in active video game sessions but these were not as effective as traditional motor skill interventions. The effects of active video games on body composition were mixed. One of the main problems with the evidence base on active video games was a lack of 'process evaluation'. As a result limited insight could be gained about participation and compliance, self-efficacy (in teachers and students), implementation strategies including health and safety, equipment/resource availability, teaching styles and approaches and assessment of learning. Given limitations in the current literature Norris and colleagues (Norris et al., 2016) concluded that there was insufficient evidence for active video games to be used as physical activity and health promoting interventions in school settings.

Not only has technology such as active video games been used to augment teaching, Giblin, Collins and Button (2014) propose that they have application in assessment. They contend that exer-gaming technological platforms have the potential to help physical educators monitor learning along the journey of becoming physically literate. Low-cost motion capture devices used in physical education could enhance the quality of movement testing procedures, provide individualised and detailed feedback and allow longitudinal data gathering to monitor motor skill development. In some of our recent work we have used 'sensors' to characterise the quality of children's movement (Barnes, Clark, Holton, Stratton, & Summers, 2016; Clark et al., 2017). Working alongside engineers we have generated 'heat maps' of movement quality (see Figure 22.1). The heat map provides a fingerprint of a

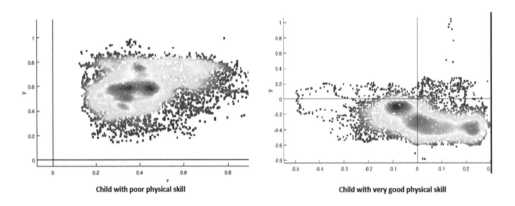

Child with poor physical skill   Child with very good physical skill

Figure 22.1 Sensor derived performance of high and low skilled children completing the Dragon Challenge V1.0 assessment of physical competency

child's fundamental movement skill as measured using the Dragon Challenge V1.0 (Stratton, Foweather, Rotchell, English, & Hughes 2016). These heat maps provide powerful visual information that will be used to assess the 'quality of movement' of children. Subsequently a physical educator will use their pedagogical skills to seek ways of moving the fingerprint towards the gold standard. For example in Figure 22.1 the child with poor skill has the majority of heat in the mid to left section of the graphic whereas the child with very good skill has their heat in the bottom right side of the heat map. Using this technology linked to smartphones or tablets the physical educator would aim to use a range of 'teachalogical' skills to shift the heat in the child who has poor skills closer to the heat in the map from the child with vey good skills. In future these heat maps will be part of a physical educator's assessment toolkit and will be transmitted wirelessly to handheld devices in real time for immediate analysis during the teaching assessment pedagogical process.

Chapter summary

In conclusion the health related benefits of physical activity have been recognised for centuries but the best approach to delivering a health related exercise curriculum are hampered by a curriculum dominated by team games and competition. Health related exercise focused curricula are available but these are only recognised later in a children's physical education curriculum. Pedagogical changes that focus on the psychomotor, cognitive and affective domains integrated with a re-emergence of physical literacy and a broad spectrum of teaching styles have resulted in a more inclusive curriculum that seeks to promote positive healthy and active behaviours in students. Where curricula have been researched, there are positive effects on physical competence, physical fitness, physical activity and academic achievement and related constructs. These improvements have been achieved when the teaching focuses on the dimension of interest be it physical activity, fitness, motor competence and so on. The integration of technology to augment teaching and assessment in the physical education curriculum has had a positive effect even though results are limited. Information technology and the 'internet of things' will significantly influence teaching and learning approaches in physical education and change the process by which the curriculum is delivered, how children are assessed and how their achievement is reported to parents and other interested parties. Finally whilst physical education positively influences the quality and quantity of health related physical activity the evidence base is susceptible to bias and significantly more research is required before the clear benefits of physical education on the physical literacy and health of children across the life course can be unequivocally supported.

- The relationship physical education and health has been recognised through history by Plato, John F. Kennedy and Nelson Mandela.
- Changes in teaching approaches and styles prompted by Mosston and Ashworth (1988) have resulted in a more inclusive physical education curriculum that aims to develop physical literacy in all children.
- Health related exercise is an essential component of the physical education curriculum yet the most effective of delivery mode is still open to debate amongst physical educators.
- Behaviour change approaches are important aspects to consider by physical educators particularly related to student's physical competence and physical literacy.

- The number of systematic reviews on the effectiveness of physical education has grown over recent times. These demonstrate that physical education is effective at:

  1. Increasing physical activity
  2. Increasing cardiorespiratory fitness
  3. Increasing motor competence
  4. Improving concentration, cognition and academic achievement.

- There has been an increase in the use of technology to augment teaching resources and approaches in physical education. There is some evidence that the use of technology maintains currency, promotes a motivational climate (edutainment) and helps develop children's physical literacy and physical activity.
- The internet of things (IoT) has a significant amount of resources in the form of apps, media and curriculum tools to augment teaching and assessment in physical education. For example the Dragon Challenge (Figure 22.1) is an excellent example of the potential of future tools available to the physical educator to assess fundamental movement skills.

References

Barnes, C.M., Clark, C.C.T., Holton, M.D., Stratton, G., & Summers, H.D. (2016). Quantitative time-profiling of children's activity and motion. *Medicine and Science in Sports and Exercise*, (August). http://doi.org/10.1249/MSS.0000000000001085

Bloom, B. (1957). Learning domains or Bloom's taxonomy. Retrieved November, 6, 2007. Retrieved from http://users.manchester.edu/Student/GJTribbett/Webpage/Bloom's Taxonomies.pdf%5Cnpapers3://publication/uuid/1053A1D1-15BC-4ED9-AEBE-DF89FD0E81A9

Boddy, L.M., Fairclough, S.J., Atkinson, G., & Stratton, G. (2012). Changes in cardiorespiratory fitness in 9- to 10.9-year-old children: Sportslinx 1998–2010. *Medicine and Science in Sports and Exercise, 44*, 481–486. http://doi.org/10.1249/MSS.0b013e3182300267

Cale, L., & Harris, J. (2006a). Interventions to promote young people's physical activity: issues, implications and recommendations for practice. *Health Education Journal, 65*(4), 320–337. http://doi.org/10.1177/0017896906069370

Cale, L., & Harris, J. (2006b). School-based physical activity interventions: Effectiveness, trends, issues, implications and recommendations for practice. *Sport, Education and Society*. http://doi.org/10.1080/13573320600924890

CDC. (2016). CDC | Physical Activity | Facts | Healthy Schools. Retrieved from www.cdc.gov/healthyschools/physicalactivity/facts.htm%5Cnhttp://www.cdc.gov/healthyschools/physicalactivity/facts.htm

Clark, C.C.T., Barnes, C.M., Holton, M., Summers, H.D., & Stratton, G. (2016). Profiling movement quality and gait characteristics according to body-mass index in children (9–11 y). *Human Movement Science, 49*, 291–300. http://doi.org/10.1016/j.humov.2016.08.003

Clark, C.C.T., Barnes, C.M., Stratton, G., McNarry, M.A., Mackintosh, K.A., & Summers, H.D. (2017). A review of emerging analytical techniques for objective physical activity measurement in humans. *Sports Medicine*. http://doi.org/10.1007/s40279-016-0585-y

Corbin, C.B. (2016). Implications of physical literacy for research and practice: a commentary. *Research Quarterly for Exercise and Sport*. http://doi.org/10.1080/02701367.2016.1124722

Donnelly, J.E., Hillman, C.H., Castelli, D., Etnier, J.L., Lee, S., Tomporowski, P., . . . Szabo-Reed, A.N. (2016). Physical activity, fitness, cognitive function, and academic achievement in children: a systematic review. *Medicine and Science in Sports and Exercise, 48*(6), 1197–1222. http://doi.org/10.1249/MSS.0000000000000901

Dudley, D., Okely, A., Pearson, P., & Cotton, W. (2011). A systematic review of the effectiveness of physical education and school sport interventions targeting physical activity, movement skills and enjoyment of physical activity. *European Physical Education Review, 17*(3), 353–378. http://doi.org/10.1177/1356336X11416734

Edwards, L.C., Bryant, A.S., Keegan, R.J., Morgan, K., & Jones, A.M. (2017). Definitions, foundations and associations of physical literacy: a systematic review. *Sports Medicine.* http://doi.org/10.1007/s40279-016-0560-7

Fairclough, S., & Stratton, G. (2005). 'Physical education makes you fit and healthy'. Physical education's contribution to young people's physical activity levels. *Health Education Research, 20*(1), 14–23. http://doi.org/10.1093/her/cyg101

Giblin, S., Collins, D., & Button, C. (2014). Physical literacy: importance, assessment and future directions. *Sports Medicine* (Auckland, N.Z.), *44*(9), 1177–1184. http://doi.org/10.1007/s40279-014-0205-7

Hollis, J.L., Williams, A.J., Sutherland, R., Campbell, E., Nathan, N., Wolfenden, L., . . . Wiggers, J. (2016). A systematic review and meta-analysis of moderate-to-vigorous physical activity levels in elementary school physical education lessons. *Preventive Medicine.* http://doi.org/10.1016/j.ypmed.2015.11.018

Jurbala, P. (2015). What is physical literacy, really? *Quest, 67*(4), 367–383. http://doi.org/10.1080/00336297.2015.1084341

Lavay, B., Sakai, J., Ortiz, C., & Roth, K. (2015). Tablet technology to monitor physical education IEP goals and benchmarks. *JOPERD: The Journal of Physical Education, Recreation & Dance, 86*(6), 16–23. http://doi.org/10.1080/07303084.2015.1053633

Lonsdale, C., Rosenkrantz, R.R., Peralta, L.R., Bennie, A., Fahey, P., & Lubans, D.R. (2013). A systematic review and meta-analysis of interventions designed to increase moderate-to-vigorous physical activity in school physical education lessons. *Preventive Medicine, 56*(2), 152–161. http://doi.org/10.1016/j.ypmed.2012.12.004

Lubans, D.R., Lonsdale, C., Cohen, K., Eather, N., Beauchamp, M.R., Morgan, P.J., . . . Smith, J.J. (2017). Framework for the design and delivery of organized physical activity sessions for children and adolescents: rationale and description of the 'SAAFE' teaching principles. *International Journal of Behavioral Nutrition and Physical Activity, 14*(1), 24. http://doi.org/10.1186/s12966-017-0479-x

Lundvall, S. (2015). Physical literacy in the field of physical education – A challenge and a possibility. *Journal of Sport and Health Science.* http://doi.org/10.1016/j.jshs.2015.02.001

Michie, S., & West, R. (2013). Behaviour change theory and evidence: a presentation to government. *Health Psychology Review, 7*(1), 1–22. http://doi.org/10.1080/17437199.2011.649445

Minatto, G., Barbosa Filho, V.C., Berria, J., & Petroski, E.L. (2016). School-based interventions to improve cardiorespiratory fitness in adolescents: systematic review with meta-analysis. *Sports Medicine* (Auckland, N.Z.), 1–20. http://doi.org/10.1007/s40279-016-0480-6

Morgan, P.J., Barnett, L.M., Cliff, D.P., Okely, A.D., Scott, H.A., Cohen, K.E., & Lubans, D.R. (2013). Fundamental movement skill interventions in youth: a systematic review and meta-analysis. *PEDIATRICS, 132*(5), e1361–e1383. http://doi.org/10.1542/peds.2013-1167

Morris, J.N., Heady, J.A., Raffle, P.A., Roberts, C.G., & Parks, J.W. (1953). Coronary heart-disease and physical activity of work. *Lancet* (London, England), *265*(6796), 1111–20; concl.

Mosston, M., & Ashworth, S. (1988). *Teaching Physical Education.* First Online Edition.

Norris, E., Hamer, M., & Stamatakis, E. (2016). Active video games in schools and effects on physical activity and health: a systematic review. *The Journal of Pediatrics, 172,* 40–46.e5. http://doi.org/10.1016/j.jpeds.2016.02.001

Papastergiou, M. (2009). Digital game-based learning in high school computer science education: impact on educational effectiveness and student motivation. *Computers & Education, 52*(1), 1–12. http://doi.org/10.1016/j.compedu.2008.06.004

Parikh, T., & Stratton, G. (2011). Influence of intensity of physical activity on adiposity and cardiorespiratory fitness in 5–18 year olds. *Sports Medicine.* http://doi.org/10.2165/11588750-000000000-00000

Powell, E., Woodfield, L.A., & Nevill, A.M. (2016). Increasing physical activity levels in primary school physical education: the SHARP Principles Model. *Preventive Medicine Reports, 3*, 7–13. http://doi.org/10.1016/j.pmedr.2015.11.007

Ryan, R.M., & Deci, E. (2000). Self-determination theory and the facilitation of intrinsic motivation, social development, and well-being. *American Psychologist, 55*, 68–78.

Sparkes, A.C. (1991). Toward understanding, dialogue, and polyvocality in the research community. *Journal of Teaching in Physical Education, 10*, 103–133.

Stratton, G. (1995). Dearing or derailing health related exercise in the National Curriculum? Tracking physical education's changing role in the promotion of public health. *British Journal of Physical Education, 26*(1), 21–25.

Stratton, G. (1997). Children's heart rates during British physical education lessons. *Journal of Teaching in Physical Education, 16*, 357–367. Retrieved from http://articles.sirc.ca/search.cfm?id=415211%5Cnhttp://search.ebscohost.com/login.aspx?direct=true&db=s3h&AN=SPH415211&site=ehost-live&scope=site%5Cnhttp://www.humankinetics.com/ DP - EBSCOhost DB - s3h

Stratton, G., Canoy, D., Boddy, L.M., Taylor, S.R., Hackett, A.F., & Buchan, I.E. (2007). Cardiorespiratory fitness and body mass index of 9–11-year-old English children: a serial cross-sectional study from 1998 to 2004. *International Journal of Obesity, 31*(7), 1172–1178. http://doi.org/10.1038/sj.ijo.0803562

Stratton, G., Foweather, L., Rotchell, J., English, J., Hughes, H. (2016). Dragon Challenge Manual. Retrieved October 5, 2017, from www.Dragon Challenge Manual. activehealthykidswales.com/. . ./Dragon_Challenge_Manual.pdf accessed

Thomas, A., & Stratton, G. (2006). What we are really doing with ICT in physical education: a national audit of equipment, use, teacher attitudes, support, and training. *British Journal of Educational Technology.* http://doi.org/10.1111/j.1467-8535.2006.00520.x

Tomkinson, G., & Olds, T. (2007). Pediatric fitness. Secular trends and geographic variability. *Med Sport Sci Basel., 50*, 168–182. http://doi.org/10.1159/000101391

Tremblay, M.S., Barnes, J.D., González, S.A., Katzmarzyk, P.T., Onywera, V.O., Reilly, J.J., . . . Wong, S.H. (2016). Global Matrix 2.0: Report card grades on the physical activity of children and youth comparing 38 countries and the Global Matrix 2.0 Research Team. *Journal of Physical Activity and Health, 13*(Suppl 2), 343–366. http://doi.org/10.1123/jpah.2016-0594

Trost, S. (2004). School physical education in the post-report era: an analysis from public health. *Journal of Teaching in Physical Education, 23*, 318–337.

United Nations. (2015). United Nations Millennium Development Goals. Retrieved from www.un.org/millenniumgoals/

van Sluijs, E.M.F., & Kriemler, S. (2016). Reflections on physical activity intervention research in young people – dos, don'ts, and critical thoughts. *International Journal of Behavioral Nutrition and Physical Activity, 13*(1), 25. http://doi.org/10.1186/s12966-016-0348-z

Whitehead, M. (2010). Physical literacy. *Physical Literacy: Throughout the Lifecourse*, 21–29. http://doi.org/10.4324/9780203881903

Whitehead, M. (2013). Definition of physical literacy and clarification of related issues. *Journal of the International Council of Sport Science and Physical Education, 65*, 29–34. http://doi.org/1728-5909

WHO. (2010). Global recommendations on physical activity for health. *Geneva: World Health Organization*, 60. http://doi.org/10.1080/11026480410034349

Williams, A. (1988). Historiography of health and fitness in physical education. *British Journal of Physical Education, 3* (Research Supplement), 1–4.

23 Physical activity and older adults

Gladys Onambele-Pearson, Declan Ryan, David Tomlinson and Jorgen Wullems

Keywords: Diurnal rhythm, fall prevention, limitations, optimal protocol, exercise palatability

Introduction

Based on the multitude of sources of information and recommendations pertaining to health recommendations for older persons, we would think that today's individuals (at least in the 1st world) aged 65 and over, are fully informed in the concept of, and engaged in the process of, maintaining physical and mental health in their later years. In broad terms, the current recommendations for physical activity tend to share the following principal attributes as summarised by the World Health Organization (WHO) (World Health Organization, 2015):

1. They are neither gender, ethnic nor disease specific.
2. A minimum of 150 minutes of moderate physical activity (MPA) or 75 minutes of vigorous physical activity (VPA) per week, inclusive of leisure time activities, housework, transportation and/or planned structured exercise.
3. Where physical activity involves an aerobic element, this should be carried out in a continuous bout of 10 minutes or more, as opposed to start and stop shorter bouts, for any health benefits to be imparted.
4. Postural balance exercises should be an integral part of the physical activities undertaken.
5. Resistance training of large muscle groups, must be at least a twice weekly undertaking.
6. Even in the presence of co-morbidities and frailty, physical activity to a person's capacity must be pursued.

The degree to which the recommendations are fit for purpose is somewhat under recent scrutiny, with poor health factors still appearing in many individuals who self-report as adhering to the recommendations.

The impact of exercise in the older person

The WHO proposes that the benefits to the individual who adheres to this lifestyle, include:

1. Decreased rates of all-cause mortality, coronary heart disease, high blood pressure, stroke, type 2 diabetes, colon cancer and breast cancer;

2. A higher level of cardiorespiratory and muscular fitness, healthier body mass and composition;
3. A 'biomarker profile' that modulates the prevention of cardiovascular disease, type 2 diabetes and the enhancement of bone health;
4. Higher levels of functional health, a lower risk of falling, and better cognitive function;
5. Reduced risk of moderate and severe functional limitations and role limitations.

There is no doubt to the general value of these recommendations in terms of the favourable health effects. It is however striking that no degree of individualisation is taken into account, given the known impact of socio-economic factors on the type and frequency of physical activity. Indeed it is recognised that in adolescents for instance, being female, of a lower social class, are key determinants of the variance in total physical activity undertaken (Raudsepp, 2006). Similarly, the physiological responses to exercises are also modulated by gender and/ or decade of life. Thus, to advise on a physical activity programme in later life, influences on, and determinants of, activity levels need to be specifically considered. Indeed later life physical activity is a complex behaviour determined by many factors. Socio-economic status, social support from family and friends, and aspects of the geographical environment, are likely to influence physical activity participation (Farrell, Hollingsworth, Propper, & Shields, 2013), in a not dissimilar way to that seen in adolescents (Santos, Esculcas, & Mota, 2004). It would be expected that a socio-economic status link to physical activity would include instrumental and direct (transportation, logistics, payment of fees), motivational (encouragement), and/or observational (explicit modelling leading to improving intrinsic motivation) support.

This chapter gathers information from the most up-to-date literature on the known impact (benefits and risks), and leads informed discussions on the palatability and adherence of older persons to popular physical activity regimes.

Structured exercise

Physical activity is a modifiable health behaviour. Whilst the importance of physical activity is extensively documented and well accepted by health professionals, how specific exercise affects known outcome measures in persons aged 65 and over is not clear. Physical activity is defined as any body movement produced by skeletal muscles that results in energy expenditure (Caspersen, Powell, & Christenson, 1985). Current recommendations for physical activity in the over 65s is 150 minutes of moderate activity or 75 minutes of vigorous activity (Bull & the Expert Working Group, 2010). The categorisation of physical activity is commonly intertwined with structured exercise as both terms have similar characteristics. Yet, exercise is a different concept as it is usually planned and time limited, and with the specific aim of increasing an aspect of physical fitness (Caspersen et al., 1985) (see Figure 23.1). Structured exercise can be categorised by intensity including: a) medium to vigorous exercise such as resistance or aerobic exercise, and b) low impact low-intensity exercise such as yoga or seated exercise classes. Whilst the modality and intensity of exercise can differ, the focus of increasing/ maintaining physical function in the elderly is the main aim in all protocols.

Resistance exercise training

The most beneficial intervention to increase muscle structure and function and reduce age-related muscle weakness in the older person is resistance training. The effects of

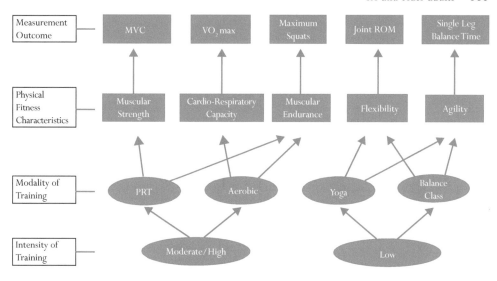

Figure 23.1 The links between structured modalities of training and physical fitness characteristics targeted in over 65s. (PRT = progressive resistance training; MVC = maximum voluntary contraction; ROM = range of motion)

progressive resistance exercise (PRT) in the older person are well documented (Table 23.1). Intervention studies have shown significant gains in muscle strength (Taaffe et al., 1996), muscle size (Harridge, Kryger, & Stensgaard, 1999), muscle activation capacity (Morse et al., 2005), specific force (Morse et al., 2007), tendon stiffness (Onambele-Pearson & Pearson, 2012; Reeves, Narici, & Maganaris, 2003) and bone density (Nelson et al., 1994) following twice or thrice weekly sessions of PRT. The functional implications of these adaptations translates to increases in efficient sit-to-stand transitions (Fahlman, McNevin, Boardley, Morgan, & Topp, 2011), walking speed (Henwood & Taaffe, 2005), balance (Nelson et al., 1994; Onambele-Pearson, Breen, & Stewart, 2010a; Onambele et al., 2008) in a long list of other functional benefits. Improvements reported in these functional tasks play a leading role in the maintenance of independent later life. Whilst the main adaptations of PRT centre on structural changes to skeletal muscle, there have been several studies demonstrating improvements in decreasing systemic inflammation bio-markers that are upregulated in ageing such as interlukin-6 (Onambele-Pearson, Breen, & Stewart, 2010a; Onambele-Pearson, Breen, & Stewart, 2010b; Prestes et al., 2009) and tumour necrosis factor α (Greiwe, Cheng, Rubin, Yarasheski, & Semenkovich, 2001). The inflamed endocrine milieu seen with increased age is in fact negatively associated with a variety of morbidities (e.g. cardiovascular disease), thus the impact of such co-morbidities is expanded upon later in this chapter.

It should nevertheless be noted that there are some risks associated with PRT in the older person, particularly the nature of high-intensity activity and the familiarity with the tasks for the individual. PRT places high stress levels on active muscles and joint structures, requires potentially uncomfortable physical positioning during repetitive loading, thus potentially increasing the risk of injury (Kolber, Beekhuizen, Cheng, & Hellman, 2010).

Table 23.1   Adaptations associated with a variety of modalities of exercise in the elderly

Modality of exercise	Intensity	Adaptations	Functional Tasks
Resistance exercise	Moderate to High	↑ Muscle Strength ↑ Muscle Power ↑ Muscle Size ↑ Activation Capacity ↑ Tendon Stiffness ↓ Systemic Inflammatory Biomarkers	↑ Gait Speed ↑ Postural Balance ↑ Sit to Stand ↓ Risk of Falling
Aerobic exercise	Moderate to High	↑ Capillary Density ↑ Mitochondrial Density ↑ Lipid Profile ↑ Blood Glucose Uptake ↓ Systemic Inflammatory Biomarkers ↑ Aerobic Power	↑ Gait Speed ↑ Postural Balance ↑ 6 Minute Walk Time
Dance	Low/Moderate/High	↑ Muscle Strength ↑ Joint Range of Motion	↑ Gait Speed ↑ Flexibility
Yoga	Low	↑ Muscle Strength ↑ Joint Range of Motion	↓ Risk of Falling ↑ Postural Balance ↑ Flexibility
Balance themed exercise	Low	↑ Muscle Strength	↓ Risk of Falling ↑ Postural Balance
Pilates/core based exercise	Low	↑ Muscle Strength ↑ Joint Range of Motion	↓ Risk of Falling ↑ Postural Balance ↑ Flexibility

Aerobic exercise training

Aerobic/endurance training can be characterised by numerous activities that range from recreational walking to high-intensity running. The stimulus placed on skeletal muscle here is different to that in resistance/strength-based training, with repeated muscle contractions placing a greater demand on the cardiovascular system. The benefits with this modality of training are the central and peripheral adaptations of the cardiovascular system, increasing the capacity to deliver oxygen (O_2) to working muscles during activity (Holloszy & Coyle, 1984) and improving the capability of skeletal muscles to generate energy via oxidative metabolism (Cadore, Pinto, Bottaro, & Izquierdo, 2014). These effects are achieved through structural increases in both mitochondrial and capillary density (Iversen et al., 2011) and a shift in fibre type towards oxidative slow twitch muscle fibres (Howald, Hoppeler, Claassen, Mathieu, & Straub, 1985).

There are two types of traditional aerobic exercise: (i) **continuous**, based on training at one uninterrupted level throughout the protocol or (ii) **interval**, based on training delivered in short high-intensity bursts. Training intensity for over 65s tends to be set using varying methodologies. First, the subjective intensity assessment uses a 10-point scale with 0 classed as sitting and 10 being classed as an all-out effort for a minimum of 30 minutes, 5 days/week (Nelson et al., 2007a). Second, the more objective assessments either use heart rate, the participant's aerobic threshold or VO_2 max, or both in conjunction (Emerenziani et al., 2015). Whilst a traditional structured aerobic session increases functional capacity, unconventional dance based exercise classes also increase cardiorespiratory endurance, strength/endurance, body agility, flexibility, body fat, and balance in elderly women (Hopkins, Murrah, Hoeger, & Rhodes, 1990; Serra et al., 2016; Wu, Tu, Hsu, & Tsao, 2016). This demonstrates that to improve physical fitness, health and functional ability in over 65s, a variety of structured and semi-structured aerobic based training methods may be used.

Notably, an important factor to consider when choosing between training methodologies is whether the exercise meets the individual's physical, social and emotional requirements to effect a long-term lifestyle change. With moderate-/vigorous-intensity training in particular, the over 65s tend to present poor exercise tolerance especially when they are frail, and with no previous history of structured exercise. In addition, blood pressure increases acutely during physical activity (Palatini, 1988). Therefore medical and training history should be taken into account when prescribing moderate/vigorous training intensity to this age group.

Low intensity low impact exercise

Previous research has shown the benefit of low impact structured exercise sessions such as yoga, tai chi, pilates and balance themed classes and their positive effect on functional measures including flexibility (Geremia, Iskiewicz, Marschner, Lehnen, & Lehnen, 2015; Grabara & Szopa, 2015), lowering the risk of falling (Schmid, Van Puymbroeck, & Koceja, 2010), increasing postural balance (Taylor et al., 2012) and improving quality of life (Woodyard, 2011). Low-intensity exercise is more likely to be palatable to over 65s and especially to those who are either frail or have no previous history of structured physical exercise. Further, low-intensity exercise presents lower injury incidence by minimising high levels of stress and strain on both the cardiovascular, musculoskeletal and endocrine systems (Onambele-Pearson et al., 2010a, 2010b).

Physical activity and its impact on a key physical functioning marker: falls

One in three adults in the UK over the age of 65 years fall at least once a year. In these individuals, falls that result in injury result in loss of independence (Piirtola & Era, 2006), and are one of the leading causes of death from injury (Rubenstein, 2006). The number of over 65s will increase by 2 million by 2021 and with over £2 billion currently spent every year by the NHS on falls, this will undoubtedly infer a significant burden on the NHS.

The key modifiable risk factors associated with increased risk of falling include muscle weakness, balance and gait abnormalities (Granacher, Muehlbauer, & Gruber, 2012; Maki, Holliday, & Topper, 1994; Rubenstein & Josephson, 2002). Postural balance is an important prerequisite for independent and successful performance of daily living activities (Prata & Scheicher, 2012) including for instance, stairs negotiations and standing up from a chair (Granacher et al., 2012). With the obligatory aspect of ageing-related decrement in muscular performance and functional capacity, it is increasingly understood that lifestyle, and in particular habitual ambulation/physical activity, may modulate the rate and magnitude of these deleterious changes. For instance, a sedentary lifestyle (participation in activities characterised by an energy expenditure ≤ 1.5 metabolic equivalents and a sitting or reclining posture (Owen, Healy, Matthews, & Dunstan, 2010), has been shown to reduce the functional reserve capacity of older individuals or the excess above that needed for normal functioning. Such reserves are key, as they would normally allow for adaptations and responses to changes in the environment. Older adults aged >65+ years are the most sedentary in society with a sedentary time representing 65–80% of their waking day, with over 8.5 hours of that time spent sitting (Harvey, Chastin, & Skelton, 2015). Arguably, this lifestyle may contribute to elderly individuals being physically weaker, slower and having a reduced motor coordination in comparison to their younger counterparts (Enoka, 1994).

On the other side of the lifestyle spectrum lies physical activity. Participation in regular physical activity elicits a number of favourable responses that are understood to contribute to healthy ageing. Studies show that training counteracts ageing-related postural impairments (Perrin, Gauchard, Perrot, & Jeandel, 1999) by acting on the motor response or on balance sensors (Gauchard, Gangloff, Jeandel, & Perrin, 2003; Howe, Rochester, Neil, Skelton, & Ballinger, 2011). Researchers report that a progressive heavy-resistance training programme combined with explosive types of exercises leads to great gains not only in maximal isometric and dynamic strength but also in explosive force production characteristics of the leg extensor muscles in both middle-aged and elderly men and women (Häkkinen et al., 1998). The strength gains are accompanied by considerable increases in the voluntary neural activation of the agonist muscles in middle-aged and elderly subjects of both genders, with significant reductions taking place in the antagonist co-activation of the maximal extension action in older persons. Such adaptations are key for adequate/steady postural balance maintenance. In parallel, through a systemic review and meta-analysis (Thibaud et al., 2012), it is evident that physical activity in individuals over 60 years acts as a protecting factor against falls. Physically active older people are less at risk of falling (OR of 0.75 [95% CI of 0.64, 0.88]) than those who are physically inactive or sedentary (OR of 1.41 [95% CI of 1.10, 1.82]).

Physical activity and its impact on a key psychological marker: cognitive function

Cognitive function is an essential component of daily living and makes a significant contribution to quality of life (Williams & Kemper, 2010). Human ageing can lead to cognitive decline (Brehmer, Kalpouzos, Wenger, & Lovden, 2014), often termed dementia, and affecting an estimated 36 million people, with Alzheimer's disease being the most common form (Larson, Yaffe, & Langa, 2013). Polypharmacy being an issue with the older person, non-pharmacological interventions that could help individuals maintain their cognitive capacity in older age and reduce levels of morbidity are therefore highly desirable.

There is growing evidence that exercise could protect against ageing-related dementia (Boots et al., 2015; Liu-Ambrose & Donaldson, 2009) as it has been associated with improved cognitive performance especially in tasks involving executive control (Komulainen et al., 2010; Prakash et al., 2011), which are the processes involved in selecting, scheduling and coordinating perception, memory and action (Pontifex, Hillman, Fernhall, Thompson, &

Valentini, 2009). Table 23.2, summarises further research in this area. Similarly, research suggests that higher cardiorespiratory fitness in middle-aged adults correlates with a lower risk of dementia later in life (Defina et al., 2013). In support of this theorem, studies in mice demonstrate that chronic exercise can reduce the risk of Alzheimer's disease, delaying its onset and progression (Cho et al., 2015; García-Mesa et al., 2011; Liu, Zhao, Zhang, & Shi, 2013). Interestingly, a community-based research study links cardiorespiratory fitness response with cognitive gains rather than the exercise dose (i.e., duration) itself (Vidoni et al., 2015).

Several theories have been proposed to explain the mechanisms underlying the exercise–cognition relationship. These include, but are not limited to, reduced levels of homocysteine (Chang, Tsai, Huang, Wang, & Chu, 2014; Garcia, Haron, Pulman, Hua, & Freedman, 2004), increased event-related brain potentials (Kamijo, Nishihira, Higashiura, & Kuroiwa, 2007; Szucs & Soltesz, 2010), the transient hypofrontality theory (Del Giorno, Hall, O'Leary, Bixby, & Miller, 2010; Dietrich, 2006) and increased cerebral blood flow (A.D. Brown et al., 2010; Querido & Sheel, 2007). Whilst it is beyond the scope of this chapter to examine these in detail, the roles of brain-derived neurotrophic factor (BDNF) which is linked with neurogenesis in the brain thus plays an important role in brain plasticity, and insulin-like growth factor 1 (IGF-1) which is linked to protein synthesis stimulation, are arguably key. Exercise is associated with increased BDNF levels (Griffin et al., 2011; Komulainen et al., 2010). This is significant because low levels of BDNF have been linked to Alzheimer's disease. Importantly also, exercise increases IGF-1 concentrations (Chang et al., 2014; Sonntag, Ramsey, & Carter, 2005). This is potentially relevant since lower IGF-1 concentrations correlate with ageing-related cognitive decline (Al-Delaimy, von Muhlen, & Barrett-Connor, 2009; Voss, Nagamatsu, Liu-Ambrose, & Kramer, 2011).

Aerobic exercise and resistance training represent distinct forms of exercise with different physiological and metabolic demands (Pontifex et al., 2009). If interventions to improve cognitive function are to be recommended, it is essential to understand how these exercise modalities affect cognition. It is also important to consider the effect of ageing on the responsiveness of the cognitive function system (Defina et al., 2013).

In recent studies of older persons, cognitive function was positively correlated with fitness (VO_{2max}) in older women aged 50–90 years (A.D. Brown et al., 2010). Similarly, higher fitness levels in older adults are correlated with improved Stroop test performance (Prakash et al., 2011), whereby during an executive function enabling task, irrelevant information or interference is inhibited so that an appropriate response can be selected (Etnier & Chang, 2009). In fact, meta-analytic reviews conclude a positive effect of aerobic exercise on cognition.

A meta-analysis previously concluded that combinations of aerobic exercise and resistance training positively affected cognitive performance in older adults more than aerobic exercise alone (Colcombe & Kramer, 2003). However, studies that directly compare aerobic exercise and resistance training and their effect on cognition are in fact scarce. A study compared the effects of different exercise modalities on cognition among older persons aged 62–95 during a six-month intervention (A.K. Brown, Liu-Ambrose, Tate, & Lord, 2009). Participants were randomly assigned to either a group-exercise programme including twice-weekly resistance training and balance components, a twice-weekly flexibility and relaxation group or a control group. Participants were assessed for several aspects of cognition including fluid intelligence, with the Stroop test used to assess executive function. Executive function did not improve in any of the three groups. Fluid intelligence results increased significantly in the resistance-training group only. Therefore the authors concluded that resistance training and balance exercises could reduce age-related cognitive decline in senior adults. However given that no aerobic

Table 23.2 Summary of studies investigating the effects on cognition of chronic resistance training

Date	Study	Sample population	Intervention period	Cognitive test	Cognitive test outcome
1997	Tsutsumi et al.	Senior adults (Mage = 68 y)	12 weeks	Various tests of executive function	No improvement
2006	Lachman et al.	Senior adults	3 and 6 months	WAIS Backward Digit Span	Improvement
2007	Cassilhas et al.	Senior men (65–75 y)	6 months	Various Tests of Working Memory	Improvement
2008	Liu-Ambrose et al.	Senior adults (over 70 y)	6 months	Stroop Test and Trail Making Test	Improvement
2010	Kimura et al.	Senior adults (over 65 y)	12 weeks	Task-switching Test	No improvement

training was in fact included, this leaves the door open for further research to confirm the contribution of aerobic exercise to cognitive function maintenance in older people.

Evaluation of the impact of the exercise context

Low levels of physical activity and socio-economic status in middle-aged and older adults are associated with poor musculoskeletal, metabolic, cardiovascular and psychological health and this ultimately leads to loss of independent living and quality of life in old age. Interventions designed to increase physical activity levels and promote social interaction, particularly those with either peer-mentor/lifestyle coaches, or an outdoors community-spirited emphasis such as walking groups, should lead to improved health status, owing to longer lasting uptake.

Indoor vs. outdoor exercise prescription

A common reason for an older person to start exercising is to increase their physiologic reserves and hence reduce the risk of frailty. To achieve this, 50 hours of cumulative exercise is needed (Sherrington et al., 2008). In other words, long-term exercise participation is important, but unfortunately not a common habit in older people (World Health Organization, 2007). Although evidence on the (causal nature of the) relationship between the physical setting of exercise and health benefits in older persons is limited (Kerr, Sallis, et al., 2012), there are some clear differences between both settings which may affect the impact and long-term adherence of the exercise behaviour.

Unlike outdoor exercise, an indoor environment allows an older person to exercise in a clean and safe setting all year-round, independent of the weather or season (Hug, Hartig, Hansmann, Seeland, & Hornung, 2009). Additionally, these settings are most often equipped for both resistance and endurance training (Hug et al., 2009). Hence, indoor facilities are likely to be the optimal setting for optimal training in all including the older person. However, indoor exercise also presents a few disadvantages. Firstly, older adults often have vitamin D deficiency which is related to chronic conditions such as cardiovascular disease and bone health (Lauretani, Maggio, Valenti, Dall'Aglio, & Ceda, 2010). Therefore, it is suggested that by going outdoors, older adults may experience physical and mental benefits (e.g. reduced depression) and an improved sense of well-being from a combination of exercise and vitamin D (Buman & King, 2010; Frumkin, 2001; Kerr, Sallis, et al., 2012; Nelson et al., 2007b; St Leger, 2003; Thompson Coon et al., 2011). The fact that exercising outdoors occurs at a higher intensity but with a lower perceived exertion makes it different from indoor exercising, which may influence the beneficial effect of exercise ultimately (Ceci & Hassmén, 1991; Teas, 2007). In addition, poor long-term adherence of exercising indoors is a well-recognised issue (Thompson Coon et al., 2011). Studies have shown that outdoor exercise can have long-term health benefits in older adults (Jacobs et al., 2008; Kono, Kai, Sakato, & Rubenstein, 2004), since engaging in it is an important factor for behavioural maintenance (Hekler et al., 2013; Maas, van Dillen, Verheij, & Groenewegen, 2009). It is suggested that outdoor exercisers may enjoy the exercise more, and perform it for longer and/or more frequently (Maas et al., 2009). For example, previous research shows that over a period of time outdoor exercisers accumulate significantly more minutes of intense exercise than indoor exercisers (Takano, Nakamura, & Watanabe, 2002). The presence of social interaction may play a key role in enjoyment and adherence to exercise (Gladwell, Brown, Wood, Sandercock, & Barton, 2013; Hug et al., 2009; Maas et al., 2009; Takano et al., 2002; Teas et al., 2007). In fact, research suggests that socialising opportunities appear to be more persuasive for persons to engage in exercise sessions than actual health benefits (Schasberger et al., 2009).

Despite the beneficial effects of outdoor exercise for older persons, it may also adversely affect health through exposure to pollutants and a challenging neighbourhood design in a built-outdoor environment (Kerr, Marshall, et al., 2012). The latter may prevent older persons with impaired physical function and fear of falling from engaging in exercising outdoors (Michael, Green, & Farquhar, 2006; Murayama, Yoshie, Sugawara, Wakui, & Arami, 2012; Rantakokko et al., 2009). Therefore, this sub-population would probably benefit with initially engaging in indoor exercise, e.g. to improve lower-extremity physical function and self-confidence, before going outdoors (Kerr, Sallis, et al., 2012). In that case, indoor settings are a viable temporary alternative to outdoors. Moreover, exercising in an appealing and supportive indoor environment may have better psychological effect and adherence than exercising in a busy, and hence perceived as threatening, urban environment (Thompson Coon et al., 2011). Hence, should the benefits of outdoor exercise be conclusively shown to outweigh those of indoor activities, it will become crucial for communities to provide both safe and attractive outdoor exercise locations for older persons (Murayama et al., 2012; Takano et al., 2002). Even further, we would also argue that natural green, rather than built-outdoor environments might be the preferable option, since current evidence suggests that nature-based exercise provides greater physiological and psychological health benefits in adults (Bowler, Buyung-Ali, Knight, & Pullin, 2010; Gladwell et al., 2013; Pretty, Griffin, Sellens, & Pretty, 2003; Thompson Coon et al., 2011). However, it must be noted that subgroups of the population, and in particular the older person, might have different responsiveness to exercising in green spaces (Richardson & Mitchell, 2010). Future research should therefore specifically investigate any age-sensitivity to/preference for, outdoors green environment-based physical activities.

Whilst the duration of participation prior to measureable psycho-physical effects is unclear, based on available literature, outdoor exercise might be preferred for older persons (Figure 23.2), even if outdoor pursuits may not necessarily be accessible/appealing to all (Thompson Coon et al., 2011). Nevertheless, as the older person tends to struggle to achieve optimal

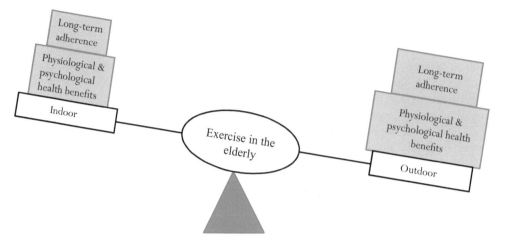

Figure 23.2 A balance representing the overall findings of indoor vs. outdoor exercise in the elderly

levels of activity for a number of intrinsic and extrinsic reasons, any exercise participation is encouraged as it will likely induce health benefits regardless of the physical setting for the exercises (Nelson et al., 2007b).

Energy balance

Energy cannot be created or destroyed, it can only be transformed. Within human physiology, the equation: Energy Stores = Energy Intake (EI) − Energy Expenditure (EE) is commonly used. When EI = EE then body mass is likely to be maintained. EE is comprised of Resting Metabolic Rate (RMR) (60–70% contribution), thermic (8–13% contribution), brown adipose tissue (2–3% contribution) and physical activity (15–30% contribution) (Wilson & Morley, 2003). The RMR of young males (18–33 years) is 1785.6 ± 43.2 kcal·day^{-1} and decreases approximately 3.50% per decade of ageing (69–89 years: 1497.6 ± 28.8 kcal·day^{-1}) (Fukagawa, Bandini, & Young, 1990). This is mainly due to reductions in fat-free mass (FFM) (explaining 82.8% and 45.3% of the variance in young adults' and older adults' RMR, respectively (Bosy-Westphal et al., 2003)). With this decline in RMR, there is a subsequent decline in EI, known as physiological anorexia. Declined RMR can be attenuated with engagement in exercise, and is unlikely to be due to the preservation of dietary intake. Indeed, the difference in dietary intake between pre- and post-menopausal runners is found to be similar to that of pre- and post-menopausal sedentary women (Van Pelt et al., 1997).

With exercise for weight loss, most interventions do not meet the expected weight loss as over half of the groups compensate for the increased EE with increased EI (King, Hopkins, Caudwell, Stubbs, & Blundell, 2008; Thomas et al., 2012). When body mass is broken down into its components, partaking in exercise only (60 mins @ 75% of maximum oxygen utilisation, 5 times a week for 12 weeks) results in a lower reduction in fat mass compared to partaking in a dietary calorie control regime or dieting (500 kcal·day^{-1} reduction) plus exercise (Solomon et al., 2008). More importantly, dieting plus exercise does improve cardiometabolic variables that are associated with cardiovascular disease, by a greater amount compared to dieting or exercise alone. Improving health biomarkers in older adults is more important than weight loss *per se* because increasing BMI is not associated with an increased hazard risk (HR) of three-year follow-up mortality (BMI > 35.0 kg·m⁻² relative to 'healthy' BMI). On the other hand, being underweight (< 18.5 kg·m⁻² BMI relative to a 'healthy' BMI population), the older person may simply be the phenotypic expression of another underlying comorbidity since nearly 50% of this age group reported that weight loss had been unintentional (Locher et al., 2007). In view of the above, it therefore appears that exercise and diet for weight loss should not be the focus in older adults, rather exercise and diet for improved health and physical functioning.

Physical status associated limitations to exercise

Frailty as a limitation to exercise

Currently, there is no consensus on the definition of frailty, though it is acknowledged that it incorporates the degradation of several physiological parameters, increased risk of falling, feelings of vulnerability, and is highly prevalent in older adults (Fried et al., 2001; Viña, Salvador-Pascual, Tarazona-Santabalbina, Rodriguez-Mañas, & Gomez-Cabrera, 2016). Engagement in physical activity, specifically walking and stair climbing, accounts for 30.0% and 20.0% of non-syncopal falls in older adults (Nevitt, Cummings, & Hudes, 1991). Therefore, consideration for the participant's physical limitations is needed prior to a physical activity intervention. Moderate-vigorous physical activity (MVPA, $3.0 - \geq 6.0 \times$ RMR) is the recommended aerobic intensity for health improvements. In the NHANES cohort of older adults (50+ years), an hour a day increase in older adult's MVPA was associated with a 0.045 point (95% CI 0.028, 0.063) reduction in the 46-item frailty index score (possible score range 0–1) (Blodgett, Theou, Kirkland, Andreou, & Rockwood, 2015). However, attaining and maintaining this intensity of physical activity is difficult for older adults. Therefore, a focus towards functional and light-intensity physical activity (LIPA, $1.50–3.00 \times$ RMR) would seem more appropriate. For example, three months thrice weekly, 'posture transition' training (sitting to standing, prone to supine) led to improvements in a physical performance test. These tests comprised placing a book on an overhead shelf, putting on a coat, picking up a penny from the floor, walking 50.0 feet, turning 360°, ascending stairs, rising from a chair, and the Romberg tests (M. Brown et al., 2000) which are all essential movements for daily function. The relationship between LIPA and physical and psychological health is also documented in epidemiology, predicting that the 30 minute substitution of sitting for LIPA can lead to similar improvements compared to MVPA (physical: b 0.46 95%CI 0.37,0.54, b 0.37 95%CI 0.28, 0.46, psychosocial: b 0.24 95%CI 0.12,0.36, b −0.02 95%CI −0.13, 0.10, respectively) (Buman et al., 2010).

Cardiovascular disease and cancer as limitations to exercise

Cardiovascular disease (CVD) mortality, after cancer, is most prevalent in older adults, increasing nearly two-fold per decade of life after the age of 55 (Figure 23.3). Those who already suffer with CVD may be hesitant to participate in physical activity, however the rate of cardiovascular events during supervised exercise is reported to range from 1/50000–1/20000 patient hours of exercise (Franklin, Bonzheim, Gordon, & Timmis, 1998) with evidence to suggest participation will in fact reduce total and cardiac mortality by 27.0% (95%CI −2.00, 40.0) and 31.0% (95%CI −6.00, 49.0), respectively (Jolliffe et al., 2001).

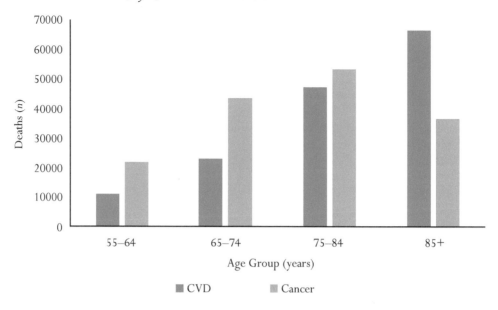

Figure 23.3 The number of CVD and cancer deaths in the United Kingdom for 2014 throughout older age
Source: Adapted from Townsend et al. 2015

The maintenance of physical activity is essential following a cardiac event in older adults as patients who attend more than 24 rehabilitation sessions were 19.0% relatively less likely to die within five years after a cardiac event compared to those with 24 sessions or fewer (Suaya, Stason, Ades, Normand, & Shepard, 2009).

Along with CVD, cancer is one of the greatest causes of mortality in the UK (Townsend, Bhatnagar, Wilkins, Wickramasinghe, & Rayner, 2015). Cancer comes in many forms and therefore it is not possible to recommend the same levels of exercise for everyone. For example, those with immunity cancers should avoid the use of public fitness facilities due to the increased contraction risk of bacterial and viral infections through bodily fluid contact. Cancer and its treatment inflicts psychological distress (e.g. feelings of fatigue, anxiety, depression) and has been the focus of physical activity research. A systematic review by Luctkar-Flude, Groll, Tranmer, and Woodend (2007) found that older adults have reduced feelings of fatigue and improved quality of life when exercise is taken up either during or following cancer treatment. Overall, research into the effects of physical activity on older cancer survivors is limited and requires further investigation (Daum, Cochrane, Fitzgerald, Johnson, & Buford, 2016). For now, the general consensus appears to be similar to that of healthy older adults, interventions should have a focus on functional and quality of life improvement.

Should the diurnal rhythm be a consideration for exercise in the older person?

Skeletal muscle is a highly plastic tissue that readily adapts to changes during and following a loading state (Campos et al., 2002). Increased load imposed on the skeletal muscle elicits adaptations that result in changes in the contractile characteristics of the muscle, ultimately leading to muscle hypertrophy (Hulmi et al., 2009). More specifically, when skeletal muscle is subjected to an overload stimulus, the resultant micro-injuries in the myofibers and extracellular matrix (Hulmi et al., 2009), leads to a chain of myogenic events (Housh, Housh, Johnson, & Chu, 1992). These events culminate in the enlargement of the diameter of individual fibres, thus resulting in an increase in muscle cross sectional area (CSA) and fascicle length, ultimately causing muscle hypertrophy (Seynnes, de Boer, & Narici, 2007).

Research into the different intensities, volume and load used in resistance training allow conclusions to be drawn on what may yield the best results when hypertrophy is the main emphasis for this of training. Researchers examined bodybuilders using a programme involving moderate load (65–75% 1RM), high volume (6–8 reps) with short rest periods (1–2 minutes). Results showed that this produces a greater testosterone response than a high load (> 85% 1RM), low volume with long rest periods (3 minutes) (Kraemer et al., 1991; Kraemer et al., 1990). This type of training has also been shown to illicit the greatest increase in Growth Hormone (GH) response (Kanaley, Weltman, Pieper, Weltman, & Hartman, 2001; Kraemer et al., 1991; Kraemer et al., 1990) which inevitably increases insulin growth factor-1 (IGF-1) secretion allowing for greater protein synthesis (Borst et al., 2001). In addition, GH has mainly anabolic properties which spike after various forms of exercise (Crewther, Keogh, Cronin, & Cook, 2006). Resistance training promotes the increase of GH isoforms allowing for sustained action on target tissues (Ahtiainen, Pakarinen, Alen, Kraemer, & Häkkinen, 2003), as well as enhanced interaction with muscle cell receptors which facilitate exercise recovery and the hypertrophic response (Crewther et al., 2006). The increase in GH is thought to be associated with a concurrent increase in IGF-1, thereby enabling further myogenic promotion (Velloso, 2008). Hormones such as testosterone, cortisol, GH and IGF-1 have been extensively examined as to their role in the muscles' hypertrophic response to resistance training (Fry, 2004; Kraemer & Ratamess, 2005; Schoenfeld, 2013).

Research is pointing to an optimal timing for maximal exercise-induced gains. The premise is that testosterone has considerable anabolic effects, binding with androgen receptors and interacting with DNA, subsequently causing an increase in skeletal muscle cell size (Kraemer & Ratamess, 2005). It can also have indirect effects on protein accretion through the release of GH (Kraemer et al., 1991), as well as promoting satellite cell replication and activation, at least in the first 20 weeks of use (for a review read Kadi, 2008). Data previously identified significant correlations between training-induced increase in testosterone and muscle cross-sectional area (Ahtiainen et al., 2003). Interestingly, data also highlights diurnal variation in testosterone, with a peak between 7 and 9 am (Diver, Imtiaz, Ahmad, Vora, & Fraser, 2003). On the other hand, as cortisol increases protein metabolism, it could be suggested that the reduction of circulating cortisol levels would allow for a greater hypertrophic response, when the timing for exercise is optimised (Burley, Whittingham-Dowd, Allen, Grosset, & Onambele-Pearson, 2016). Cortisol levels peak during the early hours just before awakening with levels progressively decreasing throughout the day, reaching its lowest level between 5 and 7 pm (Kanaley et al., 2001). Whilst exercise results in a decrease in cortisol and greater reductions appear to be prevalent in the morning (Burley et al., 2016; Pledge, Grosset, & Onambele-Pearson, 2011; Sedliak, Finni, Peltonen, & Häkkinen, 2008), interestingly in terms of 'muscle growth promoting' endocrine milieu, the testosterone:cortisol ratio is at its peak in the evening. In view of the above, and in view also of the fact that androgen levels naturally decrease with age (Kaufman & Vermeulen, 2005), some research now associates the diurnal fluctuations in these hormones to an optimisation of training routines, and hence tentatively point to training in the evening as the most favourable endocrine environment (Burley et al., 2016; Teo, Newton, & McGuigan, 2011).

Chapter summary

In summary, the primary aim of increasing physical activity in someone aged over 65 is to improve their health, fitness and quality of life, whilst managing ageing-related co-morbidities and limitations to exercise. To ensure this criterion is achieved, the selection of activities should take a multi-faceted approach through the integration of numerous structured exercise methods. Whilst it is accepted that the gold standard for increasing muscle size and resultant strength is through PRT, both aerobic and balance-focused training should be incorporated into a structured exercise programme alongside PRT, not least for holistic health benefits. However, to ensure adherence and compliance to a structured exercise programme, the focus should be individualised and programmed to fit the specific needs and lifestyle of the individual, taking into account their physical status, group versus lone exercise preferences, including inclination or otherwise for activities in green outdoor spaces. The necessity to conduct conventional structured exercise is less of an issue in over 65s given that leisure-based dance classes are shown to increase both functional fitness and numerous physiological outcome measures.

- The adherence and **palatability** of exercise is an important factor to consider when choosing the correct modality for older individuals.
- The dropout rate from **structured exercise** programmes after 6 months has shown to be as high as 50% in this age group (Hong, Hughes, & Prohaska, 2008; Picorelli et al., 2014).
- When comparing the compliance to, and palatability of, PRT vs. aerobic/endurance training, PRT is reported to be more **retentive** in elderly participants (Hong et al., 2008).
- It is suggested that the **lower impact forces** on joints during PRT compared to aerobic training and hence relatively lower discomfort, especially in participants who had osteoarthritis, may explain this retention (Picorelli et al., 2014).
- Further research should focus on understanding the **key to exercise adherence** in elderly individuals to ensure structured exercise continues for long-term sustainable success
- It is clear that a **holistic approach** (i.e. understanding the individual's physical, social and emotional reasoning for taking up or dropping out) is required in any exercise prescription in the elderly.

References

Ahtiainen, J.P., Pakarinen, A., Alen, M., Kraemer, W.J., & Häkkinen, K. (2003). Muscle hypertrophy, hormonal adaptations and strength development during strength training in strength-trained and untrained men. *European Journal of Applied Physiology, 89*(6), 555–563. doi: 10.1007/s00421-003-0833-3

Al-Delaimy, W.K., von Muhlen, D., & Barrett-Connor, E. (2009). Insulinlike growth factor-1, insulin-like growth factor binding protein-1, and cognitive function in older men and women. *Journal of the American Geriatrics Society, 57*(8), 1441–1446. doi: 10.1111/j.1532-5415.2009.02343.x

Blodgett, J., Theou, O., Kirkland, S., Andreou, P., & Rockwood, K. (2015). The association between sedentary behaviour, moderate–vigorous physical activity and frailty in NHANES cohorts. *Maturitas, 80*(2), 187–191.

Boots, E.A., Schultz, S.A., Oh, J.M., Larson, J., Edwards, D., Cook, D., . . . Okonkwo, O.C. (2015). Cardiorespiratory fitness is associated with brain structure, cognition, and mood in a middle-aged cohort at risk for Alzheimer's disease. *Brain Imaging Behav, 9*(3), 639–649. doi: 10.1007/s11682-014-9325-9

Borst, S.E., De Hoyos, D.V., Garzarella, L., Vincent, K., Pollock, B.H., Lowenthal, D.T., & Pollock, M.L. (2001). Effects of resistance training on insulin-like growth factor-I and IGF binding proteins. *Medicine and Science in Sports and Exercise, 33*(4), 648–653.

Bosy-Westphal, A., Eichhorn, C., Kutzner, D., Illner, K., Heller, M., & Müller, M.J. (2003). The age-related decline in resting energy expenditure in humans is due to the loss of fat-free mass and to alterations in its metabolically active components. *The Journal of Nutrition, 133*(7), 2356–2362.

Bowler, D.E., Buyung-Ali, L.M., Knight, T.M., & Pullin, A.S. (2010). A systematic review of evidence for the added benefits to health of exposure to natural environments. *BMC Public Health, 10*, 456. doi: 10.1186/1471-2458-10-456

Brehmer, Y., Kalpouzos, G., Wenger, E., & Lovden, M. (2014). Plasticity of brain and cognition in older adults. *Psychol Res, 78*(6), 790–802. doi: 10.1007/s00426-014-0587-z

Brown, A.D., McMorris, C.A., Longman, R.S., Leigh, R., Hill, M.D., Friedenreich, C.M., & Poulin, M.J. (2010). Effects of cardiorespiratory fitness and cerebral blood flow on cognitive outcomes in older women. *Neurobiology of Aging, 31*(12), 2047–2057. doi: 10.1016/j.neurobiolaging.2008.11.002

Brown, A.K., Liu-Ambrose, T., Tate, R., & Lord, S.R. (2009). The effect of group-based exercise on cognitive performance and mood in seniors residing in intermediate care and self-care retirement facilities: a randomised controlled trial. *British Journal of Sports Medicine, 43*(8), 608–614. doi: 10.1136/bjsm.2008.049882

Brown, M., Sinacore, D.R., Ehsani, A.A., Binder, E.F., Holloszy, J.O., & Kohrt, W.M. (2000). Low-intensity exercise as a modifier of physical frailty in older adults. *Archives of Physical Medicine and Rehabilitation, 81*(7), 960–965.

Bull, F.C., & the Expert Working Group. (2010). *Physical activity guidelines in the U.K.: review and recommendations.* Loughborough University.

Buman, M.P., Hekler, E.B., Haskell, W.L., Pruitt, L., Conway, T.L., Cain, K.L., . . . King, A.C. (2010). Objective light-intensity physical activity associations with rated health in older adults. *American Journal of Epidemiology, 172*(10), 1155–1165.

Buman, M.P., & King, A.C. (2010). Exercise as a treatment to enhance sleep. *American Journal of Lifestyle Medicine, 4*, 500–514. doi: 10.1177/1559827610375532

Burley, S.D., Whittingham-Dowd, J., Allen, J., Grosset, J.F., & Onambele-Pearson, G.L. (2016). The differential hormonal milieu of morning versus evening may have an impact on muscle hypertrophic potential. *PLoS ONE, 11*(9), e0161500. doi: 10.1371/journal.pone.0161500

Cadore, E.L., Pinto, R.S., Bottaro, M., & Izquierdo, M. (2014). Strength and endurance training prescription in healthy and frail elderly. *Aging Dis, 5*(3), 183–195. doi: 10.14336/AD.2014.0500183

Campos, G.E., Luecke, T.J., Wendeln, H.K., Toma, K., Hagerman, F.C., Murray, T.F., . . . Staron, R.S. (2002). Muscular adaptations in response to three different resistance-training regimens: specificity of repetition maximum training zones. *European Journal of Applied Physiology, 88*(1–2), 50–60. doi: 10.1007/s00421-002-0681-6

Caspersen, C.J., Powell, K.E., & Christenson, G.M. (1985). Physical activity, exercise, and physical fitness: definitions and distinctions for health-related research. *Public Health Rep, 100*(2), 126–131.

Cassilhas, R.C., Viana, V.A., Grassmann, V., Santos, R.T., Santos, R.F., Tufik, S., & Mello, M.T. (2007). The impact of resistance exercise on the cognitive function of the elderly. *Medicine and Science in Sports and Exercise, 39*, 1401–1407. doi:10.1249/ mss.0b013e318060111f

Ceci, R., & Hassmén, P. (1991). Self-monitored exercise at three different RPE intensities in treadmill vs field running. *Medicine and Science in Sports and Exercise, 23*, 732–738.

Chang, Y.K., Tsai, C.L., Huang, C.C., Wang, C.C., & Chu, I.H. (2014). Effects of acute resistance exercise on cognition in late middle-aged adults: general or specific cognitive improvement? *Journal of Science and Medicine in Sport/Sports Medicine Australia, 17*(1), 51–55. doi: 10.1016/j.jsams.2013.02.007

Cho, J., Shin, M.K., Kim, D., Lee, I., Kim, S., & Kang, H. (2015). Treadmill running reverses cognitive declines due to Alzheimer disease. *Medicine and Science in Sports and Exercise, 47*(9), 1814–1824. doi: 10.1249/MSS.0000000000000612

Colcombe, S., & Kramer, A.F. (2003). Fitness effects on the cognitive function of older adults: a meta-analytic study. *Psychol Sci, 14*(2), 125–130. doi: 10.1111/1467-9280.t01-1-01430

Crewther, B., Keogh, J., Cronin, J., & Cook, C. (2006). Possible stimuli for strength and power adaptation: acute hormonal responses. *Sports Medicine, 36*(3), 215–238.

Daum, C., Cochrane, S., Fitzgerald, J., Johnson, L., & Buford, T. (2016). Exercise interventions for preserving physical function among cancer survivors in middle to late life. *The Journal of Frailty & Aging, 5*(4), 214.

Defina, L.F., Willis, B.L., Radford, N.B., Gao, A., Leonard, D., Haskell, W.L., . . . Berry, J.D. (2013). The association between midlife cardiorespiratory fitness levels and later-life dementia: a cohort study. *Annals of Internal Medicine, 158*(3), 162–168. doi: 10.7326/0003-4819-158-3-201302050-00005

Del Giorno, J.M., Hall, E.E., O'Leary, K.C., Bixby, W.R., & Miller, P.C. (2010). Cognitive function during acute exercise: a test of the transient hypofrontality theory. *J Sport Exerc Psychol, 32*(3), 312–323.

Dietrich, A. (2006). Transient hypofrontality as a mechanism for the psychological effects of exercise. *Psychiatry Res, 145*(1), 79–83. doi: 10.1016/j.psychres.2005.07.033

Diver, M.J., Imtiaz, K.E., Ahmad, A.M., Vora, J.P., & Fraser, W.D. (2003). Diurnal rhythms of serum total, free and bioavailable testosterone and of SHBG in middle-aged men compared with those in young men. *Clin Endocrinol* (Oxf), *58*(6), 710–717.

Emerenziani, G.P., Gallotta, M.C., Meucci, M., Di Luigi, L., Migliaccio, S., Donini, L.M., . . . Guidetti, L. (2015). Effects of aerobic exercise based upon heart rate at aerobic threshold in obese elderly subjects with type 2 diabetes. *Int J Endocrinol, 2015*, 695297. doi: 10.1155/2015/695297

Enoka, R.M. (1994). *Neuromechanical basis of kinesiology* (2nd ed.): Human Kinetics.

Etnier, J.L., & Chang, Y.K. (2009). The effect of physical activity on executive function: a brief commentary on definitions, measurement issues, and the current state of the literature. *J Sport Exerc Psychol, 31*(4), 469–483.

Fahlman, M.M., McNevin, N., Boardley, D., Morgan, A., & Topp, R. (2011). Effects of resistance training on functional ability in elderly individuals. *Am J Health Promot, 25*(4), 237–243. doi: 10.4278/ajhp.081125-QUAN-292

Farrell, L., Hollingsworth, B., Propper, C., & Shields, M.A. (2013). The socioeconomic gradient in physical inactivity in England. Centre for Market and Public Organisation: University of Bristol.

Franklin, B.A., Bonzheim, K., Gordon, S., & Timmis, G.C. (1998). Safety of medically supervised outpatient cardiac rehabilitation exercise therapy: a 16-year follow-up. *Chest, 114*(3), 902–906.

Fried, L.P., Tangen, C.M., Walston, J., Newman, A.B., Hirsch, C., Gottdiener, J., . . . Burke, G. (2001). Frailty in older adults evidence for a phenotype. *The Journals of Gerontology Series A: Biological Sciences and Medical Sciences, 56*(3), M146–M157.

Frumkin, H. (2001). Beyond toxicity: human health and the natural environment. *Am J Prev Med, 20*, 234–240.

Fry, A.C. (2004). The role of resistance exercise intensity on muscle fibre adaptations. *Sports Medicine, 34*(10), 663–679.

Fukagawa, N.K., Bandini, L.G., & Young, J.B. (1990). Effect of age on body composition and resting metabolic rate. *American Journal of Physiology-Endocrinology And Metabolism, 259*(2), E233–E238.

Garcia, A., Haron, Y., Pulman, K., Hua, L., & Freedman, M. (2004). Increases in homocysteine are related to worsening of stroop scores in healthy elderly persons: a prospective follow-up study. *J Gerontol A Biol Sci Med Sci, 59*(12), 1323–1327.

García-Mesa, Y., López-Ramos, J.C., Giménez-Llort, L., Revilla, S., Guerra, R., Gruart, A., . . . Sanfeliu, C. (2011). Physical exercise protects against Alzheimer's disease in 3xTg-AD mice. *J Alzheimers Dis, 24*(3), 421–454. doi: 10.3233/JAD-2011-101635

Gauchard, G.C., Gangloff, P., Jeandel, C., & Perrin, P.P. (2003). Influence of regular proprioceptive and bioenergetic physical activities on balance control in elderly women. *J Gerontol A Biol Sci Med Sci, 58*(9), M846–850.

Geremia, J.M., Iskiewicz, M.M., Marschner, R.A., Lehnen, T.E., & Lehnen, A.M. (2015). Effect of a physical training program using the Pilates method on flexibility in elderly subjects. *Age, 37*(6), 119. doi: 10.1007/s11357-015-9856-z

Gladwell, V.F., Brown, D.K., Wood, C., Sandercock, G.R., & Barton, J.L. (2013). The great outdoors: how a green exercise environment can benefit all. *Extreme Physiology & Medicine, 2*, 3. doi: 10.1186/2046-7648-2-3

Grabara, M., & Szopa, J. (2015). Effects of hatha yoga exercises on spine flexibility in women over 50 years old. *J Phys Ther Sci, 27*(2), 361–365. doi: 10.1589/jpts.27.361

Granacher, U., Muehlbauer, T., & Gruber, M. (2012). A qualitative review of balance and strength performance in healthy older adults: impact for testing and training. *Journal of Aging Research, 2012*, 708905. doi: 10.1155/2012/708905

Greiwe, J.S., Cheng, B., Rubin, D.C., Yarasheski, K.E., & Semenkovich, C.F. (2001). Resistance exercise decreases skeletal muscle tumor necrosis factor alpha in frail elderly humans. *FASEB Journal: Official Publication of the Federation of American Societies for Experimental Biology, 15*(2), 475–482. doi: 10.1096/fj.00-0274com

Griffin, E.W., Mullally, S., Foley, C., Warmington, S.A., O'Mara, S.M., & Kelly, A.M. (2011). Aerobic exercise improves hippocampal function and increases BDNF in the serum of young adult males. *Physiol Behav, 104*(5), 934–941. doi: 10.1016/j.physbeh.2011.06.005

Häkkinen, K., Newton, R.U., Gordon, S.E., McCormick, M., Volek, J.S., Nindl, B.C., . . . Kraemer, W.J. (1998). Changes in muscle morphology, electromyographic activity, and force production characteristics during progressive strength training in young and older men. *J Gerontol A Biol Sci Med Sci, 53*(6), B415–423.

Harridge, S.D., Kryger, A., & Stensgaard, A. (1999). Knee extensor strength, activation, and size in very elderly people following strength training. *Muscle Nerve, 22*(7), 831–839.

Harvey, J.A., Chastin, S.F., & Skelton, D.A. (2015). How sedentary are older people? A systematic review of the amount of sedentary behavior. *Journal of Aging and Physical Activity, 23*(3), 471–487. doi: 10.1123/japa.2014-0164

Hekler, E.B., Buman, M.P., Poothakandiyil, N., Rivera, D.E., Dzierzewski, J.M., Morgan, A.A., . . . Giacobbi, P.R. (2013). Exploring behavioral markers of long-term physical activity maintenance: a case study of system identification modeling within a behavioral intervention. *Health Education & Behavior: The Official Publication of the Society for Public Health Education, 40*, 51S–62S. doi: 10.1177/1090198113496787

Henwood, T.R., & Taaffe, D.R. (2005). Improved physical performance in older adults undertaking a short-term programme of high-velocity resistance training. *Gerontology, 51*(2), 108–115. doi: 10.1159/000082195

Holloszy, J.O., & Coyle, E.F. (1984). Adaptations of skeletal muscle to endurance exercise and their metabolic consequences. *J Appl Physiol Respir Environ Exerc Physiol, 56*(4), 831–838.

Hong, S.Y., Hughes, S., & Prohaska, T. (2008). Factors affecting exercise attendance and completion in sedentary older adults: a meta-analytic approach. *J Phys Act Health, 5*(3), 385–397.

Hopkins, D.R., Murrah, B., Hoeger, W. W., & Rhodes, R.C. (1990). Effect of low-impact aerobic dance on the functional fitness of elderly women. *Gerontologist, 30*(2), 189–192.

Housh, D.J., Housh, T.J., Johnson, G.O., & Chu, W.K. (1992). Hypertrophic response to unilateral concentric isokinetic resistance training. *Journal of Applied Physiology, 73*(1), 65–70.

Howald, H., Hoppeler, H., Claassen, H., Mathieu, O., & Straub, R. (1985). Influences of endurance training on the ultrastructural composition of the different muscle fiber types in humans. *Pflugers Archiv: European Journal of Physiology, 403*(4), 369–376.

Howe, T.E., Rochester, L., Neil, F., Skelton, D.A., & Ballinger, C. (2011). Exercise for improving balance in older people. *Cochrane Database Syst Rev, (11)*, CD004963. doi: 10.1002/14651858. CD004963.pub3

Hug, S.-M., Hartig, T., Hansmann, R., Seeland, K., & Hornung, R. (2009). Restorative qualities of indoor and outdoor exercise settings as predictors of exercise frequency. *Health & Place, 15*, 971–980. doi: 10.1016/j.healthplace.2009.03.002

Hulmi, J.J., Kovanen, V., Selanne, H., Kraemer, W.J., Häkkinen, K., & Mero, A.A. (2009). Acute and long-term effects of resistance exercise with or without protein ingestion on muscle hypertrophy and gene expression. *Amino Acids, 37*(2), 297–308. doi: 10.1007/s00726-008-0150-6

Iversen, N., Krustrup, P., Rasmussen, H.N., Rasmussen, U.F., Saltin, B., & Pilegaard, H. (2011). Mitochondrial biogenesis and angiogenesis in skeletal muscle of the elderly. *Experimental Gerontology, 46*(8), 670–678. doi: 10.1016/j.exger.2011.03.004

Jacobs, J.M., Cohen, A., Hammerman-Rozenberg, R., Azoulay, D., Maaravi, Y., & Stessman, J. (2008). Going outdoors daily predicts long-term functional and health benefits among ambulatory older people. *J Aging Health, 20*, 259–272. doi: 10.1177/0898264308315427

Jolliffe, J., Rees, K., Taylor, R.R., Thompson, D.R., Oldridge, N., & Ebrahim, S. (2001). Exercise-based rehabilitation for coronary heart disease. *The Cochrane Library*.

Kadi, F. (2008). Cellular and molecular mechanisms responsible for the action of testosterone on human skeletal muscle. A basis for illegal performance enhancement. *Br J Pharmacol, 154*(3), 522–528. doi: 10.1038/bjp.2008.118

Kamijo, K., Nishihira, Y., Higashiura, T., & Kuroiwa, K. (2007). The interactive effect of exercise intensity and task difficulty on human cognitive processing. *Int J Psychophysiol, 65*(2), 114–121. doi: 10.1016/j.ijpsycho.2007.04.001

Kanaley, J.A., Weltman, J.Y., Pieper, K.S., Weltman, A., & Hartman, M.L. (2001). Cortisol and growth hormone responses to exercise at different times of day. *The Journal of Clinical Endocrinology and Metabolism, 86*(6), 2881–2889. doi: 10.1210/jcem.86.6.7566

Kaufman, J.M., & Vermeulen, A. (2005). The decline of androgen levels in elderly men and its clinical and therapeutic implications. *Endocr Rev, 26*(6), 833–876. doi: 10.1210/er.2004-0013

Kerr, J., Marshall, S., Godbole, S., Neukam, S., Crist, K., Wasilenko, K., . . . Buchner, D. (2012). The relationship between outdoor activity and health in older adults using GPS. *International Journal of Environmental Research and Public Health, 9*, 4615–4625.

Kerr, J., Sallis, J.F., Saelens, B.E., Cain, K.L., Conway, T.L., Frank, L.D., & King, A.C. (2012). Outdoor physical activity and self rated health in older adults living in two regions of the U.S. *Int J Behav Nutr Phys Act, 9*, 89. doi: 10.1186/1479-5868-9-89

Kimura, K., Obuchi, S., Arai, T., Nagasawa, H., Shiba, Y., Watanabe, S., & Kojima, M. (2010). The influence of short-term strength training on health-related quality of life and executive cognitive function. *Journal of Physiological Anthropology, 29*, 95–101. doi:10.2114/jpa2.29.95

King, N.A., Hopkins, M., Caudwell, P., Stubbs, R., & Blundell, J.E. (2008). Individual variability following 12 weeks of supervised exercise: identification and characterization of compensation for exercise-induced weight loss. *International Journal of Obesity, 32*(1), 177–184.

Kolber, M.J., Beekhuizen, K.S., Cheng, M.S., & Hellman, M.A. (2010). Shoulder injuries attributed to resistance training: a brief review. *Journal of Strength and Conditioning Research / National Strength & Conditioning Association, 24*(6), 1696–1704. doi: 10.1519/JSC.0b013e3181dc4330

Komulainen, P., Kivipelto, M., Lakka, T.A., Savonen, K., Hassinen, M., Kiviniemi, V., . . . Rauramaa, R. (2010). Exercise, fitness and cognition – A randomised controlled trial in older individuals: The DR's EXTRA study. *European Geriatric Medicine, 1*(5), 266–272.

Kono, A., Kai, I., Sakato, C., & Rubenstein, L.Z. (2004). Frequency of going outdoors: a predictor of functional and psychosocial change among ambulatory frail elders living at home. *J Gerontol A Biol Sci Med Sci, 59*, 275–280.

Kraemer, W.J., Gordon, S.E., Fleck, S.J., Marchitelli, L.J., Mello, R., Dziados, J.E., . . . Fry, A.C. (1991). Endogenous anabolic hormonal and growth factor responses to heavy resistance exercise in males and females. *International Journal of Sports Medicine, 12*(2), 228–235. doi: 10.1055/s-2007-1024673

Kraemer, W.J., Marchitelli, L., Gordon, S.E., Harman, E., Dziados, J.E., Mello, R., . . . Fleck, S.J. (1990). Hormonal and growth factor responses to heavy resistance exercise protocols. *Journal of Applied Physiology, 69*(4), 1442–1450.

Kraemer, W.J., & Ratamess, N.A. (2005). Hormonal responses and adaptations to resistance exercise and training. *Sports Medicine, 35*(4), 339–361.

Lachman, M.E., Neupert, S.D., Bertrand, R. and Jette, A.M. (2006) The effects of strength training on memory in older adults. *J Aging Phys Act, 14*(1), pp. 59–73.

Larson, E.B., Yaffe, K., & Langa, K.M. (2013). New insights into the dementia epidemic. *N Engl J Med, 369*(24), 2275–2277. doi: 10.1056/NEJMp1311405

Lauretani, F., Maggio, M., Valenti, G., Dall'Aglio, E., & Ceda, G.P. (2010). Vitamin D in older population: new roles for this 'classic actor'? *The Aging Male: The Official Journal of the International Society for the Study of the Aging Male, 13*, 215–232. doi: 10.3109/13685538.2010.487551

Liu, H.L., Zhao, G., Zhang, H., & Shi, L.D. (2013). Long-term treadmill exercise inhibits the progression of Alzheimer's disease-like neuropathology in the hippocampus of APP/PS1 transgenic mice. *Behav Brain Res, 256*, 261–272. doi: 10.1016/j.bbr.2013.08.008

Liu-Ambrose, T., & Donaldson, M.G. (2009). Exercise and cognition in older adults: is there a role for resistance training programmes? *British Journal of Sports Medicine, 43*(1), 25–27. doi: 10.1136/bjsm.2008.055616

Liu-Ambrose, T., Donaldson, M.G., Ahamed, Y., Graf, P., Cook, W.L., Close, J., . . . Khan, K. (2008). Otago home-based strength and balance retraining improves executive functioning in older fallers: a randomized controlled trial. *Journal of the American Geriatrics Society, 56*, 1821–1830. doi:10.1111/j.1532-5415.2008.01931.x

Locher, J.L., Roth, D.L., Ritchie, C.S., Cox, K., Sawyer, P., Bodner, E.V., & Allman, R.M. (2007). Body mass index, weight loss, and mortality in community-dwelling older adults. *The Journals of Gerontology Series A: Biological Sciences and Medical Sciences, 62*(12), 1389–1392.

Luctkar-Flude, M.F., Groll, D.L., Tranmer, J.E., & Woodend, K. (2007). Fatigue and physical activity in older adults with cancer: a systematic review of the literature. *Cancer Nursing, 30*(5), E35–E45.

Maas, J., van Dillen, S.M.E., Verheij, R.A., & Groenewegen, P.P. (2009). Social contacts as a possible mechanism behind the relation between green space and health. *Health & Place, 15*, 586–595. doi: 10.1016/j.healthplace.2008.09.006

Maki, B.E., Holliday, P.J., & Topper, A.K. (1994). A prospective study of postural balance and risk of falling in an ambulatory and independent elderly population. *Journal of Gerontology, 49*(2), M72–84.

Michael, Y.L., Green, M.K., & Farquhar, S.A. (2006). Neighborhood design and active aging. *Health & Place, 12*, 734–740. doi: 10.1016/j.healthplace.2005.08.002

Morse, C.I., Thom, J.M., Mian, O.S., Birch, K.M., & Narici, M.V. (2007). Gastrocnemius specific force is increased in elderly males following a 12-month physical training programme. *Eur J Appl Physiol, 100*(5), 563–570. doi: 10.1007/s00421-006-0246-1

Morse, C.I., Thom, J.M., Mian, O.S., Muirhead, A., Birch, K.M., & Narici, M.V. (2005). Muscle strength, volume and activation following 12-month resistance training in 70-year-old males. *European Journal of Applied Physiology, 95*(2–3), 197–204. doi: 10.1007/s00421-005-1342-3

Murayama, H., Yoshie, S., Sugawara, I., Wakui, T., & Arami, R. (2012). Contextual effect of neighborhood environment on homebound elderly in a Japanese community. *Arch Gerontol Geriatr, 54*, 67–71. doi: 10.1016/j.archger.2011.03.016

Nelson, M.E., Fiatarone, M.A., Morganti, C.M., Trice, I., Greenberg, R.A., & Evans, W.J. (1994). Effects of high-intensity strength training on multiple risk factors for osteoporotic fractures. A randomized controlled trial. *JAMA, 272*(24), 1909–1914.

Nelson, M.E., Rejeski, W.J., Blair, S.N., Duncan, P.W., Judge, J.O., King, A.C., . . . Castaneda-Sceppa, C. (2007a). Physical activity and public health in older adults: recommendation from the American College of Sports Medicine and the American Heart Association. *Medicine and Science in Sports and Exercise, 39*(8), 1435–1445. doi: 10.1249/mss.0b013e3180616aa2

Nelson, M.E., Rejeski, W.J., Blair, S.N., Duncan, P.W., Judge, J.O., King, A.C., . . . Castaneda-Sceppa, C. (2007b). Physical activity and public health in older adults: recommendation from the American College of Sports Medicine and the American Heart Association. *Medicine and Science in Sports and Exercise, 39*(8), 1435–1445. doi:10.1249/mss.0b013e3180616aa2

Nevitt, M.C., Cummings, S.R., & Hudes, E.S. (1991). Risk factors for injurious falls: a prospective study. *Journal of Gerontology, 46*(5), M164–M170.

Onambele-Pearson, G.L., Breen, L., & Stewart, C.E. (2010a). Influence of exercise intensity in older persons with unchanged habitual nutritional intake: skeletal muscle and endocrine adaptations. *Age, 32*(2), 139–153. doi: 10.1007/s11357-010-9141-0

Onambele-Pearson, G.L., Breen, L., & Stewart, C.E. (2010b). Influences of carbohydrate plus amino acid supplementation on differing exercise intensity adaptations in older persons: skeletal muscle and endocrine responses. *Age, 32*(2), 125–138. doi: 10.1007/s11357-009-9129-9

Onambele-Pearson, G.L., & Pearson, S.J. (2012). The magnitude and character of resistance-training-induced increase in tendon stiffness at old age is gender specific. *Age, 34*(2), 427–438. doi: 10.1007/s11357-011-9248-y

Onambele, G.L., Maganaris, C.N., Mian, O.S., Tam, E., Rejc, E., McEwan, I.M., & Narici, M.V. (2008). Neuromuscular and balance responses to flywheel inertial versus weight training in older persons. *Journal of Biomechanics, 41*(15), 3133–3138. doi: 10.1016/j.jbiomech.2008.09.004

Owen, N., Healy, G.N., Matthews, C.E., & Dunstan, D.W. (2010). Too much sitting: the population health science of sedentary behavior. *Exercise and Sport Sciences Reviews, 38*(3), 105–113. doi: 10.1097/JES.0b013e3181e373a2

Palatini, P. (1988). Blood pressure behaviour during physical activity. *Sports Medicine, 5*(6), 353–374.

Perrin, P.P., Gauchard, G.C., Perrot, C., & Jeandel, C. (1999). Effects of physical and sporting activities on balance control in elderly people. *British Journal of Sports Medicine, 33*(2), 121–126.

Picorelli, A.M., Pereira, D.S., Felicio, D.C., Dos Anjos, D.M., Pereira, D.A., Dias, R.C., . . . Pereira, L.S. (2014). Adherence of older women with strength training and aerobic exercise. *Clinical Interventions in Aging, 9*, 323–331. doi: 10.2147/CIA.S54644

Piirtola, M., & Era, P. (2006). Force platform measurements as predictors of falls among older people – a review. *Gerontology, 52*(1), 1–16. doi: 10.1159/000089820

Pledge, D., Grosset, J.F., & Onambele-Pearson, G.L. (2011). Is there a morning-to-evening difference in the acute IL-6 and cortisol responses to resistance exercise? *Cytokine, 55*(2), 318–323. doi: 10.1016/j.cyto.2011.05.005

Pontifex, M.B., Hillman, C.H., Fernhall, B., Thompson, K.M., & Valentini, T.A. (2009). The effect of acute aerobic and resistance exercise on working memory. *Medicine and Science in Sports and Exercise, 41*(4), 927–934. doi: 10.1249/MSS.0b013e3181907d69

Prakash, R.S., Voss, M.W., Erickson, K.I., Lewis, J.M., Chaddock, L., Malkowski, E., . . . Kramer, A.F. (2011). Cardiorespiratory fitness and attentional control in the aging brain. *Front Hum Neurosci, 4*, 229. doi: 10.3389/fnhum.2010.00229

Prata, M.G., & Scheicher, M.E. (2012). Correlation between balance and the level of functional independence among elderly people. *Sao Paulo Med J, 130*(2), 97–101.

Prestes, J., Shiguemoto, G., Botero, J.P., Frollini, A., Dias, R., Leite, R., . . . Perez, S. (2009). Effects of resistance training on resistin, leptin, cytokines, and muscle force in elderly post-menopausal women. *J Sports Sci, 27*(14), 1607–1615. doi: 10.1080/02640410903352923

Pretty, J., Griffin, M., Sellens, M., & Pretty, C. (2003). *Green Exercise: Complementary Roles of Nature, Exercise and Diet in Physical and Emotional Well-being and Implications for Public Health Policy, 1.*

Querido, J.S., & Sheel, A.W. (2007). Regulation of cerebral blood flow during exercise. *Sports Medicine, 37*(9), 765–782.

Rantakokko, M., Mänty, M., Iwarsson, S., Törmäkangas, T., Leinonen, R., Heikkinen, E., & Rantanen, T. (2009). Fear of moving outdoors and development of outdoor walking difficulty in older people. *Journal of the American Geriatrics Society, 57*, 634–640. doi: 10.1111/j.1532-5415.2009.02180.x

Raudsepp, L. (2006). The relationship between socio-economic status, parental support and adolescent physical activity. *Acta Pædiatrica, 95*, 93–98.

Reeves, N.D., Narici, M.V., & Maganaris, C.N. (2003). Strength training alters the viscoelastic properties of tendons in elderly humans. *Muscle Nerve, 28*(1), 74–81. doi: 10.1002/mus.10392

Richardson, E.A., & Mitchell, R. (2010). Gender differences in relationships between urban green space and health in the United Kingdom. *Social Science & Medicine, 71*, 568–575. doi: 10.1016/j.socscimed.2010.04.015

Rubenstein, L.Z. (2006). Falls in older people: epidemiology, risk factors and strategies for prevention. *Age Ageing, 35 Suppl 2*, ii37–ii41. doi: 10.1093/ageing/afl084

Rubenstein, L.Z., & Josephson, K.R. (2002). The epidemiology of falls and syncope. *Clinics in Geriatric Medicine, 18*(2), 141–158.

Santos, M.P., Esculcas, C., & Mota, J. (2004). The relationship between socioeconomic status and adolescents' organized and nonorganized physical activities. *Ped Exerc Sci, 16*, 210–218.

Schasberger, M.G., Hussa, C.S., Polgar, M.F., McMonagle, J.A., Burke, S.J., & Gegaris, A.J. (2009). Promoting and developing a trail network across suburban, rural, and urban communities. *Am J Prev Med, 37*, S336–344. doi: 10.1016/j.amepre.2009.09.012

Schmid, A.A., Van Puymbroeck, M., & Koceja, D.M. (2010). Effect of a 12-week yoga intervention on fear of falling and balance in older adults: a pilot study. *Arch Phys Med Rehabil, 91*(4), 576–583. doi: 10.1016/j.apmr.2009.12.018

Schoenfeld, B.J. (2013). Postexercise hypertrophic adaptations: a reexamination of the hormone hypothesis and its applicability to resistance training program design. *Journal of Strength and Conditioning Research/National Strength & Conditioning Association, 27*(6), 1720–1730. doi: 10.1519/JSC.0b013e31828ddd53

Sedliak, M., Finni, T., Peltonen, J., & Häkkinen, K. (2008). Effect of time-of-day-specific strength training on maximum strength and EMG activity of the leg extensors in men. *J Sports Sci, 26*(10), 1005–1014. doi: 10.1080/02640410801930150

Serra, M.M., Alonso, A.C., Peterson, M., Mochizuki, L., Greve, J.M., & Garcez-Leme, L.E. (2016). Balance and muscle strength in elderly women who dance samba. *PLoS ONE, 11*(12), e0166105. doi: 10.1371/journal.pone.0166105

Seynnes, O.R., de Boer, M., & Narici, M.V. (2007). Early skeletal muscle hypertrophy and architectural changes in response to high-intensity resistance training. *Journal of Applied Physiology, 102*(1), 368–373. doi: 10.1152/japplphysiol.00789.2006

Sherrington, C., Whitney, J.C., Lord, S.R., Herbert, R.D., Cumming, R.G., & Close, J.C.T. (2008). Effective exercise for the prevention of falls: a systematic review and meta-analysis. *Journal of the American Geriatrics Society, 56*, 2234–2243. doi: 10.1111/j.1532-5415.2008.02014.x

Solomon, T.P., Sistrun, S.N., Krishnan, R.K., Del Aguila, L.F., Marchetti, C.M., O'Carroll, S.M., . . . Kirwan, J.P. (2008). Exercise and diet enhance fat oxidation and reduce insulin resistance in older obese adults. *Journal of Applied Physiology, 104*(5), 1313–1319.

Sonntag, W.E., Ramsey, M., & Carter, C.S. (2005). Growth hormone and insulin-like growth factor-1 (IGF-1) and their influence on cognitive aging. *Ageing Research Reviews, 4*(2), 195–212. doi: 10.1016/j.arr.2005.02.001

St Leger, L. (2003). Health and nature – new challenges for health promotion. *Health Promotion International, 18*, 173–175.

Suaya, J.A., Stason, W.B., Ades, P.A., Normand, S.-L.T., & Shepard, D.S. (2009). Cardiac rehabilitation and survival in older coronary patients. *Journal of the American College of Cardiology, 54*(1), 25–33.

Szucs, D., & Soltesz, F. (2010). Stimulus and response conflict in the color-word Stroop task: a combined electro-myography and event-related potential study. *Brain Res, 1325*, 63–76. doi: 10.1016/j.brainres.2010.02.011

Taaffe, D.R., Pruitt, L., Pyka, G., Guido, D., & Marcus, R. (1996). Comparative effects of high- and low-intensity resistance training on thigh muscle strength, fiber area, and tissue composition in elderly women. *Clin Physiol, 16*(4), 381–392.

Takano, T., Nakamura, K., & Watanabe, M. (2002). Urban residential environments and senior citizens' longevity in megacity areas: the importance of walkable green spaces. *Journal of Epidemiology and Community Health, 56*, 913–918.

Taylor, D., Hale, L., Schluter, P., Waters, D.L., Binns, E.E., McCracken, H., . . .Wolf, S. L. (2012). Effectiveness of tai chi as a community-based falls prevention intervention: a randomized controlled trial. *Journal of the American Geriatrics Society, 60*(5), 841–848. doi: 10.1111/j.1532-5415.2012.03928.x

Teas, J., Hurley, T., Ghumare, S., & Ogoussan, K. (2007). Walking outside improves mood for healthy postmenopausal women. *Clinical Medicine Insights. Oncology, 1*, 35–43.

Teo, W., Newton, M.J., & McGuigan, M.R. (2011). Circadian rhythms in exercise performance: implications for hormonal and muscular adaptation. *J Sports Sci Med, 10*(4), 600–606.

Thibaud, M., Bloch, F., Tournoux-Facon, C., Brèque, C., Rigaud, A.S., Dugué, B., & Kemoun, G. (2012). Impact of physical activity and sedentary behaviour on fall risks in older people: a systematic review and meta-analysis of observational studies. *Eur Rev Aging Phys Act, 9*(1), 5–15. doi: 10.1007/s11556-011-0081-1

Thomas, D., Bouchard, C., Church, T., Slentz, C., Kraus, W., Redman, L., . . . Westerterp, K. (2012). Why do individuals not lose more weight from an exercise intervention at a defined dose? An energy balance analysis. *Obesity Reviews, 13*(10), 835–847.

Thompson Coon, J., Boddy, K., Stein, K., Whear, R., Barton, J., & Depledge, M.H. (2011). Does participating in physical activity in outdoor natural environments have a greater effect on physical and mental wellbeing than physical activity indoors? A systematic review. *Environmental Science & Technology, 45*, 1761–1772. doi: 10.1021/es102947t

Townsend, N., Bhatnagar, P., Wilkins, E., Wickramasinghe, K., & Rayner, M. (2015). *Cardiovascular disease statistics 2015*. British Heart Foundation. London.

Tsutsumi, T., Don, B.M., Zaichkowsky, L.D., & Delizonna, L.L. (1997). Physical fitness and psychological benefits of strength training in community dwelling older adults. *Journal of Physiological Anthropology, 16*, 257–266. doi:10.2114/jpa.16.257

Van Pelt, R.E., Jones, P.P., Davy, K.P., DeSouza, C.A., Tanaka, H., Davy, B.M., & Seals, D.R. (1997). Regular exercise and the age-related decline in resting metabolic rate in women 1. *The Journal of Clinical Endocrinology & Metabolism, 82*(10), 3208–3212.

Velloso, C.P. (2008). Regulation of muscle mass by growth hormone and IGF-I. *Br J Pharmacol, 154*(3), 557–568. doi: 10.1038/bjp.2008.153

Vidoni, E.D., Johnson, D.K., Morris, J.K., Van Sciver, A., Greer, C.S., Billinger, S.A., . . . Burns, J. M. (2015). Dose-response of aerobic exercise on cognition: a community-based, pilot randomized controlled trial. *PLoS ONE, 10*(7), e0131647. doi: 10.1371/journal.pone.0131647

Viña, J., Salvador-Pascual, A., Tarazona-Santabalbina, F.J., Rodriguez-Mañas, L., & Gomez-Cabrera, M.C. (2016). Exercise training as a drug to treat age associated frailty. *Free Radical Biology and Medicine, 98*, 159–164.

Voss, M.W., Nagamatsu, L.S., Liu-Ambrose, T., & Kramer, A.F. (2011). Exercise, brain, and cognition across the life span. *Journal of Applied Physiology, 111*(5), 1505–1513. doi: 10.1152/japplphysiol.00210.2011

Williams, K.N., & Kemper, S. (2010). Interventions to reduce cognitive decline in aging. *J Psychosoc Nurs Ment Health Serv, 48*(5), 42–51. doi: 10.3928/02793695-20100331-03

Wilson, M.-M.G., & Morley, J.E. (2003). Invited review: aging and energy balance. *Journal of Applied Physiology, 95*(4), 1728–1736.

Woodyard, C. (2011). Exploring the therapeutic effects of yoga and its ability to increase quality of life. *Int J Yoga, 4*(2), 49–54. doi: 10.4103/0973-6131.85485

World Health Organization (2007). *WHO Global Report on Falls Prevention in Older Age*. Geneva: World Health Organization.

World Health Organization (2015). *Global Reference List of 100 Core Health Indicators*. Geneva: World Health Organization.

Wu, H.Y., Tu, J.H., Hsu, C.H., & Tsao, T.H. (2016). Effects of low-impact dance on blood biochemistry, bone mineral density, the joint range of motion of lower extremities, knee extension torque, and fall in females. *Journal of Aging and Physical Activity, 24*(1), 1–7. doi: 10.1123/japa.2014-0088

Suggested further reading

A key aspect of physical exertion that has not been discussed in this book chapter to any extent is the engagement in sedentary behaviours. Indeed, it is increasingly becoming evident that engagement in sedentary behaviours has distinct health effects, regardless of any concurrent participation in physical activity the rest of the time. This effect is significant, not least since sedentary behaviours tend to take up a greater proportion of modern daily living. The publications below are readily available and provide up-to-date overviews of this relatively new research area:

- Gladys Onambele-Pearson, Emma Bostock, Christopher Morse, Keith Winwood, Islay McEwan, & Claire Stewart, 2015. Chapter: Sedentarism and the endo-metabolic system. In *Sedentary Lifestyle: Predictive Factors, Health Risks and Physiological Implications*. (Ed.) Ahmad Alkhatib. Nova Science Publishers, New York [book in press].
- Gladys Onambele-Pearson, Jodi Ventre, & Jon Adam Brown, 2017. Reducing sedentary behaviour among older people. Chapter 7.2. In *The Palgrave Handbook of Ageing and Physical Activity Promotion*. (Ed.) Samuel Nyman. Palgrave Macmillan, UK.
- Jorgen A. Wullems, Sabine M.P. Verschueren, Hans Degens, Christopher I. Morse, & Gladys L. Onambele, 2016. A review of the prevalence of sedentarism in older adults, its physiology/health impact and non-exercise mobility counter-measures. BSRA Special issue of the journal *Biogerontology*, *17*(3), 547–565. doi: 10.1007/s10522-016-9640-1
- D. Ryan, G. Stebbings, & G.L. Onambele, 2015. The emergence of sedentary behaviour physiology and its effects on the cardiometabolic profile with ageing. *Age* (Dordr.), *37*(5), 89. doi: 10.1007/s11357-015-9832-7. Epub 2015 Aug 28.

24   Public health policy and physical activity

Justin Varney, Michael Brannan and Kevin Fenton

Keywords: Policy, government, global, national, strategy, impact

Introduction

Inactivity remains the fourth leading cause of death worldwide (Kohl et al., 2012) and one of the top 20 risk factors for disability adjusted life years. As more countries tackle infectious diseases and child and maternal malnutrition, and with generational reductions in smoking, the proportion of death and disability attributable to physical inactivity has, and will continue to increase (Forouzanfar et al., 2015).

Within the UK context inactivity sits in the top ten risk factors for preventable death and disease (Newton et al., 2015) and there has been an overall downward trend in activity, particularly in relation to utility-based short journeys by foot or bicycle.

There is a strong and growing evidence base demonstrating the significant impact of moderate or intense physical activity on a broad range of clinical conditions. But there is limited evidence or evaluation of how to systematically increase population and national levels of activity in a sustained and significant manner through national and local action.

Few countries have achieved measurable and embedded increases in physical activity at a population level, and those that have shown progress have done so through on-going national leadership, whole system approaches and routine data and evaluation – all of which support an iterative evolution of approaches that reflect cultural and societal change.

Many of the key aspects of moving a nation to regular physical activity are governed through national policy and therefore the ability of practitioners to influence the policy-making cycle is fundamental to achieving sustained reform in the short and long term.

National physical activity campaign in Finland (1980–2012)

In the 1960s, Finnish men had the highest level of mortality from coronary heart disease in the world (Thom, Epstein, Feldman, Leaverton, & Wolz, 1992). Finland passed its first Sport Act in 1980, starting a 30-year journey that bucked the international trend in declining physical activity. It took a systematic, multi-level approach of: developing the evidence base; national legislation; sectoral and multi-sector policies; national, local and community programmes, with specific foci on supporting grass roots and targeting specific population groups; re-orientating decision making towards local level; and specific funding. Monitoring, evaluation and research were incorporated across the programme to inform planning and delivery, including the quantity and quality of services and public perceptions (Vuori, Lankenau, & Pratt, 2004). Its success is demonstrated not just in the increasing population-level leisure time physical activity, but in increases across all life stages (i.e. children and young people, working age adults and older adults). In 2013, Finland renewed its commitment through a new national strategy (Ministry of Social Affairs and Health, 2013).

Formation of policy – theory and practice

Policy formation is key to the national and local response to inactivity. Moving from political intention and research into policy requires a clear articulation of evidence for impact by the agency leading the policy development and those leading implementation. However, policy is not formed in a vacuum and political and social contexts are central to embedding and supporting policy implementation. Policy formation, and subsequent implementation, requires the breadth of public health skills and demonstrates the art and science of the discipline of addressing societal challenges.

Establishing the evidence base

The initial stage of any policy formation is to understand the rationale for change. This may be based on political imperatives or commitments, emerging evidence of deficit or economic drivers based on public spending pressures.

For physical activity, the evidence base for action has been clearly stated by the World Health Organization (2010). Agreed international guidelines outline the level of physical activity that is most beneficial for health at different stages of the life course, and the level of inactivity associated with significant increases in the risk of death and disease.

Countries vary in the amount and quality of data they collect in relation to these guidelines and how routinely the information is collected for different age groups and the level of demographic detail collected. The Global Matrix Scorecard on Children and Young People's Physical Activity demonstrates, through the number of countries where a lack of data led to inconclusive scores, the international variation in data collection for children and young people for physical activity, sedentary behaviour and play.

This information is key to understanding the baseline for population activity levels and managing political expectations of changes in trends and performance. The level of detail available is key to being able to develop policy that addresses need effectively at both national and local level and allows inequalities as well as trends to be identified (Figure 24.2).

Although the evidence base is strong for the relationship between physical activity and health risks, consensus is weaker on systematic evidence for specific interventions, particularly in areas such as infrastructure or social and cultural movement.

Policy makers may also question the transferability of some evidence between countries with radically different social and cultural contexts. This is particularly relevant in relation to reducing inactivity in minority communities, such as people living with disabilities and impairments, where the social and legislative context may have a significant bearing on the impact of interventions.

However, the evidence drivers go beyond research and data and usually policy makers will move from evidence gathering into a period of stakeholder (and sometimes public) engagement, to explore policy options and the most effective way to move things forward.

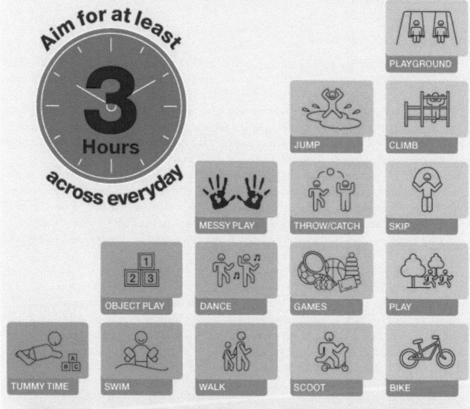

Figure 24.1 UK Chief Medical Officers' Guidelines on Physical Activity across the life course infographics

Physical activity
for children and young people
(5–18 Years)

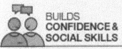
BUILDS CONFIDENCE & SOCIAL SKILLS

MAINTAINS HEALTHY WEIGHT

DEVELOPS CO-ORDINATION

STRENGTHENS MUSCLES & BONES

IMPROVES SLEEP

IMPROVES CONCENTRATION & LEARNING

IMPROVES HEALTH & FITNESS

MAKES YOU FEEL GOOD

Be physically active

Spread activity throughout the day

Aim for at least 60 minutes everyday

All activities should make you breathe faster & feel warmer

PLAY

RUN/WALK

BIKE

ACTIVE TRAVEL

SWIM

SKATE

Include muscle and bone strengthening activities

SPORT

PE

SKIP

CLIMB

3 TIMES PER WEEK

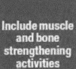
WORKOUT

DANCE

Sit less

LOUNGING

Move more

Find ways to help all children and young people accumulate at least 60 minutes of physical activity everyday

UK Chief Medical Officers' Guidelines 2011 **Start Active, Stay Active: www.bit.ly/startactive**

Figure 24.1 Continued

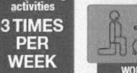

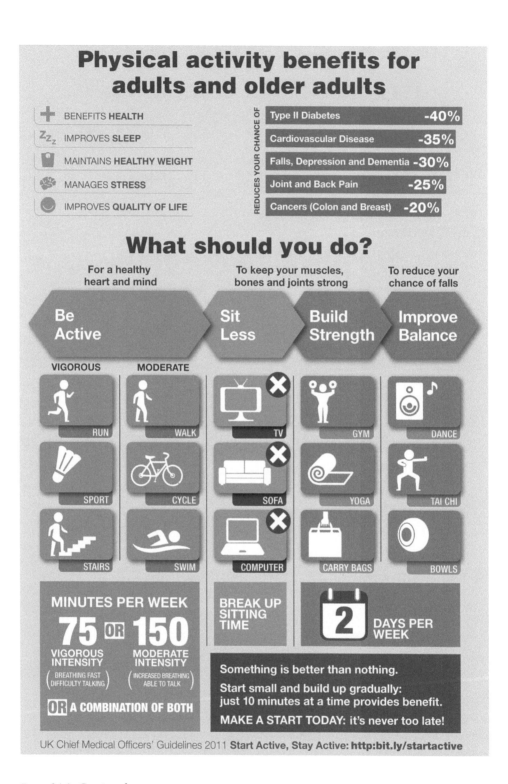

Figure 24.1 Continued

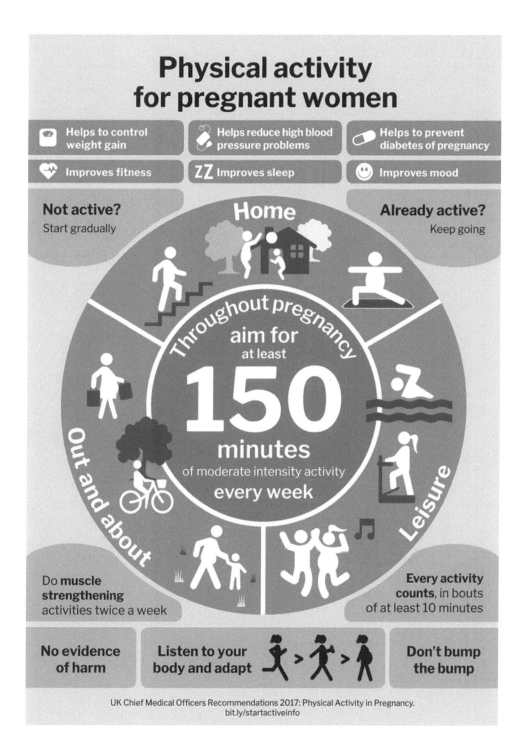

Figure 24.1 Continued

Table 24.1 Total countries scored inconclusive or A grade in Global Matrix 1.0 and 2.0 for physical activity for children and youth

	Global Matrix 1.0 2014		Global Matrix 2.0 2016	
	Inconclusive	A grade	Inconclusive	A grade
Overall physical activity			1	1
Organised sport participation	2		7	1
Active play	10		21	
Active transport	1		3	2
Sedentary behaviour	2		3	
Family & peers	9		17	
School	1	1	4	1
Community & built environment	3	1	11	3
Government strategies & investments	5		6	1
Number of countries participating	15		38	

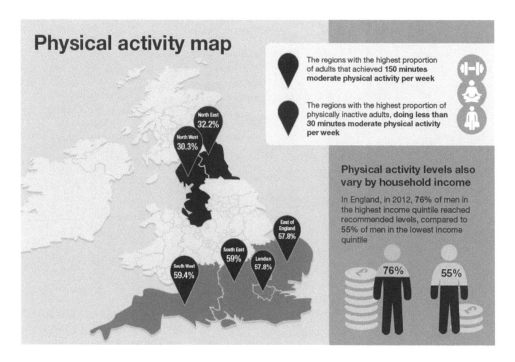

Figure 24.2 Infographic of geographical inequalities in physical activity in England in 2016

Engagement and consultation

Physical activity stakeholders cover a broad range of international, national and local organisations, and include academics, private and public sector organisations, providers of physical activity interventions and professional groups who influence behaviour choices and the built environment in which we live.

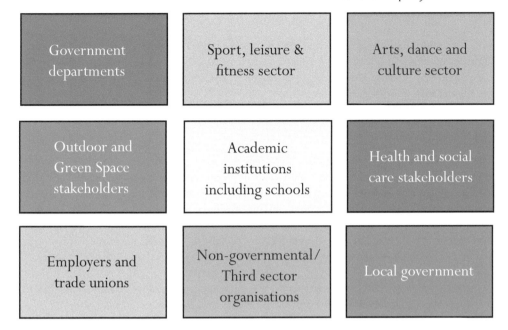

Figure 24.3 Outline of some of the key stakeholders for physical activity

Stakeholder engagement can be facilitated directly face-to-face, but this is usually focused in the early stages of policy development. Once there are more structured policy options in place this moves into more formal consultation at scale, usually through web portals. Different tiers of government may have different agreed protocols for the duration and specifications of public consultation in policy formation and this will form the framework for any specific consultation on physical activity policy.

One aspect of stakeholder engagement that may be important to consider is how the process reflects the views and experiences of minority communities and those who are most inactive in society. Some groups may require additional support to engage during this phase of policy development. This is often considered during the impact assessment phase of policy formation, but it is also important to bear in mind during the engagement phase as these stakeholders may bring different perspectives to the policy formation, particularly related to the interconnected nature of identity and health risks.

Political context

Although at a headline level promoting physical activity is a positive political move and supported by most administrations, the detail of mechanisms to enable physical activity are more political sensitive, especially in areas like transport and urban planning. Understanding the broad range of political contexts in relation to physical activity is important during policy development.

Economic and equality impact assessment

In many countries there are standardised approaches to assessing new policy or policy alterations in the context of economic impacts and effects on equality and diversity. This process is normally undertaken in the second half of policy formation and can help identify potential pitfalls and missed opportunities in the policy approach.

Spectrum of policy areas for action on inactivity

The policy enablers for tackling inactivity range across a series of departments and professional areas. A national system wide approach will require influencing policy in multiple areas simultaneously although some changes will take years to come into effect because of procurement timelines, for example travel infrastructure realignment.

In working with different policy areas it is important to consider the priority of the lead department and their deliverables and objectives. Against this context the argument for inclusion of action on physical inactivity has to be made and tailored to the language and approach of the lead department.

Although many would argue for a single cross-cutting strategy or policy on physical activity, the reality of government department processes and timescales mean that this is often difficult to achieve, and is potentially more vulnerable to political change than when action to reduce inactivity and promote physical activity is embedded across key policies in relevant departments. This disseminated approach can be more time consuming and harder to recognise, but can help reinforce the need for individual departmental leadership and ownership of actions and helps demonstrate more clearly the individual connection between reducing inactivity and that department's objectives and outcomes.

Figure 24.3 illustrates some key departments/areas to consider in taking a whole system approach, although names and designations may vary between administrations:

Education

The focus of education policy is often primarily on educational attainment, where there is a reasonable evidence base for impact, especially at primary school level. There is also evidence supporting the role of physical activity in the form of active play in motor and social skills development in early years which are fundamental developmental foundations to give every child the best start in life.

Case study: Slovenia education policy

Physical education (PE) is a compulsory subject for both primary and secondary schools requiring a minimum number of core PE hours in the curriculum as well as the option for students to opt into additional teaching on sport and dance. As well as the PE core curriculum there is a requirement for a minimum of five sports days at each grade of primary school and there is local flexibility to increase the physical activity offer during class time based on need. All primary schools are required to offer free extracurricular sports programmes for children. This combination of compulsory and optional PE, sport, dance and extracurricular physical activity provides children with between 77 and 39 minutes of activity per school day in primary school. Over 86% of boys and 76% of girls meet WHO PA guidelines in Slovenia, and although the proportion achieved during week day school time is significant the proportion of children remaining active at the weekends is similar (Sember et al., 2016).

Sport, leisure and fitness

The focus may be more on sport participation than physical activity. It may be useful to stress the contribution of sport and fitness leisure activity to regular everyday activity and work within national sports strategies to join community sport with utility and leisure physical activity.

Case study: Sporting Future

The UK Government published *Sporting Future – A New Strategy for an Active Nation* in 2015. This cross-government strategy focused on both increasing sport participation and reducing physical inactivity. The strategy set out five key outcome measures for sport: physical well-being, mental well-being, individual development, social and community development, and economic development. These five outcome measures underpin the funding strategy for sport and were reflected in Sport England's strategy 'Towards An Active Nation' and their subsequent funding streams. The strategy included a specific strand around volunteer and professional development which has been an important opportunity to embed behaviour change and brief advice skills across this workforce from baseline qualifications up.

Business development and economic productivity

This is often the highest priority for a national government and therefore an important lever for potential change. The evidence base around inactivity and economic productivity for employers could be strengthened, but there is a link between sickness absence and activity rates amongst employees (van Amelsvoort et al., 2006). The policy context for this rationale will vary between countries based on the level of employer financial responsibility for employee health coverage i.e. contrast between insurance based vs. public funded health economies.

Case study: WHO Guidelines on Improving Physical Fitness of Employees

The World Health Organization has a significant global programme of activity on occupational health and well-being through a network of collaborating centres. In 1999 the WHO published guidelines to improve physical fitness of employees (Kelly, 1999). This highlighted the correlation between physical inactivity and productivity, presenteeism and sickness absence and used case studies and evidence to set out an approach for implementing action. This was then built on in 2008 by the WHO report, *The workplace as a setting for interventions to improve diet and promote physical activity* (Quintilliani, Sattelmair, & Sorensen, 2008). At a member state level, these guidelines supported in the UK by National Institute for Health and Care Excellence, through public health guidelines (NICE, 2008) on physical activity in the workplace setting out the specific evidence-based actions required at national, local and employer level which then informed development of tools and resources to support employer led implementation (NHS Employers, 2015).

In addition to the direct employer/business impact there is some evidence of economic collateral benefits from active travel planning, cycling and walking impacting on local high street economies and provision enabling low cost travel options for those on low incomes to travel more easily to work destinations, these can be usefully articulated to help support transport policy shift.

Case Study: UK Department for Transport Sustainable Access Fund

In 2016 the UK Department for Transport launched a £60 million sustainable access revenue fund for 2017–2020 to support local government in England to invest in projects that boost the local economy through encouraging walking and cycling participation and increasing access to training, skills development and employment opportunities (HMG, 2016a). Although it is too early to judge the impact of this approach, the requirement of local transport authorities to articulate in their application to the fund the project plans to increase cycling and walking and demonstrate how this will grow employment opportunities and economic sustainability is a significant step change in the local understanding of the connection between economic sustainability and active travel planning.

Health and social care

There is growing evidence that for people with health conditions the influence of health and social care professionals can be key in motivating and sustaining behaviour change. Therefore integrating education on physical activity behaviour change into routine clinical and social care training is as important as explicit integration of physical activity into clinical care pathways and commissioning of residential and nursing care services. The evidence base for inactivity and health impact is strong and therefore this is an area where policy integration should be most accessible, but will still require consideration of how best to embed it within core departmental and political priorities.

Case study: NHS England Five Year Forward View

NHS England, the national health service lead organisation in England, published a national document in 2014 setting out the strategic forward direction in order to achieve financial sustainability and improve service outcomes (NHS England, 2014). Embedded within the document was a strong emphasis on the role of healthcare professionals in delivering primary, secondary and tertiary prevention into routine clinical practice. This has been supported by developing an education and operational approach called 'Making Every Contact Count' (MECC) (PHE, 2016) which incorporates skills for behaviour change and brief advice into routine contact conversations for all healthcare professionals. MECC is supported in explicit contract requirements for all NHS services and through a broad educational support offer including specific resources on promoting physical activity. The Forward View also highlighted that the health of staff working in the NHS is important to the organisational viability and sustainability and part of supporting their health is about addressing physical inactivity in the workforce, which has been supported by including within the NHS Quality Improvement financial incentive programme (CQUIN) a specific incentive on workforce health and well-being, highlighting physical activity as a key area for action.

Transport, planning and urban design

There is significant potential for gains through utility-based activity if policies can rebalance the focus between cars, cycling and pedestrians. However, drivers for these policies are often complex and highly political and the evidence base is often observational with potential for significant cultural confounding. Internationally there is growing recognition of a shared objective of more integrated active travel supporting increased physical activity, as well as reduced car-based carbon emissions and improved environmental sustainability (European Commission, 2014).

Case study: Active Travel (Wales) Act 2013

The Active Travel (Wales) Act (HMG, 2013a) is a piece of legislation in Wales that requires local authorities to continuously improve facilities and routes for cyclists and walkers and to publish route maps. The Act also requires new road schemes to explicitly consider the needs of pedestrians and cyclists at the design stage, and the Welsh Government to publish an annual report on Active Travel. The Act came into effect in September 2014 supported by statutory guidance for local government and focused on designated areas with populations greater than 2,000 people. A review by National Assembly for Wales Enterprise and Business Committee in 2016 highlighted the support for the ambition in the Act and recognised implementation is still in its infancy but also highlighted the need for fundamental building blocks in resources, skills and capacity to realise this ambition in practice and at scale (National Assembly for Wales Enterprise and Business Committee, 2016).

Examples of integration of physical activity into national policy

There are many examples of how physical activity has been integrated into international and national policy. These examples highlight some specific dimensions of this integration or national integrated approaches that cut across government departments to generate interconnected policies on which local action can be built.

International policy and context: Bangkok Declaration on Physical Activity for Global Health and Sustainable Development (2016) and WHO Global Non-communicable Disease Goals (2013)

Launched at the International Society for Physical Activity and Health (ISPAH) 2016 Congress held in Bangkok, the Bangkok Declaration sets outs the importance of physical activity for global health, the prevention of non-communicable diseases and how co-benefits of population-based actions on physical activity can contribute to achieving eight of the 2030 Sustainable Development Goals (SDGs). The Declaration outlines six strategic areas for investment and action at country, regional and global levels, which if implemented in all countries, would advance progress towards achieving the 2020 global voluntary target of increasing relative population levels of physical activity by 10% set out in the WHO Global Non-communicable Disease Action Plan.

National Policy Integration in England (2012–2016)

Developing a physical activity and health legacy was part of the bid to the International Olympic Committee to host the 2012 Olympic and Paralympic Games in London. Levels of inactivity were higher than comparable countries like France and Germany (Hallal et al., 2012), so a national ambition was established in 2013 to increase physical activity and reduce inactivity (HMG, 2013b). A national framework for action, Everybody Active Every Day, was coproduced with over 1,000 national and local cross-sectors based on international evidence of what works at population level to increase physical activity (Public Health England, 2014). It set out four domains for local and national action upon which policies and programmes have been overlaid. Physical activity has been integrated within a matrix of cross-sector national policies, including: Sporting Future – the first national sport strategy in 13 years focuses on reducing inactivity and improving health, rather than just participation and elite sport achievements (HMG, 2015); Childhood obesity – placing daily physical activity across settings at the heart of the national approach (HMG, 2016b); and Improving Lives: Health and work Green Paper – employer support for physical activity included with work to close the disability employment gap (HMG, 2016c).

Local policy integration: Move More Sheffield (2014–2019)

The city of Sheffield established an aim to become 'the most active city in the UK by 2020' and set out a five-year Plan to achieve it (Sheffield City Council, 2014). Its vision is to deliver city-wide cultural change based on 12 principles: bottom up; reduce participation inequalities; equal and inclusive; connecting people; whole system approach; making the easy choice; creating habits; fun; communications; visibility; working together; and evidence and evaluation. The strategy has been endorsed by cross-sector partners to deliver across six people and place outcomes. A city-wide 'Move More month' held in July 2016 was supported by more than 50 local organisations through promotions and activities in communities, schools and workplaces. A total of 6.5 million minutes of activities was recorded by participants using an associated mobile phone app.

Measuring impact and driving progress

An important part of the policy development process is being able to demonstrate the baseline, a trajectory for change in population level data for inactivity and the proportion achieving the recommended guidelines of regular activity for their age group. This data will need to be captured on a regular basis to demonstrate the impact of policy on outcomes and provide a feedback loop for future development and refresh of policy content.

Impact can be evaluated through direct measures in national and representative population surveys, such as the Health Survey for England and the Active People Survey in England, or through indirect measures that represent proxy measures or partial indicators linked to specific policy measures, for example population level survey data on individual transport modality of short distance journeys.

European network for the promotion of Health Enhancing Physical Activity (HEPA Europe)

Established in 2005, HEPA Europe aims to 'strengthen and support efforts and actions that increase participation and improve the conditions favourable to a healthy lifestyle' (HEPA Europe, 2005). It brings together members from regional, national and sub-national levels for activities based on relevant WHO policies, such as the Global Strategy for Diet, Physical

Activity and Health, the European Charter on Counteracting Obesity and the NCD Action Plan. The Network aims to be a source of knowledge, advocacy and evidence across Europe. Guiding principles are: population-based approaches based on the best scientific evidence; systematic and standardised monitoring and evaluation; sharing of practical experience and knowledge; and supporting cooperation and collaboration across sectors, networks and approaches.

Supporting policy into action requires implementation tools, guidelines and advice for both commissioners and providers within local public health systems. These vary between administrations but there are several examples of practical tools to support translation of evidence based policies and guidelines into effective action.

Building the cross-sector economic case: Return on Investment (ROI) tools

An increasing number of tools help decision makers understand where and how to invest, and calculate what and where economic returns are likely within and across sectors. The Physical Activity Return on Investment Tool models the potential health benefits of 13 evidence-based interventions in a defined geographic area and the economic payback over different time-scales (NICE, 2014). The Model for estimating the Outcomes and Values in the Economics of Sport (MOVES) estimate the economic and health benefits of a sport programme in a specific population group with a defined participation rate (Sport England, 2014). The WHO Health Economic Assessment Tool (HEAT) for walking and cycling enabled planners, practitioners and academics across transport, health and physical activity to calculate the likely mortality and associated economic benefits of real or estimated increases in walking or cycling (WHO, 2014).

Conclusions

Developing and implementing effective public health policy is an essential tool to support population level activation on, and increases in, physical activity. However the emerging evidence is clear: There is no single 'magic bullet' policy that will achieve this goal. In contrast our experience in the UK and increasingly in other countries suggests that to be most effective such policies need to be comprehensive: operating at different levels (national, regional and local and individual); across multiple sectors (health, environment, transport); involving varied disciplines; facilitating a range of evidence-based interventions (individual, family, workplace, healthcare, community and societal); addressing the social and structural determinants of health and physical activity (cultural, psychosocial, ethnic and economic); and ensuring the evaluation of different types of interventions and combinations of interventions. It is only through implementing interventions at each of the levels that we will be able to achieve the maximum possible sustained population level impact. Therefore it is important that such public policies are developed and implemented within the context of a national programme that is well resourced, governed, monitored and evaluated. There remains much to learn from cross-national comparisons of physical activity programmes, despite differences in social and cultural context, as countries are at different phases of implementation and are learning through implementation and innovation.

Effective public health policy can also help to create supportive local environments, for example within healthcare or workplace settings, to promote physical activity and support individual behaviour change. While changing behaviour is ultimately up to the individual, we now know that employers (within and outside of healthcare) have a tremendous opportunity to help their employees see the value of adopting healthier behaviours so that they can live healthier lives. A workplace culture sets the tone for its employees and workplace wellness and incentive programmes can be used to drive and reinforce healthy behaviours, bringing benefits to the employer, the employee, and to the community. Similarly healthcare and many other professionals, by virtue of their contact with the public every day, can help spread the word and help make physical activity the social norm. Public policy can facilitate and incentivise healthcare and other employers to use a range of wellness initiatives such as on-site physical activity programmes, gym memberships, walk to work schemes, incentives, and more. What's most important is to commit to wellness and physical activity promotion in the organisation and to maximise opportunities for public policy to support this.

Finally, we now understand that public health policy to promote physical activity tends to be more effective when adequately governed, implemented, monitored and resourced, as it reaches broader segments of society and require less individual effort. However, since demonstrating and evaluating real change in population levels of physical activity can take time, it is critical that there is a commitment to sustain the leadership, activation, communication, funding and evaluation to ensure that interventions are in place for long enough, and at the sufficient intensity, to achieve their goals. The case study from Finland provides an excellent example of the benefits of long-term planning and evaluation. Too often initiatives and programmes are launched without due consideration and investment being given to developing the metrics for demonstrating how, where, with whom and why such policies may or may not work. This is critical not only for the long-term sustainability of programmes, but also to contribute to the evidence base on what works in promoting physical activity. This remains an area of significant underdevelopment and a huge opportunity for national, regional and international collaboration in the next decade.

References

van Amelsvoort, L.G.P.M, Spigt, M.G, Swaen, G.M.H., & Kant, I. (2006) Leisure time physical activity and sickness absenteeism; a prospective study, *Occupational Medicine, 56*(3), 210–212.

European Commission (2014) *Planning for People: Guidelines for developing and implementing a sustainable urban mobility plan.* www.eltis.org/mobility-plans (accessed 13/12/2016).

Forouzanfar, M.H., Alexander, L., Anderson H.R., Bachman, V.F., Biryukov, S., Brauer, M., . . . Murray, C.J. (2015) Global, regional, and national comparative risk assessment of 79 behavioural, environmental and occupational, and metabolic risks or clusters of risks in 188 countries, 1990–2013: a systematic analysis for the Global Burden of Disease Study 2013. *The Lancet, 386*(10010), 2287–2323.

Hallal, P.C., Andersen, L.B., Bull, F.C., Guthold, R., Haskell, W., & Ekelund, U. for the Lancet Physical Activity Series Working Group (2012) Global physical activity levels: surveillance progress, pitfalls, and prospects. *The Lancet, 380*(9838), 247–257.

HEPA Europe (2005) The European Network for the Promotion of Physical Activity. 1st meeting of the Network, Gerlev, Denmark, 26–27 May 2005 (report on the Internet). HEPA Europe, Rome. Available from: www.euro.who.int/hepa/meetings/20050615_9

HMG (2013a) Active Travel (Wales) Act.

HMG (2013b) *Moving More, Living More.*

HMG (2015) *Sporting Future: A New Strategy for an Active Nation.*

HMG (2016a) Access Fund for Sustainable Travel: Guidance.

HMG (2016b) *Childhood Obesity Action Plan.*

HMG (2016c) *Work, Health and Disability Green Paper: Improving Lives.*

Kelly F (1999) *Guidelines on improving physical fitness in employees.* World Health Organization.

Khol, H.W., Craig, C.L., Lambert, E.V., Inoue, S., Alkandari, J.R., Leetongin, G., Kahlmeier, S., Lancet Physical Activity Series Working Group (2012) The pandemic of physical inactivity: global action for public health. *The Lancet, 380*(9838), 294–305.

Ministry of Social Affairs and Health (2013) *On the move - National strategy for physical activity promoting health and wellbeing 2020.*

National Assembly for Wales Enterprise and Business Committee (2016) Active Travel: The Start of the Journey.

Newton J.N. et al. (2015) Changes in health in England, with analysis by English regions and areas of deprivation, 1990–2013: a systematic analysis for the Global Burden of Disease Study 2013. *The Lancet 386(10010)*, 2257–2274.

NHS Employers (2015) Creating healthy NHS workplaces – A toolkit to support the implementation of the NICE workplace guidance.

NHS England (2014) NHS Five Year Forward View.

National Institute for Health and Clinical Excellence (NICE) (2014) *Physical activity return on investment tool.* www.nice.org.uk/About/What-we-do/Into-practice/Return-on-investment-tools/Physical-activity-return-on-investment-tool

NICE (2008) PH13: *Physical activity in the workplace.*

PHE (2016) Making Every Contact Count (MECC): Consensus statement.

Public Health England (2014) *Everybody active, every day: An evidence-based approach to physical activity.*

Quintilliani, L., Sattelmair, J., & Sorensen, G. (2008) *The workplace as a setting for interventions to improve diet and promote physical activity.* World Health Organization.

Sember, V., Starc, G., Jurak, G., Golobič, M., Kovač, M., Samardžija, P.P., & Morrison, S.A. (2016) Results from the Republic of Slovenia's 2016 Report Card on Physical Activity for Children and Youth. *Journal of Physical Activity and Health, 13*(11 Suppl 2), S256–S264.

Sheffield City Council (2014) *The Move More Plan: A framework for increasing physical activity in Sheffield 2014–2019.*

Sport England (2014) *Model for estimating the Outcomes and Values in the Economics of Sport (MOVES).*

Thom, T., Epstein, F., Feldman, J., Leaverton, P., & Wolz, M. (1992) Total mortality and mortality from heart disease, cancer and stroke from 1950 to 1987 in 27 countries: highlights of trends and their interrelationships among causes of death. National Institutes of Health Report No. 92–3088.

Vuori, I., Lankenau, B., & Pratt, M. (2004) Physical activity policy and program development: the experience in Finland. *Public Health Reports, 119*, 331–345.

World Health Organization (2010) *Global recommendations on physical activity for health.* www.who.int/dietphysicalactivity/factsheet_recommendations/en/

World Health Organization (2014) *Health Economic Assessment Tool (HEAT) for walking and cycling.* www.heatwalkingcycling.org/

25 Improving policy to promote physical activity

Getting to grips with health inequalities

Tess Kay

Keywords: Physical activity, health inequalities, policy, public health

Introduction

Policy to promote physical activity (PA) is increasingly 'evidence-based' – but is it based on the *right* evidence? This chapter argues that PA policy should make more use of scientific knowledge on the patterns and processes that produce structural inequalities in health. This will counter current weaknesses in PA guidance, which is selective in its use of scientific knowledge and gives disproportionate emphasis to health behaviourist approaches. This results in PA interventions which mainly focus on motivating individuals to adopt more active lifestyles while giving limited attention to important contextual factors which may affect their capacity to do so.

   This chapter makes the case for expanding the evidence base, and examines how this might be done. It overviews patterns of health inequalities and explains the importance of PA policy in addressing them. It then compares how different theoretical perspectives can inform this, and draws attention to the value of Social Determinants of Health (SDH) frameworks to the PA community. Using the example of current UK PA guidance, the chapter explores the implications of neglecting social context and discusses how a wider evidence base that addresses structural influences on health behaviour might be mobilised to inform and enhance future PA policy and practice.

Why physical activity and health inequalities are connected

Patterns of global health are changing: non-communicable diseases (NCDs), once primarily associated with high-income countries, are now the main causes of ill-health worldwide. Their rise reflects three global developments that promote unhealthy environments and limit healthy behaviours: population ageing, rapid unplanned urbanisation, and globalisation (WHO, 2008a) – structural trends that lie outside the control of individuals but impact on their lives and living conditions. The rise of NCDs is important for the PA community. NCDs are non-infectious and non-transmissible and include both physical ailments (such as heart disease, asthma, cancer and diabetes) and mental, neurological and substance use disorders (e.g. depression, dementia and alcoholism). As physical inactivity is a risk factor for NCDs, the promotion of active lifestyles is a policy priority for preventative health care.

Table 25.1   Health inequalities: the relationship between deprivation, health and life expectancy, England, 2009–11

	Least deprived 10% of areas	Most deprived 10% of areas
Total life expectancy, males	83 years	73 years
Total life expectancy, females	86 years	79 years
Years of healthy life, males	71 years	52 years
Years of healthy life, females	72 years	53 years

Source: Office for National Statistics, 2013

Although inactivity can therefore be regarded as a 'universal' challenge, the disease burden it is associated with is not uniformly distributed: every nation, regardless of its overall economic status, displays strong patterns of health inequalities with poorer groups having the highest risk of physical and mental ill-health. The impact is evident in varied life expectancies associated with levels of affluence and deprivation (Table 25.1): in 2011 men and women living in the wealthiest 10% of neighbourhoods in England could expect to live for 10 years longer than those in its poorest 10%. They could also expect almost 20 more years of healthy life – staying in good health into their 70s rather than their early 50s (ONS, 2013). Exposure to stressors in the social and physical environment is associated with both short-term changes in physiology, perceptions and behaviour; and longer-term risk of adverse outcomes including cardiovascular disease, diabetes and anxiety disorders (Thompson et al., 2015, p. 18). Little wonder that the WHO views health inequity as a form of social injustice that is killing people 'on a grand scale' (WHO, 2008b, Executive Summary n.p.).

The WHO's comprehensive report *Closing the gap in a generation* (WHO, 2008a) demonstrates how health inequalities are inextricably bound to wider processes of inequity that can only be addressed through action on the way in which power and resources are distributed in society. While this approach has been widely endorsed in principle, progress has been limited. In Europe, for example, the widespread adoption of policies to address health inequalities has not been matched by action, and there remains 'a clear gap between policymaking and the actual implementation of policies' (European Commission, 2013, p. viii).

The difficulty in addressing health inequalities may go some way to explaining why they do not feature in UK physical activity guidance. The UK is however particularly well positioned to access relevant expertise, being especially prominent in the scholarship that has informed global policy guidance on health inequalities. It is therefore worthwhile to study what this body of knowledge might offer to the PA evidence base, and how it might be accessed.

The challenges of addressing structural influences on individuals' health behaviour

The health behaviour theories that currently inform PA policy emanate from psychology and focus strongly on motivating individuals to become active. While individual action is clearly essential to raising physical activity levels, viewing people as wholly self-determining does not give sufficient recognition to how individuals are social actors interacting with their social context. Narrowly applied, health behaviourist approaches prevent external influences being identified, and can produce strategies that overlook constraints that affect those in unfavourable situations (Kay, 2016).

Health behaviourists do recognise these concerns. In fact, there is a long tradition of conceptual models of health behaviour that attempt to address wider contextual factors. The 'Social Ecological' models (SEMs) used to underpin analyses of physical activity behaviour specifically acknowledge the existence of multiple influences on individuals. First expounded in McLeroy et al.'s (1988) Ecological Model of Health Behaviours, SEMs bring together two concepts: that health behaviour is affected by *multiple levels of influence*, and that it is shaped through *reciprocal causation* between individuals and these levels.

While they vary in detail, SEMs recognise multiple spheres of influence beyond the individual, including family, community and neighbourhood; multiple policy environments; and various depictions of 'social' dimensions, including social environment, social factors, social cultural environment, and macro-level environment. McLeroy and colleagues' initial SEM specified five levels of influence (intrapersonal, interpersonal, organisational, community and public policy); subsequent versions include Stokols (1992, 1996; six levels), Story et al. (2008; four), and Sallis (2009; six).

If SEMs do indeed directly address social influences, where do they fall short? Limitations are recognised, and not only by the social science community. Health psychologists Golden and Earp (2012) warn that approaches that claim to address social influences are in fact underpinned by theories that depict individuals as self-determining, unaffected by external influences. Similarly, Burke and colleagues suggest that for all their emphasis on context and multi-level social influences, SEMs remain rooted in individual theories, despite their intentions of addressing wider influencing factors (Burke, Joseph, Pasick & Barker, 2009).

These individualistic theoretical underpinnings help explain why the representation of 'social' factors in SEMs differs so markedly from social science conceptualisations (Kay, 2016). In SEMs, constructs such as gender, age, ethnicity and social class are not conceptualised as structuring social processes; instead, they appear only as individual ('demographic' or 'biological') characteristics, devoid of any 'social' dimension. 'Gender', for example, was omitted from McLeroy et al.'s (1988) original SEM, and classed as 'biological' (with 'age' and 'genes') by Story et al. (2008). (The inclusion of a separate category of 'demographic' factors in Story et al.'s model, in which 'race/ethnicity' and 'income' were located, further emphasises how wholly 'gender' was construed as biological and shorn of social significance.) Age is also treated in SEMs as a biological process only, while references to culture generally allude only to overt and conscious actions and practices (e.g. requirements for single-sex provision for some faith groups) and do not address wider issues of identity, diversity or discrimination.

SEMs nonetheless recognise other factors as 'high' level social influences beyond individuals' own characteristics. Again, these differ from broadly sociological conceptualisations of meso- and macro-level structures. In SEMs, 'social' most often refers to direct social interaction and/or to immediate social context – e.g. social networks, social settings (community, school etc.), and social environments. At the 'highest' levels, SEMs focus on institutional structures, such as public policy, rather than social structures (McLeroy, Bibeau, Steckler & Glanz, 1988; Glanz, Sallis, Saelens & Frank, 2005). Overall, therefore, social structural phenomena are absent, including the wider social trends such as urbanisation that international authorities recognise as important influences on public health.

Beyond the conceptual level, Golden and Earp (2012) provide further insight into factors that limit the scope of SEMs by examining how they operate at the implementation level. Their review of published reports of more than 150 interventions over 20 years uncovered two important limiting factors. Firstly, they simply found that SEMs were seldom used: fewer than 10% of the interventions were based on SEMs, with the great majority instead underpinned by traditional behaviour change theories focused on changing individual moti-vations. Secondly, and perhaps even more importantly, they found that even interventions that were underpinned by SEMs rarely addressed collective and structural factors; in prac-tice they tended to focus only on individual levels of influence. Golden and Earp suggested that this partly reflected the practical challenges of targeting 'upper' levels of SEMs, which 'is likely more challenging than adapting intrapersonal- and interpersonal-level programs'. They noted the potential difficulty of translating theories about 'higher level social and behavioural change' into action at intervention level (Golden and Earp, 2012, p. 370).

On the one hand, therefore, the burgeoning literature on SEM indicates increased recog-nition of the importance of external factors as influences on health behaviour. In practice, the application of this is confounded at both the theoretical and practical level. The result is very limited capacity to address negative structural influences on health behaviour. To do so is import-ant, as addressing health inequalities among the least healthy groups is not a narrow strategy, but offers the greatest aggregate gains to population health. As Marmot emphasises:

> This link between social conditions and health is not a footnote to the 'real' concerns with health – health care and unhealthy behaviours – it should become the main focus.
>
> (Marmot, 2010b, p. 4)

The next section now considers alternative theories that address this, focusing on the poten-tial of social determinants of health frameworks for understanding health behaviour.

A framework for understanding external influences on health behaviour: introducing the Social Determinants of Health framework

There are alternatives to SEMs for addressing how health behaviour is influenced by social factors beyond the individual: Golden et al. (2015), for example, propose overcoming the individualistic bias of the SEM by 'upending' it, placing social policy at its centre, rather than at its outer reaches. A more established approach is outlined in the Social Determinants of Health (SDH) framework. The SDH framework draws on a long tradition – 'analysts have long observed that social and environmental factors decisively influence people's health' (Irwin & Scali, 2007, p. 236). It underpins much contemporary health policy, providing the theoretical underpinning for *inter alia* the World Health Organization's Commission on the Social Deter-minants of Health (cf. *Closing the gap in a generation*; WHO, 2008a), the UK Marmot Review (*Fair society, healthy lives*; Marmot, 2010a), and the European Commission's Commission on *Health inequalities in the EU* (European Commission, 2013).

The core premise of the SDH framework is that individual health outcomes are influ-enced by a range of social structural factors which reflect the wider organisation of power and resources in society. The resulting inequalities underpin the 'determinants' of health – the range of interacting factors that shape health and well-being. These include material circum-stances, the social environment, psychosocial factors, behaviours, and biological factors, which are 'in turn . . . influenced by social position, itself shaped by education, occupation, income, gender, ethnicity and race' (Marmot, 2010b, p. 11). Health inequalities do not, therefore, arise by chance, nor are they attributable to individual behaviour or characteristics or indeed by access to health care; while these are important, 'Social and economic differences in health status reflect, and are caused by, social and economic inequalities in society' (Marmot, 2010b,

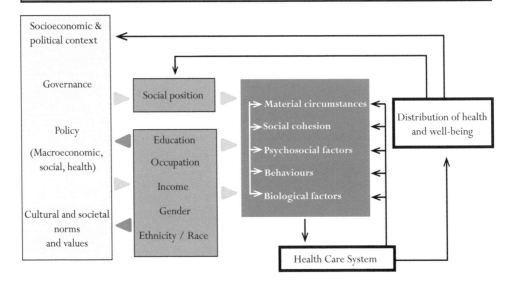

Figure 25.1 Conceptualising the social determinants of health
Source: adapted Solar & Irwin 2010

p. 12). It is therefore *necessary* to address social structural factors in order to address health inequalities and improve population health, making it important that these are incorporated in the theory that informs health interventions.

As with SEMs, there are multiple variants of 'social determinants of health' frameworks and conceptual models. The model used in WHO and EU policy analyses is built around the core concept of 'social position' as playing a central role in the social determinants of health inequalities (Solar & Irwin, 2010, pp. 4–5). It recognises three forms of 'mechanism' which interact with each other to influence exposure to health risk (Figure 25.1) – two categories of structural determinants ('socioeconomic and political context', and 'social position'), and a third – 'intermediary determinants' – which are directly experienced by individuals. Like SEMs, the framework therefore adopts a 'multi-level' approach. While SEMs take the individual as the starting point for their analysis and from there move 'up' to higher influences, the SDH framework 'begins' its analysis at the structural level and works 'down' to the individual. By doing this, much greater recognition is given to influencing factors originating beyond the individual, and specific attention is given to tracing the processes through which these macro- and meso-level factors connect to and affect individuals.

It is evident that the SDH framework has considerable common ground with the SEMs discussed previously. The two approaches address similar factors at individual, household, community and policy levels; in fact there are few factors named in one approach that are not included in the other – or could be. The main distinction is that the SDH framework displays coherence across the three categories: any factor referred to in one domain can be linked to corresponding elements in the other two. This contrasts with SMEs where, as in the example of gender, individual factors are not considered in relation to their structural properties.

One of the benefits of the SDH framework is that it directs attention to those in hardship, including groups linked by their shared experiences (e.g. of low income). The SDH is not, however, an approach confined to those on the margins. The Marmot review emphasised that the gradient of health affects the entire social spectrum, and proposed the concept of 'proportionate universalism': the notion that interventions should be both universal and targeted to where there is more need (Graham & Kelly, 2004; Bambra, Smith, Garthwaite, Joyce & Hunter, 2011, p. 401). Nonetheless, by highlighting structural variation in social position, it can inform work with priority groups for PA. Secondly, by highlighting how structural influences shape individual circumstances, it provides a valuable counterbalance to the SEM focus on individual agency. Both of these have potential to contribute to the evidence base for PA, and the next section provides an illustration of how this might occur.

Using Social Determinants of Health approaches to enhance PA guidance: the example of the UK *Start Active, Stay Active* report

The Start Active, Stay Active *report*

The *Start Active, Stay Active* (SASA) report (Department of Health, 2011) on which this example focuses is the publication in which current UK guidance was presented. SASA was a joint endeavour by the CMOs of the UK's four home countries (England, Scotland, Wales and Northern Ireland) to update and synthesise available evidence on PA and develop guidance from it. The report drew on a wide evidence base on physical activity to update previous national guidance, and established 'a UK-wide consensus on the amount of physical activity we should all aim to do at each stage of our lives' (Department of Health, 2011, p. 6). The report adopted a life course approach and stated the importance of physical activity for all ages, and for the first time provided age-appropriate guidance. It also highlighted the risk of sedentary behaviour and provided information on how different levels of physical activity ('moderate' and 'vigorous') could be combined to achieve recommended daily totals, emphasising the importance of being active on a daily basis.

The SASA report contains seven chapters. These define physical activity and explain its contribution to health (chapter 1); outline the approach taken to developing the guidance (chapter 2); present evidence and guidance about physical activity for four phases in the life course (chapters 3–6); and offer conclusions about how the guidelines can be applied, including suggestions for 'new opportunities' for action by different organisational actors (chapter 7). The four age groups are 'early years' (under 5s; chapter 3); 'children and young people' (5–18 years; chapter 4); 'adults' (19–64 years; chapter 5); and 'older adults' (65+ years; chapter 6). The report also contains appendices which detail the methodology adopted to produce the guidelines, including the evidence base used and the work undertaken by the five expert sub-groups – one for each of the four SASA age groups, and a fifth focused on sedentary behaviour. Membership overlapped between groups.

Illustrating physical activity in everyday life: the SASA report examples

The four age group chapters set out the developmental and health characteristics of the relevant age group, present the guidelines for recommended levels and types of PA, and provide a summary of the scientific evidence on which they are based. Each then offers a section on 'Understanding the guidelines', which discusses how they may translate into practice. Each of these sections contains two or three ~200 word 'boxed' examples of physical activity being incorporated in daily life by individuals in the relevant age group. In total there are ten examples, which vary in their content and detail – for example, some mention individuals' employment status while others do not. In total the examples describe 15 adults and 8 children and young people.

The inclusion of the examples is consistent with the principles underpinning SEMs: it recognises the importance of contextualising individuals' behaviour. As the report is intended as the 'first link' in a communication chain, the examples have potential practical utility in illustrating how physical activity can be incorporated into the varied lifestyles of individuals at different points in the life course. It is therefore instructive to examine how these lifestyles are portrayed in the examples.

- *Early years (0–4 yrs):* The examples focus on two children, each living with their two parents. All four parents are employed, with one mother on maternity leave. The families facilitate their children's physical activity in the context of full employment and financial security, living in neighbourhoods that give them excellent access to facilities for being active.
- *Child/youth (5–18 yrs):* The examples focus on three young people (one 7-year-old male and two 14-year-old females), all attending school; two live with both parents and one female with a lone parent; other siblings are mentioned. The two-parent teenager has a disability (deafness). All three attend school and live in their parental home in financially secure households. The physical activity opportunities include visiting National Trust properties (historic properties maintained by a national heritage charity in the UK) and walking on coastal paths.
- *Adult (18–64 yrs):* The three adult examples are focused on two men and one woman, aged 27, 37 and 22, respectively; two are in employment and one is a recent graduate who has obtained employment which she is waiting to start. The younger male is a wheelchair user. All are childless and single. All are active members of gyms and/or attend organised exercise classes.
- *Older adults (65+ yrs):* one married man aged 70 and one widow aged 81, both retired from previous paid employment and living in their own home. The two older adults are both retirees; the male worked until age 51 and the woman until age 76. They live in their own homes and lead active, sociable and apparently unconstrained lives. They are highly active – the man is a basketball referee and gardener (including gardening for others), while the woman is a member of a local walking group where she takes part in the 'fast' walks. Both have secure living conditions, good access to services and strong social networks. They display high levels of social confidence – the woman set up the walking group she participates in, while the man leads local walking tours.

The SASA report offers deliberately upbeat descriptions of individuals' living conditions and of their opportunities to be active. The ten examples emphasise opportunity and capability and most individuals appear unconstrained. Those with disabilities overcome them, and the older adults defy stereotypes of ageing through their vibrant lives incorporating being quite vigorously active. While this positivity has value, it also raises questions about how adequately the situations of less favoured groups in the population are addressed – or more fundamentally, whether they are in fact recognised. The SASA examples exclude those in the lower reaches of the social gradient – yet these are the population sectors which have the poorest health status, have most to gain from becoming more active, and are those with whom health professionals are likely to work. In fact, given the significance of physical activity to redressing health inequalities, there is even an argument that low-income and marginalised groups should be a primary focus for PA guidance.

Improving understanding of physical activity in everyday life: addressing social structural influences

It is here that adopting the social determinants of health framework could prove productive. This would expand the underpinning evidence base for PA guidance to include expert knowledge on the social structural influences that SEM models of health struggle to address. Applied to the four age groups addressed in UK PA guidance, this would enhance understanding of the characteristics of the population, draw attention to its diversity, and identify social structural processes that impact on population groups. This additional evidence could identify significant issues to be taken into account in promoting physical activity in each of the SASA age groups, such as:

- *Early years (0–4 yrs):* Data on the social determinants of health would draw attention to vulnerable children in this age group – including single-income households, and households with one or more unemployed parents. The situation of low-income families offers multiple challenges to healthy lifestyles for children and adults. In 2009, when the SASA guidelines were being developed, even government statistics recognised that more than three million of the nation's children were living in poverty (Brewer, Browne & Joyce 2009a; Brewer, Muriel, Phillips & Sibieta, 2009b).
- *Child/youth (5–18 yrs):* Data on the social determinants of health for this age group would reveal heterogeneity among older teenagers that the SASA focus on school-age young people conceals, A demographic profile would demonstrate how diverse young people are by the age of 18 in terms of their family, marital, parenting, education and employment status. Social statistical and qualitative data would also provide evidence of constraining circumstances and negative behaviours affecting many youth, including truancy, delinquency, crime, teen pregnancy, high unemployment, alcohol consumption and substance abuse (Wright, Lodge & Jacobson, 2012).
- *Adult (18–64 yrs):* Data on the social determinants of health would also produce more diverse examples of adult life across this wide age range. The SASA examples only include adults up to the age of 37, and only those without children. This overlooks how patterns of family formation, parenting and employment vary across the life course, and how differences are associated with the social gradient. Issues including the impact of parenthood on men and women's activity patterns, the challenges of achieving work-life balance, and the impact of family breakdown and reconstitution would also be identified.
- These data would be especially valuable in highlighting the way in which different family structures can be related to social disadvantage. This is demonstrated by the situation of lone parent households, which in the UK double a child's risk of living in poverty (ONS, 2015). In 2010 mothers headed more than 90% of these households (ONS, 2015) and were the most economically insecure of the working-age population, especially constrained by the absence of affordable child-care. This contrasts with the SASA report's

sole example of a lone parent family, headed by a father in full-time employment as a physiotherapist.

- *Older adults (65+ yrs):* Data on the social determinants of health would generate a very different profile of the older population from that illustrated by the SASA case studies. They would identify the constraints of ageing that are national and global policy concerns, including low income, social isolation and dependency on care services. They would also highlight the reductions in physical and mental capacities associated with biological ageing, including chronic illness (Banks, Nazroo & Steptoe, 2012).

Widening the evidence base on physical activity

Evidence-based PA policy has been diligent in its use of psychosocial theorisations of health behaviour that can inform practice. There is value in building on this to also include evidence on the social determinants of health and their effect on people's capacities to behave in healthy ways. External contextual influences are already recognised by SEMs, but these seldom draw on the very substantial, long-standing and relevant literature that examines how social disadvantage maps on to poor health, and how structural factors exert influence on health status at the individual level. Use of this expertise should be valuable in equipping practitioners to work with those who have most to gain from becoming active, but may face the biggest barriers to doing so.

While the dynamics of health inequalities are complex, there is nonetheless plentiful evidence available to ensure PA guidance is better informed about them. This includes:

- Social statistical data, including analyses of population characteristics, socio-economic variables, characteristics and dynamics of poverty and disadvantage, and patterns of health including the association of PA with health outcomes. In 2016 the UK Office for National Statistics held over 1,600 'health' datasets, 2,000 on 'society', and 4,000 on 'the environment'. Downloadable reports providing detailed data on key variables recognised in SEMs – e.g. 'family', analyses of which reveal diversity in structure, size and composition, and variation across the social gradient – e.g. higher incidences of young mothers, lone parent households and larger families in low-income groups. This category also includes substantial data on sub-groups rising in importance on the PA agenda, such as the living and health conditions of older people.
- Research that demonstrates how people are affected by adverse circumstances. Evidence on the effects of material deprivation in the UK and internationally has a long tradition (e.g. Haan, Kaplan & Camacho, 1987; Wilson et al., 2004; Thompson et al., 2015, p. 18), especially in periods of economic downturn or policy priority (mass unemployment in the 1980s; child poverty in the 1990s; post-2008 austerity), and includes research into income poverty, food insecurity, low quality housing and poor living environments. Among this work are also bodies of research addressing the complex and interrelated effects of deprivation on particular population groups, including e.g. women; lone parents; minority ethnic communities; and of course older age adults. There is a strong strand of psychosocial work which holds particular interest for PA behaviourists: it consistently shows that material hardship induces high levels of stress that are disabling and are associated with increases in depressive illnesses, suicide and para suicide. 'As a result, coping mechanisms and capacity for agency are reduced – not through inadequacy, but as a rational, and involuntary, response to hardship' (Tomlinson & Walker, 2009).

- Research, which examines the constraints affecting inactive people in everyday life. Sport England's major programmes (*Get healthy, get into sport*, 2013–16; *Get healthy, get active* (from 2016)) have had a remit to improve the evidence base. Other detailed analyses include Hills, Bradford and Johnston's (2013) study of national charity StreetGames' legacy-building programmes in disadvantaged areas; Edwards et al.'s (2015) analysis of poverty and access to young people; and Mansfield et al.'s (2015) evaluation of a complex community intervention to encourage inactive people to be active.

Expanding the evidence base in this way is most likely to be effective if it is accompanied by corresponding expansion of the PA knowledge community (Kay, 2016). This may include diversifying the disciplinary base, to include participation from social scientists; making use of a wider range of professional expertise, by including professionals from outside the research community; and obtaining lay knowledge, through consultative approaches that provide mechanisms for individuals to tell their complex stories, inform decision making and contribute to the development of interventions. This is especially important for ensuring that new knowledge is relevant and usable for practice. Engaging with non-academic and lay partners can contribute to this process and further move physical activity guidance from a hierarchical chain of communication to a collaborative partnership in which knowledge is co-produced.

Conclusion

There is little question that guidance for promoting physical activity is scientifically informed. It can become more informed by drawing on expert analysis of social determinants of health. PA policy that is informed by such research will be better equipped to address the complexities of people's situations and the factors that constrain them from being active.

This has implications for practice – for once the importance of social structural influences are recognised, PA interventions have to extend their focus beyond individual behaviour modification, to also address factors external to the individual. Connecting PA to health inequalities would lead to the use of evidence on the characteristics, situations and experiences of different population groups, and produce more informed guidance for interventions to increase physical activity levels. It would also recognise that individuals face difficulties to behaving in 'healthy' ways. Such analyses are more likely to have relevance to those with whom health workers engage than the portrayals given in guidance such as the SASA report, in which no-one is deprived, disadvantaged or constrained.

Chapter summary

Physical activity has a central role to play in addressing the dominant forms of global ill-health in our time – non-communicable diseases. NCDs are a universal challenge but unevenly distributed, creating differences in life expectancy of a decade or more among people living in the same country – and in some cases, the same city. To be effective, PA policy and practice therefore needs to recognise and confront the causes that underpin discriminatory health inequalities.

PA interventions that support inactive individuals to become more active in daily life are essential elements of this strategy. They are not sufficient by themselves, however, as they are limited in their capacity to address structural factors that materially affect individuals' behaviour but lie outside their control.

The importance of these contextual factors has long been recognised in socioecological models of health behaviour, and it is timely to revisit these approaches. This chapter has suggested that drawing on internationally recognised knowledge of the dynamics of health inequalities is an appropriate way to do so. This body of academic scholarship, professional and lay knowledge will allow the challenges and difficulties of becoming active to be given more attention, and equip global, national and local actors to support individuals to overcome inactivity.

- Physical activity has an important role to play in reducing the burden of non-communicable diseases (NCDs). The impact of non-communicable diseases is however unequal: in all countries of the world, regardless of their overall level of social and economic development, poorer sectors of the population are more affected by NCDs than more affluent citizens.
- Physical activity therefore needs to address the mechanisms of health inequalities to bring maximum benefit to those with most to gain from becoming more active. This can be achieved through an evidence base in which social determinants of health perspectives are centred, reducing the dominance of behaviour change theories. This has implications for policy, practice and promotion of physical activity.
- Policy guidance underpinned by social determinants of health perspectives would recognise that:
  o individuals are affected by constraining factors that reduce both their opportunities and their *capacity* to be active
  o constraints are most acute at the lower end of the social gradient – among the least healthy people living the most difficult lives
  o motivating individuals and changing the collective 'culture' surrounding PA are both important, but not solutions in themselves as they do not address constraints.
- Practitioner guidance would emphasise the need to identify and understand the constraints affecting inactive people, and equip deliverers to address these.
- Finally, public health messaging informed by social determinants of health perspectives would acknowledge that becoming active can be difficult and rather than chastising people for their inactivity, recognise the obstacles they face and the need for support to overcome them.

Acknowledgement: This chapter develops analysis previously explored in Kay 2016.

References

Bambra, C., Smith, K.E., Garthwaite, K., Joyce, K.E. & Hunter, D.J. (2011). A labour of Sisyphus? Public policy and health inequalities research from the Black and Acheson Reports to the Marmot Review. *Journal of Epidemiology and Community Health, 65*, 399–406.

Banks, J., Nazroo, J. & Steptoe, A. (2012). *The dynamics of ageing: evidence from the English Longitudinal Study of Ageing 2002–10*. London: Institute for Fiscal Studies.

Brewer, M., Browne, J. & Joyce, R. (2009a). *Child and Working-Age Poverty from 2010 to 2020, Commentary 121*. London: Institute for Fiscal Studies.

Brewer, M., Muriel, A., Phillips, D. & Sibieta, L. (2009b). *Poverty and Inequality in the UK: 2009, Commentary 109*. London: Institute for Fiscal Studies.

Burke, N., Joseph, G., Pasick, R.J. & Barker, J.C. (2009). Theorizing social context: rethinking behavioral theory, *Health Education & Behavior, 36*, 55S–70S.

Department of Health (2011). *Start Active, Stay Active: a report on physical activity from the four home countries' Chief Medical Officers.* London: HMSO.

Edwards, G., Grubb, B., Power, A. & Serle, N. (2015). *Moving the Goal Posts: poverty and access to sport for young people. CASE report 95.* London: London School of Economics.

European Commission (2013). *Health inequalities in the EU – Final report of a consortium. Consortium lead: Sir Michael Marmot.* Available from: http://ec.europa.eu/health/social_determinants/docs/healthinequalitiesineu_2013_en.pdf

Glanz, K., Sallis, J.F., Saelens, B.E. & Frank, L.D. (2005). Healthy nutrition environments: concepts and measures. *American Journal of Health Promotion, 19*, 330–333.

Golden, S.D. & Earp, J.A.L. (2012). Social ecological approaches to individuals and their contexts: twenty years of health education & behavior health promotion interventions. *Health Education & Behavior, 39*, 364–372.

Golden, S.D, McLeroy, K.R., Green, L., Earp, J.A. & Lieberman, L.D. (2015). Upending the social ecological model to guide health promotion efforts toward policy and environmental change. *Health Education & Behavior, 42*, 8S–14S.

Graham, H., & Kelly, M.P. (2004). *Health inequalities: concepts, frameworks and policy.* London: HAD.

Haan, N., Kaplan, G.A. & Camacho, T. (1987). Poverty and health: prospective evidence from the Alameda County Study. *American Journal of Epidemiology, 125*, 989–998.

Hills, L., Bradford, S. & Johnston, C. (2013). *Building a participation legacy from the London 2012 Olympic and Paralympic games in disadvantaged areas. Report for StreetGames.* London: Brunel University London.

Irwin, A. & Scali, E. (2007). Action on the social determinants of health: a historical perspective. *Global Public Health, 2*, 235–256.

Kay, T.A. (2016). Bodies of knowledge: connecting the evidence bases on physical activity and health inequalities. *International Journal of Sport Policy and Politics, 8*, 539–557.

Mansfield, L., Anokye, N., Fox-Rushby, J. & Kay, T.A. (2015). The Health and Sport Engagement (HASE) Intervention and Evaluation Project: protocol for the design, outcome, process and economic evaluation of a complex community sport intervention to increase levels of physical activity. *BMJ Open, 5*, pp. e009276–e009276.

Marmot, M. (2010a). The Marmot Review: *Fair society, healthy lives Strategic Review of Health Inequalities in England Post 2010.* Marmot Review Final Report. London: University College London.

Marmot, M. (2010b). The Marmot Review: *Fair society, healthy lives Strategic Review of Health Inequalities in England Post 2010.* Marmot Review Executive Summary. London: University College London.

McLeroy, K.R., Bibeau, D., Steckler, A. & Glanz, K. (1988). An ecological perspective on health promotion programs. *Health Education Quarterly, 15*, 351–377

ONS (2013). *Life expectancy at birth and at age 65 for local areas in England and Wales: 2009–11.* London: HMSO.

ONS (2015) *Families and households (2015).* London: HMSO.

Sallis, J.F. (2009). *Using research to create a less obesogenic world.* Presentation to the Texas Obesity Research Center, April 9. Accessed on 9th December 2015 at http://sallis.ucsd.edu/Documents/Pubs_documents/Slides_HoustonObesity_040909.pdf

Solar, O. & Irwin, A. (2010). *A conceptual framework for action on the social determinants of health.* Geneva: World Health Organization.

Stokols, D. (1992). Establishing and maintaining healthy environments: toward a social ecology of health promotion. *American Psychologist, 47*, 6–22.

Stokols, D. (1996). Translating social ecological theory into guidelines for community health promotion. *American Journal of Health Promotion, 10*, 282–298.

Story, M., Kaphingst, K., Robinson-O'Brien, R. & Glanz, K. (2008). Creating healthy food and eating environments: policy and environmental approaches. *Annu. Rev. Public Health, 29*, 253–272.

Thompson, C., Lewis, D.J., Greenhalgh, T., Smith, N.R., Fahy, A.E. & Cummins, S. (2015). 'Everyone was looking at you smiling': East London residents' experiences of the 2012 Olympics and its legacy on the social determinants of health. *Health and Place, 36*, 18–24.

Tomlinson, M. & Walker, R. (2009). *Coping with complexity: child and adult poverty*. London: Child Poverty Action Group.

WHO (2008a). *Closing the gap in a generation: health equity through action on the social determinants of health*. Commission on Social Determinants of Health Report. Geneva: World Health Organization.

WHO (2008b). *Closing the gap in a generation: health equity through action on the social determinants of health – Executive Summary* Commission on Social Determinants of Health Executive Summary. Geneva: World Health Organization.

Wilson, K., Elliot, S., Law, M., Eyles, J., Jerrett, M. & Keller-Olaman, S. (2004). Linking perceptions of neighbourhood to health in Hamilton, Canada. *J. Epidemiol. Commun. Health, 58*, 192–198.

Wright, C., Lodge, H. & Jacobson, B. (2012). *Childs Play? The antenatal to adolescent health legacy in the Olympic boroughs*. London: London Health Observatory.

26 International perspectives on physical activity

Adrian Bauman

Keywords: International, physical activity, global health, non-communicable disease, policy

Inactivity is a major global problem

Physical inactivity is a major public health problem, contributing to global morbidity and mortality. A 2009 WHO report ranked physical inactivity as the fourth leading risk factor (after tobacco, hypertension and high blood sugar levels), and ahead of obesity is contributing to global deaths (WHO, 2009). Inactivity contributed to around 3.5 million deaths/year, of which two-thirds were in middle and low-income countries (WHO, 2009). This is less than the subsequent estimate from the *Lancet* physical activity series (Lee et al., 2012) which estimated around 5 million deaths per year were attributable to inactivity; this was a total similar to the number of global deaths attributable to tobacco, and substantially more than were attributable to obesity (Lee et al., 2012). These analyses indicate that the burden of disease from physical inactivity is substantial, and not confined to high-income developed countries alone; changes in middle and low-income countries have led to declines in physical activity in recent decades, leading to physical inactivity becoming one of the major global risk factors for non-communicable disease (Sallis et al., 2016). Further, many other health problems are partly preventable through increased physical activity, including improving mental health, reducing falls in the elderly (and maintaining functional capacity), preventing dementia and other chronic conditions (Bauman, Merom, Bull, Buchner & Fiatarone Singh, 2016). Conservative economic estimates suggest an annual cost of at least $67B (USD) due to physical inactivity (Ding et al., 2016), although the real cost is probably much greater than this, especially in relation to premature morbidity and work absenteeism among inactive working-aged adults.

The prevalence of physical inactivity remains high. Globally around a third of adults and nearly 80% of children and adolescents (Hallal et al., 2012) fail to meet the minimum recommended levels of physical activity (150 mins/week of moderate vigorous physical activity for adults, and 60 mins per day for children and adolescents, WHO PA guidelines, 2010). The updated global prevalence in the 2016 *Lancet* series, using slightly modified criteria, estimated that 23% of adults and 80% of adolescents did not meet the physical activity guidelines for health (Sallis et al., 2016).

International perspectives on the history of physical activity and its benefits

The earliest observations of physical activity and health were made in antiquity (Berryman, 1989), where moderation in diet and exercise were recommended for good health. This notion was repeated in general medical recommendations over the ensuing two thousand years. By the 19th century the concepts of 'a fit nation' or 'fit youth' were prevalent in Northern Europe, both as part of nationalism and also for a fit military and civilian workforce (Redmond, 1988). These were nationalistic sentiments, based upon mass fitness training, physical education and physical culture among adolescents and young adults (Redmond, 1988). Only one example of national government physical activity policy can be identified; this was the Australian National Fitness Act (Collins & Lekkas, 2011), providing a comprehensive set of programmes to increase fitness and provide a training regimen for young Australians (noting that this was in the middle of World War 2, and was part of producing military fitness, and that this initiative was not sustained long term).

Although the first epidemiological evidence for physical activity (exercise) and health was published in the UK (Morris, Heady, Raffle, Roberts & Parks, 1953), much of the recent decades of epidemiological research has been conducted in the USA, some from Europe and Australia, and less evidence from other countries. Nonetheless, the relationships between physical activity and health outcomes, in the available literature, appear identical in middle- and lower to middle-income countries (Milton, Macniven & Bauman, 2014), suggesting the potential for health gain exists in all countries with, or at risk of obesity, non-communicable and other chronic diseases.

The problem of physical inactivity differs across national contexts

Understanding the health consequences of physical inactivity has occurred at different rates in different regions and countries. NCD prevention strategies have variably adopted physical activity, and have varied in the degree to which they understood physical activity as more than 'prescribing exercise as therapy in clinical settings'. Further, the declines in activity levels and development of 'inactive populations' has occurred at different rates within and between countries, making policy development more challenging.

In most high-income countries, declines in energy expenditure occurred following industrialisation, and thus during the 19th century energy expenditure at work declined, followed by declines in active travel with the rise of public transport systems and motor vehicles in the early 20th century (Hardman & Stensel, 2003). Leisure time activity remained (and possibly increased) as the main form of daily energy expenditure in wealthy industrialised nations. By contrast, the pattern in many middle-income countries was quite different. As countries in East Asia, South Asia and Latin America rapidly industrialised and urbanised, rapid declines in occupational and transport activity was not always replaced by LTPA. The rapidity of development, the lack of leisure time opportunities, climate factors and high work pressures in rapidly developing countries all contributed (Ng & Popkin, 2012). This has led to declines in physical activity in just a few decades, alongside increases in sedentary time at work (Ng & Popkin, 2012). These same countries are also in the middle of the epidemiological transition to developing NCDs and obesity, both of which could be attenuated by maintaining population physical activity levels. Challenges in maintaining activity are difficult in countries with new wealthy populations seeking to buy and use cars, dismissing previous active transport (walking and cycling) and living in (crowded) high density cities with limited accessible physical activity facilities or opportunities.

As well as differences in changes in physical activity over time, countries have adopted the concepts of 'physical activity' as a risk factor at different stages in national preventive efforts. In some countries, the more medically focused risk factors, hypertension, obesity and blood sugar levels are first mentioned, although tobacco prevention is usually recognised. Physical activity (and its need for cross-sectoral actions, not just through the health sector) is more challenging to recognise as a risk factor and more difficult to implement relevant public health actions, especially in countries where the NCD prevention strategies are health sector-centric. This has also led to different rates of development of national physical activity plans, strategies and guidelines (see below, p. 437).

WHO and international developments in physical activity policy and strategy

The international context for physical activity policies, reports and surveillance has become more prominent since around 2000. Before that time, there were sporadic World Health Organization statements about NCDs, but little that specifically targeted physical activity. The seminal change occurred globally with the release of the 2004 WHO Global Diet and Physical Activity Strategy (DPAS, WHO, 2004). This document defined the role of health and other agencies in physical activity, and urged countries to develop clear physical activity plans as part of NCD prevention. This has been followed by a range of WHO and UN statements on NCDs that mentioned and recommended physical activity as part of the solution to the global NCD crisis (row 1, Figure 26.1).

The epidemiological evidence base also matured during this period. Although there had been evidence since the 1950s that exercise was beneficial to health, there was a movement during the 1990s that made clear statements synthesising the physical activity evidence, and developing the '30 minutes a day' message (which is now characterised as '150 minutes of MVPA per week'). These syntheses led to the United States Surgeon General's report on physical activity and health in 1996 (USSG, 1996), which contributed to increasing global interest in this issue. This has been followed by guidance from national governments and from professional bodies such as the International Society of Physical Activity and Health (ISPAH, row 2, Figure 26.1). These have started to move from simply recommending physical activity to describe 'best practice guidance' in physical activity programmes. Some WHO regions have also developed clear physical activity statements, and in the case of WHO/Euro, a clear policy framework for action was published (WHO/Euro, 2016).

From the WHO perspective, there have been consistent statements and documents over the past 15 years, particularly through WHO global action plans 2008–2013 and from 2013 onwards (row 1, Figure 26.1). This most recent WHO action plan also includes the global monitoring framework with the 2025 indicator that countries need to achieve a relative 10% reduction in physical inactivity, as measured through their population surveys. Broader policy support also occurred through the UN declaration on NCDs in 2011, and the WHO NCD reports in 2014 (UN, 2011; WHO, 2013b). In 2018, the WHO produced the global action plan for physical activity (WHO, 2018), one of the strongest and most well developed cross-sectoral statements by the WHO in this area to date.

Additional supportive frameworks and evidence reviews were led by the International Society for Physical Activity and Health (ISPAH) through the 2010 Toronto Charter and subsequent '7 best investments for physical activity' two years later. There have also been regional physical activity statements from some WHO regions, and in 2016 a well-developed European region physical activity plan (WHO/Euro, 2016). These were supported by the *Lancet*

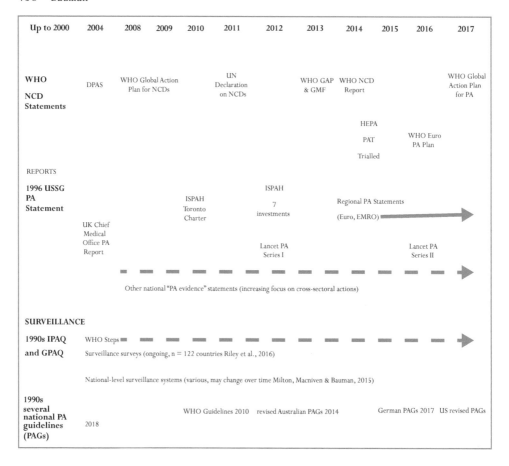

Figure 26.1 History of physical activity international policy and national-level efforts since 2000

Physical Activity Series which were released to coincide with the Summer Olympic Games which focused on a global perspective on physical activity (*Lancet*, 2012, *Lancet*, 2016).

Some countries have released specific physical activity guidelines on the dose, volume and intensity of physical activity for health (last row, Figure 26.1), including the WHO in 2010, through which guidelines for children, adults and older adults were released. Australia and the USA released such guidelines in the late 1990s, many European countries in the early 2000s, the WHO released global guidelines in 2010, and recently comprehensive German PA guidelines were released (Füzéki, Vogt & Banzer, 2017). Updates to PA guidelines have been published in Australia and Canada, and are in progress in the USA during 2018.

WHO surveys on NCDs – progress in national physical activity policy and plans

Since 2000, the WHO has conducted surveys to assess NCD prevention capacity, including physical activity actions at national and regional levels. Surveys were conducted of key national

WHO focal points in each country in 2000, 2005, 2010, 2013 and 2015. Key physical activity data were extracted from 2005 and 2015 reports (WHO, 2007; WHO, 2015) to show progress over a decade.

In 2005, engagement with physical activity was less well developed than others as one of the risk factors listed in overall NCD strategies. Oftentimes, physical activity was nested in national-level obesity prevention strategies, which excludes the plethora of non-NCD benefits of populations being more active. In the 2005 WHO surveys of countries, 23% reported national regulation or legislation relevant to physical activity, compared to over 80% for diet/nutrition and tobacco (WHO, 2007). Similarly reported physical activity policy, physical activity action plans and physical activity programmes (33% in 2005) were all half to two-thirds of the rates of policy and plans for diet and tobacco control (WHO, 2007). Nonetheless, interest in physical activity improved substantially between 2005 and 2015 (Table 26.1), with increases in physical activity policy, action plans and strategies, moving physical activity actions towards the levels reported for other primary prevention risk factors by 2015 (WHO, 2016). However, this was limited by the 'implementation gap', where the presence of policies or national strategies did not guarantee their organisational structure, funding or delivery. This gap means that many of the countries with PA plans still are delivering little in terms of population-wide programmes to promote more active adults and children.

The situation with respect to PA surveillance has substantially improved. More than two-thirds of countries had physical activity prevalence estimates from national representative surveys, indicating the potential for monitoring ongoing physical activity trends to indicate the net sum of public health preventive efforts. The presence of specific physical activity guidelines is less clear. In 2005, 30% of countries reported physical activity guidelines, but in 2015 guidelines were only asked about NCDs, not risk factors. One new question in 2015 indicated 7% of countries had fiscal incentives for promoting physical activity, a new strategy (not previously reported).

These indicators from the WHO country capacity surveys are a useful source of information for assessing progress in international efforts to increase physical activity. These will provide important intermediate indicators in progress towards achieving the WHO 2025 targets, described in the WHO Global Monitoring Framework (WHO, 2013a). This document was presented at the World Health Assembly and accepted by WHO member states. It recommended targets for all NCD risk factors, including a relative 10% decrease in the proportion of the adult population not meeting the recommended levels of physical activity for health This 10% target will be challenging to achieve in many countries, as the existing physical

Table 26.1 Trends in physical activity related policy and national surveillance

	2005 N=133 countries (69%)	2015 N=177 countries (91%)
National regulation for Physical Activity	23%	NA
National Physical Activity policy	29%	(91%)*
National action plan Physical Activity	32%	71%
National Surveys Physical Activity	62%	70%

* *'policy, plan and strategy' asked in 2015*

activity plans and strategies need to be fully operationalised and implemented in order to reduce the prevalence of inactivity. To achieve this, many countries will need to divert greater resources to physical activity promotion, and to develop and implement cross-agency work to promote physical activity (in partnership with sport, education, urban planning, transport and other sectors beyond health).

International perspectives on physical activity surveillance

Physical activity surveillance internationally is a complex and variably implemented action. A comprehensive national physical activity surveillance system should include collection of physical activity prevalence data in representative population samples. In addition, it should also include organisational and system level indicators that provide ongoing monitoring of physical activity capacity, institutional change, environmental and regulatory change that are likely to support physical activity. Many countries have some level of physical activity prevalence estimates, but few have routine comprehensive and integrated surveillance systems. One example of such a system has been developed and used in Canada and implemented at the national and provincial level (Craig, Cameron & Bauman, 2017).

Nonetheless many estimates of physical activity are available. The WHO reports these through the STEPS surveillance system, now implemented in more than 100 countries. Periodic surveys assess population physical activity levels among adults using the GPAQ instrument (Bull, Maslin & Armstrong, 2009) administered to representative population samples. These surveys collect information by questionnaire (self-report) as well as objective measures of height and weight, blood pressure, cholesterol and blood sugar levels (Riley et al., 2016). Prevalence data are stored in the WHO 'global health Observatory', and physical activity estimates of the proportion of many populations meeting physical activity recommendations are stored there (http://apps.who.int/gho/data/view.main.2463?lang=en).

A quite different and more recent compilation of PA prevalence estimates has been compiled through the International Society for Physical Activity and Health; this 'global physical activity compendium' provides an inventory of recent physical activity estimates among adults in many countries (www.globalphysicalactivityobservatory.com/). Note that these estimates may differ from those provided by the WHO; for example, an estimate for Australia in the WHO global health observatory describes a 2003 estimate using IPAQ where only 23% of adults were not meeting the PA guidelines; by contrast, the Australian Bureau of Statistics national health surveys uses older physical activity questions, and reports in 2014/15 that 44% did not meet guidelines. These differences are often due to even small differences in the questions asked (Macniven, Bauman & Abouzeid, 2012). This poses challenges for cross-national comparisons, with some countries using their own national level surveillance systems, others using the GPAQ measures from STEPS surveillance, and some using both; these measures often assess different or more limited domains of physical activity. Furthermore in several countries questions or survey methods have changed over time, such as in the UK, reducing the comparability of prevalence of physical activity estimates (Milton & Bauman, 2015).

Several research groups have collaborated to produce a report card for physical activity amongst children, and this also describes the presence of policies and programmes in some detail, so provides useful information for advocacy within and between countries to provide physical education and physical activity opportunities for children and adolescents (www. activehealthykids.org/). This started in Canada, where for over a decade, annual 'grades' were awarded to indicate regional and national progress in physical activity related indicators (Tremblay, Barnes & Bonne, 2014). These report cards were widely disseminated in Canada, and gradually adopted in other countries. They described successful implementation of physical activity programmes in different dimensions in 38 countries (Tremblay et al., 2016). These included 'grades' awarded for overall physical activity and sedentary behaviour rates, active transportation, active play, sport participation, and school programmes, as well as community and the built environment indicators (Tremblay et al., 2016). The best overall grades for children and youth physical activity programmes and policies were reported in Denmark, Slovenia and the Netherlands.

Challenges in international perspectives are made more difficult by the use of different physical activity instruments, infrequent use of objective measurement in population surveys, and differences in cultural meanings of physical activity questions, and in the survey sampling frames used. Furthermore, different domains of physical activity contribute differently across countries. For example, changes in countries undergoing economic development often remove active travel as the major form of physical activity, but failed to replace it with leisure time activity (Ng & Popkin, 2012). Population surveys that measure only leisure time activity will miss these major behavioural epidemiological trends. Changes in work practices in many countries indicate reduced energy expenditure in occupational time, contributing to a reduction in total daily physical activity (Church et al., 2011). This means that comparing population levels of physical activity, defined as the proportion meeting established guidelines, vary substantially according to the measure used and the research environment in which adult and children's population surveys are conducted (Macniven, Bauman & Abouzeid, 2012; Pedišić et al., 2017). Future directions in the international arena may involve the WHO piloting objects of measure in the STEPS surveillance system, and increased use of wearable devices, portable activity trackers and smartphones where aggregated data may reflect population-level and internationally comparable physical activity behaviour (Althoff, Hicks, King, Delp & Leskovec, 2017).

Examples and case studies of effective population physical activity initiatives

There have been thousands of physical activity programmes conducted internationally, in different settings, with different target populations. Many intensive small-scale or individual exercise programmes, targeting individual behaviour change, provide benefits to people with specific health problems, such as those with diabetes or following a cardiac event or an injurious fall. Some are at a larger scale, and are conducted in workplaces, in schools or in targeted population settings, and these will reach more individuals. However, few programmes are scaled up to the whole community or population level, and exist as evidence-based and comprehensive physical activity efforts that have demonstrable links to population level PA participation rates. Some are discussed in the *Lancet* physical activity series paper on 'scale up' (Reis et al., 2016); other examples are presented in a scale-up review of interventions for NCD prevention (Indig, Lee, Grunseit, Milat & Bauman, 2017). These programmes are important for influencing population physical activity, and extend earlier chapters' discussions of smaller scale interventions to increase activity. Here, international examples of these scaled-up and comprehensive programmes are provided, which illustrate examples or case studies that embody several to all of the elements of best practice PA programmes (Trost, Blair & Khan, 2014).

Some areas are widely discussed as having 'great potential', but remain to be evidence-based in reaching and influencing populations. Three areas are discussed below that have the potential to influence the population, but are still limited in the scientific basis for scaled-up action. For example, 'Exercise is Medicine' has become a theme promoted globally by the American College of Sports Medicine (Duperly et al., 2014; Lobelo, Stoutenberg & Hutber, 2014), and is an extension of several decades of primary care trials to promote brief advice for physical activity (Lamming et al., 2017). The setting of primary care or general practice is an obvious one for the promotion of PA to the inactive population, but trials to date have produced small and short-term effects, and usually from selected practices or practitioners, with few examples of scale-up to be adopted by the majority of primary care and healthcare practitioners and systems (Lamming et al., 2017).

Table 26.2   Case studies of broad reach or national physical activity programmes

Programme, setting, time period	Intervention components	Programme effects
Project Agita, Brazil mid 1990s–present (Matsudo et al., 2002, 2003, 2010, 2017)	Started as grassroots local PA campaign, in one region of São Paulo; developed a brand and mass media campaign, programmes targeting GPs; spread throughout Brazil, fostered environmental changes, PA programmes targeting elderly, all schoolchildren, marginalised groups; across other regions in Brazil and beyond	Well recognised campaign 'half hour man' adopted across Latin America; principles generalised to other countries and the WHO. Decrease in population prevalence of inactivity among adults in São Paulo region
Football Fans In Training, Europe, 2012–present (Wyke, 2015)	Using elite football clubs and venues as a vehicle to access middle-aged overweight men to enrol in a 12-week programme of weight loss and physical activity	Good uptake shown in Scottish study (Gray et al., 2013), with positive effects (Gray et al., 2013a), and scaled up in Scotland and in Europe (Hunt et al., 2014; van de Glind et al., 2017)
Push Play, New Zealand 2001–2010	Integrated mass media campaign (Push Play, Bauman et al., 2003) combined with distribution of GP active prescription pad intervention, and in later years, youth physical activity; focus on linking to regional sports organisations throughout NZ	Limited comparable PA surveillance data collected in NZ, but effects of delivery and sustained efforts noteworthy
Trim and Fit, Singapore 1992–2007	Part of Singapore Health Promotion Board efforts at obesity prevention; multiple PA and healthy nutrition programmes mandated in all schools; implementation and reach very high	Students' measured fitness threshold levels increased from 61% in 1993 to 81% in 2006 (Foo et al., 2013)

Another international example with 'great potential' are city-based 'bike share' schemes (also known as public bicycle programmes), where bicycles are made available for short trips, to add to the number of short active transport trips that are carried out. Although bike share schemes are well developed in cities such as London, Paris, Barcelona and Montreal, they tend to attract younger adults who are already active or attract tourists for short-term use, and evidence of population physical activity impact is limited (Bauman, Crane, Drayton & Titze, 2017). Perhaps it is the largest scale for implementing bike share schemes, such as in Hangzhou, China, which may encourage active transport by inactive adults; to date, although enthusiastically adopted in policy documents, this mode of intervention is not conclusively evidence-based for increasing population PA levels.

The third international example with 'great but unproven potential' is the use of wearable technologies, smart watches and smartphone apps to track, monitor and encourage physical activity. Recent data suggests around 50 million wearables and smart watches were sold in 2016 (Forbes, 2017), with over a billion smartphones (Forbes, 2016). Their immense global reach mean that access to these devices or phones is becoming nearly universal, but the evidence that they are useful in the long term to encourage inactive people to become and stay active is still lacking. Nonetheless, their capacity for surveillance and for intervention remains a tantalising challenge (Althoff et al., 2017).

International examples of comprehensive physical activity programmes are shown in Table 26.2. These have cross-national reach, were innovative, and have influenced or are likely to influence physical activity levels. There are few programmes that meet these criteria and are well published or documented, so only four examples are shown. Efforts were made to obtain geographic diversity, using different strategies and in diverse regions. These case studies are described below and in Table 26.2.

Case studies (Table 26.2)

1. Project Agita was a community-based programme launched by Celafiscs, an academic sport and physical activity centre, in the mid-1990s in São Paulo, Brazil. They had received minimal funding, but have developed a clear brand, an unfunded social marketing campaign that spread rapidly and attracted huge amounts of unpaid media attention, and a comprehensive cross-agency partnership that implemented numerous programmes with diverse population targets (Matsudo et al., 2002, 2003). Annual walking parades in São Paulo continue to the present, and attract tens of thousands of participants, with the aim of drawing attention to physical activity for health. The programme was scaled up to the province of São Paulo, and adapted nationally in Brazil and by many neighbouring countries in Latin America. Serial population surveys demonstrated substantial declines in inactivity among adults in the region, at least partly attributable to the Agita-related programs (Matsudo et al., 2010).

2. Football Fans in Training used the sport sector and prestigious football clubs and their venues to attract middle-aged male fans who were inactive and overweight to participate in a 12-week behaviour change programme. Using sport and fandom as facilitators, good feasibility and adoption was demonstrated in Scotland (Gray et al., 2013). The pilot RCT showed clear effects on weight loss (6 kg), and an increase of around 1700 Met-mins on average each week (which equates to more than an additional hour a day of physical activity, Gray, Hunt, Mutrie, Anderson, Treweek & Wyke, 2013a). Then project was scaled-up in Scotland (Hunt et al., 2014), and then further scaled-up to multiple European sites,

attracting 1,000 middle-aged males to participate in this programme (called EuroFit, van de Glind et al., 2017). This indicates a nexus between sports fans and the potential for health promotion, as well as a scalable intervention that is likely to be generalisable in many countries.

3. 'Push Play' in New Zealand was a national physical activity and sport programme that was implemented from 2001 to around 2010. Interestingly, it was led by the national sport agency (the Hillary Commission, later SPARC, NZ), but delivered a comprehensive suite of programmes and public health activities. The spearhead was a mass media campaign targeting all population segments, focusing on getting more active. Specific programmes and resources were developed for the Maori (indigenous New Zealanders) and Pacific Islander populations. An evidence-based general practice green prescription programme (Elley, Kerse, Arroll & Robinson, 2003) was then distributed through the regions by the sport agency to all GPs, encouraging them to promote activity in primary care. A strong link to regional sport organisations also linked physical activity and sport. Although New Zealanders are generally quite physically active, no serial surveillance or evaluation of the overall initiative was undertaken; however, it is included here as a case study of comprehensive programming, national reach and good implementation.

4. Trim and Fit was a nation-wide programme introduced in Singapore in the early 1990s as part of obesity prevention efforts. The programme was mandated, with high levels of government support for implementation. It achieved clear benefits on fitness and obesity rates, but was modified after 2007 because of potential for perceived obesity stigma among overweight children. Other programmes were then developed, including sport as a co-curricular option in schools, and mandatory physical education increased from 0.5 to 1.5 hrs/week (Foo, Vijaya, Sloan & Ling, 2013). For adults, increased attention to physical activity followed the national PA guidelines in 2011, with promotion of mass transit, increase in workplace programmes (fitness@work), and a proliferation of walking groups and sport clubs, with increased membership (Foo et al., 2013). These initiatives also resulted in serial reported increases in physical activity levels among adults over a decade (Macniven, Bauman & Abouzeid, 2012).

Chapter summary

The issue of physical inactivity remains a major contributor to global ill-health, morbidity and mortality; nonetheless, it attracts less attention than other risk factors in approaches to NCD prevention, and has therefore been described as the 'Cinderella' of risk factors (Bull & Bauman, 2011). Furthermore, even in international reviews of NCD prevention and frameworks for action, physical activity is less often mentioned than obesity, tobacco and biomarker risk factors for chronic disease (Bauman et al., 2015). The practical corollary of this is that international advocacy efforts remain a priority to re-position efforts to address physical inactivity to become commensurate with its health consequences.

The evidence base for action has evolved over six decades, and physical activity poses similar health risks across countries at all levels of development. However, the patterns and development of inactivity in populations differ across and between countries, and vary by domain of activity. Countries also vary by the degree to which they have developed physical activity guidelines and implemented physical activity plans. Differences in measurement tools may produce apparently different prevalence rates of the proportions meeting health-enhancing levels, suggesting the need for standardisation of measurement methods. One example of this has been through the World Health Organization STEPS surveillance system, now used in over 100 countries.

Strategies to increase activity levels may need to be country-specific, and require local partnerships to coordinate appropriate actions to create relevant physical activity opportunities, environments and facilities. The case studies presented here identify the elements of effective population-level programmes; these include comprehensive and cross-sectoral approaches, multiple intervention components and long-term political support and resources. Without these integrated large-scale approaches, current low physical activity levels will remain unchanged in many countries, and the opportunity for prevention practice will be missed.

- Physical inactivity causes 3.5–5 million deaths and has a global economic burden amounting to $67bn
- Physical inactivity is increasing in low- to middle-income countries where motorised transport and migration to densely populated cities has increased at a faster rate than the provision of activity enhancing infrastructures.
- The scientific base supporting the benefits of physical activity on health has increased over the past 15 years that has prompted more physical activity policies worldwide.
- To close the gap between policy and implementation, physical activity promotion programmes require equal importance to obesity, pregnancy, tobacco, alcohol and substance abuse.
- Large-scale comprehensive and cross-sectoral approaches, multiple intervention components and long-term political support and resources are now required to reduce the significant global health burden of physical inactivity.

References

Althoff, T., Hicks, J.L., King, A.C., Delp, S.L., & Leskovec, J. (2017). Large-scale physical activity data reveal worldwide activity inequality. *Nature, 547*(7663), nature23018.

Bauman, A., McLean, G., Hurdle, D., Walker, S., Boyd, J., van Aalst, I., & Carr, H. (2003). Evaluation of the national 'Push Play' campaign in New Zealand – creating population awareness of physical activity. *The New Zealand Medical Journal* (Online), *116*(1179).

Bauman, A., McGill, B., Powell, K., Lee, I.M., Heath, G., Pratt, M., Kohl, H.W., & Hallal, P. (2015). Tackling obesity: challenges ahead. *The Lancet, 386*(9995), 741–742.

Bauman, A., Merom, D., Bull, F.C., Buchner, D.M., & Fiatarone Singh, M.A. (2016). Updating the evidence for physical activity: summative reviews of the epidemiological evidence, prevalence, and interventions to promote 'Active Aging'. *The Gerontologist, 56*(Suppl_2), S268–280.

Bauman, A., Crane, M., Drayton, B.A., & Titze, S. (2017). The unrealised potential of bike share schemes to influence population physical activity levels – a narrative review. *Preventive Medicine.* 2017.

Berryman, J.W. (1989). The tradition of the 'six things non-natural': exercise and medicine from Hippocrates through ante-bellum America. In: J.O. Holloszy (Ed.). *Exercise and Sport Sciences Reviews*. Vol. 17 (pp. 515–559). Baltimore, MD: Williams & Wilkins.

Bull, F.C., Maslin, T.S., & Armstrong, T. (2009). Global Physical Activity Questionnaire (GPAQ): nine country reliability and validity study. *Journal of Physical Activity and Health, 6*(6), 790–804.

Bull, F.C., & Bauman, A.E. (2011). Physical inactivity: the 'Cinderella' risk factor for non-communicable disease prevention. *Journal of Health Communication, 16*(sup2), 13–26.

Bull, F.C., Milton, K., & Kahlmeier, S. (2014). National policy on physical activity: the development of a policy audit tool. *J Phys Act Health, 11*, 233–240.

Church, T.S., Thomas, D.M., Tudor-Locke, C., Katzmarzyk, P.T., Earnest, C.P., Rodarte, R.Q., . . . Bouchard, C. (2011). Trends over 5 decades in US occupation-related physical activity and their associations with obesity. *PLoS ONE, 6*(5), e19657.

Collins, J.A., & Lekkas, P. (2011). Fit for purpose: Australia's National fitness campaign. *Med J Aust, 195*, 714–716.

Craig, C.L., Cameron, C.A., & Bauman, A. (2017). Utility of surveillance research to inform physical activity policy: an exemplar from Canada. *Journal of Physical Activity and Health, 14*(3), 229–239.

Ding, D., Lawson, K.D., Kolbe-Alexander, T.L., Finkelstein, E.A., Katzmarzyk, P.T., van Mechelen, W., Pratt, M., Lancet Physical Activity Series 2 Executive Committee (2016). The economic burden of physical inactivity: a global analysis of major non-communicable diseases. *The Lancet, 388*(10051), 1311–1324.

Duperly, J., Collazos, V., Paez, C., Donado, C., Pratt, M., & Lobelo, F. (2014). 'Exercise is Medicine' in Latin America: training health care professionals in physical activity prescription. *Schweizerische Zeitschrift fur Sportmedizin und Sporttraumatologie, 62*(2), 38–41.

Elley, C.R., Kerse, N., Arroll, B., & Robinson, E. (2003). Effectiveness of counselling patients on physical activity in general practice: cluster randomised controlled trial. *BMJ, 326*(7393), 793.

Foo, L., Vijaya, K., Sloan, R., & Ling, A. (2013). Obesity prevention and management: Singapore's experience. *Obesity Reviews, 14*(S2), 106–113.

Forbes (2016) www.forbes.com/sites/eladnatanson/2016/09/12/2016-a-pivotal-year-for-the-smart phone-industry/#3b2f9c89386e

Forbes (2017) www.forbes.com/sites/paullamkin/2017/03/03/fitbits-dominance-diminishes-but-wearable-tech-market-bigger-than-ever/#5e1d83b77f4d

Füzéki, E., Vogt, L., & Banzer, W. (2017). German national physical activity recommendations for adults and older adults: methods, database and rationale. *Gesundheitswesen (Bundesverband der Arzte des Offentlichen Gesundheitsdienstes (Germany)), 79*(S 01), S20.

Gray, C.M., Hunt, K., Mutrie, N., Anderson, A.S., Leishman, J., Dalgarno, L., & Wyke, S. (2013). Football Fans in Training: the development and optimization of an intervention delivered through professional sports clubs to help men lose weight, become more active and adopt healthier eating habits. *BMC Public Health, 13*(1).

Gray, C.M., Hunt, K., Mutrie, N., Anderson, A.S., Treweek, S., & Wyke, S. (2013a). Weight management for overweight and obese men delivered through professional football clubs: a pilot randomized trial. *International Journal of Behavioral Nutrition and Physical Activity, 10*.

Hallal, P.C., Andersen, L.B., Bull, F.C., Guthold, R., Haskell, W., Ekelund, U., Lancet Physical Activity Series Working Group (2012). Global physical activity levels: surveillance progress, pitfalls, and prospects. *The Lancet, 380*(9838), 247–257.

Hardman, A., & Stensel, D. (2003). *Physical activity and health – the evidence explained*. London: Routledge.

Hunt, K., Gray, C.M., Maclean, A., Smillie, S., Bunn, C., & Wyke, S. (2014). Do weight management programmes delivered at professional football clubs attract and engage high risk men? A mixed-methods study. *BMC Public Health, 14*(1).

Indig, D., Lee, K., Grunseit, A., Milat, A., & Bauman, A. (2017). Pathways for scaling up public health interventions. *BMC Public Health, 18*(1), 68.

Lamming, L., Pears, S., Mason, D., Morton, K., Bijker, M., Sutton, S., . . . VBI Programme Team. (2017). What do we know about brief interventions for physical activity that could be delivered in primary care consultations? A systematic review of reviews. *Preventive Medicine, 99*, 152–163.

Lancet 2012 www.thelancet.com/series/physical-activity

Lancet 2016 www.thelancet.com/series/physical-activity-2016

Lee, I.M., Shiroma, E.J., Lobelo, F., Puska, P., Blair, S.N., Katzmarzyk, P.T., Lancet Physical Activity Series Working Group (2012). Effect of physical inactivity on major non-communicable diseases worldwide: an analysis of burden of disease and life expectancy. *The Lancet, 380*(9838), 219–229.

Lobelo, F., Stoutenberg, M., & Hutber, A. (2014). The exercise is medicine global health initiative: a 2014 update. *British Journal of Sports Medicine, 48*(22), 1627–1633.

Macniven, R., Bauman, A., & Abouzeid, M. (2012). A review of population-based prevalence studies of physical activity in adults in the Asia-Pacific region. *BMC Public Health, 12*(1), 41.

Matsudo, V., Matsudo, S., Andrade, D., Araujo, T., Andrade, E., de Oliveira, L.C., & Braggion, G.F. (2002). Promotion of physical activity in a developing country: the Agita São Paulo experience. *Public Health Nutrition, 5*(1a), 253–261.

Matsudo, S.M., Matsudo, V.R., Araujo, T.L., Andrade, D.R., Andrade, E.L., Oliveira, L.C., & Braggion, G.F. (2003). The Agita São Paulo Program as a model for using physical activity to promote health. *Revista panamericana de salud pública, 14*(4), 265–272.

Matsudo, V., Matsudo, S.M., Araújo, T.L., Andrade, D.R., Oliveira, L.C., & Hallal, P.C. (2010). Time trends in physical activity in the state of São Paulo, Brazil: 2002–2008. *Med Sci Sports Exerc, 42*(12), 2231–2236.

Matsudo, V.K., & Lambert, E.V. (2017). Bright spots, physical activity investments that work: Agita Mundo global network. *Br J Sports Med*, bjsports-2016-097291.

Milton, K., Macniven, R., & Bauman, A. (2014). Review of the epidemiological evidence for physical activity and health from low- and middle-income countries. *Global Public Health, 9*(4), 369–381.

Milton, K., & Bauman, A. (2015). A critical analysis of the cycles of physical activity policy in England. *International Journal of Behavioral Nutrition and Physical Activity, 12*(8). https://doi.org/10.1186/s12966-015-0169-5.

Morris, J.N., Heady, J.A., Raffle, P.A., Roberts, C.G., & Parks, J.W. (1953). Coronary heart-disease and physical activity of work. *The Lancet, 262*(6796), 1111–1120.

Ng, S.W., & Popkin B. (2012). Time use and physical activity: a shift away from movement across the globe. *Obesity Reviews, 13*(8), 659–680.

Pedišić, Ž., Zhong, A., Hardy, L.L., Salmon, J., Okely, A., Chau, J., van der Ploeg, H.P., & Bauman, A. (2017). Physical activity prevalence in Australian children and adolescents: why do different surveys provide different estimates? *Kinesiology, 49*(2).

Redmond, G. (1988). Historical aspects of fitness in the modern world. In R.M. Malina & H.M. Eckert (Eds). *Physical activity in early and modern populations*, NAK Academy Papers (pp. 22–33). Champaign, IL: Human Kinetics.

Reis, R.S., Salvo, D., Ogilvie, D., Lambert, E.V., Goenka, S., Brownson, R.C., Lancet Physical Activity Series 2 Executive Committee (2016). Scaling up physical activity interventions worldwide: stepping up to larger and smarter approaches to get people moving. *The Lancet, 388*(10051), 1337–1348.

Riley, L., Guthold, R., Cowan, M., Savin, S., Bhatti, L., Armstrong, T., & Bonita, R. (2016). The World Health Organization STEPwise approach to noncommunicable disease risk-factor surveillance: methods, challenges, and opportunities. *American Journal of Public Health, 106*(1), 74–78.

Sallis, J.F., Bull, F., Guthold, R., Heath, G.W., Inoue, S., Kelly, P., Oyeyemi, A.L., Perez, L.G., Richards, J., Hallal, P.C., Lancet Physical Activity Series 2 Executive Committee (2016). Progress in physical activity over the Olympic quadrennium. *The Lancet, 388*(10051), 1325–1336.

Tremblay, M.S., Barnes, J.D., & Bonne, J.C. (2014). Impact of the active healthy kids Canada report card: a 10-year analysis. *Journal of Physical Activity and Health, 11*, S3–S20.

Tremblay, M.S., Gray, C.E., Akinroye, K., Harrington, D.M., Katzmarzyk, P.T., Lambert, E.V., . . . Tomkinson, G. (2014). Physical activity of children: a global matrix of grades comparing 15 countries. *Journal of Physical Activity and Health, 11*, S113–S25.

Tremblay, M.S., Barnes, J.D., González, S.A., Katzmarzyk. P.T., Onywera, V.O., Reilly, J.J., . . . Global Matrix 2.0 Research Team (2016). Global matrix 2.0: report card grades on the physical activity of children and youth comparing 38 countries. *Journal of Physical Activity and Health, 13*(11), S343–S66.

Trost, S.G., Blair, S.N., & Khan, K.M. (2014). Physical inactivity remains the greatest public health problem of the 21st century: evidence, improved methods and solutions using the '7 investments that work' as a framework. *British Journal of Sports Medicine, 48*, 169–170.

UN General Assembly. *Political declaration of the high-level meeting of the general assembly on the prevention and control of non-communicable diseases*. New York: United Nations, General Assembly, 2011.

USSG (1996). *U.S. Department of Health and Human Services. Physical activity and health: a report of the US Surgeon General*. Atlanta, GA: Centers for Disease Control.

van de Glind, I., Bunn, C., Gray, C.M., Hunt, K., Andersen, E. Jelsma, J., . . . Wyke, S. (2017). The intervention process in the European Fans in Training (EuroFIT) trial: a mixed method protocol for evaluation. *Trials, 18*(356).

DPAS, WHO (2004). *Global strategy on diet, physical activity and health*. Geneva: World Health Organization.

WHO (2007). *Report of the 2005 global survey on the progress in national chronic diseases prevention and control*. Geneva: WHO.

WHO (2009). *Global health risks: mortality and burden of disease attributable to selected major risks*. Geneva: WHO.

WHO (2010) *Global recommendations on physical activity for health*. www.who.int/dietphysicalactivity/factsheet_recommendations/en/

WHO (2011). *66/2 Political Declaration of the High-level Meeting of the General Assembly on the Prevention and Control of Non-communicable Diseases*. www.who.int/nmh/events/un_ncd_summit2011/political_declaration_en.pdf

WHO (2013a). *WHO NCD Global Monitoring Framework*. Geneva: WHO. www.who.int/nmh/global_monitoring_framework/en/

WHO (2013b). *Global action plan for the prevention and control of NCDs, 2013–2020*. Geneva, Switzerland: World Health Organization.

WHO (2015). *Assessing national capacity for the prevention and control of non-communicable diseases: report of the 2015 global survey*. Geneva: WHO.

WHO/Euro (2016). *Physical activity strategy for the WHO European region 2016–2025*. Copenhagen: WHO.

WHO (2018), *Global action plan on physical activity (2018–2030): more active people for a healthier world*. Geneva: WHO.

Wyke, S., Hunt, K., Gray, C., Fenwick, E., Bunn, C., Donnan, P., . . . Treweek, S. (2015). Football Fans in Training (FFIT): a randomised controlled trial of a gender-sensitised weight loss and healthy living programme for men. *Public Health Research, No. 3.2*.

Appendix: figure 8.1

GIRLS UK
Body mass index (BMI)
2-20 years

RCPCH
Royal College of
Paediatrics and Child Health

(DH) Department
of Health

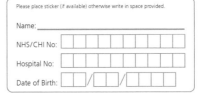

Please place sticker (if available) otherwise write in space provided.

Name: _____

NHS/CHI No:

Hospital No:

Date of Birth:

The BMI centile is a simple and reliable indicator of thinness and fatness in childhood. Where severe over- or underweight is a concern, or where there is a need for monitoring over time, BMI can be calculated and plotted on this chart. It is important also to plot the height and weight separately on the main 2-18 chart. There is also a BMI centile look-up on the standard 2-18 chart for less complex cases.

BMI is calculated by dividing weight (in kg) by the square of height (in metres e.g. 1.32 m, not centimetres e.g. 132 cm).
A simple way to do this on a calculator or mobile phone is:
1. Enter the weight. 2. Divide by height. 3. Divide the result by height.
The result can then be plotted on the chart below.

Overweight and obesity
A BMI above the 91st centile suggests overweight. A child above the 98th centile is very overweight (clinically obese) while a BMI above the 99.6th centile is severely obese. In addition to the usual nine centile lines, the BMI chart displays high lines at +3, +3.33, +3.66 and + 4 SD, which can be used to monitor the progress of children in overweight treatment programmes.

Thinness
A BMI below the 2nd centile is unusual and may reflect undernutrition, but may simply reflect a small build. The chart also displays low lines at -4 and -5 SD for those who are severely underweight. Children whose BMI lies below the 0.4th centile are likely to have additional problems and if not already receiving medical or dietetic attention should be referred.

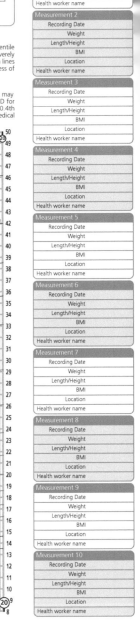

© Copyright RCPCH 2013

Figure 8.1   UK body mass index growth charts for girls and boys aged 2–20 years

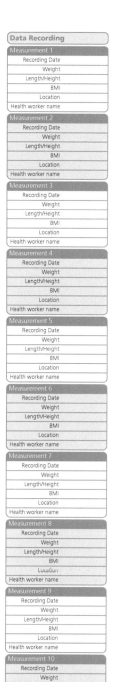

BOYS UK
Body mass index (BMI)
2-20 years

RCPCH (DH) Department of Health

Royal College of
Paediatrics and Child Health

Please place sticker (if available) otherwise write in space provided.

Name: _____

NHS/CHI No:

Hospital No:

Date of Birth:

The BMI centile is a simple and reliable indicator of thinness and fatness in childhood. Where severe over- or underweight is a concern, or where there is a need for monitoring over time, BMI can be calculated and plotted on this chart. It is important also to plot the height and weight separately on the main 2-18 chart. There is also a BMI centile look-up on the standard 2-18 chart for less complex cases.

BMI is calculated by dividing weight (in kg) by the square of height (in metres e.g. 1.32 m, not centimetres e.g. 132 cm).
A simple way to do this on a calculator or mobile phone is:
1. Enter the weight. 2. Divide by height. 3. Divide the result by height.
The result can then be plotted on the chart below.

Overweight and obesity
A BMI above the 91st centile suggests overweight. A child above the 98th centile is very overweight (clinically obese) while a BMI above the 99.6th centile is severely obese. In addition to the usual nine centile lines, the BMI chart displays high lines at +3, +3.33, +3.66 and + 4 SD, which can be used to monitor the progress of children in overweight treatment programmes.

Thinness
A BMI below the 2nd centile is unusual and may reflect undernutrition, but may simply reflect a small build. The chart also displays low lines at -4 and -5 SD for those who are severely underweight. Children whose BMI lies below the 0.4th centile are likely to have additional problems and if not already receiving medical or dietetic attention should be referred.

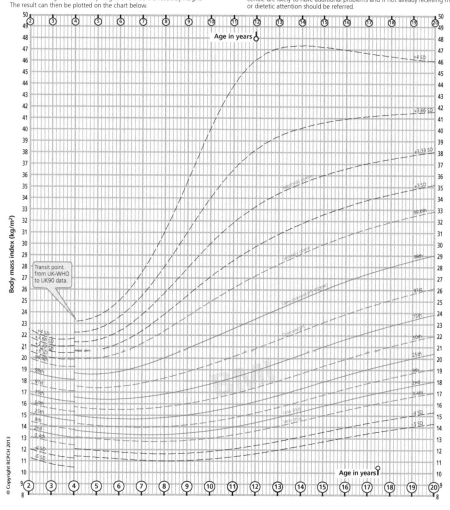

Figure 8.1 (Continued)

Notes on contributors

1. Physical activity: a multi-disciplinary introduction

Nick Draper and Gareth Stratton

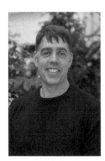

Nick Draper is a Professor of Sport and Exercise Science at the University of Canterbury, Christchurch, New Zealand. His teaching is in the area of exercise physiology and he is Programme Director for the Master of Sport Science programme. His research interests focus on psychophysiology in relation to rock climbing, rugby performance and physical activity. He is Chair of SESNZ, the national organisation for Sport and Exercise Science in New Zealand and a founder member of the International Rock Climbing Research Association.

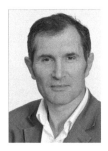

Gareth Stratton is Head of the School of Sport and Exercise Sciences and Director of the Applied Sports Exercise Technology and Medicine (A-STEM) Research Centre at Swansea University and adjunct Professor at the University of Western Australia. Professor Stratton began his career as a physical education teacher that led him to his main areas of academic interest, child maturation and physical activity and physical activity, fitness and health. He has been involved in physical activity measurement studies for nearly 30 years and he continues his interest in the development of novel sensor technologies to detect and stimulate changes in physical activity and sedentary behaviour. Professor Stratton also co-founded the E-BASE (Engineering Behaviour Analytics in Sport and Exercise) that exploits the close integration with engineering and computer sciences at Swansea. Professor Stratton also leads the physical activity pillar in PEVIEW an €8.9 million, 15-partner worldwide diabetes prevention project. In addition to his empirical work Professor Stratton has devoted time to translating research and chaired the Children and Young Peoples sub group for the Start Active Stay Active Physical Activity Guidance. He is currently a member of the Physical Literacy Framework Group for Sport Wales, an Expert Member of the National Institute for Health and Clinical Excellence

(NICE) quality standards advisory committee for childhood obesity and Chair of the PH17 Promoting physical activity programme development and evidence update group. He was also the European Representative on the Canadian 24-hour movement guidelines. Professor Stratton co-directs the Sportslinx Programme that won the Louis Bonduelle, European Childhood Obesity Group award in 2011.

2. Foundations in the science of physical activity

Helen Marshall and Louise Sheppard

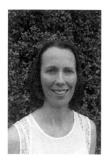

Helen Marshall is the Physical Activity and Health Promotion coordinator at Ara Institute of Canterbury, Christchurch, New Zealand. With a background in exercise physiology, her main interests include environmental physiology, the health benefits of physical activity, and health promotion. Helen is part of a steering group at Ara with a focus on promoting a healthy environment for both staff and students.

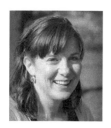

Louise Sheppard is a New Zealand Registered Physiotherapist and also holds a Master's degree in Health Sciences from the University of Otago. Louise lives in Christchurch, New Zealand where she teaches in the areas of physical activity and health. Louise is specifically interested in the role of physical activity and exercise in the management of chronic pain.

3. Historical aspects of physical activity

David Broom

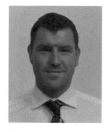

David Broom is a Reader of Physical Activity and Health at Sheffield Hallam University, UK. He teaches on the exercise prescription, physical activity promotion and physiology related modules of the physical activity related degrees. He is an appointed Fellow of the Higher Education Academy and British Association of Sport and Exercise Sciences. David's research interests include the effects of exercise on appetite, food intake and appetite related hormones but he has broader interests in physical activity and health having formerly worked for the British Heart Foundation's National Centre for Physical Activity and Health. David supervises numerous doctoral research students and has presented at many national and international conferences including invited keynotes.

4. Physical inactivity and ill health

Duck-chul Lee and Laura Ellingson

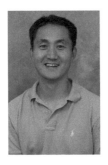

Duck-chul Lee (D.C. Lee), PhD, FACSM, is an associate professor and the director of the Physical Activity Epidemiology Laboratory at Iowa State University. His research focuses on the associations and effects of exercise, physical activity, sedentary behaviour and fitness with chronic disease prevention and longevity using comprehensive epidemiological approaches including large cohort studies and randomised controlled trials of exercise. Since his post-doctoral fellowship in 2009 at the University of South Carolina, he has published more than 80 peer-reviewed research articles in medical journals. Dr. Lee serves as principal investigator on research projects investigating the health benefits of aerobic and resistance exercise on cardiovascular health and sarcopenia, supported by the US National Institutes of Health (NIH) and several research organisations. Dr. Lee serves as a principal investigator on research projects investigating the health benefits of aerobic and resistance exercise on cardiovascular health and sarcopenia, supported by the US National Institutes of Health (NIH) and several research organizations. Dr. Lee is a Fellow of the American College of Sports Medicine (ACSM) and serves as a reviewer for NIH grant applications and major medical journals including the *Journal of the American Medical Association (JAMA)*, *Journal of the American College of Cardiology (JACC)*, and *Circulation*.

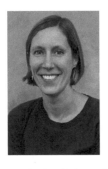

Laura Ellingson, PhD, FACSM, is an assistant professor in the Exercise Psychology and Physical Activity and Health Promotion Laboratories at Iowa State University. Her research focuses on investigating the effects of physical activity and sedentary behaviors on the mental health and quality of life of healthy individuals and those with, or at risk for developing, chronic health conditions. Dr Ellingson serves as the principal investigator on several intervention trials investigating effective ways to implement physical activity behaviour change (e.g. increasing lifestyle physical activity, decreasing sedentary time) as a potential treatment for individuals with chronic pain conditions as well as projects focusing on refining methods of physical activity and sedentary measurement. She is an active member of the Society for Behavioral Medicine, the American Pain Society, and the American College of Sports Medicine where she is a Fellow and Chair of the Psychobiology and Behavior Interest Group.

5. Physical activity and health

Ian Lahart, George Metsios and Chris Kite

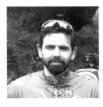

Ian Lahart is a Senior Lecturer in Exercise Physiology, a committee member of HEAT CiC, and the course leader for BSc Sport and Exercise Science at the University of Wolverhampton. Ian completed his PhD on physical activity and breast cancer in 2014. He has a number of publications in peer-reviewed journals with high impact factors in the area of exercise and chronic disease, and has presented his work at a number of research conferences, including the British Association of Sport and Exercise Science, American College of Sports Medicine and Physiology Society annual conferences. He is currently working on a Cochrane Collaboration Systematic Review on exercise and breast cancer. Through his role as a Research Fellow at Russells Hall Hospital, Dudley, he works with cardiovascular disease, cancer and rheumatoid arthritis patients. He was involved in the setting up of and helps manage a Macmillan funded exercise-based cancer rehabilitation service in Action Heart, a cardiac rehabilitation centre in Russells Hall Hospital. Ian provides exercise testing and sports science support to athletes, including runners, triathletes, cyclists, and football players.

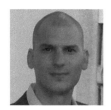

George Metsios is a Professor in Clinical Exercise Physiology at the University of Wolverhampton. His work evolves around physical activity, exercise and health and specifically how physical activity and/or exercise can be used to improve – via specific physiological and molecular/genetic mechanisms – disease symptoms and health parameters in patients with different chronic diseases. George has led randomised controlled trials and epidemiological studies and has published more than 80 peer-reviewed scientific publications in his field. His work has had a significant scientific impact since it has helped the formation of position statements and improves existing guidelines for treating different chronic diseases. His work has been used, amongst others, by the World Health Organization, the British Heart Foundation, the National Health Service and the European League Against Rheumatism. George has also received both national and international grants (Medical Research Council, FP-7, Horizon 2020) and he is an expert evaluator in multiple funding bodies and peer-reviewed journals.

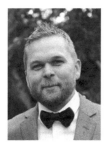

Chris Kite is currently working towards a PhD at Aston University; as a member of the Cell and Tissue Biomedical Research Group his research project is centred around the effectiveness of exercise, or exercise and diet, in the treatment and management of polycystic ovary syndrome. Following a lifelong interest in sport, Chris was awarded a first-class honours degree in Sport and Exercise science, and a distinction in the Masters (Research) programme he undertook. Previous projects have focused on improving sporting performance; most recently working as a performance analyst at a professional football team. Since working as a lecturer, Chris's research interests have slightly shifted; projects now investigate the potential of physical activity to prevent, treat and manage the symptoms of chronic disease. Aside from his PhD project, he has been involved in numerous exercise-based studies. Most notably, Chris has worked alongside departmental colleagues as a research assistant and contributed to several projects with the BBC.

6. Measuring physical activity behaviours and outcomes in children and adults

Stuart J. Fairclough, Robert J. Noonan andWhitney B. Curry

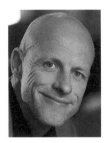

Stuart J. Fairclough, PhD, MSc, BEd (Hons) is Associate Head of the Sport and Physical Activity Department at Edge Hill University and Leader of the Physical Activity and Health Research Group there. He is primarily interested in children's physical activity, sedentary behaviour, and health, and in particular interventions to modify behaviours. Within this area his work focuses on physical activity measurement and the role of multidimensional correlates in the promotion of physically active lifestyles among young people. A core setting to this work is the school environment.

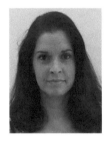

Robert J. Noonan is a Lecturer in Physical Education and Children's Physical Activity at Edge Hill University and is a member of the Physical Activity and Health Research Group there. He is broadly interested in children's physical activity and the social determinants of health. Within this area his work adopts a multi-methods approach to explore family and environmental influences on children's lifestyle behaviours.

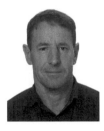

Whitney B. Curry, PhD, MPH, BA is a Senior Lecturer in Physical Education and Sport Pedagogy at Edge Hill University and is a member of the Physical Activity and Health Research Group there. She is primarily interested in measuring physical activity and sedentary time using a mixed methods approach. Within this area her work focuses on using objective measurement and self-report methods among culturally and linguistically diverse groups to accurately and reliably measure physical activity and sedentary time

7. Physical activity prescription

Michael J. Hamlin

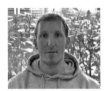

Michael J. Hamlin is Associate Professor of Exercise and Sport Science at Lincoln University, New Zealand's leading centre for sport scholarships. Mike has over 17 years' experience in university teaching and research, has published widely, given invited lectures in many countries and has contributed to the promotion of physical activity in New Zealand. A member of numerous professional societies, Mike received his BPhEd degree (1990) in exercise prescription from

Otago University, Dunedin, his MHMS degree (1995) in exercise physiology from the University of Queensland, Brisbane, and his PhD degree (1999) from Otago University, Dunedin.

8. Growth and development and physical activity

Lynne Boddy and Gareth Stratton

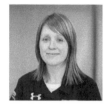

Lynne Boddy is a Reader in Children's Physical Activity based at the Physical Activity Exchange within the Research Institute for Sport and Exercise Sciences. Lynne is involved in a number of research programmes within the Physical Activity Exchange including population level fitness and physical activity surveillance studies, methodological studies examining physical activity measurement, projects investigating the links between fitness, physical activity and disease risk in children, physical activity interventions and work investigating and promoting physical activity in special populations. Lynne is particularly interested in the links between fitness, physical activity, body composition and disease risk in children. Lynne is also interested in physical activity measurement and more accurately quantifying physical activity 'dose'. Current long-term goals are to develop novel and effective interventions studies to reduce disease risk in children through the promotion of physical activity and cardiorespiratory fitness.

Gareth Stratton (see: 1. Physical activity: a multi-disciplinary introduction)

9. Motor skill development and physical activity

Jenny Clarke

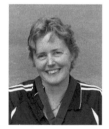

Jenny Clarke completed a DPhil in Theoretical Elementary Particle Physics at the University of Oxford, UK in 2000. She returned to New Zealand in 2005 to lead the University of Canterbury involvement in the Swiss-based Large Hadron Collider project, and discovered a new world of opportunity in education and research in sport and physical activity. Since beginning her career as a Sport Science lecturer at the University of Canterbury, Jenny has taught and carried out research in such diverse areas as biomechanics, motor learning, anatomy and sport science education. She has delivered presentations and workshops around the world on these topics, and uses coaching pedagogies informed by this research to coach croquet to beginners, elite youth and expert players, most recently developing a coaching programme around Game Sense and Positive Pedagogy.

10. Exercise physiology and physical activity

Mike Duncan

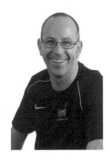

Mike Duncan is Processor of Sport and Exercise Science in the School of Life Sciences at Coventry University, UK. His research interests include the association between motor competence and physical activity in children, effects of exercise and physical activity on body fatness in children and adolescents and understanding the effect of physical activity on functional performance in older adults.

11. Paediatric physical activity and aerobic fitness

Neil Armstrong

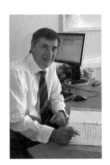

Neil Armstrong is Professor of Paediatric Physiology and the Inaugural Provost of the University of Exeter. His research on children's physical activity, physical fitness and health won the only Queen's Anniversary Prize (QAP) for Higher Education to be awarded for research in sports medicine. The QAP was presented by the Queen at Buckingham Palace for '*world class work which is of outstanding quality and importance to the nation*'. Neil has received honorary doctorates from universities in Europe and North America. He has twice chaired the Sport Science Panel in the UK Research Assessment Exercise. He is a former Chair/ President of both BASES and PEAUK. He has chaired the European Group of Pediatric Work Physiology since 1995 and serves as a member of the International Olympic Committee's expert group on sport, health and exercise in youth. He was the first scientist to be awarded Fellowship of the British, European, and American Colleges of Sport Science/Medicine.

12. Nutrition and physical activity

Daniel Bailey, Julia Zakrzewski-Fruer and Faye Powell

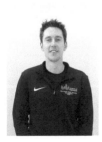

Daniel Bailey is a Senior Lecturer in Health, Nutrition and Exercise and member of the Institute for Sport and Physical Activity Research (ISPAR) at the University of Bedfordshire. He completed his undergraduate degree in Applied Sports Science in 2008 at the University of Bedfordshire and subsequently commenced a PhD programme in Physical Activity and Health at the University of Bedfordshire, submitting his PhD thesis in 2011. Dr Bailey has been lecturing in the area of physical activity, nutrition and health since 2012 and is a Registered Nutritionist (Public Health) with the Association for Nutrition. His primary research interest is the impact of sedentary behaviour (prolonged sitting) on appetite control and cardiometabolic disease risk markers. His research examines the benefits of breaking up prolonged sitting on these markers of disease risk and interventions to reduce prolonged sitting in the workplace and in the treatment of type 2 diabetes with the aim of influencing public health policy and clinical care guidelines to reduce the burden of this lifestyle risk factor on human health and disease. Dr Bailey has disseminated his findings in a number of peer-reviewed international journals, international conferences and has secured multiple funding awards in the physical activity and nutrition field.

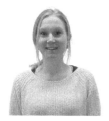

Julia Zakrzewski-Fruer is a Lecturer in Health, Nutrition and Exercise and an active member of the Institute for Sport and Physical Activity Research (ISPAR) at the University of Bedfordshire. Her research focuses on how manipulations in physical activity and nutrition can improve health and prevent obesity in children and adolescents. After gaining an undergraduate degree in Sport and Exercise Science from Loughborough University (2004–2007) and an MSc by Research from the University of Gloucestershire (2007–2008), Dr Zakrzewski-Fruer completed a PhD at Loughborough University (2008–2011) in the area of paediatric exercise metabolism. Dr Zakrzewski-Fruer then worked as a Research Officer on the International Study of Childhood Obesity, Lifestyle and the Environment (ISCOLE) at the University of Bath and continues to collaborate with an international team of experts on this project to examine associations between breakfast frequency, physical activity and obesity in children from 12 countries across the world. Dr Zakrzewski-Fruer's work has resulted in numerous publications in peer-reviewed international journals, international conference presentations and funding awards within the areas of exercise metabolism, breakfast consumption and childhood obesity.

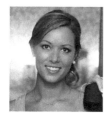

Faye Powell is a Chartered Psychologist with specialist expertise in Developmental Psychology and Health Psychology. She completed her PhD within Loughborough Centre for Research into Eating Disorders (LUCRED) at Loughborough University in 2012. Her doctoral theses explored family environmental influences on children's eating behaviour across early childhood. Since then, she has been working at The University of Bedfordshire (UoB) as a Lecturer in Developmental Psychology. Dr Powell is an active member of the UoB's Research Centre for Applied Psychology (RCAP) and Institute for Health Research (IHR). Her research interests focus around health promotion in children and their parents with particular interest in eating behaviour, physical activity and weight management. Her wider interests include diversity in public health and health inequalities. Dr Powell enjoys engaging in research and consultancy in collaboration with local partners and she is a member of Luton Flying Start 'Expert Nutrition Group' and Public Health Luton 'Obesity Steering Group'. Dr Powell has published work in international journals such as *Maternal and Child Nutrition*, *European Eating Disorders Review* and *Appetite* and has acted as a peer reviewer for a number of high impact journals.

13. Biochemistry and physical activity

Angus Lindsay and Chris Chamberlain

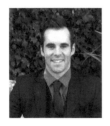

Angus Lindsay is a post-doctoral associate in the Department of Rehabilitation Medicine at the University of Minnesota. He primarily investigates the physiological function of therapeutically relevant truncated dystrophins and urinary metabolites for genetic treatment and mechanistic investigation into Duchenne Muscular Dystrophy. Prior to joining the University of Minnesota Angus completed his PhD in New Zealand, studying the psychophysiological stress response of Olympic cyclists, elite MMA fighters and professional rugby players with a scholarship from St George's Hospital. He subsequently lectured in exercise physiology at the University of Canterbury before pursuing a career in medical research. Angus has a passion for exercise that developed from a young age. He has competed at a national level in cricket, soccer and track cycling whilst simultaneously providing coaching and mentoring support for younger athletes. The combination of his passion for competitive sport and exercise research allows him unique insights into the relationship of exercise-induced biochemical perturbations and adaptations.

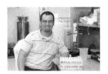

Chris Chamberlain grew up in the small town of Clontarf, MN. As a teenager, Chris's two younger brothers were diagnosed with myotonic muscular dystrophy. After graduating summa cum laude with honors in biology from Hamline University in St Paul, MN, Chris decided to pursue graduate studies focused on muscular dystrophy. Chris's dissertation work was completed at both the University of Minnesota and the University of Florida where he studied under Dr Laura P.W. Ranum, who has published seminal work elucidating the genes and mechanisms involved in both myotonic dystrophy and spinocerebellar ataxia types, 1, 5, and 8. For his graduate research, Chris generated mouse models to study the potential of Muscleblind-like 1 upregulation as a therapy for myotonic dystrophy. After finishing his thesis research in 2012, Chris moved back to the University of Minnesota to pursue postdoctoral studies with Dr James Ervasti, whose work has identified the mechanistic role of the dystrophin glycoprotein complex in many forms of muscular dystrophy. As a postdoc, Chris uses metabolomics to study Duchenne muscular dystrophy. His work focuses on both biomarkers and novel mechanistic insights into DMD.

14. Psychology and physical activity

Brad H. Miles

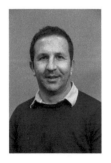

Brad H. Miles is a Lecturer in the School of Health Sciences at the University of Canterbury, Christchurch, New Zealand where he teaches and researches sport and exercise psychology. Brad received a PhD in psychology from the University of Canterbury and has been the recipient of a number of teaching and research awards. His research is primarily directed at the intersection between sport and psychology with a focus on social-cognitive mechanisms of sport performance and engagement.

15. Neurophysiology and physical activity

Michael J. Grey, Simon Franklin and Nick Kitchen

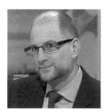

Michael J. Grey is a Reader in Rehabilitation Neuroscience at the University of East Anglia. He obtained a PhD in Biomedical Science and Engineering from the Centre for Sensory-Motor Interaction, Denmark. Subsequently, he has held research appointments in Denmark, Finland and the United Kingdom. Whilst employed at the University of Birmingham, he was a theme lead (Motor Control and Motor Neuroscience) at the MRC Arthritis Research UK Centre for Musculoskeletal Ageing Research. Michael's research is focused on neurorehabilitation following acquired brain injury. He has a particular interest in neuroplasticity in the ageing brain.

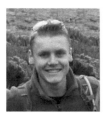

Simon Franklin completed an undergraduate degree in Sport, Exercise and Rehabilitation Sciences at the University of Birmingham graduating with First Class Honours in 2012. Through developing a keen interest in Neurophysiology, Biomechanics and Motor Control he then progressed into doctoral research completing his PhD with a particular focus on the sensorimotor system of older adults. His primary question is to determine if walking barefoot or in minimal footwear improves proprioceptive sensory feedback and foot muscle strength potentially improving the balance and gait performance of older adults.

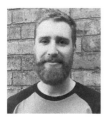

Nick Kitchen studied his undergraduate degree in Sport and Exercise Sciences at the University of Birmingham with a focus in sensorimotor control, before completing an MSc by Research in the field of neurorehabilitation and neuroplasticity. He is now in the final year of a PhD investigating how proprioceptive deficits contribute to age-related impairments in movement control. His work typically involves upper limb reaching movements and has extended to studying movement adaptations to novel force perturbations. He regularly lectures in the field of age-related neurophysiological decline with a focus towards the sensory and neuromuscular systems, and has enjoyed having the opportunity to present his work to a range of audiences during public engagement and at international conferences.

16. Biomechanics and physical activity

Neil D. Reeves and Steven J. Brown

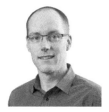

Neil D. Reeves is Professor of Musculoskeletal Biomechanics at the Manchester Metropolitan University. His main research interests include understanding the biomechanical mechanisms of gait impairment in clinical conditions, particularly in diabetes and knee osteoarthritis. He also studies alterations to musculoskeletal system mechanical properties with altered loading conditions, clinical conditions and exercise interventions. He has published over 70 papers in international journals on topics related to human movement and musculoskeletal biomechanics.

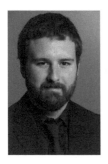

Steven J. Brown is a post-doctoral researcher of Musculoskeletal Biomechanics at the Manchester Metropolitan University. His main interests lie in gait impairment in clinical conditions, understanding the biomechanical alterations and their implications upon quality of life. His research seeks insight into the impact of diabetes upon gait during daily activities, and the potential use of exercise interventions to alter the biomechanical strategies of patients.

17. Sociology and physical activity

Ross Neville

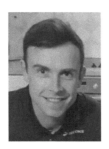

Ross Neville is with the Centre for Sport Studies within the School of Public Health, Physiotherapy and Sports Sciences, UCD, where he is an Assistant Professor and Programme Coordinator for the BSc in Sport and Exercise Management. His research expertise is within Sociology, which he applies to management contexts within the field of sport and exercise, and have been published across a range of applied sociology and interdisciplinary sports and leisure journals, including: *Quest*; *Qualitative Research in Sport, Exercise and Health*; *Sociology of Sport Journal*; *Sociology of Health & Illness*; *Medicine, Health Care and Philosophy*; *Leisure Sciences*.

His most recent research has been in the sociology of professions, and has dealt with issues such as professional qualifications, professional competencies, role boundaries and continuing professional development – across both commercial and educational contexts.

18. Physical activity in natural environments

Carly Wood, Miles Richardson and Jo Barton

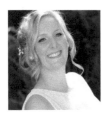

Carly Wood is a Lecturer in Exercise and Nutritional Sciences at the University of Westminster. Her primary research interests are focused on the role of natural environments in promoting physical activity and the use of GE in promoting mental wellbeing amongst both the general population and vulnerable groups. She is specifically interested in the role of GE in modifying the physiological response to stress.

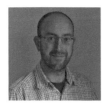

Miles Richardson is a Chartered Psychologist and Chartered Ergonomist. He founded and leads the Nature Connectedness Research Group at the University of Derby. Current research activity is focused on understanding connection to nature and interventions to improve it.

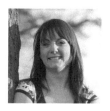

Jo Barton is a Lecturer in Sports and Exercise Science at the University of Essex and the Director of the Green Exercise Research Team. Current research focuses on how the outdoors can be used as a vehicle to drive behavioural change and promote health and well-being. The research agenda also targets vulnerable groups such as 'youth at risk' or adults with mental ill-health to explore the potential therapeutic benefits of nature-based activities.

19. Urban physical activity

Brad Harasymchuk and Chris North

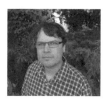

Brad Harasymchuk began his career as a teacher. He has taught in elementary, secondary and post-secondary institutions in Canada and New Zealand. He completed his Master's thesis at the University of Saskatchewan, which focused on place-based education (PBE). This research evoked a passion for social justice and PBE, which led him to pursue a PhD at the University of Canterbury in New Zealand where he delved deeper into critical pedagogies of place and decolonisation. Brad is currently a Learning Strategist in the Faculty of Student Development at Thompson Rivers University.

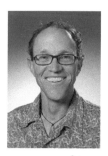

Chris North is a Senior Lecturer in outdoor and environmental education at the University of Canterbury, Christchurch, New Zealand. His teaching background includes secondary and tertiary institutions in New Zealand and North America. He has worked as a teacher, tourist guide and outdoor instructor for a range of organisations. Chris's research is in the areas of outdoor education practices, adventure education, environmental education and initial teacher education. He is a recipient of the national Environmental Leadership award and the University of Canterbury, College of Education, Health and Human Development teaching excellence award. Chris is a founder of Leave No Trace New Zealand. In his spare time, Chris enjoys family adventures in the outdoors.

20. School Gym and physical activity

Dylan Blain and Mark Bellamy

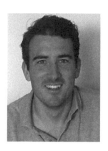

Dylan Blain is programme director of the BA Physical Education degree at the University of Wales Trinity Saint David and Lecturer in Physical Education with the Coleg Cymraeg Cendlaethol. Previously Dylan has taught physical eduction in a range of secondary schools. He regularly consults with local authorities in delivering professional development opportunites for physical education teachers at both primary and secondary level. Currently he is studying for his PhD where he is exploring the relationships among adolescent motivation, physical literacy, physical activity and well-being. He also has an interest in exploring the role of technology within physical education and has presented internationally on the topic.

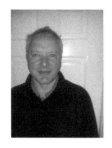

Mark Bellamy has a PhD, is a Chartered Psychologist and Associate Fellow of the British Psychological Society. Mark has been active in support and development with sportspeople and the military over the previous 25 years. During this time he has worked with UK-Athletics across three Olympic Games providing psychological support to their Olympic athletes. Mark has also worked with high level sports in a wide variety of disciplines, with athletes ranging from development to world class and world champion. Mark has also supported the work of the Armed Forces providing the external education for the PT Core over a 5-year period and also has developed key training equipment that is used by the Armed Forces and high level sports across the world. Over the previous five years or so Mark has been heavily involved with the development of physical education in the UK, is a member of a number of cross parliamentary groups on fitness and health for young people and has co-authored a report into physical education in the UK for the British Government. This work has largely been based on a PE programme that has been successfully running in Wales and has been widely recognised as a beacon of good practice. Mark also mentors a number of young people through their work and sport and provides this same role with small businesses. Mark has a particular interest in the psychology of injury and has worked closely with injury teams at UK-Athletics, Premiership Football and the Physical Training Core of the British Army.

21. Physical activity promotion strategies

Clover Maitland and Michael Rosenberg

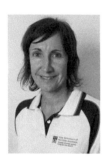

Clover Maitland is a Research Fellow with the Health Promotion Evaluation Unit within the School of Human Sciences at the University of Western Australia. Prior to commencing at UWA, Clover held a senior management position with the Heart Foundation in Western Australia, managing mass media leading social marketing campaigns and health promotion programmes to address physical inactivity and unhealthy weight. A passion for the promotion of physical activity and keen interest in the role of research and evaluation to inform policy and practice, led her to a PhD at UWA investigating home environmental influences on children's activity. Since joining UWA, Clover has worked across a number of research and teaching roles in her interest areas of physical activity, health promotion and public health.

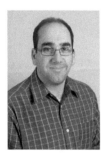

Michael Rosenberg is a health and exercise scientist and Director of the Health Promotion Evaluation Unit at the University of Western Australia. He has 20 years of experience in community-based health programme evaluation and applied research on population-based prevention of NCD risk factors (physical inactivity, unhealthy diet, alcohol and tobacco use). Dr Rosenberg has a broad range of research interests focused around: public health epidemiology; health promotion programme evaluation; children's physical activity; and the use of integrative technologies to measure and improve human health. Michael has been a lead investigator on research assessing the prevalence of health behaviours at state and national level in children and adults, lead evaluator of West Australian state-wide physical activity, healthy weight, youth tobacco control, and workplace health community campaigns; and lead of innovative research using technologies to address NCD risk factors.

22. School physical education and physical activity

Gareth Stratton and Nick Draper
See: 1. Physical activity: a multi-disciplinary introduction

23. Physical activity and older adults

Gladys Onambele-Pearson, Declan Ryan, David Tomlinson and Jorgen Wullems

Gladys Onambele-Pearson is a Reader in Human Muscle & Tendon Physiology and Co-Director of the Musculoskeletal Sciences and Sport Medicine (previously Health Exercise & Active Living) Research Centre at the Manchester Metropolitan University. Her research is concerned with lifestyle-based strategies towards increased vitality in older age. Her research links with institutions around the globe are maintained through her roles as grant reviewer for 12 awarding bodies worldwide, peer-reviewed for 32 journals, research theme lead for the British Physiological Society (Human & Exercise Physiology), national health provider Governor as well as co-organising numerous international conferences. Her most recent research funds are via an EU programme entitled MOVE-AGE, in which she assesses the impact of sedentary lifestyle on the muscle-tendon, cardiovascular and genetics signatures of sarcopenia.

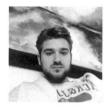

Declan Ryan is a PhD student at the 'Health Exercise & Active Living' Research Centre of Manchester Metropolitan University. His current research explores the impact of sedentary behaviour and physical activity on the cardio-metabolic health of older adults under the supervision of his Director of Studies, Dr Gladys Onambele-Pearson. Declan's research has been internationally recognised, receiving bursary awards from the Wellcome Trust and the Physiological Society to present at their respective conferences. His future ambition is to progress and contribute to the research area of physical behaviour in older adults, driving changes in public health policy to help inform the general public about the impact of sedentary behaviour and physical activity.

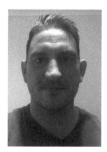

David Tomlinson is a Postdoctoral Researcher within the 'Exercise and Ageing Physiology' Research Group, part of the 'Health, Exercise & Active Living' Research Centre at Manchester Metropolitan University. His PhD documented the combined effects of ageing and body composition on skeletal muscle structure and function. After completion of his PhD, his main research foci cover topical areas on sedentarism, ageing, obesity and nutrition and document their subsequent effects on skeletal muscle characteristics. Future research will target the development of successful (non-pharmaceutical) interventions to reverse known adverse effects of ageing, inactivity and adiposity.

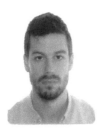

Jorgen Wullems holds a BSc degree in Health Sciences for which he studied at both Maastricht University, Netherlands and University of Jyväskylä, Finland. During his undergraduate studies he specialised in Human Movement Sciences and Bioregulation & Health. He also has an MSc degree in Physical Activity and Health from Maastricht University, Netherlands. In 2014 he was awarded a European Commission-funded MOVE-AGE fellowship to obtain a doctorate, under the supervision of Dr Gladys Onambele-Pearson at both Manchester Metropolitan University, United Kingdom and University of Leuven, Belgium. His doctoral research is in muscle physiology and focuses on how sedentary behaviour affects muscle-tendon properties in the elderly.

24. Public health policy and physical activity

Justin Varney, Michael Brannan and Kevin Fenton

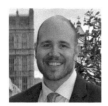

Justin Varney leads Public Health England's work to improve the health and well-being of working age adults and reduce health inequalities in this group. This portfolio includes leading PHE's work on physical activity, health and worklessness and workplace health as well as managing the teams leading our work on sexual, reproductive health and HIV prevention, community pharmacy and allied health professionals. Dr Varney is PHE's senior liaison for the Department of Culture, Media and Sport, leading our work to support the implementation of the Sport Strategy and working closely with colleagues in Sport England and Arts Council England towards our shared aim of getting everybody active every day. He sits on the WHO Technical Advisory Group for the Global Action Plan on Physical Activity and is an advisor to the Council of the Faculty of Sports and Exercise Medicine and the Council for Health and Work. Prior to joining Public Health England, Dr Varney was a Joint Deputy Director of Public Health in East London working between the Primary Care Trust and Local Authority. He trained in General Practice before specialising in Public Health Medicine and has worked across both primary and secondary care settings. Justin has a special interest in lesbian, gay, bisexual and trans health inequalities and domestic violence as a public health issue.

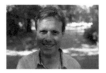

Michael Brannan is Deputy National Lead for Adult Health and Well-being at Public Health England. His portfolio includes physical activity and work and health. He was an author of the national physical activity framework, *Everybody Active Every Day*. Mike has worked in the public, private, academic and voluntary sectors and has over a decade of experience as a public health professional at national, regional and local levels. He has held leadership roles on health inequalities, transport, sustainability, housing, employment, health and work and physical activity. Prior to public health, Mike had an eclectic background as a biochemist and a public relations consultant.

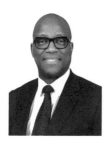

Kevin Fenton is the Director for Health and Wellbeing at the London Borough of Southwark. In this role, which incorporates the statutory functions of the Director for Public Health, he works across the entire Council to champion and promote health, well-being, sustainability and equity in all policies and programmes. Key priorities include social regeneration, developing and supporting sustainable, high-quality and integrated health and social care systems, and improving health and reducing inequalities for all of Southwark's residents. Professor Fenton is on secondment to Southwark Council from Public Health England (PHE), where he was the National Director for Health and Wellbeing leading PHE's national prevention programmes including screening for cancer and other conditions, health checks, public mental health, sexual and reproductive health, and a range of well-being programmes for infants, youth, adults and older adults. He also led PHE's health equity portfolio with a range of programmes and activities focused on addressing the social determinants of health and promoting place-based approaches to health improvement. Professor Fenton was previously the director of the National Centre for HIV/AIDS, Viral Hepatitis, STD, and TB Prevention (NCHHSTP), Centres for Disease Control and Prevention (CDC), a position he held for seven years from November 2005. He also served as chief of CDC's National Syphilis Elimination Effort and has worked in research, epidemiology, and the prevention of HIV and other STDs since 1995. Previously he was the director of the HIV and STI Department at the United Kingdom's Health Protection Agency. He attended medical school in Jamaica, obtained his Master's in public health at the London School of Hygiene and Tropical Medicine, and PhD in Infectious Disease Epidemiology at University College London. He has authored or co-authored more than 250 peer-reviewed scientific articles and policy reports.

25. Improving policy to promote physical activity

Tess Kay

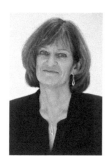

Tess Kay is Dean of Research at Brunel University London and Professor of Sport and Social Sciences. She leads the Brunel Sport, Health and Wellbeing research group (B.SHaW) in undertaking social science-led research into sport, health and physical activity. She has more than 30 years' experience of researching the processes and outcomes of engaging marginalised groups in sport for diverse funders including ESRC, PHE, Macmillan Cancer Support, DFID, UKSport, Sport England and sportscotland. She is a Fellow of the Academy of Social Sciences and an advocate for the co-production of knowledge by researchers, policy-makers and practitioners.

26. International perspectives on physical activity

Adrian Bauman

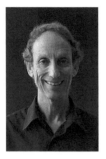

Adrian Bauman is involved in a diverse research programme on chronic disease prevention and methods research. He leads the Prevention Research Collaboration, a specialised research group within the Sydney School of Public Health with expertise in non-communicable disease prevention and other aspects of applied research in primary prevention, epidemiology and health promotion. The group conducts population-wide research and translational research, particularly evaluating population-wide prevention programmes and the subsequent dissemination of relevant programmes. As leader of the Physical Activity, Exercise and Energy Expenditure Theme at the Charles Perkins Centre, Professor Bauman chairs the university-wide physical activity network (PLANET), bringing together inter-faculty collaborations on physical activity and exercise. Additionally, as co-Director of the WHO Collaborating Centre on Physical Activity, Nutrition and Obesity he oversees the centre's global role in physical activity, sedentary behaviour, nutrition, obesity and diabetes. The centre provides technical support to countries on measurement, surveillance, evidence synthesis and policy-related research. Current projects include physical activity surveillance projects conducted around the world (as part of the WHO centre). His research studies are focused on evaluating complex public health programmes, for example evaluating the Get Healthy Service in NSW, the free NSW Health information and coaching service and obesity prevention programme. He is leading several projects on sitting-reduction interventions in different workplaces and worksites. Epidemiological studies of the health consequences of sitting on various chronic diseases and on mortality also are underway. Additionally, he is studying the outcomes of research-funded public health interventions and the impact on policy and practice.

Index

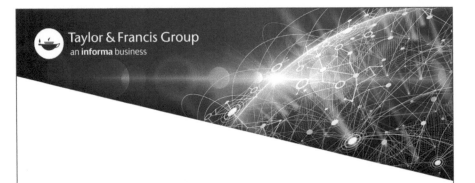

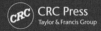